O
Disaster Medicine

About the Oxford American Handbooks in Medicine

The Oxford American Handbooks are pocket clinical books, providing practical guidance in quick reference, note form. Titles cover major medical specialties or cross-specialty topics and are aimed at students, residents, internists, family physicians, and practicing physicians within specific disciplines.

Their reputation is built on including the best clinical information, complemented by hints, tips, and advice from the authors. Each one is carefully reviewed by senior subject experts, residents, and students to ensure that content reflects the reality of day-to-day medical practice.

Key series features

- Written in short chunks, each topic is covered in a concise format to enable readers to find information quickly. They are also perfect for test preparation and gaining a quick overview of a subject without scanning through unnecessary pages.
- Content is evidence based and complemented by the expertise and judgment of experienced authors.
- The Handbooks provide a humanistic approach to medicine—they are more than just treatment by numbers.
- A "friend in your pocket," the Handbooks offer honest, reliable guidance about the difficulties of practicing medicine and provide coverage of both the practice and art of medicine.
- For quick reference, useful "everyday" information is included on the inside covers.

Published and Forthcoming Oxford American Handbooks

Oxford American Handbook of
  Clinical Medicine
Oxford American Handbook of
  Anesthesiology
Oxford American Handbook of
  Cardiology
Oxford American Handbook of
  Clinical Dentistry
Oxford American Handbook of
  Clinical Diagnosis
Oxford American Handbook of Clinical
  Examination and Practical Skills
Oxford American Handbook of
  Clinical Pharmacy
Oxford American Handbook of
  Critical Care
Oxford American Handbook of
  Disaster Medicine
Oxford American Handbook of
  Endocrinology and Diabetes
Oxford American Handbook of
  Emergency Medicine
Oxford American Handbook of
  Gastroenterology and Hepatology
Oxford American Handbook of
  Geriatric Medicine
Oxford American Handbook of
  Hospice and Palliative Medicine
Oxford American Handbook of
  Infectious Diseases

Oxford American Handbook of
  Nephrology and Hypertension
Oxford American Handbook of
  Neurology
Oxford American Handbook of
  Obstetrics and Gynecology
Oxford American Handbook of
  Oncology
Oxford American Handbook of
  Ophthalmology
Oxford American Handbook of
  Otolaryngology
Oxford American Handbook of
  Pediatrics
Oxford American Handbook of
  Physical Medicine and Rehabilitation
Oxford American Handbook of
  Psychiatry
Oxford American Handbook of
  Pulmonary Medicine
Oxford American Handbook of
  Reproductive Medicine
Oxford American Handbook of
  Rheumatology
Oxford American Handbook of
  Sports Medicine
Oxford American Handbook of
  Surgery
Oxford American Handbook of
  Urology

Oxford American Handbook of
Disaster Medicine

Edited by

Robert A. Partridge, MD, MPH, FACEP

Department of Emergency
Medicine, Emerson Hospital
Concord, Massachusetts and
Department of Emergency
Medicine, Rhode Island
Hospital
Adjunct Associate Professor of
Emergency Medicine
Warren Alpert Medical School of
Brown University
Providence, Rhode Island

Lawrence Proano, MD, DTMH, FACEP

Department of Emergency
Medicine, Rhode Island Hospital
Clinical Associate Professor of
Emergency Medicine
Warren Alpert Medical School of
Brown University
Providence, Rhode Island

David Marcozzi, MD, MHS-CL, FACEP

Office of the Assistant Secretary
of Preparedness and Response
Department of Health and Human
Services
Washington, DC

With
Alexander G. Garza, MD, MPH

Director of Military Programs,
Department of Emergency
Medicine
Washington Hospital Center
Georgetown University School of
Medicine
Washington, DC

Ira Nemeth, MD, FACEP

Assistant Professor and Director
of EMS and Disaster Medicine
Section of Emergency Medicine,
Department of Medicine
Baylor College of Medicine
Houston, Texas

Kathryn Brinsfield, MD

Department of Homeland Security
Washington, DC and
Associate Professor of Emergency
Medicine, Boston University
Associate Medical Director,
Boston EMS
Boston, Massachusetts

Eric S. Weinstein, MD

Attending Physician, Carolinas
Hospital System
Emergency Department
Florence, South Carolina

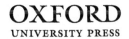

OXFORD
UNIVERSITY PRESS

OXFORD
UNIVERSITY PRESS

Oxford University Press, Inc. publishes works that further
Oxford University's objective of excellence
in research, scholarship and education.

Oxford New York

Auckland Cape Town Dar es Salaam Hong Kong Karachi
Kuala Lumpur Madrid Melbourne Mexico City Nairobi
New Delhi Shanghai Taipei Toronto

With offices in

Argentina Austria Brazil Chile Czech Republic France Greece
Guatemala Hungary Italy Japan Poland Portugal
Singapore South Korea Switzerland Thailand Turkey Ukraine Vietnam

Copyright © 2012 by Oxford University Press, Inc.

Published by Oxford University Press Inc.
198 Madison Avenue, New York, New York 10016
www.oup.com

Oxford is a registered trademark of Oxford University Press

Materials appearing in this book prepared by United States government
employees were not prepared in the individuals' official capacity as
U.S. government employees. Therefore, any views expressed therein do not
represent the views of the United States government and such individuals'
participation in the Work is not meant to serve as an official endorsement
by the United States government. Dr. Kathryn Brinsfield was not an
employee of the US government while serving as co-editor of this book.

Library of Congress Cataloging in Publication Data

Oxford American handbook of disaster medicine / edited by Robert A. Partridge
... [et al.].
p. ; cm. — (Oxford American handbooks in medicine)
Handbook of disaster medicine
Includes bibliographical references and index.
ISBN 978-0-19-537906-8
I. Partridge, Robert A. II. Title: Handbook of disaster medicine. III. Series: Oxford
American handbooks.
[DNLM: 1. Disaster Planning—Handbooks. 2. Disaster Medicine—Handbooks. WA 39]
363.348—dc23
2011039724

Dedicated to my parents, Raymond and Alison, and my beloved wife and children, Karen, Rachel, Sarah, and Alexander. You have all given me endless support, encouragement, and love.

Robert Partridge

This book is dedicated to the mentors who have been role models in my professional career, and to all those who selflessly respond to help others when disaster strikes.

Lawrence Proano

To those who have helped me along the way—my wife, my parents, my brother and sister, Dr. Robert Kadlec, Dr. Kevin Yeskey, Mrs. Heidi Avery, Mr. Richard Reed, Dr. Kathleen Clem, Dr. Michael Hocker, Dr. Selim Suner, and all my colleagues and friends—I dedicate this text to your love, mentorship, and unwavering support. Thank you.

David Marcozzi

Foreword

With the incidence of natural and intentional disasters–and the number of people affected by such events–on the increase, the importance of disasters as a public-health problem has captured the attention of the world. This situation represents an unprecedented challenge to the medical and public-health community. Ten years have now passed since the catastrophic events of September 11, 2001. Since then, periodic reviews of the medical and public-health impact of disasters have appeared in a number of publications, with updates on the "state of the art" of disaster science. As a result, a considerable body of knowledge and experience related to the adverse health effects of disasters is now accumulating that requires regular updating so that we can apply the lessons learned during one disaster to the management of the next. These historical lessons will not be implemented, however, unless they are supported by adequate preparedness planning, coordination, communications, logistics, personnel management, and training of physicians and other health-care providers.

By blending the comprehensiveness of a weighty full-length text with the convenience of a field guide, the *Oxford American Handbook of Disaster Medicine* skilfully addresses these challenges and more. With years of experience, editors Robert Partridge and Lawrence Proano, along with a distinguished list of co-authors, give the reader ample technical descriptions of each kind of disaster, pertinent summaries of previous disasters, and copious information useful for health-care providers in the field, the classroom, or the ward. Unique chapters address topics such as the political and ethical issues in disaster response; urban versus rural approaches; effective media relations; interfaces between disaster medicine and military, operational, and wilderness medicine; and the evolving priorities of the Department of Homeland Security (example, the NRP and an NIMS). In view of recent catastrophic events and newly recognized threats, specific elements such as tsunamis and pandemic influenza that are usually included as part of other chapters (for example, earthquakes and communicable diseases) are now covered in their own chapters. Deserving of special attention are crosscutting chapters in the handbook that integrate information across hazards, such as communications, lessons learned, exercises and drills, and disaster informatics.

In addition, while always emphasizing the use of proven and evidence-based medical methods and practices, Drs. Partridge and Proano challenge health professionals with questions that must still be answered for them to respond effectively in emergency situations. Approached from a real-world perspective, designed and written by clinical and public-health providers with disaster experience, this handbook provides realistic, hands-on experiences that challenge the reader to apply information provided in every chapter. The inclusion of "key messages" and "essential concepts" that introduce each chapter, plus practical information such as protocols, clinical tools, and unique case studies, has resulted in the creation of a major resource that will serve as a timely and comprehensive text for health providers. It will be an important resource in the education of hospital, community, state, and national health and emergency managers, as well as medical students and residents who will assume mass emergency preparedness responsibilities soon, if not immediately after graduation.

All disasters are unique because each affected community has different social, economic, cultural, and baseline health conditions. The *Oxford American Handbook of Disaster Medicine* will serve as the most up-to-date field manual and course textbook available not only for medical professionals responsible for preparing their hospitals to respond effectively to disasters, pandemics, and other public health crises, but also for emergency managers and other decision makers charged with ensuring that disasters are well managed.

Eric K. Noji, MD
Washington, DC

Preface

Disasters happen—anywhere, anytime, and frequently. In the United States, in response to numerous recent man-made and natural catastrophes, disaster preparation efforts have become widespread. Over time, they have also become more complex and broader in scope.

Added layers of complexity make it more difficult to stay on top of best practices, but it is essential to do so. The public expects a rapid, well-coordinated and effective response when disaster strikes. The media will cover the disaster and the response with extensive detail and analysis. After a disaster, recovery and mitigation of future disasters are critical elements of the disaster cycle that will be an ongoing challenge for disaster planners and providers.

Preparation for disasters has occurred at the federal, state, and regional levels, with active involvement of health professionals, law enforcement, rescue and recovery personnel, and relief organizations, as well as ordinary citizens. However, even with the most careful preparation and planning, a disaster will overwhelm all standard resources. Responders have an opportunity to save lives, limit damage and maintain public confidence by doing their jobs well. To manage a disaster effectively, health practitioners must be ready to think on the fly, make rapid and unfamiliar decisions and know where to obtain key knowledge and resources.

This handbook is intended to be one such resource. It can be pulled out of a pocket, off a desktop, or out of the glove compartment of a rescue vehicle, to provide immediate, accessible information on a wide range of topics. By covering critical areas of disaster preparation, planning, and response for the types of disasters that are most likely to occur in the United States and around the world, this book gives health-care responders a first-line tool for ensuring their own preparedness. It is designed to assist involved health practitioners on any aspect of disaster management at any point along the disaster timeline.

Although this handbook is thorough, it is not comprehensive. Readers are encouraged to consult other texts, peer-reviewed literature, web sites and suggested readings at the end of each chapter for additional information and detail. It is our hope that this handbook will be an essential part of a larger library of information to help health practitioners limit the impact of disasters through effective preparation and response.

Robert Partridge
Lawrence Proano

Acknowledgments

The authors are grateful for the efforts of many people who worked very hard to make this book possible. Foremost, we would like to thank all of our co-authors. The depth and quality of this book are a testament to their dedication and interest in the study of disaster medicine.

Thanks also go out to our co-editors, David Marcozzi, Alex Garza, Kathy Brinsfield, Ira Nemeth, and Eric Weinstein, whose vision guided the development of this project.

In addition, we are indebted to the team at Oxford University Press, particularly Andrea Seils and Staci Hou, who have worked diligently to bring this book to fruition.

Finally, we would like to acknowledge disaster responders everywhere, whom we all rely on but often don't have the opportunity to thank. Their work has not only informed and inspired us but also left us better prepared to respond to the next disaster.

Robert Partridge
Lawrence Proano

Contents

Part 6: Specific Hazards in Disasters
Human Caused Disasters

Biological Disasters

Chemical Disasters

Contributors

D. Adam Algren, MD
Assistant Professor of Emergency
Medicine and Pediatrics
Truman Medical Center/Children's
Mercy Hospital
University of Missouri-Kansas City
School of Medicine
Kansas City, MO
and
Medical Director
University of Kansas Hospital
Poison Control Center
Kansas City, KS

Evan Avraham Alpert, MD
Attending Physician
Emergency Department
Sheba Medical Center, Israel

Michael Sean Antonis, DO, RDMS, FACEP
Assistant Professor of Clinical
Emergency Medicine
Department of Emergency
Medicine
Georgetown University Medical
School
MedStar Health: Washington
Hospital Center and Georgetown
University
Washington, DC

Christian Arbelaez, MD, MPH
Assistant Residency Director,
Department of Emergency
Medicine
Associate Director, Office for
Multicultural Faculty Careers
Brigham and Women's Hospital
Assistant Professor of Medicine
Harvard Medical School
Boston, MA

James J. Augustine, MD
Director of Clinical Operations,
EMP Management
Canton, OH
and
Assistant Clinical Professor
Department of Emergency
Medicine
Wright State University
Dayton, OH

Kavita Babu, MD
Assistant Professor
Division of Medical Toxicology
Department of Emergency
Medicine
Warren Alpert Medical School of
Brown University
Providence, RI

Jennifer Bahr, MD
Medical College of Wisconsin
Milwaukee, WI

Cindy Baseluos, MD
Staff Physician
Richmond University Medical
Center
Staten Island, NY

Jeff Beeson, DO, FACEP
Medical Director
Emergency Physicians Advisory
Board
Fort Worth, TX
and
Clinical Assistant Professor
Emergency Medicine
University of Texas Southwestern
Medical
Dallas, TX

Jason Bellows, MD, FACEP
Lutheran Medical Center
Denver, CO

Gerald W. Beltran, DO
Department of Emergency
Medicine
Carilion Clinic
Roanoke, VA

Matthew Bitner, MD
Director, Prehospital Education
and Research
Associate Director, Prehospital
Medicine
Section of Prehospital and
Disaster Medicine
Division of Emergency Medicine
Duke University Health System
Durham, NC

Leila Blonski, RN
Madigan Army Medical Center
Department of Emergency
Medicine
Tacoma, WA

**David Bouslough, MD, MPH,
DTM&H**
Clinical Assistant Professor
Division of International
Emergency Medicine
Department of Emergency
Medicine
Warren Alpert Medical School of
Brown University
Providence, RI

**Susan Miller Briggs, MD,
MPH, FACS**
Associate Professor of Surgery
Harvard Medical School
Co-Director, Office of Disaster
Response, Center for Global
Health
Massachusetts General Hospital
Boston, MA

John Broach, MD, MPH
Assistant Professor, Emergency
Medicine
Division of Disaster Medicine &
Emergency Management
Department of Emergency
Medicine
University of Massachusetts
Medical School
UMass Memorial Medical Center
Worcester, MA

Tracy Buchman, DHA
Madison, WI

**Frederick M. Burkle, Jr.,
MD, MPH, DTM**
Senior Fellow & Scientist
Harvard Humanitarian Initiative
Harvard School of Public Health
Cambridge, MA

John D. Cahill, MD
Assistant Professor of Clinical
Medicine
Columbia University College of
Physicians & Surgeons
and
Adjunct Assistant Professor of
Emergency Medicine
Warren Alpert Medical School of
Brown University
and
Director, Global Health
Fellowship
Senior Attending in Infectious
Disease & Emergency Medicine
Saint Luke's Roosevelt Hospital
Center
New York, NY

Dinah Cannefax
Cannefax Consulting
Emergency Management in
Healthcare
Dallas, TX

John T. Carlo, MD, MS
Program Director
Chemical and Biological Early
Detection (BioWatch) Program
Center for Infectious Disease
Research and Policy (CIDRAP)
The University of Minnesota
Minneapolis, MN

Jimmy Cooper, MD, FACEP
San Antonio, TX

Peter John Cuenca, MD
Lieutenant Colonel, Medical
Corps
United States Army
Assistant Professor of Military/
Emergency Medicine
Uniformed Services University of
the Health Sciences
Department of Emergency
Medicine
Brooke Army Medical Center
Fort Sam Houston, TX

**Michelle Daniel, MD,
FACEP**
Assistant Professor (Clinical),
Department of Emergency
Medicine
Warren Alpert Medical School of
Brown University
Attending Physician Rhode Island
The Miriam and Hasbro Children's
Hospitals
Providence, RI

Christopher Daniel, MA
Safer Institute
Providence, RI

**Michelle M. Darcy, BSN,
RN, CEN**
Madigan Army Medical Center
Department of Emergency
Medicine
Tacoma, WA

Siri Daulaire, MD
Department of Emergency
Medicine
Warren Alpert Medical School of
Brown University
Rhode Island Hospital
Providence, RI

Diane DeVita, MD, FACEP
Assistant Chief, Administration
and Operations
Department of Emergency
Medicine
Madigan Healthcare System
Tacoma, WA

**Constance J. Doyle, MD,
FACEP**
Core Faculty
University of Michigan/St. Joseph
Mercy Emergency
Medicine Residency
Deputy Medical Director
Washtenaw/ Livingston Medical
Control
Authority Attending Emergency
Physician
St. Joseph Mercy Hospital
Ann Arbor, MI

**Brenda O'Connell Driggers,
RN, BSN**
Trauma/Chest Pain Center
Coordinator
Carolinas Hospital System
Florence, SC

Mazen El Sayed, MD
Instructor of Emergency
Medicine
Department of Emergency
Medicine
Boston University School of
Medicine
Boston MA

Daniel B. Fagbuyi, MD, FAAP
Medical Director, Disaster Preparedness and Emergency Management
Children's National Medical Center
Assistant Professor, Pediatrics and Emergency Medicine
The George Washington University School of Medicine
Washington, DC

Michelle A. Fischer, MD, MPH, FACEP
Assistant Professor
Department of Emergency Medicine
Penn State Hershey Medical Center
Hershey, PA

Bryan Fisk, MD, MSc
Assistant Chief, Critical Care Medicine
Walter Reed Army Medical Center
Washington, DC

John L. Foggle, MD, MBA
Assistant Professor, Department of Emergency Medicine
Warren Alpert Medical School of Brown University
Providence, RI

Rachel L. Fowler, MD, MPH
Assistant Professor
Department of Emergency Medicine
Warren Alpert Medical School of Brown University
Providence, RI

Ray Fowler, MD, FACEP
Professor of Emergency Medicine, Surgery, Health Professions, and Emergency Medical Education
Chief of EMS Operations
Co-Chief in the Section on EMS, Disaster Medicine, and Homeland Security
The University of Texas Southwestern Medical Center
and
Attending Emergency Medicine Faculty
Parkland Memorial Hospital
Dallas, TX

Tyeese Gaines Reid, DO, MA
Attending Physician
Raritan Bay Medical Center
Perth Amboy, NJ

Justin S. Gatewood, MD
Assistant Professor of Emergency Medicine
Department of Emergency Medicine
Georgetown University School of Medicine
Washington Hospital Center
Washington, DC

James Geiling, MD
Professor of Medicine
Dartmouth Medical School
Hanover, NH
and
Chief, Medical Service
VA Medical Center
White River Junction, VT

Steven Go, MD
Associate Professor of Emergency
Medicine
Department of Emergency
Medicine
University of Missouri, Kansas City
School of Medicine
Kansas City, MO

Robert Gougelet, MD
Assistant Professor of Medicine
(Emergency Medicine)
Director, New England Center for
Emergency Preparedness
at Dartmouth Medical School
Director, Northern New England
MMRS
Dartmouth Medical School
Hanover, NH

Matthew Gratton, MD
CAPT MC USN (ret)
Associate Professor and Chair
Emergency Medicine
University of Missouri at Kansas
City School of Medicine
Truman Medical Center
Kansas City, MO

Michael Gray, MD
Chief Resident
UMass Emergency Medicine
Residency Program
Worcester, MA

Ian Greenwald, MD, FACEP
Chief Medical Officer
Duke Preparedness and Response
Center
Duke University Health System
Durham, NC

Jason Hack, MD
Division Director, Medical
Toxicology
UEMF Director, Educational
Program in Medical Toxicology
Associate Professor
Warren Alpert Medical School of
Brown University
Attending Physician, Department
of Emergency Medicine
Rhode Island Hospital, Miriam
Hospital
Providence, RI

**Lori L. Harrington, MD,
MPH**
Associate Medical Director
Boston EMS
Assistant Professor of Emergency
Medicine
Department of Emergency
Medicine
Boston Medical Center
Boston, MA

**Alison Schroth Hayward,
MD**
Department of Emergency
Medicine
Mayo Clinic College of Medicine
Rochester, MN

Kwa heri Heard, MA
Metropolitan Medical Response
System Program Manager
Emergency Management Specialist
City of Dallas Office of Emergency
Management
Dallas, TX

John L. Hick, MD
Associate Professor of Emergency Medicine
University of Minnesota
Medical Director for Emergency Preparedness
Hennepin County Medical Center
Minneapolis, MN

Korin Hudson, MD, FACEP, NREMT-P
Assistant Professor of Emergency Medicine
Georgetown University School of Medicine
Georgetown University Hospital & Washington Hospital Center
Washington, DC

Alexander P. Isakov, MD, MPH
Executive Director
Office of Critical Event Preparedness and Response
Associate Professor of Emergency Medicine
Emory University
Atlanta, GA

Irving "Jake" Jacoby, MD
Clinical Professor of Medicine and Surgery
University of California San Diego School of Medicine
and
Attending Physician, Department of Emergency Medicine
UC San Diego Medical Center
San Diego, CA

Gabrielle Jacquet, MD
Department of Emergency Medicine
Denver Health Medical Center
Denver, CO

Liudvikas Jagminas, MD, FACEP
Associate Professor and Vice Chair
Department of Emergency Medicine
Yale School of Medicine
New Haven, CT

Ashika Jain, MD
Emergency Ultrasound Fellow
Department of Emergency Medicine
Maimonides Medical Center
Brooklyn, NY

Melinda Johnson, MPP
Denver Metropolitan Medical Response System
Denver Health & Hospital Authority
Denver, CO

Ramon W. Johnson, MD, FACEP
Department of Emergency Medicine
Mission Hospital Regional Medical Center
Mission Viejo, CA

Jerrilyn Jones, MD
Emergency Medicine Resident
Boston Medical Center
Boston, MA

Robert A. Jones, MD
Department of Emergency Medicine
Madigan Army Medical Center
Tacoma, WA

Peter Kemetzhofer, MD, FACEP
Department of Trauma Surgery
University of Vienna
Vienna, Austria

Jake Kesterson, MD
Department of Emergency
Medicine
Truman Medical Center
Kansas City, MO

Kelly R. Klein, MD, FACEP
Staff Physician
Department of Emergency
Medicine
Hospital Emergency Preparedness
Medical Director
Eastern Maine Medical Center
Bangor, ME

Deborah L. Korik, MD
Attending Physician
Northeast Emergency Associates
Beverly Hospital
Beverly, MA

David R. Lane, MD
Assistant Professor, Department
of Emergency Medicine
Georgetown University School of
Medicine
Washington Hospital Center and
Georgetown University Hospital
Emergency Medicine Residency
Program
Washington, DC

David C. Lee, MD
Associate Professor of Emergency
Medicine
Hofstra School of Medicine
North Shore University Hospital
Manhasset, NY

Adam C. Levine, MD, MPH
Assistant Professor of Emergency
Medicine
Division of International
Emergency Medicine
Department of Emergency
Medicine
Warren Alpert Medical School of
Brown University
Providence, RI

Alexis Lieser, MD
Department of Emergency
Medicine
University of California, Irvine
Irvine, CA

David C. Mackenzie, MD, CM
Assistant Clinical Instructor
Department of Emergency
Medicine
Warren Alpert Medical School of
Brown University
Providence, RI

**William Mastrianni, MA,
EMT-P**
Team Leader, SC-1 DMAT
HHS/ASPR/OPEO/NDMS

**Paul T. Mayer, MD, MBA,
FACEP**
Director, Department of Combat
Medic Training
Army Medical Department Center
and School

Kerry K. McCabe, MD
Assistant Professor of Emergency
Medicine
Boston University School of
Medicine
Associate Residency Director
Department of Emergency
Medicine
Boston Medical Center
Boston, MA

**COL John McManus, MD,
MCR, FACEP, FAAEM**
Director, U.S. Army EMS
EMS Fellowship Program Director
San Antonio Uniformed Services
Health Education Consortium
Medical Clinical Associate
Professor, Emergency Medicine
University of Texas Heath Science
Center
San Antonio, TX

Bryan F. McNally, MD, MPH
Assistant Professor of Emergency
Medicine
Emory University School of
Medicine
Atlanta, GA

David A. Meguerdichian, MD
Instructor of Medicine
Harvard Medical School
Department of Emergency
Medicine
Brigham and Women's Hospital /
Faulkner Hospital
Boston, MA

**Andrew Milsten, MD, MS,
FACEP**
Associate Professor, Emergency
Medicine
Director, Disaster Medicine &
Emergency Management
Fellowship
Department of Emergency
Medicine
University of Massachusetts
Medical School
UMass Memorial Medical
Center
Worcester, MA

Peter Moffett, MD
Staff Physician
Department of Emergency
Medicine
Carl R. Darnall Army Medical
Center
Fort Hood, TX

**Krithika M. Muruganandan,
MD**
International Emergency Medicine
Fellow
Department of Emergency
Medicine
Warren Alpert Medical School of
Brown University
Providence, RI

Helen Ouyang, MD, MPH
Department of Emergency Medicine
Brigham and Women's Hospital
and
Department of Emergency Medicine
Massachusetts General Hospital
Boston, MA

Kobi Peleg, PhD, MPH
Director, National Center for
Trauma & Emergency Medicine
Research
The Gertner Institute for Health
Policy & Epidemiology
Head, Disaster Medicine
Department
Head, The Executive Master
Program for Emergency and
Disaster Management
School of Public Health, Tel-Aviv
University
Tel-Aviv, Israel

**Zaffer Qasim, MBBS, MRCS,
MCEM**
Specialty Registrar in Emergency
Medicine/Critical Care Medicine
Manchester, United Kingdom

**Lou E. Romig, MD, FAAP,
FACEP**
Pediatric Emergency Physician
Miami Children's Hospital
Miami, FL

Megan L. Salinas, MD
Division of Emergency Medicine
Huntington Memorial Hospital
Pasadena, CA

**Joseph A. Salomone, III,
MD, FAAEM**
Associate Professor
Department of Emergency Medicine
EMS Medical Director
Truman Medical Centers/UMKC
School of Medicine
Kansas City, MO

Carl H. Schultz, MD, FACEP
Professor of Emergency Medicine
Director of Research, Center for
Disaster Medical Sciences
Director, EMS and Disaster
Medical Sciences Fellowship
University of California Irvine
School of Medicine
Director, Disaster Medical Services
Department of Emergency
Medicine
University of California Irvine
Medical Center
Orange, CA

**Richard B. Schwartz, MD,
FACEP**
Professor and Chairman
Department of Emergency Medicine
Georgia Health Sciences
University
Augusta, GA

Sachita Shah, MD
Assistant Professor of Emergency
Medicine
Division of Emergency Medicine
Department of Internal Medicine
University of Washington School
of Medicine
Seattle, WA

**Wayne Smith, BSc, MBChB,
EMDM, FCEM (SA)**
Head, Disaster Medicine
Division of Emergency Medicine
Stellenbosch University &
University of Cape Town
Provincial Government of the
Western Cape
Cape Town, South Africa

Amy M. Stubbs, MD
Assistant Professor of Emergency
Medicine
Associate Residency Program
Director
Truman Medical Center
University of Kansas City-Missouri
Kansas City, MO

Payal Sud, MD
Medical Toxicology Fellow
Department of Emergency Medicine
North Shore University Hospital
Manhasset, NY

**Ramona Sunderwirth, MD,
MPH, FAAP**
Director, Global Health
Fellowship
Attending, Pediatric Emergency
Medicine
Department of Emergency
Medicine
St Luke's/Roosevelt Hospital
New York, NY

**Selim Suner, MD, MS,
FACEP**
Associate Professor of Emergency
Medicine, Surgery and Engineering
Warren Alpert Medical School of
Brown University
Providence, RI

Ryan Tai
Warren Alpert Medical School of
Brown University
Providence, RI

**Deepti Thomas-Paulose,
MD, MPH**
St.Luke's Roosevelt Hospital Center
Department of Emergency Medicine
Global Health Division
Instructor of Clinical Medicine
Columbia University College of
Physicians and Surgeons
New York, NY

**Anthony J. Tomassoni, MD,
MS, FACEP, FACMT**
Department of Emergency Medicine
Yale University School of Medicine
Medical Director
Yale New Haven Health
System Center for Emergency
Preparedness and Healthcare
Solutions
New Haven, CT

Henry H. Truong, MD
Staff Physician
Salem Emergency Physicians
Salem, OR

Claire Uebbing, MD
Emergency Medicine Global
Health Fellow
St. Luke's Roosevelt Hospital
New York, NY

Lee Wallis, MBChB, FCEM, MD
Professor of Emergency Medicine
Stellenbosch University
Cape Town, South Africa

Adam Webster, BS
Safety & Emergency Preparedness
Coordinator
Facilities Management
Las Colinas Medical Center
Irving, TX

Melissa White
Emory University
Atlanta, GA

Alexander Wielaard, MD
Department of Emergency
Medicine
Shore Health System
Baltimore, MD

Kenneth A. Williams, MD, FACEP
Associate Professor of Emergency
Medicine (Clinical)
Department of Emergency
Medicine
Warren Alpert Medical School of
Brown University
Providence, RI

Bradley Younggren, MD
Assistant Clinical Professor of
Medicine
University of Washington
Evergreen Hospital Medical
Center
Kirkland, WA

Richard D. Zane, MD, FAAEM
Associate Professor
Harvard Medical School
Department of Emergency
Medicine
Brigham and Women's Hospital
Boston, MA

Part 1

Introduction

Definition of a disaster

Peter Moffett

Overview

Defining a disaster is not a simple academic exercise. A "disaster" to one organization could be a routine event for others. In addition, there is a distinction between the medical definition of a disaster and the lay definition of a disaster. What is often defined as a "disaster" by the layperson might be better described as "tragic."

Defining a disaster is important for any organization planning on when and how to initiate its disaster plans. Only after defining the problem can a plan be formulated. The definition of the disaster dictates the degree of response and will often be communicated across a variety of specialties and agencies.

As Gregory Ciottone mentions in his textbook on disaster medicine, "Unlike other areas of medicine...the care of casualties from a disaster requires the healthcare provider to integrate into the larger, predominantly non-medical multidisciplinary response."

"Basic" definition of a disaster

There is no one single definition of a disaster that has been agreed upon by experts or groups. A quick glance at the Emergency Management Institute's document that defines terms for their training lists 79 separate definitions for a disaster. The following list suggests some basic definitions of a disaster.

Disaster

A disaster is an event that results in a demand for services that exceeds available resources.

Example: A single-vehicle collision with three serious casualties may be a disaster for a small rural emergency department with single-physician coverage. However, this situation would be easily managed in an urban trauma system.

UN Disaster Management Training Program's definition

A disaster is a serious disruption of the functioning of a society, causing widespread human, material, or environmental losses that exceed the ability of the affected society to cope using only its own resources.

The Joint Commission (TJC) definition

A disaster is a natural or man-made event that suddenly or significantly disrupts the environments of care; disrupts care or treatment; or changes or increases demands for the organization's services.

Internal versus external disaster

This hospital-centered model of disasters distinguishes between an "internal" and an "external" disaster. The advantages of this distinction include the ability for an institution to determine if their infrastructure has been affected by the disaster if there is an immediate threat to the safety of the patients and employees. The disadvantages of this definition are that it is not useful to other agencies, and many events are both internal and external (e.g., an earthquake, flood, or hurricane).

Internal disaster

Disaster that affects the hospital and/or hospital grounds, e.g.:

- Bomb threat
- Fire or explosion
- Power failure
- Employee strike

External disaster

Disaster that affects the surrounding community but not the hospital directly, e.g.:

- Chemical plant explosion
- Riots
- Tornado through a residential community

Etiological descriptors

Another model to describe disasters includes whether the event is man-made or natural, with subdivisions for specific causes.

One advantage to this approach is that it allows an organization to tailor its response if special resources are needed for an event—for example, collecting additional warming devices needed for a winter storm.

A disadvantage is that there may be little crossover between different types of disasters and the resources required may be different. Furthermore, extensive and complex plans for each disaster are required.

Man-made disasters

CBRNE

- **C**hemical
  - Release of sarin gas by terrorists
  - Tanker truck collision with release of chlorine gas
- **B**iological
  - Anthrax-laced letters sent through the mail
  - Release of *Yersinia pestis* (bubonic plague) by terrorists
- **R**adiological/**N**uclear
  - Explosion at a nuclear plant (Chernobyl)
  - "Dirty" bomb with dispersion of radioactive material
- **E**xplosive incidents
  - Gasoline tanker truck collision on a busy highway
  - Improvised explosive device (IED)

Dam failure

Rioting or civil unrest

Mechanical or structural

Natural disasters

- Earthquake
- Wildfire
- Flood
- Heat
- Hurricane
- Landslide
- Thunderstorms
- Tornado
- Tsunami
- Volcano
- Blizzards and ice storms

Levels of disaster

Another classification scheme for disasters is based on the resources required for a response.

An advantage of this system is that it focuses on response and is easy to use. A disadvantage of this system is that it does not facilitate preparations for specific scenarios.

Level I
Local emergency medical services (EMS) and hospital are able to respond.
• Single area hospital activated

Level II
Multijurisdictional aid is needed.
• Several local hospitals activated

Level III
State or federal aid is needed.
• Request for aid based on state and federal regulations

Potential injury-causing event (PICE)

This is a relatively new term that has been suggested as a way of eliminating the broad term "disaster" and using a multi-tiered system to instead focus on the needed response. The nomenclature is somewhat complex but may suit some institutional needs.

An event is described on the basis of three different prefixes and by a PICE stage, which includes the projected need for outside aid and the status of outside aid.

Prefix A—potential for additional casualties
- *Static:* no more potential for additional casualties
  - Motor vehicle accident
- *Dynamic:* potential for additional casualties
  - Continuing wildfires

Prefix B—ability of local resources to respond
- *Controlled:* local resources able to respond without augmentation
  - Bus accident in a large urban area with multiple hospitals
- *Disruptive:* local resources overwhelmed but able to respond with augmentation of resources
  - Bus accident in a small rural community with a single hospital (becomes controlled when two more trauma surgeons respond)
- *Paralytic:* local resources overwhelmed and augmentation alone will not suffice. Complete reconstruction of the system is needed.
  - *Destructive:* a hospital emergency department (ED) is destroyed by flooding (will need to be rebuilt or completely relocated to become controlled)
  - *Nondestructive:* power failure to a hospital emergency room (ER) (once power is restored, the event is controlled)

Prefix C—geographic involvement of event
- *Local*
  - Nursing strike at a single hospital
- *Regional*
  - City-wide flooding (Hurricane Katrina)
- *National*
  - Armenian earthquake of 1988
- *International*
  - 2004 Indian Ocean tsunami

PICE stage—projected need for and status of outside aid
- *Stage 0:* No need for outside aid and aid is inactive
  - Three-car motor vehicle collision in an urban setting
- *Stage I:* Small chance that outside aid is needed and aid should be on alert
  - 10-car motor vehicle collision in an urban setting
- *Stage II:* Moderate chance that outside aid is needed and aid should be on standby (prepared to dispatch quickly)
  - Riots that close several regional hospitals

- *Stage III:* Local resources are overwhelmed and need immediate dispatch of outside aid
  - Destruction of all of the city hospitals by flooding
  - Three-car motor vehicle collision in a small rural hospital

Examples
- Multiple-vehicle crash (rural community): static, disruptive, local PICE stage I
- Multiple-vehicle crash (urban setting): static, controlled, local PICE stage 0
- Continuing wildfires; dynamic, disruptive, regional PICE stage III

Conclusion

Only after defining a disaster can an organization move into the disaster cycle. With a variety of systems to classify a disaster, an organization can tailor definitions to meet its needs.

The etiological descriptor of disaster fits easily into the all-hazards approach discussed in Chapter 2.

However an organization defines a disaster, it must be consistent, applicable, and well understood by all participants in the disaster plan.

Suggested readings

Ciottone G (2006). Introduction to disaster medicine. In Ciottone G, ed. *Disaster Medicine*. Philadelphia: Elsevier Health Sciences, pp. 3–6..

Dallas CE, et al., eds. (2007). Chapter 1: All hazards course overview and DISASTER paradigm. In: Dallas CE, eds. *Basic Disaster Life Support Provider Manual* Version 2.6. Chicago: American Medical Association, pp. 6–7.

Koenig K, Dinerman N, Kuehl A (1996). Disaster nomenclature—a functional impact approach: the PICE system. *Acad Emerg Med* 3:723–727.

Schultz C, Koenig K, Noji E (2006). Disaster preparedness. In Marx J, ed. *Rosen's Emergency Medicine Concepts and Clinical Practice*, 6th ed., Vol. 3. Philadelphia: Elsevier Health Sciences, pp. 3010–3021.

All-hazards approach

Ira Nemeth

Introduction

The definition of all-hazards is that it describes "an incident, natural or man-made, that warrants action to protect life, property, environment, and public health or safety, and to minimize disruptions of government social, or economic activities" (FEMA NRF Resource Center).

The "all-hazards" concept of emergency management has its roots in the creation of the Federal Emergency Management Agency (FEMA). The National Governors Association made recommendations to President Carter to improve disaster response. The first recommendation was to combine all the federal disaster relief agencies into one agency—FEMA. The second recommendation was to allow civil defense funding to be used to prepare for other hazards.

FEMA developed the Integrated Emergency Management System (IEMS) to help state and local jurisdictions implement the theory of comprehensive emergency management (Fig. 2.1). The IEMS was composed of three ideas:

- Planning needed to be cross-jurisdictional and include other response partners.
- A multiyear planning cycle was needed to advance preparedness.
- Emergency operation plans should be organized around functions (capabilities), not agencies or hazards.

Homeland Security Presidential Directive–8 (HSPD-8) was issued on December 17, 2003, and directed the Secretary of Homeland Security to develop a national domestic all-hazards preparedness goal. To accomplish this task, the National Preparedness Guidelines (NPG) were published in September 2007. The NPG has four components:

- The National Preparedness Vision: a short statement of the national preparedness goals
- The National Planning Scenarios: a group of planning, training, and exercise scenarios that cover the full spectrum of emergencies. Currently, there are 15 different scenarios that are used by the federal government and made available for state, local, and tribal governments.

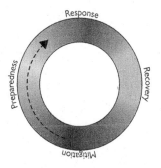

Figure 2.1 Comprehensive emergency management theory.

- The Universal Task List (UTL): a list of approximately 1600 individual tasks that are arranged into common target capabilities of prevention, protection, response, and recovery in disaster events. These tasks provide a common vocabulary and identify the highest priorities to be accomplished.
- The Target Capabilities List (TCL): a list of 37 capabilities that every community should posses to be prepared for a disaster.

The national preparedness vision

"A NATION PREPARED with coordinated capabilities to prevent, protect against, respond to, and recover from all hazards in a way that balances risk with resources and need."
—*National Preparedness Guidelines*, September 2007

The NPG are meant to provide a framework to allow all communities to best determine where to appropriately allocate disaster resources. Many of the federal planning documents will use the NPG to provide the overarching concepts.

An all-hazards approach is one of the main themes of the NPG. Preparedness must address prevention, protection, response, and recovery from terrorist attacks, major disasters, and other emergencies. The NPG is designed to allow for a risk-based approach.

It is important for communities to evaluate and tailor their approach to disaster preparedness. Risk has three components:
* Threat
* Vulnerability
* Consequence

Preparedness is a continuous cycle that is a requirement of all levels of government and agencies involved in disaster response. The NPG establishes a proposed preparedness cycle (Fig. 2.2) to helps guide all agencies involved.

Private, nonprofit, faith-based, and other nongovernmental organizations should be included in preparedness activities. All participating agencies should use the same capabilities-based metrics set out in the TCL.

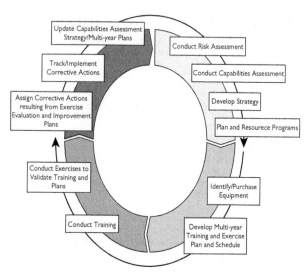

Figure 2.2 Preparedness cycle.

Capabilities

Capabilities provide "the means to accomplish a mission or function and achieve desired outcomes by performing critical tasks, under specified conditions, to target levels of performance" (Target Capabilities List).

The TCL lists 37 capabilities (Table 2.1) that are needed in an all-hazards response. These are divided into prevent, protect, respond, and recover mission capabilities. A few capabilities that apply across all missions are listed as common capabilities.

The capabilities discussed in the TCL were chosen because the local jurisdictions and states lead them with support from the federal government and the private sector.

Each capability summary has 12 parts:

- Definition of the capability
- Outcome—describes the expected results of the capability
- Relationship to the National Response Framework (NRF) Emergency Support Functions (ESF)
- Preparedness activities, critical tasks as defined by the UTL, measures and metrics. Preparedness is done before the capability is needed.
- Performance activities, critical tasks, measures, and metrics. Performance is the application of the capability.
- Activity process flow diagram
- Capability elements—resources needed to accomplish the critical tasks to the level defined by the measure and metrics. National Incident Management System (NIMS) resource typing definitions are used where available.
- Linked capabilities—a list of capabilities connected to the capability being summarized and the relationship between the two capabilities
- Planning assumptions made to pick the appropriate tasks and metrics
- National preparedness levels—a list of resources with numbers needed for each agency responsible to lead the activity supported by the resource
- References

Table 2.1 Capabilities

Common mission area	Respond mission area
<ul><li>Communications</li><li>Community preparedness and participation</li><li>Planning</li><li>Risk management</li><li>Intelligence/information sharing and dissemination</li></ul>**Prevent mission area**<ul><li>CBRNE detection</li><li>Information gathering and Recognition of indicators and warnings</li><li>Intelligence analysis and production</li><li>Counter-terror investigations and law enforcement</li></ul>**Protect mission area**<ul><li>Critical infrastructure protection</li><li>Epidemiological surveillance and investigation</li><li>Food and agriculture safety and defense</li><li>Laboratory testing</li></ul>	<ul><li>Animal health emergency support</li><li>Citizen evacuation and shelter in place</li><li>Critical resource logistics and distribution</li><li>Emergency operations center management</li><li>Emergency public information and warning</li><li>Environmental health</li><li>Explosive-device response operations</li><li>Fatality management</li><li>Fire incident response support</li><li>Isolation and quarantine</li><li>Mass care (sheltering, feeding, and related services)</li><li>Mass prophylaxis</li><li>Medical-supplies management and distribution</li><li>Medical surge</li><li>Onsite incident management</li><li>Emergency public safety and security response</li><li>Responder safety and health</li><li>Emergency triage and pre–hospital treatment</li><li>Search and rescue (land-based)</li><li>Volunteer management and donations</li><li>Weapons of mass destruction/hazardous-materials response and decontamination</li></ul>

Recover mission area
- Economic and community recovery
- Restoration of lifelines

Capabilities-based preparedness

The NPG is based on a capabilities-based approach to planning. All-hazards planning can be accomplished using a capabilities-based approach. The definition of capabilities-based preparedness is "preparing, under uncertainty, to provide capabilities suitable for a wide range of challenges while working within an economic framework that necessitates prioritization and choice" (*National Planning Guidelines*).

In 2005, 15 national planning scenarios were published to provide a diversity of high-consequence threats for disaster planning. The scenarios cover all-hazards and provide information to allow the scenario to be scaled and customized to communities' needs.

While some of the topics apply primarily to federal responses, all levels of government can use them.

National planning scenarios
Improvised nuclear device
- Aerosolized anthrax
- Pandemic influenza
- Plague
- Blister agent
- Toxic industrial chemical
- Nerve agent
- Chlorine tank explosion
- Major earthquake
- Major hurricane
- Radiological dispersal device (RDD)
- Improvised explosive device (IED)
- Food contamination
- Foreign animal disease (FAD)
- Cyber attack

The planning scenarios helped focus the creation of the UTL and the TCL. Fifteen scenarios are not enough to cover all possible major events, but were felt to provide a minimum necessary to develop the range of response capabilities needed to develop an all-hazards approach.

The preparedness cycle (Fig. 2.2) lays out the steps involved in creating a capabilities-based preparedness process.

The step needed prior to entering into the preparedness cycle is to convene a diverse working group. The working group should coordinate across disciplines, agencies, and jurisdictions. When possible, private sector and nongovernmental partners should be included.

Priorities

Another goal of the NPG was to establish the national priorities. The priorities were identified from national strategies, presidential directives, state and urban-area Homeland Security strategies, and lessons-learned reports. Eight priorities were identified initially.

The federal funds provided to local communities for preparedness activities have been directed toward the following priorities:

- Expand regional collaboration
- Implement the National Incident Management System (NIMS) and the National Response Plan (now called the National Response Framework)
- Implement the National Infrastructure Protection Plan (NIPP)
- Strengthen information-sharing and collaboration capabilities
- Strengthen communications capabilities
- Strengthen CBRNE detection, response, and decontamination capabilities
- Strengthen medical-surge and mass-prophylaxis capabilities
- Strengthen planning and citizen-preparedness capabilities

The first three priorities listed cross most capabilities. The other priorities are directed at improving specific capabilities that were identified as gaps. For example, the "strengthen medical surge" and "mass prophylaxis" capabilities address two specific capabilities.

Many federal programs have been supporting this priority, including the Hospital Preparedness Program (HPP), administered by the Assistant Secretary for Preparedness and Response in Health and Human Services, and the Centers for Disease Control (CDC)–administered Cooperative Agreement on Public Health Preparedness and Response for Bioterrorism. Both programs provide funding to local jurisdictions and states to increase medical-surge and mass-prophylaxis capacity.

Exercise and training

In any system designed to increase preparedness, exercise and training is a requirement. This is a multiyear exercise program to ensure that all capabilities needed in an all-hazards response are properly evaluated.

The Homeland Security Exercise and Evaluation Program (HSEEP) was created to help focus on performance of critical tasks in a standardized format. A five-volume set lays out the HSEEP guidance:

- *HSEEP Volume I: HSEEP Overview and Exercise Program Management* provides guidance for building and maintaining an effective exercise program and summarizes the planning and evaluation processes.
- *HSEEP Volume II: Exercise Planning and Conduct* helps planners outline a standardized foundation, design, development, and conduct process adaptable to any type of exercise.
- *HSEEP Volume III: Exercise Evaluation and Improvement Planning* offers proven methodology for evaluating and documenting exercises and implementing an improvement plan.
- *HSEEP Volume IV: Sample Exercise Documents and Formats* provides sample exercise materials referenced in HSEEP Volumes I, II, III, and V.

- *HSEEP Volume V: Prevention Exercises* contains guidance consistent with the HSEEP model to assist jurisdictions in designing and evaluating exercises that test pre-incident capabilities such as intelligence analysis and information sharing.

A standardized exercise and evaluation program that tests capabilities selected from the TCL using identified critical tasks provides a standardized pathway to improvement that can be translated across jurisdictions and agencies. HSEEP processes standardize the exercise and evaluation pieces of the preparedness cycle.

All exercises should generate an improvement plan from which corrective actions can be taken. Corrective actions will have timelines for completion. Once a corrective action has been completed, the new process should be incorporated in an exercise.

Summary

An all-hazards approach describes a philosophy of preparedness that is based on a capability framework and involves all response partners. The federal government has provided guidance and standardized terminology to help facilitate this approach. All agencies should use the federal guidelines and apply them to their individual communities.

A continuous cycle of planning, training, exercise, and evaluation helps increase the disaster preparedness of the community and the nation.

Suggested readings

Boatright CJ, Brewster PW (2010). Public health and emergency management systems. In Koenig KL, Schultz CH, eds. *Disaster Medicine: Comprehensive Principles and Practices.* New York: Cambridge University Press, pp. 133–150.

Federal Emergency Management Agency. National Response Framework Resource Center glossary/acronyms. Retrieved December 2, 2010, from http://www.fema.gov/emergency/nrf/glossary.htm

U.S. Department of Homeland Security (2007, February), *Homeland Security Exercise and Evaluation Program (HSEEP)—Volume I: HSEEP Overview and Exercise Program Management.* Washington, DC: USDHS.

U.S. Department of Homeland Security (2007, September). National Preparedness Guidelines. Washington, DC: USDHS.

U.S. Department of Homeland Security (2007, September). Target capabilities list—a companion to the national preparedness guidelines. Washington, DC: USDHS.

Chapter 3

The disaster cycle: an overview of disaster phases

Robert A. Jones

Disaster cycle

Although there are many definitions for what constitutes a disaster, one generally accepted definition is that a disaster is any event that results in a demand for services that exceeds available resources.

Disasters go through characteristic phases, defined as the *disaster cycle*. While this cycle helps to provide a framework for planning and response to a given disaster, it is important to realize that it is an artificial division with significant overlap between the phases.

Figure 3.1 illustrates the four phases of the disaster cycle that are discussed in this chapter.

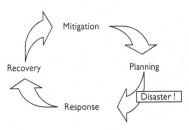

Figure 3.1 The disaster cycle.

Phases of the disaster cycle

Mitigation

The first phase of the disaster cycle is mitigation, which consists of the steps taken to minimize the effects of future disasters. The mitigation phase differs from the planning phase in that the mitigation phase is focused less on the medical or humanitarian response to a disaster and more on protecting physical structures and economic development.

The effectiveness of the mitigation phase is dependent on an accurate assessment of the kind of disasters most likely to affect the community. This continued threat analysis must include the following:

- Examination of prior disasters to look for steps that can be taken to minimize the negative outcome of future disasters
- Analysis of emerging threats
- New buildings or skyscrapers
- New industrial or chemical plants
- New rail lines, airports, seaports, or highways
- Security vulnerabilities at potential terrorist targets

Some examples of mitigation include the following:

- Governmental
- Building codes in an earthquake-prone area
- Zoning laws to prevent building in an area prone to flooding
- Personal
- Flood insurance to minimize economic impact of a disaster
- Fastening down a heavy bookcase so it doesn't fall and cause injury during an earthquake

Planning

The next phase of the disaster cycle is planning and preparation. It includes logistical planning as well as exercises necessary to effectively respond to a disaster.

The overall goal of the planning phase is to prepare the emergency response agencies and the population to minimize the loss of life and the societal impact of a disaster.

The planning phase can be divided into two different categories: general planning and event-specific planning.

General planning

This occurs throughout the interdisaster period and involves establishing an emergency operations plan (EOP).

- Planning for communications during a disaster
- Training first responders
- Stockpiling food and supplies
- Round-table exercises
- Establishing mutual aid agreements
- Planning for interagency coordination at local, state, and national levels
- Providing information to the public about personal readiness, including information on home disaster kits

Event-specific planning

This constitutes the efforts of preparing for a specific event, once an imminent threat has been identified.

- Making public announcements
- Preparing evacuation routes
- Organizing shelters
- Providing information to the public about what steps they should take to ensure their safety

Response

The response phase constitutes the immediate efforts to prevent the loss of life both during and after a disaster. The success of this phase relies heavily on preparations made during the planning phase. The disaster response will include the following:

- Alerting the public and activating the community EOP
- Providing emergency medical care as well as safety and security
- Search and rescue
- Fire protection efforts
- Evacuation and providing emergency shelters
- Suspending nonessential operations as needed to support disaster response efforts

In addition to preventing the loss of life, another goal of the response phase is to minimize the economic and societal impact of the disaster by providing basic needs to disaster victims until more comprehensive, long-term solutions can be identified.

The initial response will be lead by local first responders and community volunteers. Depending on the scope of the disaster, this may later be augmented by state and federal agencies as well as national and international nongovernmental organizations (NGOs).

Recovery

The recovery phase begins shortly after the disaster has started. It consists of rebuilding the affected area back into a functioning community. Depending on the scope and nature of a given disaster, this will require the efforts of both emergency response agencies as well as public resources.

This cooperation between the community and aid agencies will be necessary in order to

- Re-establish basic utilities such as electricity and water
- Rebuild the physical infrastructure
- Return displaced people back to their homes
- Return civil services such as police and health care to their pre-disaster roles
- Return commerce to the affected area

The recovery phase can be divided into two parts:

- *Short term recovery:* re-establishing vital needs such as food, shelter, and emergency medical treatment. This part overlaps with the response phase.
- *Long term recovery:* return to normalcy. This part may last for months to years. It can sometimes result in the complete redevelopment of an

area, which is why it is an advantageous time to consider implementing new mitigation measures.

In addition to physical, medical, and economic recovery, special attention must be given to groups within the population who may have greater difficulty coping with a disaster. Such groups include the following:
- Individuals with psychiatric illnesses
- Young children
- The elderly
- Residents of university dorms or skilled nursing facilities
- First responders who may suffer from acute stress reaction or post-traumatic stress disorder

The recovery phase deserves emphasis. Most disaster plans focus on the response phase, with less attention and less funding for the recovery phase, despite the fact that this is frequently the longest and most expensive part of the disaster cycle.

Conclusion

While it may be helpful to think of four discrete phases when planning for a disaster, the reality is that these phases often have a significant amount of overlap. In fact, different areas of a disaster zone can be in different phases despite the fact that they are dealing with the same disaster event.

In summary, the disaster cycle is helpful to consider when planning for a disaster, but the phases cannot be thought of too rigidly as they often coincide.

Suggested readings

Ciottone G (2006). Introduction to disaster medicine. In Ciottone G, ed. *Disaster Medicine.* Philadelphia: Elsevier Health Sciences, pp. 3–6.

Federal Emergency Management Agency. IS-1 Emergency Manager: An orientation to the position. FEMA independent study program. Retrieved September 5, 2008, from http://training.fema.gov/EMIWeb/IS/is1.asp.

Hogan DE, Burstein JL (2007). Basic perspectives on disaster, In Hogan DE, Burstein JL, *Disaster Medicine,* 2nd ed. Philadelphia: Lippincott Williams & Wilkins, pp. 1–11.

Nogi EK, Kelen GD (2004). Disaster medical services, In Tintinalli JE, ed. *Emergency Medicine: A Comprehensive Study Guide,* 6th ed. New York: McGraw-Hill, pp. 27–35.

Schultz C, Koenig K, Noji E (2006). Disaster preparedness. In Marx J, ed. *Rosen's Emergency Medicine Concepts and Clinical Practice,* 6th ed. Vol. 3. Philadelphia: Elsevier Health Sciences, pp. 3010–3021.

Warfield C. The disaster management cycle. Retrieved August 28, 2008, from http://www.gdrc.org/uem/disasters/1-dm_cycle.html

Mitigation phase of disasters

Kelly R. Klein

Melinda Johnson

Overview

Emergency preparedness can be defined as the activities and measures designed or undertaken to prepare for or minimize the effects of a hazard on the population, deal with the immediate emergency conditions that would be created by the hazard, effect emergency repairs, and restore vital utilities and facilities destroyed or damaged by the hazard (Stafford Act).

Mitigation, which is an integral part of emergency preparedness, is any sustained action taken to reduce or eliminate long-term risk to life and property from a hazard event. The Federal Emergency Management Agency (FEMA) defines mitigation planning as "a process for state, local, and Indian Tribal governments to identify policies, activities, and tools to implement mitigation actions." Importantly, mitigation actions involve sustained or permanent reduction of exposure to or potential loss from hazard events.

Mitigation focuses on breaking the cycle of disaster damage, reconstruction, and repeated damage seen in areas prone to disasters such as floods, hurricanes, earthquakes, which cost billions of dollars every year.

Mitigation includes the following activities:

- Complying with or exceeding floodplain management regulations
- Enforcing stringent building codes, flood-proofing requirements, seismic design standards, and wind-bracing requirements for new construction or repair of existing buildings
- Adopting zoning ordinances that steer development away from areas subject to flooding, storm surge, or coastal erosion
- Retrofitting buildings to withstand hurricane-strength winds or earthquakes

There are four phases of emergency management:

- Mitigation (prevention, protection)
- Preparedness (planning, training, exercises)
- Response
- Recovery

As the first step, mitigation involves all levels of society, the private sector, and public government. It helps organizations identify threats, determine vulnerabilities, and identify required resources needed to prevent the cycle destruction (National Incident Management System). The goal of mitigation activities is to eliminate or reduce the probability of disaster occurrence or reduce the effects of unavoidable disasters.

Mitigation can focus on the larger issues, such as where and how to build a new facility, but it can also focus on simple measures to prevent loss and injury, such as fastening bookcases to the wall in earthquake-prone areas.

The effectiveness of a mitigation strategy will depend on the availability of information on hazards and emergency risks and on the countermeasures to be taken. The mitigation phase, and indeed the whole disaster management cycle, includes the shaping of public policies and plans that either modify the causes of disasters or decrease their effects on people, property, and infrastructure.

Hazard overview

A multidisciplinary approach is necessary to create an effective mitigation plan. This requires outside resources, including emergency management and an understanding of hazards outside of the facility that would impact hospital operations.

For most organizations, the mitigation planning process begins with identifying potential hazards or emergency events by conducting a hazard vulnerability analysis (HVA). These hazards are any event that can reasonably be expected to occur within a given community and should include

- Natural events
- Technological failures
- Human threats

Technological hazards include disruption of vital services such as water, computer systems, electricity, or communications and are impacted by the density and socioeconomic structure of the surrounding community. In addition, human threats, both intentional and unintentional, should be examined (e.g., terrorist activity, mass events, and civil disturbances).

In the hospital scenario, the mitigation plan outlines the hospital's approach for identifying a realized threat, hazard, or other incident and is intended to provide a starting point for the four-step mitigation preparedness process.

The medical impact of a damaged health facility affects not just emergency care and inpatient care. A hospital's role in preventive medicine is essential, thus the long-term impact of the loss of a hospital far exceeds the impact of delayed treatment of trauma injuries.

The cost of disaster mitigation for a new facility can add 2% to the total cost. Retrofitting an existing building can add 8–15%.

Hazard vulnerability analysis (HVA)

The Joint Commission (TJC) requires that response plans identify "direct and indirect" effects that hazards may have on the hospital. After the identification of potential hazards, the facility should complete an HVA.

Questions that should be asked by the HVA team are as follows:

Is the event probable? Should consider:
- Known risk
- Historical data
- Manufacturer/vendor statistics

Issues to consider for human impact:
- Potential for staff death or injury
- Potential for patient death or injury

Issues to consider for property impact:
- Cost to replace
- Cost to set up temporary replacement
- Cost to repair
- Time to recover

Issues to consider for business impact:
- Business interruption
- Employees unable to report to work
- Customers unable to reach facility
- Company in violation of contractual agreements
- Imposition of fines and penalties or legal costs
- Interruption of critical supplies
- Interruption of product distribution
- Reputation and public image
- Financial impact and burden

Issues to consider for preparedness:
- Status of current plans
- Frequency of drills
- Training status
- Insurance
- Availability of alternate sources for critical supplies/services

Issues to consider for internal resources:
- Types of supplies on hand; will they meet need?
- Volume of supplies on hand; will they meet need?
- Staff availability
- Coordination with medical office buildings (MOBs)
- Availability of backup systems
- Internal resources' ability to withstand disasters and maintain survivability

Issues to consider for external resources:
- Types of agreements with community agencies, and drills?
- Coordination with local and state agencies
- Coordination with proximal health-care facilities
- Coordination with treatment-specific facilities
- Community resources

Each of these categories is described in semiquantitative terms: low, moderate, high, or not applicable.

Plugged into an Excel spreadsheet, the goal of the HAV is to aggregate the hazards and give the probability of each event to assist the planner in developing the emergency operations plan (EOP).

Examples of hazards

Zoning and building-code requirements for rebuilding in high-hazard areas
- Floodplain buyouts
- Analyses of floodplain and other hazard-related data to determine where it is safe to build in normal times, open shelters in emergencies, or locate temporary housing in the aftermath of a disaster.

Critical infrastructure protection
- Radiation detection
- Improvised explosive device (IED) prevention
- Hardening
- Security
- Communications security

Staff
- Availability or willingness of staff to report to work during an emergency
- Family members of staff—children and elderly parents who will need care during an emergency
- Pets
- Proper protection of staff during an event
- Pharmaceutical prophylaxis
- Personal protective equipment (PPE)

Type of natural hazards
- Hurricane
- Tornado
- Blizzard
- Earthquake
- Infections disease outbreak
- Contamination
- Flood
- Fire

Human-event hazards
- Active shooter
- Hostage situation
- Mass-casualty incident (hazardous materials [HazMat])
- HazMat incident (internal)
- Weapons of mass destruction (WMD) (biological)
- WMD (chemical)
- WMD (nuclear)
- HazMat incident (external)
- Illegal chemical Lab
- Bomb threat
- Mass-casualty incident (medical)
- Mass-casualty incident (trauma)

- Civil disturbance
- Infant abduction

Technological hazards
- Medical-vacuum failure
- Generator failure
- Medical-gas failure
- Information systems failure
- Communications failure
- Fire (internal)
- Sewer failure
- Natural gas failure
- Water failure
- Steam failure
- Flood (internal)
- Electrical failure
- Fire system failure
- Heating, ventilation, and air conditioning (HVAC) failure
- Fuel shortage

Each of these elements should be reflected in the EOP with an appropriate response plan.

For example, the mitigation plan for infant abduction would include restricted access and badging for only those employees who work in nursery, a security code specific for infant abduction—e.g., "Code Pink"—having all egress points for the nursery areas lock down with a single mechanism when the code is called, and security cameras covering the area. The EOP would indicate how each of these mitigation elements acts in concert with one another to prevent and respond to an infant abduction.

Emergency operations plan (EOP)

Once the HVA is complete, the planner must develop mitigation goals and objectives, identify and prioritize mitigation actions, formulate an implementation strategy, and assemble the planning document.

The creation of the emergency operations plan (EOP) is the final step in mitigation planning. An EOP outlining the behavior of a hospital in a disaster event must be reviewed and updated annually. Additionally, it must take into consideration the requirements of the regulatory and accreditation agencies, professional standards, and current best practices of emergency planning.

The EOP contains the steps to appropriately respond to each of the hazards identified by the HVA. While most organizations have moved to an all-hazards approach for their EOP, a plan to respond to each type of hazard must be a part of the EOP.

Financial assistance in mitigation planning

In order to encourage the use of mitigation planning, FEMA has created several grant programs that include a mitigation plan requirement.

Stafford Act grant programs
- Hazard Mitigation Grant Program (HMGP)
- Pre-Disaster Mitigation Program (PDM)
- Public Assistance (PA)

National Flood Insurance Act grant programs
- Flood Mitigation Assistance (FMA)
- Repetitive Flood Claims (RFC)
- Severe Repetitive Loss (SRL)

There are also laws, regulations, and guidance associated with mitigation planning that determine eligibility for the grants.

The Disaster Mitigation Act of 2000 provides the legal basis for FEMA's mitigation plan requirements for state, local, and Indian Tribal governments as a condition of mitigation grant assistance.

Mitigation Planning Regulations (Interim Final Rule), as published in the *Code of Federal Regulations*, provide the rules for state, local, and Indian Tribal governments to meet in order to be eligible for specified FEMA mitigation grants.

Mitigation Planning Guidance provides additional guidance for state, local, and Indian Tribal governments to meet the requirements of FEMA's Mitigation Planning Regulations. Such guidance includes the following:
- Mitigation Planning Guidance "Blue Book"
- Mitigation Planning "How-To" Guides (FEMA)

Conclusion

Mitigation efforts in hospital preparedness plans are an essential component in responding to and recovering from disasters. Mitigation is an ongoing process and must include identifying hazard vulnerabilities and what plans are needed for response. Only by appropriately identifying areas of vulnerability can these issues be properly addressed in the planning process.

However, hospital mitigation efforts cannot occur in a vacuum and must include community partners. A hospital might be unaware of hazards in the community that would impact the facility if they did not engage emergency managers and other partners in the process.

Suggested readings

Disaster Mitigation Planning Assistance Web site: http://matrix.msu.edu/~disaster/

Federal Emergency Management Agency. Developing the mitigation plan: identifying mitigation actions and implementation strategies. Retrieved March 20, 2009, from http://www.fema.gov/library/viewRecord.do?id=1886

Federal Emergency Management Agency. Guide for all hazards emergency planning, Retrieved April 22, 2009, from http://www.fema.gov/pdf/plan/slg101.pdf

Federal Emergency Management Agency. Mitigation. Retrieved March 11, 2009, from http://www.fema.gov/plan/mitplanning/index.shtm

Federal Emergency Management Agency (2007, June). Robert T. Stafford Disaster Relief and Emergency Assistance Act (Public Law 93-288). Retrieved October 15, 2008, from http://www.fema.gov/pdf/about/stafford_act.pdf

Federal Emergency Management Agency (2008, August). National Incident Management System. Retrieved October 15, 2008, from http://www.fema.gov/emergency/nims/index.shtm

Kaiser Foundation Health Plan, Inc. (2001). Kaiser Permanente HVA. Retrieved March 20, 2009, from http://www.njha.com/ep/pdf/627200834041PM.pdf

Keyes D, Carbone AJ, Burstein J, Schwartz R, Swientor R (2005). *Medical Response to Terrorism: Preparedness and Clinical Practice.* 236. Philadelphia: Lippincott Williams & Williams. Retrieved March 23, 2009, from http://www.helid.desastres.net/gsdl2/collect/who/pdf/s8283e/s8283e.pdf

Pan American Health Organization. Disaster home page. http://new.paho.org/disasters/

Pan American Health Organization. Natural disaster mitigation in drinking water and sewage systems. http://www.paho.org/english/Ped/nd-water_mit.pdf

Pan American Health Organization. Safe hospitals—reference documents. http://www.disaster-info.net/safehospitals_refdocs/

Urban Environmental Management. Disaster risk and mitigation. http://www.gdrc.org/uem/disasters/index.html

Preparedness phase of disaster

Tracy Buchman

Overview

Preparedness can be defined as the activities, tasks, programs, and systems developed and implemented prior to an emergency that are used to support the prevention of, mitigation of, response to, and recovery from emergencies (National Fire Protection Association [NFPA], 2007).

Preparedness is a continuous process and involves integration at all levels of government and between government, private sector, and nongovernmental organizations to identify threats, determine vulnerabilities, and identify required resources (National Incident Management System [NIMS]).

Emergency preparedness can be defined as the activities and measures designed or undertaken to prepare for or minimize the effects of a hazard on the civilian population, to deal with the immediate emergency conditions that would be created by the hazard, and to effectuate emergency repairs to, or the emergency restoration of, vital utilities and facilities destroyed or damaged by the hazard (Stafford Act).

The main activities in the preparedness phase revolve around planning, training, and exercising the plan.

Emergency management committee

A motivated multidisciplinary committee is essential to successful planning. This committee should meet regularly and consist of clinical and nonclinical representatives. Additionally, local agencies such as police, fire and emergency medical services, emergency management, and public health should be included in committee deliberations to help clarify roles and responsibilities and encourage personal networking (Hospital Incident Command System [HICS] Guidebook).

Committee activities should include the following:

- Creating and updating a comprehensive all-hazards emergency management program on an annual basis
- Conducting a hazard vulnerability analysis (HVA) on an annual basis
- Developing an emergency operations plan (EOP) and standard operating procedures to address the hazards identified
- Providing for continuity of operations planning by writing needed hospital operations plans
- Ensuring that all employees and medical staff receive training in accordance with hospital requirements and regulatory guidelines and understand their role(s) and responsibilities for a disaster response

All-hazards emergency operations plan

The EOP outlines the hospital's approach for responding to and recovering from a realized threat, hazard, or other incident and is intended to provide overall direction and synchronization of the response structure and processes to be used by the hospital.

Essential areas that should be comprehensively and concisely addressed include the the following:

- Initiation activities
  - Plan initiation
  - Incident phases
  - Hospital command center (HCC)
  - Hospital incident command system (HICS)
- Emergency communication and notification
  - Internal and staff notification levels
  - Notification and communication with external agencies
  - Communication with patients and family
  - Backup communications
  - Communication with purveyors
  - Communication with other health-care organizations
- Resource and asset management
  - Obtaining and replenishing of medical and nonmedical supplies
  - Managing staff support activities
  - Sharing of resources
  - Evacuation activities
- Security and safety operations
  - Security, including local support
  - Managing hazardous wastes: biological, radiological, and chemical
  - Access and egress control (facility lockdown)
  - Traffic control
- Managing staff roles and responsibilities
  - Staffing critical areas: responsibilities and identification
- Managing utilities
  - Alternative utilities
- Managing patient clinical and support activities
  - Clinical activities
  - Special patients
  - Personal hygiene and sanitation requirements
  - Mental health services
  - Patient tracking
  - Fatality management
  - Decontamination
- Recovery procedures
  - Recovery activities initiation
  - Demobilization: HCC, staff and resources
  - Department director responsibilities
  - Evaluation of events and exercises (after-action report)

Incident planning

Hospital planning for possible disaster-related incidents can be lengthy. Planning guidance from governmental agencies and professional associations is available in print form and on Web sites.

The following series of incident planning guides (IPGs) have been developed by the Hospital Emergency Incident Command System IV (HEICS IV) project to assist hospitals with evaluating existing plans or writing needed plans.

The guides were written to prompt the plan writer and reviewer(s) to consider what the EOP should address, based on the nature of the incident, available resources, and response needs, to manage 27 of the Department of Homeland Security's hospital-related national scenarios.

National planning scenarios

Internal incident planning guides (IPG)

- Bomb threat
- Evacuation
- Fire
- Hazardous material spill
- Hospital overload
- Hostage/barricade
- Infant or child abduction
- Internal flooding
- Loss of HVAC
- Loss of power
- Loss of water
- Severe weather
- Work stoppage

External incident planning guides (IPG)

- Nuclear detonation
- Biological attack—Anthrax
- Biological disease outbreak—pandemic Influenza
- Biological attack—plague
- Chemical attack—blister agent
- Chemical attack—toxic industrial chemicals
- Chemical attack—nerve agent
- Chemical attack—chlorine
- Natural disaster—earthquake
- Natural disaster—hurricane
- Radiological attack—radiological dispersion device (RDD)
- Explosives attack—improvised explosive device (IED)
- Biological attack—food contamination
- Cyber attack

Each IPG is formatted according to four specific time periods and contains planning considerations for each time period:
- Immediate: 0–2 hours
- Intermediate: 2–12 hours
- Extended: greater than 12 hours
- Demobilization and system recovery

Thorough planning and standardization among hospitals throughout the United States enhance overall efficiency and effectiveness in the response and recovery phases of an incident.

Exercising the plan

Exercising the plan is an important component in the planning phase in order to achieve and evaluate proficiency.

The Joint Commission outlines standards for exercises in the Emergency Management Standard EM.03.01.03. The Homeland Security Exercise and Evaluation Program (HSEEP) is a set of tools to help design, conduct, evaluate, and improve hospital exercises. Use of these tools can assist the organization in complying with the standards of regulatory and accrediting agencies.

An exercise approach that is often used can be referred to as the "crawl-walk-run" approach. As described in the HICS Guidebook, the "crawl-walk-run" approach is accomplished by the following:

- Tabletop exercise (**crawl**) enables participants to move through a scenario on the basis of discussions regarding the coordination of plans and procedures with other departments or agencies.
- Functional exercise (**walk**) helps participants work through plans and procedures in a real-time scenario, typically based in an operations center environment. The exercise pace can be increased or decreased depending on the participants' ability to work through their plans and procedures.
- Full-scale exercise (**run**) requires participants to move people and apparatus while working through plans and procedures in real time.

The following checklist identifies key HSEEP elements that should be included in the design, conduct, evaluation, and improvement process:

- Exercise scenarios are developed with the response partners being part of the exercise.
- Exercise scenarios are based on the hazard vulnerability assessment (HVA), including previously identified opportunities and resolved issues.
- Exercise objectives are based on minimal levels of readiness, critical areas, and/or target capabilities.
- Objectives of the exercise are to be SMART and to assess capabilities in order to identify gaps, deficiencies, and vulnerabilities.
  - **S**imple—straightforward, easy to read.
  - **M**easurable—specific and quantifiable.
  - **A**chievable —within the time of the exercise.
  - **R**ealistic—is the scenario likely to occur?
  - **T**ask-oriented—some observable action taken: incident command (IC) should be set up within 10 minutes of notification.
- The exercise is evaluated using the HSEEP After-Action Report and Improvement Plan (AAR/IP) template. Correction actions for identified gaps, deficiencies, and vulnerabilities are documented and dates for correction of corrective actions are established.
- The completion dates for assignments in the AAR/IP are monitored and reported.

Conclusion

Hospital preparedness is an essential component of the nation's preparedness against both intentional acts of terror and naturally occurring crises that have the potential to cause serious harm to the U.S. population or territory.

Planning is an ongoing process and must concentrate on regulatory standards and identified hazard vulnerabilities. Cyclic training and exercising on incident management and emergency response procedures ensures adequate staff preparation, competence, and confidence.

Furthermore, hospital-planning efforts must be integrated with other health-care organizations and external response partners. Effective hospital planning with the community also better ensures business continuity during and following an incident.

Suggested readings

California Emergency Medical Services Authority (2007). Hospital Incident Command System (HICS). Retrieved October 15, 2008, from http://www.emsa.ca.gov/HICS/default.asp

Federal Emergency Management Agency. Homeland Security Exercise and Evaluation Program. Retrieved October 15, 2008, from https://hseep.dhs.gov/pages/1001_HSEEP7.aspx

Federal Emergency Management Agency (2007, June). Robert T. Stafford Disaster Relief and Emergency Assistance Act (Public Law 93-288). Retrieved October 15, 2008, from http://www.fema.gov/pdf/about/stafford_act.pdf

Federal Emergency Management Agency (2008, May). State and Local Guide (SLG) 101: Guide for All-Hazard Emergency Operations Planning. Retrieved October 15, 2008, from http://www.fema.gov/plan/gaheop.shtm

Federal Emergency Management Agency (2008, August). National Incident Management System. Retrieved October 15, 2008, from http://www.fema.gov/emergency/nims/index.shtm

National Fire Protection Association (2007). NFPA 1600 Standard on Disaster/Emergency Management and Business Continuity Programs (2007 ed.). Quincy, MA: National Fire Protection Association.

The Joint Commission (2008). Comprehensive Accreditation Manual for Hospitals: The Official Handbook. Oakbrook Terrace, IL: Joint Commission Resources.

U.S. Department of Veterans Affairs (2008, August). 2008 Emergency Management Program Guidebook. Retrieved October 15, 2008, from http://www1.va.gov/emshg/page.cfm?pg=114

Response phase of disaster

Adam Webster

Introduction

The medical-response phase of a disaster is typically short-lived and the most chaotic period of the disaster cycle. Depending on the type of incident, the duration of the incident can last anywhere from 2 to 12 hours or 3 to 7 days. After that period, the recovery and mitigation efforts begin.

Even response issues that extend to several weeks' duration, such as search and rescue, utility restoration, or health and medical response, are brief in duration compared to the entire disaster response effort. Knowing the lifecycle of an incident will help determine this time frame.

Incident notification

The first phase of the cycle is incident notification. Frequently, hospitals will only receive short-term notice of an impending incident, as little as 5 to 10 minutes.

The emergency department (ED) will be notified through medical control of the types of trauma patient(s) it will receive. Based on this initial notification, the ED charge nurse can determine the ED's bed capacity, staff, and resources needs for disaster patients. If medical control alerts the hospital of multiple casualties as a result of an emergency or disaster, the administrator on duty (AOD) should be notified.

Hospitals should be provided the following information:

- Type of incident
- Location of the incident
- Number and type of injuries
- Special actions to be taken (decontamination, transportation of patients)
- Estimated time of arrival of first arriving EMS units

Developing an incident planning process is vital to the hospital's operations at this time. There are six essential steps in the incident planning process:

- Understanding the hospital's policies and procedures
- Assessing the situation
- Establishing incident objectives
- Determining appropriate strategies to achieve disaster management objectives
- Giving tactical direction and ensuring accountability
- Providing necessary operational changes, such as assigning more or fewer resources or changing disaster response tactics

Emergency operations plan

Once the situation has been assessed and based on the type of incident, it may be necessary to activate the hospital's emergency operations plan (EOP) and work under the hospital incident command system (HICS).

After patients begin to arrive, it may be necessary to activate the hospital's incident command (IC) center. The administrator on duty (or designee) assuming the IC role will need to call their incident management team (IMT) to report to the command center for an incident briefing.

The IMT may consist of the incident commander and an administrative assistant. In some cases, this may suffice, depending on how well versed the IMT is with HICS and the hospital's EOP.

Each section branch may not work out of the command center, but instead may work in other available sites within the hospital.

Communications

By monitoring communication with medical control, private EMS companies, and local emergency management, the number of casualties a hospital might receive can be estimated.

When the ED begins to approach its surge capacity limit, the administration will need to make the decision if the hospital wants to continue accepting patients or request that patients be diverted to other hospitals. If the hospital continues to accept patients, extra staff may be needed from other departments to assist with the triage and treatment segment.

Hospitals may need a staging area for staff to stay or meet to receive task assignments. The person managing the staging area is the personnel staging unit leader under the HICS operations section.

Reassessment

After the initial surge of trauma patients, hospitals must re-evaluate their resources and assets. Hospitals should have emergency contingency plans with their regular vendors in the event of a disaster.

Once this option is exhausted, hospitals should contact the emergency operations center (EOC) to request medical supplies and equipment. Resources should only be requested through the EOC if other hospitals or medical suppliers are unable to provide the supplies or equipment needed.

Sharing information with internal hospital staff is critical to help them understand the situation. A mass emergency notification system should be used to communicate with staff. Keeping staff, patients, and visitors informed will prevent the transmission of misinformation.

External communications with police, fire, EMS, or other hospitals should occur on a regular schedule, such as every hour or upon any sudden change in hospital status (e.g., another wave of trauma patients, critical resource shortfalls). Communication can be by phone, e-mail, hand-held radios, or amateur radio.

In a disaster event, it is best to communicate with external agencies through the Incident Message form (HICS 213). By using this form, communication is documented and easily understood by the receiving agency.

Once the transport of patients from the scene of the disaster to the hospital has been completed, the hospital can begin to make its demobilization plan. This may not take effect immediately, but there will be certain HICS positions that can be deactivated or combined with other positions in order to return to normal operations. The trigger of when to officially demobilize will be based on the amount of resources needed to treat the existing casualties. If the resource requests are manageable, then HICS and the hospital command center can be demobilized and deactivated and operations can be restored to normal.

Response actions cannot be accomplished without thorough mitigation and preparedness plans. Hospitals and treatment centers must identify the hazards and vulnerabilities in order to determine what to plan for, and then create an EOP and exercise to determine the best response.

Testing a hospital's EOP and stressing its capabilities will further advance preparedness for an emergency or disaster. This will ensure an organized and orderly disaster response and recovery.

Suggested readings

California Emergency Medical Systems Authority (2006, August). Hospital Incident Management System Guidebook. Chapter 2: Overview of the principles of the incident command system, p. 12. http://www.emsa.ca.gov/HICS/files/Guidebook_Glossary.pdf

California Emergency Medical Systems Authority (2006, August). Hospital Incident Management System Guidebook. Chapter 6: Lifecycle of an incident, pp. 51–69. http://www.emsa.ca.gov/HICS/files/Guidebook_Glossary.pdf

Cloonan C (Colonel). Mass casualty management—initial responder: tips on what to do. Accessed April 22, 2009, from http://www.brooksidepress.com/Products/OperationalMedicine/DATA/operationalmed/MilitaryMedicine/Disaster1.doc

Federal Emergency Management Agency (2008, April). FEMA ICS-300: Intermediate ICS for Expanding Incidents. http://training.fema.gov/EMIWeb/IS/ICSResource/ICSResCntr_Training.htm

Recovery phase of disasters

Rachel L. Fowler

Introduction

"[I]n seeking to move away from our emergency, humanitarian phase to a more developmental phase, our people will have to make fundamental shifts in their own attitudes—in living, in doing business, in coexisting with one another. They will have to break with time-honored traditions if, for instance, these are violations of human rights or perpetuate systemic inefficiencies."

—*Ellen Johnson Sirleaf*, President of Liberia

Preparedness. Response. Recovery. Mitigation. Originally described as the third discrete stage in a linear four-phase process of reconstruction and development, the concept of recovery is increasingly recognized as dynamic and often overlapping with all stages of emergency management, particularly mitigation. Recovery remains the least concrete and most difficult to define of all stages.

Given the multifaceted and unique nature of both natural and humanitarian disasters, it is challenging to construct a singular, algorithmic model that is applicable to all disaster settings and populations. However, common themes emerge that may be used as guides during this important process.

Recent conceptual models have increasingly emphasized the inclusion of varying degrees of mitigation, emphasizing a concept originally proposed by Haas et al. (1977) as "value choices that give varying emphasis to the early return to normalcy, the reduction of future vulnerability, or to opportunities for improved efficiency, equity, and amenity."

As both a necessary element of immediate disaster management and an opportunity to fortify populations against future catastrophe, the process of recovery is complex and longitudinal.

- Recovery should not simply focus on "return to normalcy" or a previous state of affairs, but instead a situation better equipped to manage future disasters.
- Bolstering the needs of a given population will depend significantly on the character and extent of the disaster, as well as the preexisting conditions of the setting.
- A high-impact natural disaster may necessitate recovery and mitigation efforts focused on public services infrastructure and housing needs.
- Complex humanitarian emergencies, such as war, genocide, and terrorism, will require strategies to identify and address risk factors for violent recidivism in order to prevent recurrent conflict.

Principle

The definition of recovery has evolved from its original introduction as a component of a four-stage value-added "ordered, knowable, and predictable" process, as described by Haas et al. (1977) to a fluid phase that is often interdependent on and occurring simultaneously with all others. Its primary premise is one of sustainability.

- The concept of sustainable development was originally introduced in the report of the 1987 United Nations World Commission on Environment and Development as "development that meets the needs of the present without compromising the ability of future generations to meet their own needs."
- Recovery efforts should seek to re-establish and enhance the self-sufficiency of a community and not merely to revert to a pre-disaster state.
- Given the collective desire to re-establish normalcy as quickly as possible in the aftermath of a disaster, particularly when a significant and conspicuous percentage of the population has been displaced, sustainable development is often at odds with a natural tendency to return to familiar methods and surroundings.
- Increased media exposure also places political leaders under considerable pressure to make recovery efforts rapid, visible, and tangible.

For these reasons, it is important that the preparedness phase incorporate thoughtful and conscientious pre-disaster recovery planning. In the absence of careful planning, recovery efforts easily become focused on repair rather than on development. Recovery must hinge upon development in order to remain sustainable.

Practice

To date, no recognized guidelines exist to aid the disaster manager in formulation of a specific recovery plan. In general, recovery entails the process of

- Rebuilding and reshaping the physical infrastructure
- Restoring the social, economic, and natural environment. The direct and indirect effects of a specific disaster, whether natural or humanitarian, will determine the nature of such actions.

Direct effects are those most visible and include the following:

- Death
- Disability
- Psychological trauma
- Damages to public services infrastructure, notably
- Housing
- Systems of water and sanitation
- Clinics and hospitals
- Roads and transportation

Indirect effects may be less overt but are equally destructive and include

- Loss of businesses and jobs
- Decreased spending
- Altered family units and social support systems
- Communicable disease epidemics
- Malnutrition
- Increased violence

Recovery efforts address direct and indirect effects on a continuum ranging from simple repair and restoration to sustainable development and mitigation. Ideally, the focus should remain on sustainability.

For example, a natural disaster urban expansion plan that adequately assesses vulnerability of building sites will more successfully mitigate against future catastrophe than simply offering disaster loans to repair preexisting structures.

Similarly, recovery plans can serve as opportunities for sustainable economic development by replenishing lost business inventory and working capital. At the same time they can restructure business interiors to optimally match operational needs and correct preexisting urban design flaws in pedestrian access and parking.

In the post-conflict setting, recovery efforts might include not only long-term planning for disease control programs that address increased spread of communicable illnesses but also mitigation that attempts to identify risk and protective factors for the purposes of preventive intervention and future conflict aversion.

Coordination

It is essential that recovery plans address actual rather than projected population needs.

- Failure to coordinate and match population-defined needs with the influx of external aid risks a secondary disaster in the form of poorly distributed donor resources.
- Efficient distribution of resources and development of aid programs involves implementing the concept of matching community-defined needs with the capacities of both donor and local organizations that will be designing and implementing recovery programs.
- This approach to recovery effectively allows the community to define and prioritize post-disaster development efforts. It implicitly engenders self-sufficiency and sustainability by promoting the creation of reliable, internal networks that will survive beyond the recovery phase and form the foundation of a stronger and more resilient post-disaster community.

Such networks of local community and social services organizations are described as systems of horizontal integration. Populations with high degrees of pre-disaster horizontal integration will be better equipped to coordinate recovery aid resources and less likely to fragment under duress of disaster. As such, the development of horizontal integration is an important component of both preparedness, as well as recovery and mitigation efforts.

Vertical integration describes a community's access to external resources and larger social and political institutions. Populations with high degrees of vertical integration are publicly visible, influential, and capable of easier access to external funds.

A balance between vertical and horizontal integration results in optimum coordination.

- An overdependence on vertical aid results in an approach that fails to sufficiently involve those at the community level, thereby hampering self-sufficiency.
- Too little horizontal mediation results in poorly defined needs and subsequent chaotic, unregulated application of external resources.

When the latter occurs, it is likely that recovery efforts will be unnecessarily redundant on some fronts, while leaving other areas with inadequate or no aid. Recovery should be coordinated in a manner that supports the overarching premise of doing the most good for the most people.

Conclusions and emerging themes

- Perceive disaster recovery from the outset as a long-term process spanning years or even decades.
- Develop and encourage a collective mental vision of a more resilient post-disaster community that supersedes a mere return to normalcy.
- Promote the moment of opportunity for community reshaping and future hazard mitigation.
- Involve key local, governmental, international, and humanitarian aid stakeholders early to achieve balanced, integrated management and to promote self-sufficiency.
- Secure representation for less powerful and more socially vulnerable groups.
- Prevent a secondary disaster by ensuring that provision of external aid is centrally coordinated and distributed in accordance with the "concept of fit."
- Incorporate the concept of sustainable development into every element of pre- and post-disaster recovery planning.

Suggested readings

Berke PR, Campanella TJ (2006). Planning for postdisaster resiliency. *Annals of the American Academy of Political and Social Science:* Vol. 604, *Shelter from the Storm: Repairing the National Emergency Management System after Hurricane Katrina,* pp. 192–207.

Berke PR, Kartez J, Wenger D (1993). Recovery after disaster: achieving sustainable development, mitigation and equity. *Disasters* 17(2):93–109.

Haas JE, Kates RW, Bowden MJ (1977). *Reconstruction Following Disaster.* Cambridge, MA: MIT Press.

Petterson J (1999). A review of the literature and programs on local recovery from disaster. Report No. 102. Fairfax, VA: Public Entity Risk Institute.

Reza A, Anderson M, Mercy JA (2008), Chapter 20: A public health approach to preventing the health consequences of armed conflict. In Levy BS, Sidel VW, eds. *War and Public Health,* 2nd ed. New York: Oxford University Press, pp. 339–356.

Rubin CB (2008–2009). Webmaster for Disaster Recovery Resources Web site: http://www.disasterrecoveryresources.net. Supported by the Public Entity Risk Institute.

Rubin CB (2009) Long term recovery from disasters—the neglected component of emergency management, *Journal of Homeland Security and Emergency Management:* 6(1), Article 46.

Rubin C, Saperstein M, Barbee D (1985). Community Recovery from a Major Disaster. Monograph 41. Institute of Behavioral Science, University of Colorado, Boulder, CO.

Sirleaf EJ (2009). *This Child Will Be Great: Memoir of a Remarkable Life by Africa's First Woman President.* New York: Harper Collins, p. 303.

Smith GP, Wenger D (2006), Chapter 14: Sustainable disaster recovery: operationalizing an existing agenda. In Rodriguez H, Quarantelli EL, Dynes R, eds. *Handbook of Disaster Research.* New York: Springer, pp. 234–274.

Spangle W & Associates (1991). *Rebuilding After Earthquakes: Lessons from Planners.* Portola Valley, CA: William Spangle & Associates, Inc.

Temin E (2006). Chapter 49: Rehabilitation and reconstruction. In Ciottone G, ed. *Disaster Medicine.* Philadelphia: Mosby, pp. 317–321.

Toole MJ (1997). Chapter 20: Complex emergencies: refugee and other populations. In Noji EK, ed. *The Public Health Consequences of Disasters.* New York: Oxford University Press, pp. 419–442.

World Commission on Environment and Development (1987). Our Common Future, Report of the World Commission on Environment and Development, Published as Annex to General Assembly document A/42/427, Development and International Co-operation: Environment. August 2, 1987.

Part 2

General Concepts

Components of
Disaster Response

Local-level disaster response

Michael Gray

Andrew Milsten

Introduction

The response to any disaster begins with the deployment of local resources for the initial containment and medical management of the emergency. The disaster response ultimately ends with local resources in the final act of cleaning up from the disaster.

Throughout the management of a disaster, there may be federal or state support, but these are usually delayed unless the disaster can be predicted, such as an expected hurricane. As the local response is critical in the management of any disaster, it is imperative that all resources be considered in preparation for a disaster.

This section will describe the key concepts in the medical preparation of a local disaster management plan.

Governmental operations and local disaster planning

Fundamental to understanding local components of an effective emergency management strategy is an understanding of the local governmental agencies and structures. All communities are required by the Emergency Planning and Community Right to Know Act to have established state emergency response committees and local emergency planning committees.

How these local planning committees interact and integrate within the government varies by community. A local response might be organized by town, city, municipality, county, or tribe.

The local government agency responsible for the integration an emergency action plan may be composed of elected officials, appointed officials, or a combination of both.

Three basic questions need to be addressed when organizing the emergency health care plan to a disaster.

- What agencies and officials are responsible for providing essential services that coordinate with emergency medical planning and treatment?

An understanding of the government agency involved and the hierarchy of that agency will be critical when integrating various services for medical management during a disaster.

For example, the medical staff must be aware of when a scene is safe to enter, how to obtain needed supplies, and how to coordinate the safety of medical personnel at the primary site of the disaster. The primary official who will procure additional medical supplies or activate other services may be the town manager, the incident commander, or another designated official.

- Who will be the chief medical officer (CMO) responsible for the activation and planning of the disaster medical services and who does that person answer to?

In many disaster plans, the general command structure is organized by the incident command system (ICS). Under the ICS, there needs to be a designated person whose primary responsibility is organization and deployment of medical resources. This person may be the ICS commander or someone who answers directly to the ICS commander. In either case, the CMO needs to be heavily involved with the planning of a disaster response.

- How are additional medical resources procured?

It is unreasonable and often not feasible for a single community to have both the financial resources and personnel to be consistently staffed for every disaster. As such, disaster planners need to be aware of the various options available for additional resources. A good disaster plan also describes how resources are activated.

Local resources for disaster planning

Medical preparation in disaster planning requires involvement of multiple agencies and resources. Local emergency service departments are used almost universally and are a significant part of the local response to a disaster.

However, most disasters require medical assistance beyond the capability of local responders. Therefore, to prepare for a disaster response, officials need to consider the options beyond local EMS.

Local emergency planning committees

Local emergency planning committees and state emergency response commissions were mandated by the Environmental Protection Agency (EPA) in 1986 for the purpose of improving community access to chemical hazards and planning for chemical disasters.

The limitation of the local emergency planning committee is that they are mandated, at a minimum, to prepare for chemical disasters and track hazardous chemicals in a community. There is no mandate for planning for other disasters in the EPA's law.

Many localities have emergency operation plans as directed by the Federal Emergency Management Agency (FEMA) that are incorporated into the responsibilities of the local emergency planning committee. Some of the local plans are updated on a consistent basis and others are supplied with a minimal amount of information as required by FEMA for federal funding purposes. As such, there is a wide variation in preparedness at a local level.

The medical community needs to be aware that local and state emergency committees exist and that the medical community needs to be involved with these committees.

Local and state committees are involved with more than the medical management of a disaster. They may also be planning for search and rescue preparations, cleanup, coordination with utility providers to provide electricity and water, and transportation and communication in a disaster.

The actual medical management of a disaster needs to be represented on the local and state committees for the coordination of increased hospital utilization and deployment of patients to various hospitals, EMS transportation, triage systems, medical protocols, and communication for medical providers.

Intergovernmental agreements

Intergovernmental agreements (IGAs) are agreements between neighboring communities to share resources in the event of increased demand such as a disaster.

There are many different types of IGAs. IGAs may define agreements between local law enforcement, fire department, or emergency medical services. The agreements may be written as a formal contract with payment made for the services, as a joint agreement with neighboring localities sharing the services, or as an informal understanding of mutual aid in the event that a local service's resources are overwhelmed.

The advantages of IGAs are numerous. IGAs enable smaller communities to provide a broader range of services than they would otherwise not be able to afford. They permit decreased duplication of rarely used services and allow for sharing of expensive equipment and specialized services.

As beneficial as IGAs are, there are also limitations, including the fact that many IGAs are informal in nature and poorly constructed. It is often difficult to distribute costs among communities in the event of a shared resource. There may also be a perceived or actual loss of control over services of a small community to a larger community that controls the limited resource.

Despite these limitations, IGAs are a critical component to any effective local emergency response system. A proper IGA should define the extent of the shared resources, including the operation protocols, risks and liabilities, and finances.

Other community medical resources

Most communities are unable to provide full medical disaster management resources based solely on municipal resources. In planning for disasters, the medical community has to consider all resources available and reach out to the private sector for planning.

Although small disasters may be handled entirely by the municipality without additional community resources, larger disasters may require some assistance beyond the government's ability. Resources to consider when planning for a disaster include those listed on Table 8.1.

Medical Reserve Corps (MRC)

The MRC is a volunteer organization composed of active and retired medical professionals including physicians, nurses, and allied health professionals who are available to provide additional resources in the event of an emergency. The MRC can often assist during the initial hours of a disaster response in an organized fashion during the time of maximal surge of new patients.

Table 8.1 Resources to consider when planning for a disaster

Transportation	Diagnostics	Facilities	Supplies	Personal
EMS	Hospitals	Hospitals	Pharmacies	Physicians
Taxi	Physician offices	Nursing homes	Department stores	School nurses
Air ambulance	Freestanding labs	Schools	Medical supply stores	Medical students
School buses		Hotels		Veterinarians
Regional transit authority		Gymnasiums or arenas		Physical therapists, athletic trainers

The MRC is run under the direction of the Office of the Surgeon General and is a partner of Civilian Corps. The MRC is often involved with local and state emergency planning committees.

National Voluntary Organizations Active in Disaster

NVOAD is an organization that focuses on the coordination of multiple volunteer organizations that respond to a disaster. The purpose is to coordinate better communications between organizations to more efficiently provide volunteer services in a disaster while minimizing redundancy between volunteer service organizations.

State medical societies

Many state medical societies are able to provide additional assistance and support during a disaster and often have a list serve available for communicating with physicians when needed.

Federal assistance

The federal government may be required to lend assistance to a local disaster response. Communities need to know how to activate federal assistance through their state emergency planning committees and how to integrate the federal support.

Localities need to be aware of the limitations of federal support and how to best incorporate this support into the disaster plan.

Federal assistance for medical management in the event of disasters is typically provided by Disaster Medical Assistance Teams (DMAT) and is overseen by the Department of Health and Human Services. DMATs are designed to assist the local response by providing additional medical personnel and equipment to a medical disaster.

Scene planning

Preparation and planning for a disaster involves more than gathering and cataloguing resources. Local planning committees need to consider the actual operation and deployment of resources during a disaster.

The response to a disaster goes well beyond medical management of victims; however, the focus here will be only on medical-scene planning.

The primary components of response scene planning involve those discussed below.

Containment of a disaster

Although not typically considered part of the medical response to a disaster, there are times when this will involve the medical community. Infectious disease outbreaks need to be quarantined in order to limit the spread of disease. Involvement with public health personal is critical for containment in these cases.

Search and rescue

This is usually handled by fire and EMS systems and is usually not a significant part of the medical response unless it involves treatment of the victim in a remote location.

Triage of victims

There are multiple triage systems that are available and appropriate for different situations that need to be considered in the planning phases. This includes the type of triage system used, how victims will be marked, and how victims will be cohorted.

Decontamination

Fire and EMS personnel need to be aware of decontamination prior to entering a scene or handling victims. Any potential decontamination issues need to be relayed to receiving hospitals for proper preparation for victims transported by EMS and those transported by private vehicle.

Numerous reports demonstrate that patients arrive at hospitals without any attempt at decontamination. Six hundred patients arrived at a hospital in Tokyo without decontamination after a Sarin attack in 1995. Another study showed that 18% of patients transported for HazMat exposures were never decontaminated.

On scene treatment

The initial stabilization of the critically ill to ensure reasonable, safe transport to a receiving hospital, and protocols for physicians, nurses, and EMS personnel need to be considered prior to a disaster.

On-scene treatment may consist of triage and initial stabilization for some disasters, while in other disasters it may mean care at a facility that has been converted to provide longer care in the event of a prolonged disaster response.

Transportation

Transportation considerations include how to transport patients and where to take them. The number of patients in a disaster is often more than EMS can immediately transport. Alternative transportation for those with injuries needing treatment who are otherwise stable is an important component of local planning.

Hospitals need to be able to increase to surge capacity in order to accommodate the influx of patients. Hospitals remote from the disaster may also need to surge for increased patients so that the closest hospitals will not be overwhelmed by the sudden increase.

Re-triage and reassessment of victims

Conditions can rapidly change. Patients who were stable may decompensate during a disaster. Procedures for ongoing care and re-triage need to constantly be in motion during a disaster.

Convergent volunteerism

The term used for unexpected personnel arriving at the scene of a large-scale disaster is *convergent volunteerism*.

During many recent disasters, there have been many volunteers who converge on the disaster scene with good intentions but without necessary equipment or logistics for proper execution. These volunteers may inadvertently be in the path of well-laid plans for disaster management or could become victims themselves. The possibility of convergent volunteerism must be considered when planning for a disaster.

For example, at the World Trade Center disaster there were concerns over lack of oversight, lack of accountability, patient tracking, and ability to truly credential convergent volunteers. Frequently these volunteers were unknowingly interfering with previously developed EMS protocols. Many volunteers were working in significantly hazardous conditions.

Frequently, convergent volunteers are misled by requests for help from the media that may not be required or requested by the incident commander.

As such, it is imperative the incident commander knows what resources are available and how to activate them. This way, all personnel (including convergent volunteers) can be tracked to ensure their safety and the safety of the disaster scene. They can also be properly equipped and a well-controlled response maintained.

Conclusions

All disasters require a strong local response both in the initial aftermath of a disaster and during the prolonged reconstruction period afterward. Although state, federal, and, potentially, international support may become involved with any disaster management incident, it is ultimately the municipality that will dictate the success or failure of a disaster response.

Medical management is only one aspect of the disaster response, but it needs to be carefully planned in conjunction with local planning committees. The medical staff involved with planning need to be aware of all resources available, the hierarchy of the municipality that will be directing the disaster, and how to activate all resources available.

The disaster plan should anticipate the inevitable increase in volunteers that arrive without formal requests for help and how to integrate or control this convergent volunteerism.

Suggested readings

Cone DC, Weir SD, Bogucki S (2003). Convergent volunteerism. *Ann Emerg Med* 41(4): 457–462.
Disaster Medical Assistance Team. http://www.dmat.org/
Medical Reserve Corps. http://www.medicalreservecorps.gov/HomePage
Municipal Research and Services Center of Washington Intergovernmental Agreements. http://www.mrsc.org/Subjects/Planning/intrgov.aspx. Accessed on 04/14/2010
National Voluntary Organizations Active in Disaster. http://www.nvoad.org/

Chapter 9

State-level disaster response

John Broach

Andrew Milsten

Introduction

The state-level response to disasters follows a framework established in several key pieces of federal legislation. However, the specifics of how each state responds to disasters are unique to the locale. Although some overarching principles and minimum standards have been established, the implementation of the state emergency management plan is largely defined by the individual states.

While significant differences exist among the states in terms of actual disaster management plans, the state role in general consists of at least the following five components:

- Coordination, via a state emergency operations center (EOC) of activities of multiple localities when multiple local jurisdictions are affected
- Assuming responsibility for primary incident command for events that reach a statewide level of response or participating in establishment of unified command for incidents involving multiple jurisdictions
- Mobilization of state-level resources specific to disaster response, including the state department of public health, the state emergency management office, and the state National Guard
- Accessing mutual aid agreements with other states if a disaster overwhelms the resources of the state
- Accessing and coordinating the deployment of federal resources via a declaration of a state of emergency by the office of the governor

State response structure

The state response to disasters follows the general pattern of disaster response, with local agencies being the first involved and then successively higher levels of government if a given level is unable to respond adequately. At each level, the local authorities make a decision to request resources from a higher level of government, if needed.

In general, the state emergency management agency becomes involved in the response when a locality's resources are overwhelmed or when multiple jurisdictions are involved and coordination at the state level is needed to ensure an effective response.

This system is laid out in the National Incident Management System (NIMS) as a tiered approach to disaster response. It is represented graphically in Figure 9.1.

The state-level infrastructure for emergency management is mandated by the Emergency Planning and Community Right to Know Act of 1986 (EPCRA). This act mandates creation of a state emergency response commission (SERC) and local emergency planning committees (LEPCs).

LEPCs have responsibility to plan for emergency response in given regions. The SERC has the responsibility of overseeing and coordinating the activities of the various LEPCs. More specifically, the responsibilities of the SERC are

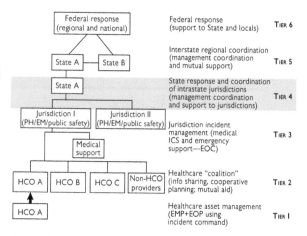

Figure 9.1 The National Incident Management System (NIMS) Tiered Approach to Disaster Response. EM, emergency management; EMP, emergency management program; EOC, emergency operations center; EOP, emergency operations plan; HCO, health care organization; ICS, incident command system; PH, public health. *Source:* United States Department of Health and Human Services.

- To supervise and coordinate the activities of the LEPCs
- To review the emergency response plans generated by the LEPCs annually
- To receive reports mandated by the EPCRA
- To make reports regarding these activities available to the public

Each state also has an agency devoted to emergency response. In most cases, this is known as the state emergency management agency.

The role of this agency is to coordinate the response to disasters or emergencies that either involve a number of local municipalities or overwhelm the resources of one municipality or state territory. The precise function and procedures followed by these agencies are specific to the individual states.

Metropolitan Medical Response System (MMRS)

The Metropolitan Medical Response System (MMRS) is an entity that is federally funded and locally controlled but that also has responsibilities within the framework of statewide disaster response.

MMRS is a regional coordinating system allowing various regions around the country to have a forum for medical professionals, EMS personnel, and others to coordinate disaster planning and medical response to disasters. MMRS committees have responsibility for assessment of resources within a region and for coordination of response with other agencies.

There are a total of 124 MMRS jurisdictions, with some states having more than one MMRS region, and some MMRS regions cover more than one state.

While not a state-specific resource, MMRS is an important example of the importance of coordination of local state and federal resources.

Additional state disaster resources

In addition to the dedicated state agency responsible for emergency management, there are a number of state-level government bodies that may be involved in a response to a disaster.

State department of public health

This department may be responsible for coordinating epidemiological surveillance through state laboratories in cases of infectious disease outbreaks; providing guidelines for patient care and forcing protection in epidemic emergencies; and coordinating syndromic or laboratory surveillance and sharing this information among points of care within the state.

Public safety organizations

Public safety organizations such as state police may be required for provision of security or for logistical support.

State emergency medical services director

The state EMS director may be involved in planning and is always involved in the preparation of protocols for disaster response.

Other specialized state resources

Other specialized resources such as urban search and rescue teams or other disaster response units may used depending on the nature of the incident.

Another state resource that deserves special mention is the state National Guard. The National Guard of each state is considered a state resource and can only be "federalized" or managed by the federal government under certain extreme circumstances.

The Insurrection Act of 1807 governs the use of the National Guard and its federalization in times of insurrection. Presidential authority was widened in 2006 to include the ability to federalize the guard in times of disaster. This amendment, however, was repealed, such that current mobilization of the guard is managed by governors.

Thus, the National Guard is considered a resource of the individual states and is often called upon to assist with security, logistics, medical care, and other functions in large-scale disasters.

National resources coordinated by states

In addition to these resources controlled directly by each state, there are a number of national-level programs, which are coordinated at least in part by each state.

The Medical Reserve Corps (MRC) is one such program that identifies medical professionals who agree to be available in some capacity to assist in disaster response, if needed. This is a federal program managed by the U.S. Public Health Service, but organization and requirements of MRC units are unique to each state, and protocols are created with state government involvement.

The Community Emergency Response Team (CERT) is another type of organization that is not under direct state control, although coordination between teams and the requirements of members are mandated by the state. This resource and the MRC units are some of the many resources that states can use in their management of emergencies before turning to the federal government for assistance.

If the resources of one state are overwhelmed by the needs created by a disaster, the state can access aid through mutual aid agreements with other states or from the federal government. State mutual aid is coordinated by the Emergency Management Assistance Compact (EMAC) system, which is a system of agreements between states to assist each other when one state's resources are overwhelmed. Under this rubric, a request is made by the governor of the affected state, and resources can be deployed directly from other states without necessitating federal assistance or involvement.

The final important role of the state government in disaster response is to act as a conduit and coordinating body for federal aid to local jurisdictions. Access to federal resources is granted when a state governor makes a declaration of a state of emergency and formally appeals for federal help. The resources available from the federal government to assist the states are discussed in Chapter 10.

The specific state procedures for making this declaration are unique to each state, but the process is governed by Public Law 93-288 (as amended by Public Law 100-707), the Robert T. Stafford Disaster Relief and Emergency Assistance Act of 1988. This legislation creates the mechanism for federal assistance to be coordinated at the state level and mandates that access to these resources be from the level of the state government instead of directly by local jurisdictions.

In summary, the role of the state government in response to disasters consists of coordination of multiple jurisdictions, the use of state-level resources such as state National Guard and management of statewide events through an office of emergency management, and coordination of federal assistance, if required. While each state has its own procedures and system for responding to disasters, this basic framework is mandated by federal law and establishes the place of the state government in the NIMS.

Suggested readings

Federal Emergency Management Agency (2007). National Incident Management System (draft May 24, 2007), Emergency Responder Field Operating Guide (ERFOG).

Public Law 93-288 (as amended by Public Law 100-707), the Robert T. Stafford Disaster Relief and Emergency Assistance Act of 1988.

U.S. Department of Health and Human Services (2007, September). MSCC Handbook: A Management System for Integrating Medical and Health Resources During Large-Scale Emergencies, 2nd ed. http://www.hhs.gov/disasters/discussion/planners/mscc/index.html

U.S. Department of Homeland Security (2008, February), MMRS target capabilities/capability focus areas and community preparedness, http://www.fema.gov/pdf/government/grant/hsgp/fy08_hsgp_guide_mmrs.pdf

Federal disaster response

Selim Suner

Introduction

Before discussing the federal components involved in disaster response in the United States, it must be reiterated that the most effective elements deployed in the initial hours to days of a significant disaster are local. This concept cannot be overstated. Initial search and rescue, first aid, and pre-hospital and hospital-level care following a disaster are carried out by the local providers.

Preparedness is not only essential for large health-care facilities, fire and EMS agencies, or other first-responder organizations but also for smaller clinics, doctor's offices, and individuals and family units. Without the initial local response, federal aid during disasters cannot effectively mitigate morbidity and mortality.

However, following the initial local response, health-care facilities in the disaster zone and adjacent locales should expect a swift and organized federal response. For the most efficient and safe handling of disaster victims in need of health care, a collaborative effort by the federal responders and local providers is essential. Knowledge of the federal response capability will facilitate early and effective collaboration.

There is a complex organization around federal disaster response, which involves many agencies at multiple levels of government. The interactions within these agencies, their roles, and their responsibilities are discussed in detail in a national response plan. Detailed and exhaustive discussion of this plan and all of its components are beyond the scope of this publication.

The organizations that will most likely interact with local health-care providers will be discussed briefly in this section.

National Disaster Medical System (NDMS)

The agency with the largest capability of medical response following a disaster is the National Disaster Medical System (NDMS). With over 8000 health-care and support personnel organized into response teams (Disaster Medical Assistance Teams [DMAT], Disaster Mortuary Operations Response Teams [DMORT], and other support elements), this organization is the "feet-on-the-ground" of U.S. medical disaster response.

Initially formed for the purposes of receiving, caring for, and transporting larger numbers of casualties expected during the first Gulf War in the late 1980s, this organization was transformed and developed to respond to natural and man-made disasters in the United States and abroad.

The NDMS was formed with the collaborative efforts of the Department of Health and Human Services (DHHS), Department of Defense (DoD), Department of Veteran's Health Administration (VHA), and the Federal Emergency Management Agency (FEMA). The major role of each component of NDMS is outlined in Table 10.1.

The principle behind the NDMS is that it is a federal–private collaborative organization. Civilian health-care providers and support staff make up the bulk of the workforce and over 1800 hospitals provide bed capacity for the system. The federal offices of NDMS provide a management structure, supply and equipment chain, training, and oversight to the individual teams, which are dispersed around the United States and are also local assets to the communities where they are based.

DMAT units are composed of physicians, mid-level providers, pharmacists, nurses, respiratory therapists, pharmacy technicians, paramedical, emergency medical technicians, and support personnel. The teams travel with their own equipment and supplies, including food, shelter, electrical, water and waste treatment facilities.

They are trained and equipped to establish operations in their tents and treat 300 patients for 72 hours without resupply. Their training not only incorporates medical care techniques in austere conditions but also self-care, mental health, cultural sensitivity, details of the national response plan, and interagency collaboration.

Table 10.1 Components of NDMS

Agency	Major Role
DHHS	Health response, mental health response
VHA	Health response, emergency management
DoD	Transportation, mobile care teams
FEMA	Emergency management, search and rescue, infrastructure and resupply

Public Health Service (PHS)

The commissioned officers of the Public Health Service, and the Commissioned Core Readiness Force (CCRF), with approximately 3000 personnel, operate similar to the DMAT contingent during disasters. The officers in the CCRF are similarly trained and equipped.

Unlike the civilian DMAT organization, these teams are operated under chain of command, and CCRF team members are often in uniform.

In past disaster operations DMAT and CCRF have worked together, often augmenting each other's operations.

Other agencies and organizations

- FEMA is instrumental in conducting assessments of disaster zones and identifying risks. Search-and-rescue and resupply operations are often coordinated and conducted through this agency.
- The VHA has a large contingent of personnel and has specialized teams to handle radiation emergencies.
- The Centers for Disease Control and Prevention (CDC) has assets to mitigate biological terrorism events. The Strategic National Stockpile (SNS), operated under the CDC, contains massive amounts of supplies, equipment, and medications, which can be deployed rapidly to a disaster zone. With the CHEMPACK program, antidotes, which are extremely time sensitive, are distributed to local communities and maintained in secured locations throughout the country.
- The Substance Abuse and Mental Health Services Administration (SAMSHA) is instrumental in maintaining mental health among responders and deploys teams to deal with mental health issues in disaster zones.
- The American Red Cross (ARC) is instrumental in disaster response. Among other duties, the ARC has the main objective of providing shelter operations for displaced persons. The ARC provides, shelter, food, health, and mental health services.

Other federal organizations maintain readiness for handling specific roles during disasters.

In addition, specialized teams within the NDMS, VHA and DoD are available to respond to specific incidents such as biological, chemical, or radiological incidents. The services of these teams can be obtained through requests made through NDMS or FEMA. Teams that are specifically trained and equipped for pediatrics, burn, crush, mental health, surgical operations, and decontamination operations can be accessed from federal resources.

There are also many local assets that can be deployed during a disaster. Some of these programs include the Metropolitan Medical Response System (MMRS) with specialized strike teams and National Guard teams equipped and trained for biological and chemical terrorist events.

There are multiple other agencies that contribute to disaster health operations. Exhaustive knowledge of each organization is not necessary to conduct health care during a disaster. Understanding the chain of support of and clearly communicating assets and needs during disaster care operations is essential to maintain health care operations after a major disaster.

Suggested readings

Ciottone G, ed. (2006) *Disaster Medicine,* Philadelphia: Elsevier Health Sciences.

Hogan DE, Burstein JL, eds. (2007). *Disaster Medicine.* Philadelphia: Lippincott.

Koenig KL, Schulz CH, eds. (2009). *Koenig and Schultz's Disaster Medicine.* New York: Cambridge University Press.

Chapter 11

Military disaster response

Paul T. Mayer

Introduction

Disaster response begins as a series of local actions. Only when local resources are overwhelmed are other tiers brought to bear.

The National Incident Management System (NIMS) directs how responders from different jurisdictions and disciplines may better cooperate and enable effective emergency response to natural and man-made disasters. NIMS affords a unified approach to incident management as well as standard command and management structures, with an emphasis on preparedness, mutual aid, and resource management.

This tiered response system should appropriately escalate the resources employed when local officials request assistance from other levels of the response system: regional, state, federal, or even international. The Department of Defense (DoD) is also a major component of the federal disaster response in the United States.

National Response Framework

In 2008, the U.S. federal government revised the National Defense Plan and codified its national disaster response into the National Response Framework (NRF). The NRF defines the principles, roles, and structures that organize how the United States responds to disasters.

The NRF
- Describes how communities, tribes, states, the federal government, private sectors, and nongovernmental partners work together to coordinate national response
- Describes specific authorities and best practices for managing incidents
- Builds upon the NIMS, which provides a consistent template for managing disaster incidents

The NRF defines emergency support functions (ESF), which provide the structure for coordinating federal interagency support for a federal response to disaster incidents. The ESF group functions are most frequently used to provide federal support to states and federal-to-federal support for declared disasters, emergencies under the Stafford Act, and non–Stafford Act incidents (see Table 11.1).

The DoD is the primary agency for ESF 9 and is a support agency for all other functions.

National Disaster Medical System

The NRF uses the National Disaster Medical System (NDMS), a cooperative, asset-sharing partnership among the Department of Health and Human Services (DHHS), the Department of Veterans Affairs (DVA), the Department of Homeland Security (DHS), and the Department of Defense (DoD), to direct a federal medical response. The NDMS provides medical resources for meeting the requirements of ESF 8 in the NRF.

The NDMS provides civilian assistance to military health care in the event of overwhelming combat casualties and provides federal health-care assistance to local resources overwhelmed by disasters.

Either a presidential declaration of a national emergency or directive from one of the secretaries of DHS, DHHS, or DoD may activate the NDMS.

Table 11.1 Roles and responsibilities of the ESFs

ESF #1 – Transportation	• Aviation/airspace management and control • Transportation safety • Restoration and recovery of transport infrastructure • Movement restrictions
ESF #2 – Communications infrastructure	• Coordination with telecommunications and information technology industries • Restoration and repair of telecommunications • Protection, restoration, and sustainment of national cyber and information technology • Oversight of communications within the federal incident management and response structures
ESF #3 – Public works and engineering	• Infrastructure protection and emergency repair • Infrastructure restoration • Engineering services and construction management • Emergency contracting of support for life-saving and life-sustaining services
ESF #4 – Firefighting	• Coordination of damage and impact assessment and of federal firefighting activities • Support to wildland, rural, and urban firefighting
ESF #5 – Emergency management	• Coordination of incident management and response efforts • Issuance of mission assignments • Resource and human capital • Incident action planning • Financial management
ESF #6 – Mass care, emergency assistance, housing, and human services	• Mass care • Emergency assistance • Disaster housing • Human services
ESF #7 – Logistics management and resource support	• Comprehensive, national incident logistics planning, management, and sustainment capability • Resource support (facility space, office equipment and supplies, contracting service, etc.)
ESF #8 – Public health and medical services	• Public health • Medical • Mental health services • Mass-fatality management

Table 11.1 (Contd.)

ESF #9 – Search and rescue	• Life-saving assistance • Search-and-rescue operations
ESF #10 – Oil and hazardous materials	• Oil and hazardous-material (chemical, biological, radiological, etc.) response • Environmental short- and long-term cleanup • Response
ESF #11 – Agriculture and natural resources	• Nutrition assistance • Animal and plant disease and pest response • Food safety and security • Natural and cultural resources and historic-properties protection and restoration • Safety and well-being of household pets
ESF #12 – Energy	• Energy infrastructure assessment, repair, and restoration • Energy industry utilities coordination • Energy forecast
ESF #13 – Public safety	• Social and economic community impact assessment • Security planning and technical resource assistance • Public safety and security support • Support to access, traffic, and crowd control
ESF #14 – Long-term community recovery	• Social and economic community impact assessment • Long-term community recovery assistance to states, local governments, and the private sector • Analysis and review of mitigation program implementation
ESF #15 – External affairs	• Emergency public information and protection action guidance • Media and community relations • Congressional and international affairs • Tribal and insular affairs

The NDMS provides three major capabilities:
- Pre-hospital medical operations
- Medical evacuation
- Definitive care

Civilian Disaster Medical Assistance Teams (DMATs) are designed to provide most of the pre-hospital medical care, with the DoD, primarily Air Force, coordinating and executing most of the medical evacuation operations to an NDMS supporting hospital.

Over 1800 hospitals support the NDMS by providing over 100,000 treatment beds for definitive care. Regional Federal Coordinating Centers (FCC) coordinate the patient movement and distribute patients throughout the NDMS system.

Department of Defense response

The Department of Defense possesses the capabilities of rapidly deployable, specialized logistical, technical, medical, recovery, HazMat, and humanitarian relief assets. The DoD maintains a well-developed logistical base and the most advanced delivery platforms on land, air, or sea in the world.

Thus the DoD is a major component of the federal response to both domestic and international incidents, given this unparalleled ability to provide readily available, highly skilled expertise rapidly throughout the world. Its integration into the unified interagency response is well delineated by the NRF.

The Quadrennial Defense Review (QDR) defines the DoD's responsibilities within this broader national framework for humanitarian assistance and disaster relief operations. The spectrum of military operations in this consequence management mission varies from delivering relief supplies to supporting civil authorities with law enforcement.

For federal military forces, command runs from the president to the Secretary of Defense to the commander of the combatant command to the DoD on-scene commander. Military forces will always remain under the operational and administrative control of the military chain of command, and these forces are subject to redirection or recall at any time. Military forces do not fall under the jurisdiction of the incident command system (ICS) or the unified command structure.

The DoD has a long tradition of supporting civil authorities while maintaining its primary mission of fighting and winning the nation's wars. The DoD, including active, reserve, and National Guard components, supports all 15 ESFs and can project that support anywhere in the world.

This support, called Defense Support to Civil Authorities (DSCA), is formally defined in the NRF and supported by a myriad of policies, statutes, and executive orders. It does not, however, apply to foreign disasters. Directives also allow the DoD to participate in international relief operations after the Department of State sends a request to the Secretary of Defense.

The DSCA process requires a lead federal agency (LFA) to request DoD support through the Federal Emergency Management Agency (FEMA) to the Joint Director of Military Support (JDOMS) on the Joint Chiefs of Staff. The JDOMS validates the request using standardized criteria (Table 11.2)

Table 11.2 Department of Defense deployment criteria

- Legality (compliance with laws)
- Lethality (potential use of lethal force by or against DoD forces)
- Risk (safety of DoD forces)
- Cost (who plays, and impact on DoD budget)
- Appropriateness (whether the requested mission is in the interest of the Department to conduct)
- Readiness (impact on DoD's ability to perform its primary mission)

and may then task a combatant command with DSCA support missions for presidentially declared emergencies.

This mission is directed through U.S. Northern Command (NORTHCOM) in Colorado Springs, CO, through either a Joint Task Force–Consequence Management (JTF-CM) or Joint Task Force–Civil Support (JTF-CS).

Defense coordinating officer (DCO)

The DoD has appointed 10 DCOs, one for each FEMA region, to serve as a single point of contact at the Joint Field Office (JFO) for requesting assistance from the DoD. With few exceptions, requests for DSCAs originating at the JFO are coordinated with and processed through the DCO.

The DCO may have a Defense coordinating element consisting of staff and military liaison officers to facilitate coordination and support to activated ESFs.

Joint Task Force (JTF) commander

Based on the complexity and type of incident, as well as the anticipated level of DoD resource involvement, the DoD may elect to designate a JTF to command federal (Title 10) military activities in support of the disaster response effort. The colocation of the JTF command and control element does not replace the requirement for a DCO/Defense coordinating element as part of the JFO unified coordination staff. The DCO remains the DoD single point of contact in the JFO for requesting assistance from the DoD.

In emphasis, the deployment of DoD assets into a civilian environment involves many legal considerations. The mission of law enforcement is particularly restricted. Following are the some of the major governances:

- **The Posse Comitatus Act**, 18 U.S.C. § 1385 (2007), prevents direct involvement by active duty military personnel in traditional law enforcement activities except as otherwise authorized by the Constitution or statute.
- **Military Support for Civilian Law Enforcement Agencies**, 10 U.S.C. §§ 371-382 (2007), authorizes the U.S. military to assist state and local law enforcement agencies without engaging in the execution of the law by sharing information and expertise; furnishing equipment, supplies, and services; and helping to operate equipment.
- **Section 2567 of Title 10, United States Code (2007)**, authorizes the Secretary of Defense (following a determination by the president to invoke 10 U.S.C. § 333(a)(1)(A) of the Restoration Act to provide supplies, services, and equipment to persons affected by a public emergency.
- **Section 382 of Title 10, United States Code and Section 831 of Title 18, United States Code (2007)**, authorizes the Attorney General to request assistance from the Secretary of Defense when both the Attorney General and the Secretary of Defense agree that an "emergency situation" involving biological, chemical, or nuclear weapons of mass destruction exists and the Secretary of Defense determines that the requested assistance will not impede military readiness.

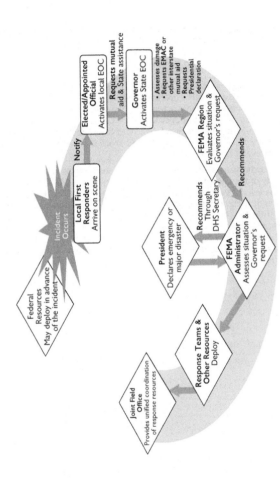

Figure 11.1 Summary of Stafford Act to support states.

National Guard assets

The National Guard is initially a crucial state (not federal) resource with expertise in communications, logistics, search and rescue, and decontamination. The governor of a state may activate elements of that state's National Guard (32 U.S.C. 904).

There is a clear distinction: *National Guard forces employed under State Active Duty or Title 32 status are under the command and control of the governor of their state and are not part of federal military response efforts.*

Title 32 is not subject to *posse comitatus* restrictions and allows the governor, with the approval of the president or the Secretary of Defense, to order a Guard member to duty to

- Perform training and other operational activities.
- Conduct homeland defense activities for the military protection of the territory or domestic population of the United States, or of the infrastructure or other assets of the United States determined by the Secretary of Defense to be critical to national security, from a threat or aggression against the United States.

In rare circumstances, invasion by a foreign nation, rebellion against the authority of the United States, or where the president is unable to execute the laws of the United States with regular forces (10 U.S.C. 12406), the president can federalize National Guard forces for domestic duties under Title 10. These forces are no longer under the command of the governor. Instead, the Department of Defense assumes full responsibility for all aspects of the deployment, including command and control. These National Guard forces then become governed by the same restrictions as other federal forces as described above.

Deployment capabilities

Mass resources

The DoD can respond with either mass resources or specialized capabilities. It provides mass resources to augment the resources that may exist within other agencies. Mass resources may include the following:

- Fixed facility military hospitals and over 100,000 public health and federal healthcare professionals
- Deployable medical platforms (teams to hospitals)
- Air evacuation assets
- Pharmaceutical and medical supply caches
- Mass vaccine programs
- Water purification systems
- Troops for maintaining order, clearing debris, delivering supplies, etc.

Specialized capabilities

The DoD may also deploy specialized resources or expertise that is limited or difficult to maintain in the civilian environment.

CBRNE

The DoD is developing improved systems to *sense*—detect and identify threats; *shape*—provide early warning; *shield*—protect the population; and *sustain*—operate in a contaminated environment. Enhanced reconnaissance systems with sensors are integrated with the DHS BIOWATCH program. Vaccines, antidotes, and better protective and detecting equipment are being developed in collaborative, interagency projects such as the National Interagency Biodefense Campus.

The DoD will rely primarily on dual-capable forces for this domestic consequence management mission. JTF-CS provides the dedicated command and control element for CBRNE civil support capabilities.

The Army National Guard Weapons of Mass Destruction (WMD) Civil Support Teams can operate under federal control in times of crisis. Additional dual-use CBRNE units include the U.S. Army Chemical And Biological Special Medical Augmentation Response Team (C/B SMART), U.S. Air Force Radiation Assessment Team (AFRAT), and U.S. Marine Corps Chemical Biological Incident Response Force (CBIRF), a 350-member rapid response unit with patient extrication, decontamination, and medical stabilization capabilities.

Preventive medicine

Displaced populations are a significant challenge with any disaster response, and preventive medicine and public health is tantamount to any response effort. The DoD has these deployable assets.

For example, the U.S. Army deploys Special Medical Augmentation Response Teams (SMART)—preventive medicine teams to provide short-duration preventive-medicine augmentation responses to disasters, civil–military cooperative action, and humanitarian and emergency incidents.

In addition, the DoD possesses deployable public health laboratories and the U.S. Navy has its Environmental and Preventive Medicine unit.

The DoD deploys and has readily available expertise from federal scientific research institutions. These institutions have processes tailored to support an expeditionary force that is remotely positioned and include the following:

- U.S. Army Medical Research Institute of Infectious Disease (USAMRIID)
- Medical Research Institute for Chemical Defense (USAMRICD)
- Armed Forces Radiobiological Research Institute (AFRRI)
- Armed Forces Institute of Pathology (AFIP)

Summary

In summary, the primary mission of the DoD is national defense, but after approval of the Secretary of Defense or under the direction of the president, the department may commit resources to disaster mitigation if requested by local authorities. The requested support is evaluated for legality, lethality, risk, cost, appropriateness, and impact on readiness.

Responding units remain under the command of the DoD but cooperate closely with operating organizations at all levels.

Key points

- The majority of disaster responses can be accomplished with local or state resources. However, a state may request the federal government for assistance. A significant portion of that response may be accomplished with DoD resources.
- There are significant legal requirements when mobilizing military assets for civilian consequence management.
- The DoD has the capabilities to provide support in all of the ESFs described in the NRF.
- The DoD mostly provides mass resource and transportation assistance in a disaster response, but has many diverse specialized capabilities.

Suggested readings

Ciottone GR, ed. (2006), *Disaster Medicine*, 3rd ed, St. Louis: Mosby.

Department of Department of Defense (2005, June), Strategy for homeland defense and civil support, Washington, DC: Government Printing Office, http://www.defenselink.mil/news/Jun2005/d20050630homeland.pdf

Office of Homeland Security (2004, March), National Incident Management System, Washington, DC: Government Printing Office, http://www.fema.gov/emergency/nrf/.

Office of Homeland Security (2008, March), National Response Framework, Washington, DC: Government Printing Office, http://www.fema.gov/emergency/nrf/.

Office of Homeland Security (2008, March), National Disaster Medical System, Washington, DC: Government Printing Office, http://www.fema.gov/emergency/nrf/.

Quadrennial Defense Review, http://www.defenselink.mil/qdr/report/Report20060203.pdf, 2006

DoD Directive 5100.46, Foreign Disaster Relief, December 4, 19DoD Directive 3025.15, Military Assistance to Civil Authorities, February 18, 1997.

Emergency management in disasters

Kwa heri Heard

Historical perspective

Two worlds collide

Inclusion of the public health and medical communities in emergency management preparedness and response is still fairly new. Prior to events such as the Oklahoma City Bombing and the September 11 terrorist attacks, the two entities had (in their view) clearly defined and rather different roles and responsibilities during emergencies. First responders (police, fire, EMS, and emergency management) responded to incidents on scene and handled all aspects of the emergency. The public health and hospital communities were responsible for caring for the sick and injured once they arrived at their facility in need of treatment.

This system functioned adequately for day-to-day emergencies. However, it became less capable once the United State began experiencing unprecedented events that included large numbers of injured and deceased.

For emergency management to be successful in responding to large-scale disaster incidents, it needed to change the way it functioned. Those involved at the planning table would have to expand to include medical and public health—disciplines that were always thought of as important, but not necessarily considered pertinent to planning for a response.

In order for public health and hospitals to be successful and protect their patients, they would have to be a part of the planning process. The two entities would have to realize that their roles were similar to that of first responders and that they would have to work together to save lives.

Local response

On a local level, emergency management is responsible for coordinating and building partnerships with all parties responsible for responding to an emergency. Emergency managers must coordinate the activities of all agencies, including public health and hospitals, involved and disseminate critical information.

For example, if a train derails and releases a hazardous chemical, hospitals would need to know that there may be an influx of patients into their emergency department, some of whom may need decontamination. This knowledge also helps emergency managers know when they can reach out to particular agencies for their specialized assistance. An example would be contacting the local health department to provide nurses in a shelter operation.

Once the agencies learn each other's capabilities, they are now ready to start the planning process. The plan should include not only major activities, such as how they will respond to large-scale events, but also how they will do very basic activities, such as sharing communications and notifying other agencies of incidents.

Once the planning is done, the document must be tested to ensure the information works. The testing of the information is done through a series of exercises. These exercises can be open discussions, called tabletop drills, or more elaborate productions, termed full-scale exercises.

Drills are low stress in nature and allow for conversations and questions. This method is an excellent way to fine-tune a plan and educate other parties of its content.

Full-scale exercises simulate an actual disaster. Through conducting such a full-scale drill, potential deficiencies can be identified, which may have gone unnoticed during the planning phase.

If done successfully, the relationship built between public health, hospitals, and first responders will be evident during an actual emergency. The participants will work seamlessly to achieve the ultimate goal of protecting life during an emergency.

This does not mean that the operation will be without mishaps or errors, but the response as a whole will be more organized, and any mishaps can be remedied more quickly than if the entities did not work together. An example of such effective coordination would be the operations in the City of Dallas during Hurricane Ike and Hurricane Gustav.

Case study

The City of Dallas was responsible for establishing a mega–shelter operation for those citizens fleeing imminent danger of a hurricane near the Houston–Harris County Gulf Coast area. The first time Dallas set up such a shelter was during Hurricanes Katrina and Rita in 2005.

The shelters were set up at the Dallas Convention Center and Reunion Arena. It included sleeping and medical accommodations for roughly 1500 people. The operation lasted for over a month and required the assistance of more than 2500 employees and volunteers.

By all accounts this was a successful operation, but there were many corrections that needed to be made. In fact, programs were created specifically in the health and medical community to improve the response if it ever happened again.

The City of Dallas Office of Emergency Management and Dallas County Health and Human Services worked diligently to correct issues identified and even created a "medical operations center" to better coordinate medical response. Plans were written and tested through drills, including both tabletop and full-scales exercises.

On August 31, 2008, Dallas tested their new shelter plan. Hurricane Gustav threatened the Louisiana and Texas coast. Many of those fleeing the area made their way to Dallas.

A mega–shelter operation was set up in the Convention Center to house approximately 1000 people. A medical clinic, including a pharmacy was also established at the shelter, similar to what was established during Katrina and Rita. This time, however, the operation worked smoothly and accommodated twice as many medical special needs.

Emergency management knew to contact public health as soon as the decision was made to set up the shelter so that they could implement their plan for setting up the clinic. Public health was included in all emergency management planning meetings to ensure that all players were on the same page. They were also included in all conference calls and briefings, again to make sure everyone was equipped with the information needed to run a successful operation.

Immediately following Gustav, Hurricane Ike occurred and the entire operation was tested once again. In both cases, all involved agencies worked well together, especially the public health, hospital, and emergency management agencies.

Federal assistance

Metropolitan Medical Response System (MMRS)

The federal government, in an effort to seek collaboration between first responders, emergency management, and the health and medical community, has created programs to help foster these relationships.

One very important step taken was the creation of the Metropolitan Medical Response System (MMRS) program. This program was founded by the Department of Health and Human Services (HHS) in 1996 in response to the increased terrorist threat evidenced by the Sarin nerve agent gas attack in the Tokyo subway system in March 1995.

The program was designed to enhance and coordinate local and regional response capabilities for highly populated areas that could be targeted by a terrorist attack using weapons of mass destruction (WMD).

The MMRS concept, organizing principles, and resources are also applicable to the management of large-scale incidents such as hazardous materials (HazMat) accidents, epidemic disease outbreaks, and natural disasters requiring specialized and carefully coordinated medical preparation and response.

The program undertakes the following:

- Integrates and enhances existing response systems to respond to a mass casualty or "surge" event
- Incorporates customized incident planning and specialized training and exercises
- Provides specialized pharmaceutical and equipment acquisition including, but not limited to, protective equipment, communications equipment, and medical supplies
- Uses an "all-hazards" planning approach
- Prioritizes the response activities and allocation of resources until significant external resources arrive and are operational (typically between 24 and 72 hours)

The MMRS program supports local jurisdictions in planning, developing, equipping, and training regionalized networks of "first responders" (e.g., law enforcement officials, medical and public health personnel, HazMat technicians, and firefighters).

MMRS planning addresses the following five areas: early recognition, mass immunization and prophylaxis, mass patient care, mass fatality management, and environment surety.

Key components of MMRS

- Planning team
- Logistics
- Forward movement of patients
- Provision of medical care
- Integration of health science
- Response structure
- Biological elements
- Training
- Equipment and pharmaceuticals
- Operational capabilities

By virtue of its integrated structure, MMRS has promoted partnerships that bring together a variety of emergency preparedness and emergency management systems. These partnerships span the local, state, and federal levels as well as the public and private sectors.

In forging close operational links between emergency responders of all types, the MMRS program has helped create a working national emergency response infrastructure in our most highly populated and most vulnerable localities.

Public Health Emergency Preparedness (PHEP) grant and the Hospital Preparedness program

Two other programs funded by the federal government to foster building relationships in planning for emergencies are the Centers for Disease Control and Prevention (CDC) Public Health Emergency Preparedness (PHEP) grant and the Hospital Preparedness program grant.

The PHEP was created to support preparedness nationwide in state, local, tribal, and territorial public health departments in 2002, shortly after the events of September 11, 2001, and subsequent anthrax attacks.

It provides funding to enable public health departments to have the capacity and capability to effectively respond to the public health consequences of terrorist threats, as well as infectious disease outbreaks, natural disasters, and biological, chemical, nuclear, and radiological emergencies. These emergency preparedness and response efforts are designed to support the National Response Framework (NRF) and the National Incident Management System (NIMS) and are targeted specifically for the development of emergency-ready public health departments.

The CDC provides PHEP funding to 62 grantees, which include 50 states, eight territories (Puerto Rico, the Virgin Islands, American Samoa, Commonwealth of the Northern Mariana Islands, Guam, Republic of the Marshall Islands, Republic of Palau, and the Federated States of Micronesia), and four metropolitan areas (Washington, D.C., Chicago, Los Angeles County, and New York City).

The Hospital Preparedness Program (HPP) enhances the ability of hospitals and health-care systems to prepare for and respond to bioterrorism and other public health emergencies. Current program priority areas include interoperable communication systems, bed tracking, personnel management, fatality management planning, and hospital evacuation planning. During the past 5 years, HPP funds have also improved bed and personnel surge capacity, decontamination capabilities, isolation capacity, pharmaceutical supplies, training, education, drills, and exercises. Hospitals, outpatient facilities, health centers, poison control centers, EMS, and other health-care partners work with the appropriate state or local health department to develop health-care system preparedness through this program.

The HPP supports priorities established by the National Preparedness Goal established by the Department of Homeland Security (DHS) in 2005. The Goal guides entities at all levels of government in the development and maintenance of capabilities to prevent, protect against, respond to, and recover from major events, including incidents of national significance. Additionally, the goal will assist entities at all levels of government in the development and maintenance of the capabilities to identify, prioritize, and protect critical infrastructure

The Pandemic and All Hazards Preparedness Act of 2006 transferred the National Bioterrorism Hospital Preparedness Program (NBHPP) from the Health Resources and Services Administration to the Assistant Secretary for Preparedness and Response (ASPR). The focus of the program is now all-hazards preparedness and not solely bioterrorism.

The Pandemic and All-Hazards Preparedness Act of 2006 (Public Law 109-417) amended section 319C-2 of the Public Health Service (PHS) Act authorizing the Secretary of Health and Human Services (HHS) to award competitive grants or cooperative agreements to eligible entities to enable such entities to improve surge capacity and enhance community and hospital preparedness for public health emergencies.

Program primary priorities

- Interoperable communications system
- Bed-tracking system
- Emergency System for the Advance Registration of Volunteer Health Professionals (ESAR-VHP)
- Fatality management plans
- Hospital evacuation plans

The creation of these programs has helped to build bridges across the public health, hospital and emergency management discipline to create a cohesive and inclusive response to emergencies.

Suggested readings

Coordinating Office for Terrorism Preparedness and Emergency Response (COTPER) funding guidance and technical assistance to states. http://www.bt.cdc.gov/cotper/coopagreement/

Federal Emergency Management Agency (2004). FY 05 Homeland Security grants announced (December 3, 2004), http://mmrs.fema.gov/Main Events/fy2005awards.aspx

MMRS National Program Office. History of the Metropolitan Medical Response System (MMRS): the first decade: 1995–2005, http://www.cabq.gov/envhealth/pdf/HistoryoftheMMRS.pdf

U.S. Department of Health and Human Services (2004). Metropolitan Medical Response System overview, DHS/FEMA/EPR Preparedness/MMRS/ April 15, 2004

U.S. Department of Health and Human Services (April 4, 2011). The Hospital Preparedness Program. http://www.phe.gov/Preparedness/planning/hpp/Pages/overview.aspx

Chapter 13

Emergency medical services

Ray Fowler

Jeff Beeson

Principle

Emergency medical services (EMS) systems, together with the fire and public safety services, are the bedrock infrastructure of disaster response in the civilian environment of the United States. This chapter describes the essential elements of EMS systems, their multiorganizational linkages in mitigating and responding to disasters, and the grades of response available by the out-of-hospital EMS systems community.

EMS conducts the practice of medicine in the out-of-hospital environment. Properly managed EMS systems must have careful medical oversight provided by the EMS medical director as designated by state law.

The National Association of EMS Physicians has stated that "the distinctive medical practice of EMS and the particular nuances of delivering out-of-hospital emergency care are clearly unique and, in turn, they require a specialized body of medical knowledge and certain discrete competencies."

They state further, "EMS medical practice still requires specialized proficiencies for a myriad of clinical care scenarios and medical conditions that generally are not approached or treated the same once inside the emergency department (ED) or other hospital settings."

Introduction

The 1966 National Academy of Sciences Report (resulting in part in the creation of the first curricula for the training of emergency medical technicians by the Department of Transportation) and the 1973 EMS Systems Act resulted in gradual improvement in clinical care in the field.

Long-term funding for EMS and a close working relationship with the growing specialty of emergency medicine were major factors in the emergence of emergency medical services as a recognized subspecialty of emergency medicine by the American Board of Medical Specialties in 2010.

Scope of practice of providers

Each state has the statutory authority and responsibility to regulate EMS within its borders and to determine the scope of practice of EMS personnel. As part of their commitment to realize the vision of the EMS agenda for the future, the National Highway Traffic Safety Administration (NHTSA) and the Health Resources and Human Services Administration (HRSA) oversaw the development of a National Scope of Practice Model (NSP Model) for all levels of EMS providers, which was released in 2007.

The NSP Model sets out four levels of providers: emergency medical responder, emergency medical technician, advanced emergency medical technician, and paramedic. These four levels were developed in consideration of the broad needs of the country, while allowing for the development of educational guidelines, teaching materials, and the establishment of certifying examinations.

The skills taught at each level increase in complexity with advancing levels. The National EMS Scope of Practice Model is a consensus-based document that was developed to improve the consistency of EMS personnel licensure levels and nomenclature among states. However, it does not have any regulatory authority.

According to the NHTSA manual, "the Scope of Practice Model should be used by the States to develop scope of practice legislation, rules and regulation. The specific mechanism that each State uses to define the State's scope of practice for EMS personnel varies. State scopes of practice may be more specific than those included in this model and may specifically identify both the minimum and maximum skills and roles of each level of EMS licensure. Scopes of practice are typically defined in law, regulations, or policy documents. Some States include specific language within the law, regulation or policy, while others refer to a separate document using a technique known as "incorporation by reference."

The National EMS Scope of Practice Model offers a contemporary replacement for incorporation by reference or language for inclusion in law, regulation, or policy.

For an EMS provider to be working clinically for an EMS agency, four criteria must be met:

- Training by a qualified program (Fig. 13.1)
- Certification by an examination process
- Licensed by the state
- Credentialed by the medical director

The NHTSA goes further to define the paramedic as an individual who "has knowledge, skills, and abilities developed by appropriate formal education and training." The paramedic has the knowledge associated with, and is expected to be competent in, all of the skills of the emergency medical responder (EMR), emergency medical training (EMT), and advanced emergency medical technician (AEMT). While the NSP Model generally defines the scope of practice of EMS personnel, states vary as to its implementation.

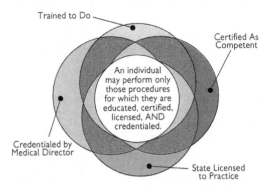

Trained to Do

Certified As Competent

An individual may perform only those procedures for which they are educated, certified, licensed, AND credentialed.

Credentialed by Medical Director

State Licensed to Practice

Figure 13.1 Certification and training.
Source: National Highway Traffic Safety Administration (NHTSA).

For example, Texas is a "delegated practice" state where the EMS medical director establishes training and credentialing standards for an EMS agency. The state of Alabama, by contrast, has both a single statewide clinical protocol and equipment list for EMS agencies, from which deviation is not permitted.

Disaster preparedness planners are obliged to become familiar with the skills to which prehospital care providers are certified in that area. Also, planners must remember that providers may not overstep the bounds of training and certification, even in the setting of a multicasualty or disaster incident.

An EMT-level provider (formerly classified as the EMT-Basic) who has not been trained, certified, and credentialed in advanced airway management and, particularly, endotracheal intubation is not certified to perform that skill under any circumstances.

Additional training and certifications are available to EMS personnel. Such additional training includes critical care, air medical training, and confined space conditions.

EMS agency system design

- Fire service
- Third service
- Private sector
- Hospital-based
- Law enforcement

The proliferation of EMS systems in the United States has resulted in diverse methods of the provision of prehospital emergency care (PEC) to different populations.

Fire service

Some EMS care in the United States is provided through fire service–based EMS operations. EMS providers in fire-based agencies are usually members of the fire service, are often certified firefighters, and commonly have multiple additional levels of training, including in hazardous materials management, swift-water rescue, and rescue from heights.

Third service

A "third-service" EMS agency is one that is established in a given municipality as a public entity existing in addition and parallel to the fire service and public safety (police and sheriff departments). The EMS providers in these agencies are typically employees of the municipality for whom they work.

A variant of the third service is the "public utility model" (PUM). In this setting, an oversight board is usually established by the municipality and then contracts to an outside EMS agency to provide EMS services according to certain performance measures.

Private providers

There is a diverse assortment of private providers of EMS services in the United States. Typically, 911 calls are distributed to such agencies that have registered in the community, have demonstrated capacity to manage emergency medical responses, and have been awarded the "response zone" for a given area.

Non-emergency responses (such as transports to dialysis or returning discharged patients from hospitals) may be supplied by a diverse group of private providers in competition in the private sector. Local regulation may, however, provide for municipal oversight of non-emergency responses and transports.

Hospital-based

In some centers, hospitals have established the infrastructure of personnel, training, certification, equipment, and supplies required to create and maintain a modern EMS system. In these systems, the EMS personnel are generally employees of the establishing hospital system or a related corporate entity.

Hospital-based EMS systems are bound by EMTALA regulations pursuant to the provision of an appropriate medical screening examination.

Law enforcement

Law enforcement agencies may also supply various EMS services, from simple "basic life support" (such as CPR and automated external defibrillators) to air transport services.

Communications in EMS systems

A complex web of real-time electronic communication underlies and permeates an EMS agency.

Public safety access points (PSAPs) provide the public the ability to call for help, usually through the use of the 911 emergency number. 911 centers can generally identify the location of the caller, although a majority of 911 calls are now placed from wireless devices that can make the location of the person in distress problematic.

PSAPs are the usually the location point for the dispatching emergency responders (though it is common that these calls are forwarded to the EMS agency that will respond to the call).

Emergency operations centers (EOCs) are the central points for the control, management, and distribution of assets responding to disasters. EOCs are usually separate from PSAPs, though many models exist as suits municipality needs and assets. PSAPs maintain a dynamic link with EOCs.

EMS providers are involved in numerous communication needs from their ambulances:

- Dispatch to and from ambulance: notification of calls, response methods ("hot or cold"), request for public safety and additional equipment
- Ambulance to supervisor: as under dispatch, plus management of difficult situations, equipment and materiel issues
- Ambulance to online medical control (OLMC, see below) for clinical consult regarding patient condition
- Ambulance to destination receiving facility (if different from OLMC): voice and data (e.g., ECG transmission)
- Ambulance to data center (for electronic medical record management)

Online medical control (OLMC) is an entity established for multiple purposes in interaction with EMS agencies and EOCs. OLMC is generally an entity always available through radio or cellular communication to provide real-time consultation to field providers during the management of difficult medical situations. This consultation includes assistance with diagnosis, management, and patient refusal situations.

OLMC can also offer assistance with electronic linking to EOCs for multicasualty incidents (MCIs). Additionally, OLMC can lend assistance in distributing patients from the field to multiple emergency medical receiving facilities so that hospitals do not become overwhelmed.

Many centers have a separate, central OLMC, which is distinct from the emergency receiving facility. In other centers it is customary for EMS providers to contact the destination hospital facility to provide OLMC.

The contacting of separate hospitals for OLMC can provide some variability in the response from OLMC from hospital to hospital. A state may address this variability by requiring training and certification of OLMC physicians.

EMS roles in disaster mitigation and response

General concepts

- All responders—public health, EOC staff, public safety officers, and all potentially responding members of the health-care community—must complete appropriate emergency incident training.
- EMS is a part of the Incident Command System (ICS) and must play a dynamic and cooperative role in the system.
- Pre-established relationships and contact individuals are mandatory for optimal preparedness.
- Use of the ICS concept in system-wide planning will break down barriers and smooth the process of cooperation in the event of an incident.

Major public health emergencies and unified command

- Emergencies affecting the public health mandate responses from many agencies and jurisdictions in public health emergencies because of the risk posed to the entire population.
- In the event that a unified command must be established, the represented agencies at the command post must include a senior staff EMS member.

EMS providers will require medical support

- Prevention and management of occupational injuries will likely be required.
- Overall monitoring of the activities and health of medical responders is necessary.

Radiological and nuclear responses

- Prompt alerting of the community to prevent exposure to ionizing radiation, including from fallout, can substantially reduce long-term illness and death.
- Efforts to prevent internal exposure through the use of N-95 or equivalent masks is the preferential approach to prevent ingestion.

Special EMS

- Disaster Medical Assistance Teams (DMAT) may be assigned to the incident location.
- Urban search and rescue teams (USAR) will be activated for incidents requiring victim rescue and recovery.
- Water rescue and recovery operations may play a role in disaster situations such as flooding and weather-related disasters.
- Tactical EMS teams may be activated.
- Medical oversight and support for hazardous material responses is required, usually provided by lead members of the responding EMS agency.
- Management of animal care is an essential part of planning. Disaster veterinary assistance teams may be activated.

Dilemmas in prehospital disaster preparedness

Supplies

Extensive commitment of public funds is needed for very rare potential disaster episodes, such as prepositioning large supplies of nerve agent antidote or antibiotics against biological attacks, all of which will expire over time.

It is difficult to know where to pre-position supplies to provide for the optimal use.

Scalability is defined as the ability to increase the positive response to a disaster situation in order to optimize citizen safety and attempt to operate within community assets. Absence of scalability threatens secondary issues, such as cholera outbreaks following earthquakes.

Triage

Numerous triage methods are found through EMS-provider training (see Fig. 13.2).

There is a linear relationship between ineffective triage and bad patient outcome. Recent CDC work on unifying triage of patients through the "SALT Triage" plan may help alleviate this disparity in training (Fig. 13.3).

MASS triage (Move, Assess, Sort, Send) is an effective method of sorting large numbers of victims in preparation for the individual assessment of victims.

Triage tags may not be available, and rescuers must be prepared to physically record documentation of triage category on the patient, typically the forehead, using a marking pen.

Types of conditions

Bio-weapons can produce symptoms that are extraordinarily difficult to diagnose until the situation is understood. Hours to days may pass from the onset of the outbreak until the causative agent is identified.

Chemical exposures will likely produce areas inaccessible to EMS personnel until cleared by HazMat personnel. Working in the field in protective suits (such as Level A protection) makes patient care very difficult and places the EMS provider at risk for injury.

Personnel

In a disaster, the EMS providers reporting to work will likely go to their full-time job. EMS agencies depending on part-time provider assistance will sustain personnel shortages, which will increase response times.

Employees scheduled for regular duty shifts may not show up because of personal issues that the disaster has caused at home. Preparations for employee no-shows should be expected.

Exposure of EMS providers to elements of the disaster may well injure the responders themselves.

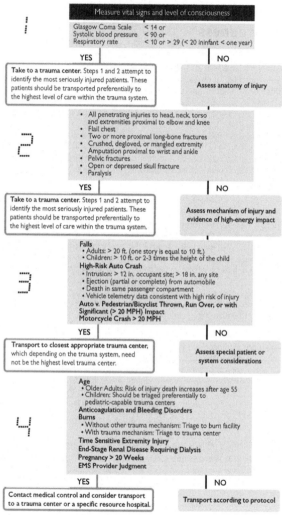

1

Measure vital signs and level of consciousness

Glasgow Coma Scale	< 14 or
Systolic blood pressure	< 90 or
Respiratory rate	< 10 or > 29 (< 20 ininfant < one year)

YES → **Take to a trauma center.** Steps 1 and 2 attempt to identify the most seriously injured patients. These patients should be transported preferentially to the highest level of care within the trauma system.

NO → **Assess anatomy of injury**

2

- All penetrating injuries to head, neck, torso and extremities proximal to elbow and knee
- Flail chest
- Two or more proximal long-bone fractures
- Crushed, degloved, or mangled extremity
- Amputation proximal to wrist and ankle
- Pelvic fractures
- Open or depressed skull fracture
- Paralysis

YES → **Take to a trauma center.** Steps 1 and 2 attempt to identify the most seriously injured patients. These patients should be transported preferentially to the highest level of care within the trauma system.

NO → **Assess mechanism of injury and evidence of high-energy impact**

3

Falls
- Adults: > 20 ft. (one story is equal to 10 ft.)
- Children: > 10 ft. or 2-3 times the height of the child

High-Risk Auto Crash
- Intrusion: > 12 in. occupant site; > 18 in. any site
- Ejection (partial or complete) from automobile
- Death in same passenger compartment
- Vehicle telemetry data consistent with high risk of injury

Auto v. Pedestrian/Bicyclist Thrown, Run Over, or with Significant (> 20 MPH) Impact
Motorcycle Crash > 20 MPH

YES → **Transport to closest appropriate trauma center,** which depending on the trauma system, need not be the highest level trauma center.

NO → **Assess special patient or system considerations**

4

Age
- Older Adults: Risk of injury death increases after age 55
- Children: Should be triaged preferentially to pediatric-capable trauma centers

Anticoagulation and Bleeding Disorders

Burns
- Without other trauma mechanism: Triage to burn facility
- With trauma mechanism: Triage to trauma center

Time Sensitive Extremity Injury
End-Stage Renal Disease Requiring Dialysis
Pregnancy > 20 Weeks
EMS Provider Judgment

YES → **Contact medical control and consider transport to a trauma center or a specific resource hospital.**

NO → **Transport according to protocol**

When in doubt, transport to a trauma center.

For more information, visit: www.cdc.gov/FieldTriage

Figure 13.2 Field triage decision scheme: the National Trauma Triage Protocol.
Source: Centers for Disease Control and Prevention

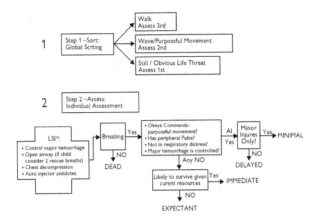

Figure 13.3 SALT triage scheme.
Source: Centers for Disease Control and Prevention.

Patient load

EMS systems typically operate at high-volume levels of response and transport during normal times. A disaster in a community will drastically overload the emergency response system with patients, requiring alternative transport methods and destinations.

Standard EMS case types will predictably increase in volume. For example, particulate releases could increase the likelihood of chronic respiratory illness exacerbation. Such patients also rise to a high triage level for emergent management and transport.

Communications

Emergency response systems will be overwhelmed by callers in a major disaster. Emergency communications may not sustain the impact of a major environmental disaster, preventing calls from reaching responders.

Conclusion

The emergency medical services teams in a geographic area provide a critical arm in community preparedness for disasters, victim rescue, patient care in the field, resuscitative maneuvers, and, most importantly, transport of the acutely ill and injured to appropriate destinations. These teams must play an integral role in the creation of operational clinical response to provide the best available outcome in the event of a disaster.

Suggested readings

American Medical Association (2007). MASS triage. Advanced Disaster Life Support. http://www. ama-assn.org/resources/doc/cphpdr/ndls_brochure.pdf

Bass R (2009). History. In Cone D, O'Connor R, Fowler R, eds. *Emergency Medical Services: Clinical Practice and Systems Oversight*, 4th ed. National Association of EMS Physicians, Vol 2:3.

Centers for Disease Control and Prevention (2009, January). CDC guidelines for the triage of injured patients. Retrieved December 29, 2010, from http://www.cdc.gov/mmwr/pdf/rr/rr5801.pdf

Lerner B, Schwartz R, McGovern J (2009). Prehospital triage for mass casualties. In Cone D, O'Connor R, Fowler R, eds. *Emergency Medical Services: Clinical Practice and Systems Oversight*, 4th ed. National Association of EMS Physicians, Vol 4(2):11–15.

National Academy of Sciences (1966). Accidental death and disability: The neglected disease of modern society, Washington, DC: National Academy Press. Retrieved December 29, 2010, from http://www.nap.edu/openbook.php?record_id=9978&page=R1

National Highway Traffic Safety Administration (2007, February). National EMS Scope of Practice Model. DOT HS 810 657. Retrieved December 29, 2010, from http://www.nhtsa.gov/people/injury/ems/EMSScope.pdf

Pepe P, Copass M, Fowler R. Racht E (2009). Medical direction of EMS systems, In Cone D, O'Connor R, Fowler R, eds. *Emergency Medical Services: Clinical Practice and Systems Oversight*, 4th ed. National Association of EMS Physicians, Vol 2:22.

White J (2009). Radiological and nuclear response for emergency medical personnel. In Cone D, O'Connor R, Fowler R, eds. *Emergency Medical Services: Clinical Practice and Systems Oversight*, 4th ed. National Association of EMS Physicians, Vol 4(5):46–57.

Public health in disasters

John T. Carlo

Essential concepts

Public health standards include safe drinking water, food, shelter, and medical care. These measures have dramatically improved life expectancy and reduced mortality over the last 100 years in the United States.

The practice of public health involves the study of risk to the health of populations and the institution of measures to remove these risks. In the United States, it is accepted that tap water and foods will be available, safe and free from disease.

Access to medical care is also an assumed principle. Such infrastructure, however, remains forever vulnerable, and disasters can pose an immediate, short-term, and long-term reduction in these standards.

The Sphere Project

The Sphere Project was created in 1997 by over 20 humanitarian groups internationally in order to alleviate human suffering arising out of calamity and conflict. The fundamental concept is that those affected by a disaster have a right to life with dignity.

The Project identifies minimum standards that should be attained during a disaster response. Included are assistance with key components.

Water, sanitation, and hygiene promotion
- 2–4 gallons of potable water per person, including intake, hygiene, and cooking needs
- A maximum of 20 persons per toilet
- Hand washing and personal hygiene
- Avoiding mosquito exposure
- Solid waste management

Food security, nutrition, and food aid
- 2,100 kcals per person per day, 10–12% by protein, 17% by fat, and adequate micronutrient intake
- Food should be
- Prepared in clean areas with all raw produce washed
- Cooked to the proper temperatures based on type of meat
- Kept at or above 140°F until eaten
- Refrigerated at or below 40°F

Shelter
- Minimum space of 38 ft² per person,
- Comfortable bedding
- Proper access for those with disabilities

Health services
- Trauma care
- Mental health care
- Chronic illness care
- Handling remains of the dead

The 1988 report on the Future of Public Health by the Institute of Medicine suggested three principles for core public health functions: assessment, policy development, and assurance. Each of these principles has distinct applications toward disaster response directives.

Assessment

Assessment should include the ability to study the public health implications of the disaster in order to better understand the risks, dangers, and needs of the community. See Table 14.1.

Post-disaster surveillance

Surveillance systems

Surveillance systems should be implemented to act as early warning systems for potential infectious disease outbreaks and to determine needs of the affected population post-disaster. A surveillance system involves the collection and interpretation of data.

Data collection

Information pertaining to the health status and risk of a population is important to collect in real time so that community leaders can mitigate potential health threats quickly. Specific information should include whether there is adequate
- Clean drinking water
- Availability of food and supplies for safely preparing food
- Safe and adequate shelter space
- Electricity, especially for vulnerable populations (see below)

Additionally, data pertaining to the types of medical illnesses seen by clinicians post-disaster should be collected and analyzed by public health officials. Information should include:
- Number of individuals seen for medical evaluations
- Percentage of vulnerable populations (see next page)
- Number of individuals with fever and/or symptoms of vomiting, diarrhea, cough, or other upper respiratory symptoms
- Number of individuals with symptoms suspicious for other infectious diseases including scabies, lice, or other infestations, conjunctivitis, jaundice, and severe headache
- Number of injuries
- Number of assault-related injuries

Table 14.1 Public health impact of selected disasters

Effect	Earthquakes	Tornados	Floods	Hurricanes
Deaths	Many	Few	Few	Many
Severe injuries	Many	Moderate	Few	Few
Evacuations	Rare	Rare	Common	Common
Risk of infectious disease	Small	Small	Varies	Small

Source: *Emergency Health Management After Natural Disaster*. Office of Emergency Preparedness and Disaster Relief Coordination: Scientific Publication No. 47. Washington, DC. Pan American Health Organization, 1981.

This data are best expressed as a percentage, with the denominator being the affected population for the given area and time.

Data interpretation

The above data should be analyzed (in real time, if possible) to determine whether appropriate responder staffing and resources are available. For example, knowing the relative percentage of pediatric visits helps determine whether additional pediatric specialists should be made available.

While it is often difficult to determine when an outbreak of infectious disease is occurring, potential indicators include the following:

- Occurrence or suspected occurrence of a novel disease, or illness not known to be endemic to an area, e.g., cholera, yellow fever, measles
- Increase in rate of illness above an expected rate of incidence (see case study, Box 14.1).

Upon recognition of any of these indicators, public health officials should further investigate in order to verify and potentially enact measures for mitigation.

Vulnerable populations

Determination of the demographics of the population affected by the disaster should be a component of the post-disaster surveillance.

Box 14.1. Case Study

Outbreak of norovirus in a large shelter following Hurricane Katrina, 2005, Dallas, TX

While housing over 46,000 individuals displaced from the New Orleans in Dallas, responding health-care workers began noticing an increase in cases of acute diarrheal illness.

Using information from clinical encounters, county epidemiologists created an epidemiological curve showing the number of cases of diarrheal illness over time (see Fig. 14.1). Initially, 42% of cases occurred in children under the age of 10. Norovirus was isolated in 2 of the 7 bulk stool samples.

Based on this information, immediate control measures were instituted, including the following:

- Increasing diligence in hand washing for responders and evacuees. Hand-washing stations were placed around restrooms and volunteers monitored areas for compliance.
- Establishing a medical recovery and isolation area. Individuals who were symptomatic were asked to reside in a separate area with their families.
- Posting of personal hygiene signs throughout the shelter.
- Establishing a more regulated play area for the children, including only allowing toys into the area that could be sanitized.
- Establishing specific baby-changing station areas and supplies.

As a result of these immediate control measures, cases of diarrheal illness diminished and further illness was avoided.

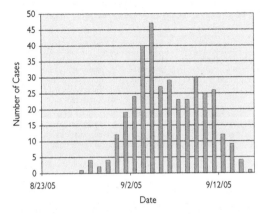

Figure 14.1 Number of cases of diarrheal illness by date.

Specific characteristics of individuals which may place them at higher risk either during or immediate after a disaster include the following:
- Children
- Older individuals
- Persons living with HIV/AIDS
- Persons with sensory deficits
- Persons who need mobility assistance or assistance with daily activities of living
- Persons with mental impairment
- Persons who require dialysis or other essential medical service
- Persons who lack financial independence

Post-disaster infectious disease risk

Disasters increase the population's risk for infectious diseases. Changes to the environment, contamination of food and water, and crowded shelter settings can all affect the epidemiology of many infectious diseases. Public health officials, first responders, and clinicians should all be aware of these risks.

In the United States, most disasters have not been associated with a post-event outbreak of infectious disease (Table 14.2). This reflects our current public health standards, relatively high immunization rates, and relatively low prevalence of infectious diseases in the community and the environment.

This is not the case elsewhere in the world. There, hepatitis A, hepatitis E, *E. coli*, cholera, malaria, measles, Chagas' disease, melioidosis, and tuberculosis have all been reported after major disasters.

Table 14.2 Reported infectious disease outbreaks after disasters in the United States

Exposure	Organism(s)	Treatment	Notes
Wounds or puncture injuries	*Staphylococci* spp and *Streptococci* spp, including MRSA	β-lactam antibiotics, clindamycin.	Trimethoprim-sulfamethoxazole (Bactrim) or vancomycin (intravenous) if MRSA is suspected
	Vibrio spp., *Aeromonas* spp, rapidly growing *Mycobacteria* spp	Ceftazidime and doxycycline, or cefotaxime or ciprofloxacin	Suspect when wound is contaminated with seawater or history of raw seafood consumption. More common in individuals with underlying liver diseases
Respiratory	Influenza, respiratory syncytial virus (RSV), adenovirus	Usually supportive	Recommend isolation of sick individuals, influenza vaccination
	Leptospirosis	Penicillin G or doxycycline	Occurs through contact with fresh water contaminated with infected animal urine
Diarrheal diseases	*Caliciviridae* family: *Norovirus*, *Sapovirus*, *Lagovirus*, *Vesivirus*	Supportive, ensure adequate hydration	Outbreaks reported during Hurricane Katrina. Recommend isolation of symptomatic persons
Vector-borne diseases	West Nile virus	Supportive	Mosquito control in endemic areas
	St. Louis encephalitis	Supportive	Mosquito control in endemic areas

Policy development

Policy development by public health officials involves use of scientific knowledge for guiding the planning and response to disasters. This includes the use of the public health model. The public health model involves the prevention of disease through numerous methods:

- Early detection
- Treatment
- Prophylaxis
- Isolation
- Quarantine
- Education
- Decontamination

The public health model ascribes to fulfill the mission of public health, which is to ensure the conditions in which people can be healthy.

After the Anthrax letter attacks in 2001, the United States developed a national plan to prepare and respond to a future bioterrorist attack. The creation of several federal programs (see Table 14.3) was completed in an attempt to increase preparedness levels across the United States.

Additionally, the creation of a national Medical Reserve Corps (MRC) with local chapters in communities was formed as a partner program under the USA Freedom Corps in 2002. The functions of MRC units are to supplement existing emergency and public health resources when needed. MRC personnel are volunteers given disaster response training.

Use of the public health model during a disaster response results in a shift from traditional medical care practice, since most medical care in the United States is treatment oriented.

Because a disaster could overwhelm the existing infrastructure of health care, a utilitarian response may become necessary. This would involve the concepts of population-based measures, such as doing the greatest good for the greatest number, treating those with a higher likelihood of survival, or prioritizing those with the greatest societal impact (e.g., health care workers).

For example, if a pandemic from a novel strain of influenza virus resulted in overwhelming numbers of patients requiring ventilators, workers would have to determine how to best allocate ventilators to those individuals thought to have the highest probability of survival.

Additionally, control measures such as the administration of chemo-prophylaxis after an Anthrax attack may result in the removal of the prescriptive requirement for these medications and the distribution of antibiotics by nontraditional volunteers or responders such as a postal worker or volunteer. Such programs are being undertaken at the national, state, and local levels across the United States.

Assurance

Historically, a core principle of public health practice has been to use legal enforcement of measures thought to be in the best interest of the community. To this end, public health officials in the United States have utilized laws to destroy property, close businesses, involuntarily treat individuals, and separate individuals who possibly could infect others.

Many of these older quarantine and isolation laws involving such police powers are at odds with citizens' expectations of civil rights and liberties today.

In an attempt to modernize and unify emergency public health law, Dr. Lawrence Gostin drafted the Model State Emergency Health Powers Act (MSEHPA) in 2001. The act defines a public health emergency as an event with imminent threat of an illness, or health condition that poses a high probability of harming a large number of people, causing death or serious long-term disabilities.

Various components or features of the MSEHPA have been passed by 33 states as of April 15, 2007.

Table 14.3 Federal preparedness programs enacted after 2001

Program	Function
Public Health Emergency Preparedness Program	Provides funding for state and local preparedness initiatives. Includes Cities Readiness Initiative, Metropolitan Medical Response System, Pandemic All-Hazards Preparedness Act
Hospital Preparedness Program	Allocates funding to hospitals for emergency preparedness. Administered by assistant secretary for preparedness and response (ASPR).
Strategic National Stockpile	Designed to provide medical supplies and medications to state and local agencies in the event of a disaster
BioWatch	An early warning detection system designed to alert officials to a possible aerosolized release of a bioterrorism agent
Postal Services Biological Detection System	Designed to detect and contain mail that contains bioterrorism agents
BioSense	Syndromic surveillance system designed to characterize variances from normal rates of hospital admissions for symptoms consistent with a possible bioterrorism attack
BioShield	Provides expedited research, procurement, and use of medical countermeasures against possible chemical, biological, radiological, or nuclear attack

Recommendations of the MSEHPA include the following:
- Establish a comprehensive plan for coordinating the response in the event of a public health emergency
- Authorize data collection and reporting, management of property, protection of persons, and access to communications
- Allow investigation by authorities by granting access to individuals' health information under specified circumstances
- Allow the use of appropriate property, as necessary, for care, treatment, vaccination, and housing of patients
- Enable authorities to destroy contaminated facilities or materials and provide measures to safely dispose of human remains
- Grant authorities to provide care, treatment, and vaccination
- Provide the above services without unduly interfering with civil rights and liberties

Suggested readings

Committee for the Study of the Future of Public Health; Division of Health Care Services (1988). *The Future of Public Health*. National Academies Press. Washington DC.

Gostin, Lawrence O, Sapsin, Jason W, Teret, Stephen P, et al. (2001). The Model State Emergency Health Powers Act. Planning for and response to bioterrorism and naturally occurring infectious diseases. *JAMA* 288:622–628.

Ivers LC, Ryan ET (2006). Infectious diseases of severe weather-related and flood-related natural disasters. *Curr Opin Infect Dis*. 19:408–414.

Pickering LK, Baker CJ, Long SS, et al. *Red Book: 2006 Report of the Committee on Infectious Diseases*. 27th ed. Elk Grove Village, IL: American Academy of Pediatrics.

Steering Committee for Humanitarian Response, InterAction with VOICE, ICVA (2004). The Humanitarian Charter and Minimum Standards in Disaster Response. The Sphere Project. Oxfam, GB.

Wetterhall, SF, Noji, EK (1997). Surveillance and epidemiology. In Noji, EK, ed. *The Public Health Consequences of Disasters*. New York: Oxford University Press, pp 37–64.

Chapter 15

International disaster response

Claire Uebbing

John D. Cahill

Ramona Sunderwirth

Introduction

During a disaster, whether natural or man-made, first response focuses on mobilizing emergency services to provide for basic humanitarian needs (adequate water, shelter, food, sanitation, security) for affected individuals and communities.

Disaster response depends on the afflicted country's prior disaster mitigation and preparation planning as well as its level of economic development (as demonstrated in the large differences in mortality and destruction after the 2010 earthquakes in Haiti and Chile).

Disaster response needs to be tailored and flexible to adapt to the local environment, whether rural or increasingly, urban settings. Responses also depend on effective warning systems and duration of the disaster.

Local, national, and global political realities are important as possible sources of disaster or as counterproductive forces to disaster response. Media awareness and coverage influence public support for disaster responses: "hidden disasters" receive far less financial support even though they may be equally or more devastating than those receiving media attention.

Complicating most disasters is the damage to the public health infrastructure as well as to the livelihoods (livestock, farmland, businesses, etc.) of many citizens. In conflict and terrorist situations, critical infrastructures may be strategically targeted, further complicating response.

Disaster response is becoming a field of trained professionals, with protocols and standardized response efforts. The UN and WHO have worked together to create the "cluster" approach to help coordinate disaster relief efforts among relief organizations (Fig. 15.1). Response agencies focus their efforts in one of the 11 clusters and coordinate activities to avoid redundancy.

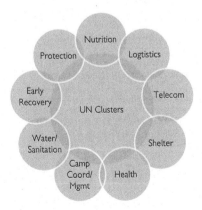

Figure 15.1 Cluster approach to coordinate disaster relief efforts.

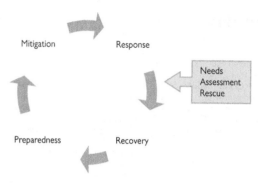

Figure 15.2 Disaster cycle.

Ideally, the initial rapid assessment and rescue occur simultaneously.

Affected communities must be involved in all states of planning and delivery of response. Equitable distribution according to need is essential to successful, sustainable recovery from a disaster.

Response is a continuous process involving individuals and groups from the affected community in the effort to rebuild, assess vulnerabilities, and initiate preparation and mitigation to reduce the damage inflicted by potential future disasters (see Fig. 15.2).

Initial rapid assessment

In any emergency, basic needs must be assessed rapidly in order to determine and direct aid efforts.
- Initiated by local, regional, or national officials and the nations' UN coordinators
- Large-scale disasters involve international humanitarian aid agencies and nongovernmental organizations (NGOs) (Médecins Sans Frontières [MSF], International Medical Corps [IMC], etc.), the UN and UN agencies, military forces, and international financial institutions (International Monetary Fund [IMF], World Bank, etc.)
- Disaster Assistance Response Teams (DARTs) are often deployed with specially trained team members to assist in six areas

Information obtained

- Victims, displaced population profile (general characteristics, health status, capacities and assets)
- Health and nutrition (demographics, vulnerable populations, pre-existing health problems, rates of malnutrition, existing facilities, staff and equipment)
- Water (needs, sources, quality)
- Food and agriculture (availability, distribution system, effect of disaster on agriculture production capabilities)
- Shelter (affected population, materials, distribution)
- Search and rescue (types of structures, equipment needed)
- Sanitation (pre-existing facilities, number of latrines, collection of garbage)
- Logistics (transportation available—airports, trucks, railroads, warehouses)
- Coordination capacity (level of discord in local government, NGOs' capabilities)
- Infrastructure (communications, electric power, fuel, water and sewage, roads and bridges)

Obtaining accurate information at this stage is critical in mobilizing the appropriate teams and supplies and equipment to deal with the situation.

Rescue

Mortality is highest in the first 72 hours post-disaster. Death often occurs from traumatic injuries, exposure, and inhospitable conditions.
- Local search and rescue: up to 90% is undertaken by local individuals; professional teams are mobilized and arrive within 24–48 hours (or longer in more remote areas).
- In the first wave, local and state first responders and core emergency workers arrive (firemen, police, EMS, and trained volunteers).
- In the second wave, national and international specialized teams arrive.

Relief

Public health remains the priority, and standards have been set to achieve adequate response efforts (SPHERE minimum standards that guide relief in health services, water and sanitation, shelter, human rights, and humanitarian behavioral standards). This phase usually lasts 3–6 months.

Essential benchmarks should be met during the emergency phase (EP) (when the crude mortality rate [CMR] is >1/10,000 deaths/day) as well as during the post-emergency phase (PEP) (when the CMR should return to local standards or <1/10,000 deaths/day).

Top ten priorities

- After initial rapid assessment, detailed, ongoing surveys of needs
- Measles immunization and routine immunization (depending on baseline immunization rates)
  - Water and sanitation
  - Water—EP: 5 L water/person/day; PEP: 15–20 L water/person/day
  - Water for consumption should contain <10 fecal coliforms/100 mL
  - Latrines—EP: 1 latrine/50–100 persons; PEP: 1 latrine per 20 persons or per family
- Food and nutrition
  - Minimum ration: 2100 kcal/person/day with 10% protein and 10% fat energy
  - Determine rates of severe malnutrition and implement therapeutic feeding program
  - Surveillance to detect micronutrient deficiencies and supplement as needed
- Shelter and site planning
  - Space: 30 m² space available per person, 3.5 m² shelter space per person
  - 250 people per water point
  - Roads, firebreaks, water supply and sanitation areas, health and nutrition facilities, security stations
- Health care in the emergency phase
  - Four levels of care: a referral hospital, a central facility, peripheral outposts, outreach activities
  - Involve local and host health authorities in medical programs and training
  - Initial trauma care, then rehabilitation
  - Primary health care for acute and chronic illness, maternal and child health , reproductive health, mental health care
  - Develop referral program, disease treatment protocols, data collection system
- Control of communicable diseases and epidemics
  - Focus on prevention
  - Health teams must be prepared to respond to epidemics
- Public health surveillance
  - Early detection of disease outbreaks
  - Data collection informs program activities and efficacy
  - Weekly or monthly meetings to analyze data and feedback to decision makers
- Human resources and training
  - Standardized recruitment, training, and security of workers
  - Establish network of community health workers and home visitors
- Coordination
  - Define leadership: Office of the United Nations High Commissioner for Refugees (UNHCR) in refugee situations; UN country coordinator and United Nations Office for the Coordination of Humanitarian Affairs (UN-OCHA) in natural

disaster or internally displaced persons (IDP) situation; NGOs organize into their assigned clusters
- Involve affected community, local government, and ministry of health in response efforts

Public health measures applied during the disaster response phase offer the best chance for low morbidity and mortality.

It is also important to recognize that the response phase is a cycle in which continual reassessment, preparation, and response are necessary in order to prevent secondary disaster.

Suggested readings

Medécins Sans Frontières (1997). *Refugee Health—An Approach to Emergency Situations.* Oxford: Macmillan.

The Sphere Project—Humanitarian Charter and Minimum Standards in Disaster Response. 4th ed. Oxford: Oxfam, 2004.

Quarantelli EL (2003). *A Half Century of Social Science Disaster Research: Selected Findings and Their Applicability.* Newark, DE: University of Delaware Press.

USAID. *Field Operations Guide for Disaster Assessment and Response.* Field Operating Guide 3.0. Washington, DC: U.S. Government Printing Office.

Warfield, C (2010, October). The disaster management cycle. http://www.gdrc.org/uem/disasters/1-dm_cycle.html.

Chapter 16

Complex humanitarian emergencies

Frederick M. Burkle, Jr.

Conventional wars

Conventional wars are declared, cross-border confrontations between nations, or blocs of nations. They arise from chronic hostilities, threats and disputes over borders, territory, or resources. Examples are World Wars I and II, and the 1991 Persian Gulf War.

Responsibilities for those providing aid and assistance to recover the destroyed health and public health infrastructures and systems are defined by the Fourth Geneva Convention, especially Articles 55 and 56.

Unconventional wars

Conflicts that provoke a variety of unconventional warfare responses are collectively referred to as *complex humanitarian emergencies* (CHEs). Hostilities range from unconventional warfare, prolonged political violence, terrorism, to wars of national liberation in the developing world. Since 9/11 they have spread to developed countries as well.

- CHEs represent the most common human-generated disasters of the past three decades. More people have been killed by elements within their own country than by outside forces.
- Of 120 armed conflicts since World War II, 80% were waged by, or against, entities that were not nations.

Definition

CHEs are defined by the United Nations (UN) as major humanitarian crises of a multi-causal nature that require a systematic response. CHEs commonly involve a long-term combination of political, conflict, and peacekeeping factors.

CHEs have a *singular ability* to erode or destroy the cultural, civil, political, and economic integrity of established societies and are internal to existing political and economic structures of the country in conflict.

Some researchers include large-scale natural disasters in their definition. While the disaster event may accelerate or catalyze the onset of a CHE, they differ from natural disasters and deserve to be understood and responded to as such.

Definition modifiers

- No two CHEs are alike; they will vary in characteristics, intensity, and duration.
- CHEs include a lethal and unpredictable mix of ethnic and religious inequities, poverty, social injustices, cultural incompatibility, pervasive ignorance, racism, oppression, and religious fundamentalism.
- Characteristically, CHEs result in more civilian victims than military personnel casualties, a level that may be as high as 10 civilians for every militant killed.

Impact on health

Heath systems are first to be destroyed and last to be recovered.

All CHEs adversely affect public health protections, denying access to the most vulnerable of populations (e.g., women, children, the elderly, and the disabled).

CHEs are recognized public health emergencies when loss of public health protections, both physical and social, result in a collapse of health services, disease control capacity, poor access to health care, outbreaks of communicable diseases, malnutrition, interrupted supplies and logistics, and environmental decay, to name but a few.

The human cost of complex humanitarian emergencies

CHEs are initially confined within nation-state borders and result in massive numbers of internally displaced populations (IDPs). Most risk affecting neighboring countries with fleeing refugees and in spreading the political turmoil and the conflict across borders.

Epidemiological studies

Epidemiological studies document the short- and long-term impact of various forms of political violence through

- Assessing consequences, including severity of the conflict;
- Measuring the impact or outcome of interventions in declining mortality and morbidity; and
- Identifying the most vulnerable of populations requiring care.

Epidemiological data and analyses

- Detect and verify continued health problems
- Confirm whether victims are benefiting from aid operations
- Facilitate major alterations in the direction of care and health recovery strategies of the international relief community and governmental donors

Assessments, data collection, and analysis

The assessment process is provided by teams that first observe, walk the territory, and talk to the survivors. This process is followed by
- Population-based cluster sampling that determines under–age 5 mortality rates (U5MR), nutritional indices, and crude mortality rates.
- Rates further disaggregated for age and gender to determine the most vulnerable of populations in need.

In circumstances where populations are rapidly shifting, less stringent methodologies such as "excess mortality" determinations are implemented.

In time, and with improved human and logistical resources available, more exact nutritional indices (weight for height, z-scores, and micronutrient deficiencies), infant mortality rates (IMR), and maternal mortality rates (MMR), among others, are assessed and monitored.

The humanitarian community relies on use of specific direct and indirect indices.

Direct indices
- Death, injury, and disabilities, including psychological; in addition the direct consequences resulting from a lack of protection from, and respect for, international humanitarian law.
- Quantitative in nature, subject to organized attempts to measure (i.e., population based cluster sampling), and easier to find and hold people accountable.

Indirect indices
- Deaths that would not have occurred without the conflict. They are seen as collateral damage resulting from population displacement, disruption of food supplies, destroyed health facilities and public health infrastructure, and the consequences, such as poverty and destroyed livelihoods.
- In contrast to direct deaths, indirect deaths are rarely measured, are more functional and abstract in nature, and frequently require qualitative or semiquantitative measures; it is difficult to determine accountability.
- They ultimately account for 90% or more of overall mortality and morbidity.
- Women and children are the most common victims, as are the elderly and those with disabilities.

Operational implications
- Intervention from outside agencies and organizations is initially driven by reports of battlefield and civilian deaths.
- Assessment teams use both direct observation and rapid assessment tools to assess the consequences of the conflict on essential public health parameters such as access to and availability of food, water, sanitation, shelter, health, and fuel.

- No existing datasets measure indirect death tolls; except for a few countries, the humanitarian community has no idea of the worldwide extent of indirect deaths from prolonged political violence.
- Baseline mortality rates (region and country-specific) are found on Web sites from the World Health Organization (WHO), UNICEF, ReliefWeb, and the Centre for Research on the Epidemiology of Disasters (CRED).

Epidemiological models

CHEs can, for planning and training purposes, be placed in one of three epidemiological models.

Developing country model

Examples include Angola, Somalia, Liberia, Afghanistan, and Congo.

Health profiles (Table 16.1) reflect acute and often severe malnutrition combined with clinical or subclinical micronutrient deficiencies (e.g., vitamins A, C, and B6 are common, but endemic regional nutritional deficiencies, such as B1-thiamine and clinical beri beri will also increase).

Seventy-five percent of all communicable-disease epidemics in the world occur in CHEs. Direct and indirect effects result in high crude mortality rates (CMRs) and case fatality rates (CFRs) (e.g., measles and malaria in malnourished children) and outbreaks of endemic diseases such as malaria, diarrheal disease and dehydration, acute upper and lower respiratory diseases, meningitis, tuberculosis, vaccine-preventable diseases such as diphtheria and tetanus, and outbreaks of other tropical diseases such as leishmaniasis and leprosy, which were recently reported in the Sudan.

Developed country model

Examples include the former Yugoslavia and Iraq.

Pre-conflict health profiles (Table 16.2) are similar to those of Western developed countries with relatively healthy populations. Baseline demographics are usually available for population-based assessments.

Established public health infrastructure has been in place for years, including education and practice of basic hygiene; epidemics are few. As violence destroys vital infrastructure and health-sector workers flee or are killed, the public health consequences rapidly surface.

Table 16.1 Developing country health profile

- 90% of deaths are preventable
- Outbreaks of communicable diseases
- Malnutrition and micronutrient diseases
- Absent protective public health infrastructure
- Major deficiencies in WHO childhood vaccine protection
- Mental health consequences are most often unmeasured and untreated
- Internally displaced and refugee populations
- Weaponry: usually small arms and machetes; account for 4–11% of deaths
- High crude mortality rates: range from 7 to 70 times normal baseline
- Higher mortality rates in orphaned and unaccompanied children
- High case fatality rates

Table 16.2 Developed country model health profile

- Conflict occurs in baseline populations who are relatively healthy
- Demographic and disease profiles similar to those of Western industrialized countries
- Excess trauma deaths from war-related advanced weaponry and small arms
- Excess age- and gender-related deaths increase during times of ethnic cleaning
- Few epidemics
- Excess mortality from untreated chronic diseases
- Significant rates of elderly with undernutrition
- Rape, abductions, and psychological traumatic exposures are common

Health profiles show high mortality from advanced weaponry that targets groups for the purpose of ethnic cleansing and genocide.

Excess mortality increases in the elderly who, until the war and conflict, enjoyed an economic status that made medications available for chronic diseases such hypertension, diabetes, and cancers. The elderly may be most vulnerable for undernutrition.

Rape and psychological exposures are common and, when promoted by a warring faction, represent yet another form of ethnic cleansing.

Chronic/smoldering country model
Examples include Haiti, Sudan, and Palestine.

The health profiles (Table 16.3) result from prolonged degradation (e.g., 55 years in Sudan) of access and availability to many basic services.

Cultures are often one of sustained violence experiencing a daily struggle to sustain basic health and public health services.

Children grow up chronically malnourished and have little access to health care and education. Children suffer both chronic stunting and acute malnutrition, which makes them more vulnerable to disease and their complications.

Health-care workers are most likely expatriates, as schools of medicine and nursing no longer exist. Reproductive services such as birth control, safe birthing, and C-section equipment are a luxury.

Table 16.3 Smoldering or chronic country model health profile

- Many years, even decades, of chronic violence
- Social and political unrest
- Poor maintenance of basic public health infrastructure
- Environmental degradation is high
- Little or no access and availability of health and education
- Below-sustenance-level economy
- Chronic malnutrition and stunted growth
- Children grow up only knowing a culture of violence
- Few indigenous health-care providers
- Lack of basic reproductive health services
- Organized mental health services are generally nonexistent
- Incidents of violent surges result in peaks in death rates from direct violence and sudden-onset consequences of chronic conditions (i.e., acute malnutrition and dehydration in children with chronic malnutrition)
- Primarily small-arms deaths and wounds, advanced weaponry increasing
- Violent surges increase internally displaced and refugee populations

Specific health issues

Epidemiological-model data may overlap. Iraq illustrates how a country at war is prone to slip rapidly from a former developed country model to that of a least developing country. Over time, deaths from inadequate public health protections exceeded those caused by violence alone.

Communicable diseases, alone or in combination with malnutrition, account for most deaths. Populations without adequate food for health have risen to 1 billion worldwide. Acts of genocide, ethnic cleansing, and torture have been reported in all models.

Psychosocial and mental health problems are widespread in CHEs. Services need to be provided through both primary health care and community settings: Presentations tend to fall into three categories:
- Disabling psychiatric illnesses (new or pre-existing illness).
- Severe psychological reactions to witnessed or experienced trauma.
- Significant but temporary problems in individuals who are able to cope and adapt once peace and order are restored. This subgroup generally represents the majority of those presenting with symptoms.

International response

Sovereignty of nations limits capacity of international bodies to protect and respond to victims under existing international laws, including the UN Charter and the fourth Geneva Convention. Only the UN has the legal authority to respond militarily with peacekeeping and peace enforcement actions. UN Charter language does not adequately address internal conflicts and genocidal actions.

A UN Security Council resolution will mandate the UN to provide for aid and assistance to the civilian population, implemented through the humanitarian response community and national governmental and international donors:

- UN agencies such as UNICEF, WHO, and Office of the United Nations High Commissioner for Refugees (UNHCR) have the mandate to protect civilian populations within conflicted countries, on their borders, and as refugees in neighboring countries.
- Field programs are implemented through nongovernmental organizations (NGOs), the Red Cross Movement (resources from both the International Committee of the Red Cross and the Federation of Red Cross and Red Crescent National Societies), and a myriad of host nation voluntary organizations.
- Despite universal neutrality provisions, attacks on and assassinations of humanitarian aid personnel have increased by more than 200% over the last decade.
- Aid and assistance provided by the militaries in conflict remain controversial.

Each CHE has unique legal exceptions and guidelines. The Western-led Coalition military campaign in Afghanistan was not specifically mandated by the UN but is widely perceived to be a legitimate form of self-defense from global terrorism under Article 51 of the UN Charter. The International Security Assistance Force (ISAF) is a NATO-led security mission established by the UN Security Council.

Anticipated end state

Acute-phase priorities of relief programs focus on the following:
- Supplementary and therapeutic feeding
- Nutritional and health assessments
- Vaccine control measures
- Essential medications
- Surveillance programs

The outcome assumption is that low-cost humanitarian aid, if properly performed and managed, will reduce the direct indicator rates to pre-war and conflict levels or better within 4–6 months.

As the direct-effect mortality rates decline, so does outside interest and relief aid from donor agencies and governments, often giving a false assurance of success. Up to 47% of CHEs return to war within a decade—a rate that can be 60+% in Africa.

CHEs have changed substantially over the last three decades, especially in the overall levels of insecurity. Iraq and Afghanistan are examples where assessments and relief strategies have not effectively dealt with worsening security and catastrophic public health failures, especially as they impact civilians and the relief community.

Suggested readings

Review chapters

Burkle FM Jr, Greenough PG (2006). Complex emergencies. In Ciottone GR, ed. *Disaster Medicine.* Philadelphia: Elsevier-Mosby. pp. 43–50.

Burkle FM Jr (2010). Complex public health emergencies. In Koenig KL, Schultz CH, eds. *Disaster Medicine: Comprehensive Principles and Practices.* New York: Cambridge University Press, pp. 361–376.

The SPHERE Project: Humanitarian Charter and Minimum Standards in Disaster Response, 2004 edition. Geneva: Oxfam Publishing.

Peer-reviewed literature

Albala-Bertrand JM (2000). What is a complex humanitarian emergency? An analytical essay. Department of Economics, Queen Mary College, University of London. Working Paper No. 420, October 2000: 1–29.

Burkle FM Jr (2006). Complex humanitarian emergencies: a review of epidemiological and response models. *J Postgrad Med.* 52(2):109–114.

Burkle FM Jr, Chatterjee P, Bass J, Bolton P (2008). Guidelines for the psycho-social and mental health assessment and management of displaced populations in humanitarian crises. In: *Public Health Guide for Emergencies.* Geneva and Baltimore: International Federation of Red Cross and Red Crescent Societies, and Johns Hopkins University Medical Institutions.

Connolly MA, Gayer M, Ryan MJ, Salama P, Spiegel P, Heymann DL (2004). Communicable diseases in complex emergencies: impact and challenges. *Lancet* 364(9449):1974–1983.

Jones L, Asare JB, El Masri M, Mohanraj A, Sherief H, van Ommeren M (2009). Severe mental disorders in complex emergencies. *Lancet* 374(9690):654–661.

Roberts L, Hofmann CA (2004). Assessing the impact of humanitarian assistance in the health sector. *Emerg Themes Epidemiol* 1(1):3.

Spiegel PB, Checchi F, Colombo S, Paik E (2010). Health-care needs of people affected by conflict: future trends and changing frameworks. *Lancet* 375(9711):341–345.

Web sites

Centre for Research on the Epidemiology of Disasters (CRED): http://www.cred.be/
International Committee of the Red Cross (ICRC): http://www.icrc.org/
ReliefWeb (countries and emergencies): http://www.reliefweb.int/rw/dbc.nsf/doc103?OpenForm
World Health Organization (health topics and health report): http://www.who.int/en/

Hospital Components of Disaster Response

Hospital administration disaster response

David Bouslough

Introduction

In the past century, the role of the hospital in society has dramatically changed. This transition has occurred as a result of the public's expectations and as a response to rapid advances in medicine. It is fueled by the external pressures of regulatory agencies and medical economics.

The expectations for hospital emergency preparedness have also changed, driven by the same external forces. Emergency preparedness now encompasses an all-hazards approach, with hospital administrations challenged to develop equally robust plans to answer a Monday afternoon patient surge in the emergency department, the need for vertical and horizontal evacuation of a clinical unit threatened by fire, or an influenza pandemic that outstrips resources nationwide.

This chapter discusses the various components and initiatives that hospital administrators must implement to ensure that the hospital is prepared to effectively respond to a disaster.

Emergency management coordinator (EMC)

In light of the heightened expectations placed on hospitals to develop all-hazards emergency operation plans, many administrators choose to hire individuals specifically trained in emergency management to lead their planning efforts. In response to this health sector–wide trend, training programs at the preprofessional, college and university, as well as postdoctoral levels have dramatically increased in the last decade.

The EMC's responsibilities often include management of the emergency preparedness committee and its objectives, development of a comprehensive emergency response strategy based on a facility hazard vulnerability analysis, and the implementation of a command and control management framework (Hospital Incident Command System).

Emergency preparedness committee (EPC)

The EPC is a group of staff, often assembled by hospital administration, tasked with the following objectives:

- Author and update the institution's emergency operations plan
- Design and upkeep of the emergency operations center
- Develop and execute preparedness exercises and training
- Serve as subject-matter experts in the event of a disaster
- Function as a liaison entity between the institution's planning and response efforts and other regulatory and/or partnering institutions (e.g., department or ministry of health, neighboring hospitals, fire, police, prehospital medical care agencies)
- Manage preparedness grant funds and meet grant requirements

Hospitals vary in their stated mission, their health-care capacity, and their responsibilities within a medical system. These factors will likely play important roles in further defining committee objectives and activities.

Committee size is variable between institutions. While smaller groups (5–10 members) may lead to greater efficiency in decision making, they lack sufficient personnel to accomplish the work of the committee and miss the valuable input of clinical and service staffs not represented in discussions.

Alternatively, large groups (20+ members) may provide a robust work force and extensive expertise upon which to draw, but are likely to suffer from "decision-making paralysis."

Hazard vulnerability analysis (HVA)

The HVA is an element of emergency preparedness that allows EMCs to set priorities as they develop their disaster preparedness, response, and recovery plans. An HVA directs attention to the regional hazards from which the hospital requires protection.

While these tools are designed to identify hazards creating the most risk for a health-care facility, it is nevertheless prudent for EMCs and EPCs to develop plans to address those hazards deemed less likely, but catastrophic in nature.

Internet links to representative HVA tools are listed in Table 17.4 (p. 150).

Emergency operations plan (EOP)

The EOP is a written document that a hospital maintains, which outlines its response to hazards identified in the facility's HVA. The plan should be based on an all-hazards approach and include measures for mitigation, preparedness, response, and recovery.

A sample EOP development tool is listed in Box 17.1 (p. 149).

Emergency operations center (EOC)

The EOC is the physical location where hospital administrators and EPC members gather to coordinate information, manage resources, and respond to an emergency. EOC design should focus on ensuring efficient and effective flow of information.

Exercises, training, and meetings held in this space can be used to test its effectiveness and improve its design.

Internet links to EOC design principles and templates are listed in Table 17.4 (p. 150).

Hospital Incident Command System (HICS)

The HICS is an example of a management tool developed for U.S. hospitals in 2006. It represents a standardized approach to small and large emergencies, as well as the nonemergent challenges of daily operations.

Incident command systems are discussed in detail in Chapter 31.

Several important command features of HICS are summarized in Table 17.1. Figure 17.1 demonstrates the HICS organizational chart for personnel just below the section chief level.

Table 17.1 Important command features

Feature	Definition
Chain of command	The orderly line of authority within the ranks of the incident management organization
Unity of command	Every individual has a designated supervisor to whom he or she reports at the scene of the incident.
Unified command	Allows agencies with different legal, geographic, and functional authorities and responsibilities to work together effectively without affecting individual agency authority, responsibility, or accountability
Span of control	Any individual with incident management supervisory responsibility should have between three and seven subordinates.

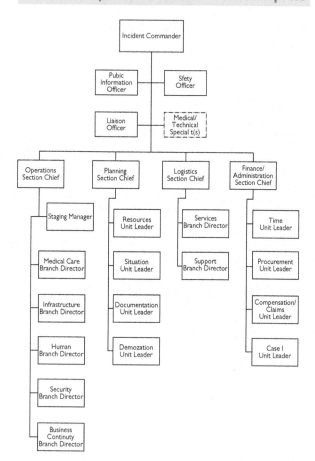

Figure 17.1 Organization of incident management personnel just below section chief.

Medical/technical specialists and specialized teams

When the scale of an emergency response grows, the incident commander may appoint a command staff comprised of a public information officer, safety officer, liaison officer, and medical/technical specialist. This final appointee serves to provide specialized expertise, insight, and recommendations during the event.

Additionally, unique characteristics of an emergency activation may require development of task forces or strike teams to provide specific skill sets to the response effort, as shown in Table 17.2.

Table 17.2 Expertise required for specific disaster events

Medical/technical specialists	Specialized teams
Emerging infectious disease	Radiation, nuclear detection
Chemical, biological, radiation, nuclear	Decontamination
Medical ethics	Bomb squad
Legal counsel	Burn care
Coroner/medical examiner	Mental health, critical incident stress management

Hospital's role in regional preparedness

Large-scale disasters often affect multiple adjacent communities, may create mass casualties in the hundreds or thousands, and far exceed the response capacity of any one institution. While many agencies may respond collaboratively to mitigate such an event, the hospital, by virtue of its medical expertise, is poised to provide health-care leadership across public and private sectors.

Hospital administration and emergency preparedness personnel often take active roles in developing regional preparedness initiatives.

Metropolitan Medical Response Systems (MMRS)

The MMRS program was developed in the United States in 1996 and is currently administered by the Department of Homeland Security. Local metropolitan areas were tasked with integrating the capacities of healthcare institutions and medical systems with public and private industry as well as government to maximize all-hazards mass casualty preparedness and response.

Evaluation of 124 successful MMRS jurisdictions since the program's inception has demonstrated several habits of effective regional teams (Table 17.3).

Table 17.3 Habits of effective regional preparedness teams

- Maximize use of federal preparedness funding, developing planning bodies to help direct spending and avoid duplication of effort
- Define the metropolitan region and stakeholders
- Use gaps in regional planning to inform priority objectives
- Secure the support and leadership of hospital executives
- Use a neutral "mediator" agency to ensure collaboration between competitors
- Partner with trade organizations and associations that can fairly represent stakeholders (e.g., departments of health, hospital associations, medical associations)
- Use regional planning efforts to implement interoperable communications
- Employ creative strategies to incentivize hospital participation
- Use electronic communication systems between hospitals and key agencies to provide situational awareness and event tracking
- Key operational functions of regional groups include the ability to coordinate the transfer, deployment, and distribution of patients, staff, and supplies and to make decisions regarding scarce medical resources and altering standards of care

Source: Maldin B, Lam C, Franco, C, et al. (2007). Regional approaches to hospital preparedness. *Biosecur Bioterror* 5(1):43–53.

Interagency collaboration and communication

When an emergency outstrips the capacity of one hospital or requires the simultaneous response of multiple agencies, collaboration and communication cannot be overemphasized.

Unified command management structures, joint information centers, and regional or state EOCs and incident management teams can be used to address the additional resources and operational support needs of expanding incidents. Hospital administrative willingness to develop lateral aid and memoranda of understanding is essential. The principles and tools of effective disaster communications are outlined in Chapter 27.

The frequency with which a hospital is required to respond to a given disaster type contributes to the training diligence or complacency of hospital administration and personnel.

Training exercises should be based on the institution's HVA, addressing response to disasters and events most likely to occur, before planning for less likely events.

Important disaster exercise design principles are listed in Box 17.1.

Additional hospital disaster exercise evaluation tools are listed in Table 17.4.

Box 17.1 Disaster exercise design principles

- Confirm budget, protected time, and administrative support for exercise.
- Address a disaster preparedness topic consistent with the institutional HVA.
- Define specific goals and objectives for the exercise.
- Choose an exercise modality (operational drill, tabletop exercise, simulation) that best supports these goals and objectives.
- Consider:
  - Method of event notification
  - Utilization of the ICS and EOC
  - Number and type of hospital personnel required
  - Methods of communication to be used
  - Activities to be completed and supplies needed
  - Safety measures for all participants
  - Plan a thorough and multifaceted evaluation of the exercise
  - Incorporate lessons learned into the emergency action plan (EAP) and further training

Table 17.4 Select hospital emergency preparedness planning resources

Planning topic	Resource agency	Internet link
HVA	Hospital Safety Center	http://www.hospitalsafetycenter.com/platinum/hazards_vulnerability_analysis.cfm
	California Hospital Association	http://www.calhospitalprepare.org/ctegory/content-area/planning-topics/healthcare-emergency-management/hazard-vulnerability-analysis
	Canadian Provincial Emergency Program	http://www.pep.bc.ca/hrva/toolkit.html
EOP	Federal Emergency Management Agency	http://www.fema.gov/pdf/plan/slg101.pdf
EOC	Davis Logic	http://www.davislogic.com/EOC.htm
	Department of Defense	http://www.wbdg.org/ccb/DOD/UFC/ufc_4_141_04.pdf
	Department of Homeland Security	http://www.icfi.com/markets/homeland-security/doc_files/eoc-design.pdf
ACS	Agency for Healthcare Research and Quality	http://www.ahrq.gov/research/altsites
POD	Agency for Healthcare Research and Quality	http://www.ahrq.gov/research/cbmprophyl/cbmpro.htm,
	New York City emergency planners	http://www.nyc.gov/html/doh/html/bhpp/bhpp-hospital.shtml#2
Exercise	Agency for Healthcare Research and Quality	http://www.ahrq.gov/prep/drillelements

ACS, alternate care site; EOC, emergency operations center; EOP, emergency operations plan; HVA, hazard vulnerability analysis; POD, point of distribution.

Suggested readings

Federal Emergency Management Agency, ICS 200 training manual, http://emilms.fema.gov/is200_ICS/ICS0101summary.htm

Maldin B, Lam C, Franco, C, Press D, Waldhorn R, Toner E, O'Toole T, Inglesby TV (2007). Regional approaches to hospital preparedness. *Biosecur Bioterrror* 5(1):43–53.

Hospital ancillary services disaster response

David Bouslough

Introduction

Hospital administration, medical staff, nursing, and ancillary services all work together to respond to an event. Hospital ancillary-services personnel perform a critical supportive role in disaster response. Inadequate disaster preparation and planning for ancillary services can limit all other aspects of hospital disaster response.

Disaster-time work assignments for ancillary services that approximate nonemergency job descriptions are optimal. Those professionals trained to provide acute care should be the first assigned to this role in an emergency. This arrangement does not guarantee that acute-care specialists will be adept at all aspects of disaster care (e.g., rationing medical supplies and services).

Ancillary-personnel challenges also arise when disaster-time needs are unique to the event, especially in terms of manpower and specialized disaster training. For example, decontamination teams should be identified well in advance, consist of interested individuals across specialties and work shifts, participate in special training sessions, and exercise their skills often.

Only as a last resort should "just in time" training sessions be used and "Job Action Sheets" be thrust into the hands of personnel who must learn their responsibilities real-time during an actual disaster.

Personnel and volunteers

Providing for staffing shortages is a key responsibility of the planning section chief. Skilled and nonskilled volunteer recruitment plans should be multi-tiered and robust. Use of an Emergency System for Advanced Registration of Volunteer Health Professionals (ESAR-VHP) pre-authorizes and credentials personnel for disaster-time assignments.

Sources of skilled volunteers
- Adjacent hospitals, urgent care, and primary care clinics
- EMS, fire and police forces
- Department of health resources: Medical Reserve Corps (MRC), alternative care sites (ACS), points of distribution (PODs)
- State response teams: emergency management agencies (EMAs), incident management teams
- Federal response teams: Disaster Medical Assistance Teams, Disaster Mortuary Teams, National Medical Burn Teams, National Pharmaceutical Response Teams, etc.
- National programs and organizations: Emergency Management Assistance Compact, American Red Cross, etc.

Sources of nonskilled volunteers
- Service organizations: Boy and Girl Scouts, Lion's and Rotary clubs, etc.
- Faith-based organizations: churches, tabernacles, mosques, YMCA/YWCA, etc.

Effective regional preparedness planning

Key operational functions of regional groups include the ability to coordinate the transfer, deployment, and distribution of patients, staff, and supplies and to make decisions regarding scarce medical resources and altering of standards of care. Planning for ancillary-services coordination in a disaster is an important component of this process.

Alternate care site (ACS) development

When an emergency situation creates mass casualties whose medical need outstrips a hospital's surge capacity, an ACS may be used to decentralize health care away from the hospital setting and decompress patient surge.

ACS geographic location, physical infrastructure, staffing and medical supply needs, patient transport, documentation, and patient-tracking aspects require careful consideration in planning.

Valuable tools for choosing and developing an effective ACS have been developed by the Agency for Healthcare Research and Quality.

Points of distribution (POD) planning

Emerging infectious disease outbreaks, the threat of bioterrorism, and our recent history of global pandemic illness combine to present emergency scenarios in which large populations of people may require mass-vaccination or treatment.

Many local and federal governments have invested in stockpiling pharmaceuticals. Accessing these stockpiles and effectively dispensing them to affected individuals require careful planning and should primarily occur at locations other than health-care facilities tasked with the treatment of acute and chronic conditions.

The functions of a POD include education, screening, and medication and vaccine dispensing.

Evacuation and sheltering

Evacuation planning requires consideration of vertical and horizontal movement of patients, predetermined muster points, the evacuation of medical supplies for continued patient care, continuity of medical records, patient and staff tracking, and facility inspection for re-inhabiting the hospital.

Training and exercise

Two of the greatest challenges facing the EPC are the dispersal of critical information in the emergency action plan (EAP) to all members of the hospital staff, and the maintenance of that knowledge over time.

As institutions, hospitals usually have educational systems built into their organizational chart. Nursing units train with nursing supervisors or nurse educators. Physicians educate themselves and each other through hospital grand rounds, lectures, continuing medical education, and mentoring activities. Support services and security personnel may have annual competency fairs, computer learning modules, and/or physical performance examinations. EPCs are advised to make use of the existing educational pathways within their facility before attempting to add or create alternate educational methods.

A new focus in disaster planning is establishing competencies through development of curricula that is evidence based, standardized, and applicable to the training of all members of the multidisciplinary health-care team.

Seven cross-cutting competencies (Box 18.1) can focus the learner on topical knowledge building, technical skill development, and decision-making capacity. Learning can be mapped according to individual staff needs, focusing on the competencies most important to their performance.

By adopting this curriculum development approach, emergency preparedness educators have the opportunity to maximize the efficiency of their training efforts and increase the penetration of information to all personnel institution-wide.

Training exercises should be based on the institution's HVA, addressing response to disasters and events most likely to occur.

Box 18.1 Cross-cutting competencies for ancillary health-care workers

- Recognize a potential critical event and implement initial actions
- Apply the principles of critical event management
- Demonstrate critical event safety principles
- Understand the institutional emergency operations plan
- Understand the incident command system and one's role in it
- Demonstrate the knowledge and skills needed to fulfill one's role during a critical event

Source: Hsu EB, Thomas TL, Bass EB, et al. (2006). Healthcare worker competencies for disaster training. *BMC Med Ed* 6:19.

Pitfalls in hospital preparedness for ancillary services

- Lack of adequate communication elements:
  - Current phone trees
  - Redundant systems
  - Interoperable capabilities
- Underestimated hospital security needs
- Insufficient decontamination supplies, personnel, training, and procedures
- Staff and volunteer management issues:
  - Quality training
  - Safety
  - Accommodations
- Exercise realism, content, and debriefing with captured lessons learned
- Not recognizing the division of institutional, local, and regional responsibilities
- Lack of hospital administrative will in provision of time, personnel, capital

Suggested reading

Hsu EB, Thomas TL, Bass EB, Whyne D, Kelen GB, Green GB (2006). Healthcare worker competencies for disaster training. *BMC Med Ed* 6:19.

Chapter 19

Hospital medical staff disaster response

Alison Schroth Hayward

Andrew Milsten

Medical staffing needs

A fully staffed disaster response will require leadership as well as all levels of personnel. An institutional response must include all branches of staffing:

- Operations
- Planning
- Logistics
- Financial/administrative

Each of these staffing needs is part of a full operational incident command system (ICS) as defined by the Department of Homeland Security and should be addressed in advance by the disaster planning committee.

Organizational charts defining leaders for each component of the response, as well as the overall response, must be created. The Federal Emergency Management Agency (FEMA) also recommends a clear line of succession in the absence of designated leaders and legal assurance that the succeeding leadership will be able to fulfill necessary duties.

Staff should be "cross-trained and vertically trained" with the goal that any staff member could fulfill the duties of their peers, as well as staff members directly above and below them. Ideally, however, staff should fill the position most similar to their own occupation.

Staffing needs should be tailored to each incident, depending on type and magnitude of incident and available staff.

Competence, training, and equipment

All key personnel with a direct role in institutional disaster management and emergency response should be trained using the appropriate courses from the National Incident Management System (NIMS) curriculum created by the Department of Homeland Security to ensure compliance with federal requirements.

The NIMS curriculum and a comprehensive library of other courses in disaster planning and response are available and open to all U.S. residents, at http://training.fema.gov.

Training for general medical staff should be formal and standardized. Recommendations have been made for a competency-based approach to staff training, based on review of the existing literature.

The following are competencies that have been identified for disaster response.

Initial actions

Staff must be able to identify a potentially critical event and notify proper authorities, including either directly activating the disaster plan or contacting a person who is authorized to activate the plan.

Staff should also have the knowledge base to be able to recognize precautions that should be taken for safety depending on the nature of the event (biological, chemical, nuclear, etc.) and mobilize resources for preparation and disaster mitigation.

Management

It is important that staff be aware of the management components necessary in each stage of disaster, including preparedness, response, and recovery.

All staff members should be familiar with how to identify and address safety concerns—for themselves, for other staff members, and for the security of the institution during a disaster response.

In order to ensure an effective, coordinated response, medical staff must be aware of how institutional emergency operations plans would affect their area of work and how to access information regarding detailed plans for any given scenario. Specifically, they must be familiar with their role in the incident command system.

Competence in critical event communications must be a part of staff training.

Staff surge capacity

Surge capacity, the ability to rapidly scale up staff capacity to meet the demands of a disaster response situation, is critical to an emergency operations plan for hospital staffing

Experience has shown that the majority of patients are expected to arrive at the closest medical facility within 90 minutes of a disaster event, that the possibility for diversion or transfer of casualties will be limited, and that prevention of casualty entry into the facility should not be considered an option because of ethical and bureaucratic concerns.

These factors combined mean that the closest medical facility is likely to bear the brunt of the responsibility for caring for casualties, and without a plan for surge capacity, medical staff may be overwhelmed.

In most disasters, the number of staff who report to the institution is in excess of what is needed. However, in the most critical situations, staff may be much less likely to report because they are unable to reach the institution or fear for personal safety.

In such situations, the following modifications to staffing protocols should be considered:
- Changing length of shifts or responsibilities
- Decreasing administrative duties, frequency of patient reassessments or certain patient care responsibilities (i.e., hygiene) in the interest of caring for greater numbers of patients
- Temporarily increasing nurse-to-patient ratios

Potential sources of staff for surge capacity include the following:
- State Emergency Systems for Advanced Registration of Volunteer Healthcare Professionals (ESAR-VHP). Local hospital staff, clinic staff, and health professional volunteers registered with an ESAR-VHP have had their credentials verified
- The Medical Reserve Corps (MRC). Local MRC units of volunteers may include medical and public health professionals, such as physicians, nurses, pharmacists, dentists, veterinarians, epidemiologists, and paramedics
- Federal public health and medical teams (e.g., National Disaster Medical System, Public Health Service)
- Trainees
- Patient family members
- Military members
- Community emergency response teams (CERTs)
- Lay volunteers

Notification of staff

Because casualties of disasters typically arrive at hospitals within 1 to 1.5 hours of the disaster's occurrence, hospitals must be ready to activate disaster plans with little advance notice.

Each institution will require a communications plan that can be put in place by a taskforce or workgroup dedicated to the issue. In order to implement such a plan, the institution must be properly prepared with central databases describing all staff members and their roles, both clinical and nonclinical.

Initial response must be carried out by staff who are on duty at the time of the disaster and should not be dependent on staff on call, whose ability to be present could be impeded by the conditions of the disaster.

Staff on duty at any given time must have the ability to activate the disaster plan and independently modify it on the basis of needs of the situation until supplemental staff arrives.

Recommendations for staff notification in disaster situations are as follows:

- Launch of a Web page accessible by staff, featuring ongoing status updates and links to relevant protocols and other logistical documentation.
- Institution of a call-in number for staff, which can be used from any location to call in and receive a current status report.
- One new modality that can be used for effective initial disaster alert and staff recall is Short Message Service (SMS) text messaging via cell phones.

Ongoing communication issues

- Staff will need to have access to ongoing updates throughout each phase of the disaster.
- Implementation of a phone alert system to determine if staff will be able to make it to their upcoming shift, to improve contingency planning, is recommended.
- A designee or group should be appointed to assess current staff needs and absenteeism rates and plan accordingly. This task can be divided into clinical and nonclinical staffing needs assessment, if necessary.
- A designee or group should also be put into place as communications liaison(s), to work with incident command and prepare status updates for Web site and phone distribution to staff in a timely manner.

Role of on-scene medical staff

- Medical staff on duty during a disaster must have had training or be able to immediately access training relevant to the disaster scenario, such as training on the use of personal protective equipment for that particular scenario.
- Medical staff working during disaster scenarios must have the knowledge and skills to implement an efficient and realistic patient triage system, as well as specific decontamination measures as needed during the triage process.
- Employee health services should be provided for medical staff on duty during the course of disaster operations.

Ethical considerations

In a disaster such as an infectious disease outbreak, bioterrorism attack, or nuclear radiation incident, conditions at work may pose a danger to medical staff. Physical disasters such as bomb attacks, earthquakes, or floods may pose threats to the families of medical staff. Either or both of these situations may contribute to a reluctance of medical staff to come to work during disaster conditions.

Both the American Medical Association Code of Ethics and the American College of Emergency Physicians' Code of Ethics agree that physicians are ethically obligated to serve patients when there is a need for such care. This imperative has been judged "prima facie," but is not an absolute moral duty.

During the SARS outbreak in Toronto and during Hurricane Katrina, the majority of physicians remained at their posts, treating patients for days after the disaster occurred.

In general, studies have shown that the desire of physicians and nurses to assist in a disaster scenario correlates directly with the degree of personal risk inherent to the type of disaster being addressed (i.e., toxicological, radiological).

Suggested readings

Agency for Healthcare Research and Quality. Mass medical care with scarce resources: the essentials. Hospital/acute care. http://www.ahrq.gov/prep/mmcessentials/mcc5.htm

Auf Der Heide C (2006). The importance of evidence-based disaster planning. *Ann Emerg Med* 47:34–49.

Bradt DA, Aitken P, Fitzgerald G, et al. (2009). Emergency department surge capacity: recommendations of the Australasian Surge Strategy Working Group. *Acad Emerg Med* 16:1350–1358.

Department of Homeland Security. Federal Continuity Directive 1 (FCD 1). http://www.fema.gov/pdf/about/org/ncp/fcd1.pdf

Epstein RH, Ekbatani A, Kaplan J, Shechter R, Grunwald Z (2010). Development of a staff recall system for mass casualty incidents using cell phone text messaging. *Anesth Analg* 110(3):871–878.

Federal Emergency Management Agency. Incident Command System (ICS) review document. http://training.fema.gov/EMIWeb/IS/ICSResource/assets/reviewMaterials.pdf

Hsu EB, et al. (2006). Healthcare worker competencies for disaster training. *BMC Med Educ* 6:19.

Iserson K, et al. (2008) Fight or flight: the ethics of emergency physician disaster response. *Ann Emerg Med* 51:345–353.

National Center for Injury Prevention and Control, Coordinating Center for Environmental Health and Injury Prevention, US Department of Health and Human Services (2007, April). In a moment's notice: surge capacity for terrorist bombings—challenges and proposed solutions. Atlanta, GA: Centers for Disease Control and Prevention.

Qureshi K, et al. (2005). Health care workers' ability and willingness to report to duty during catastrophic disasters. *J Urban Health* 82(3):378–388.

Reilly M, et al. (2009). Education and training of hospital workers: who are essential personnel during a disaster? *Prehosp Disaster Med* 24(3):239–245.

Sandrock C (2010). Chapter 4. Manpower. Recommendations and standard operating procedures for intensive care unit and hospital preparations for an influenza epidemic or mass disaster. European Society of Intensive Care Medicine's Task Force for intensive care unit triage during an influenza epidemic or mass disaster. *Intensive Care Med* 36(Suppl 1):S32–37.

Chapter 20

Hospital nursing disaster response

Diane DeVita

Michelle M. Darcy

Leila L. Blonski

Nursing role in disaster response

Registered nurses (RNs) represent the largest group of health-care professionals in the United States. Numbering over 2.7 million in 2003, they represent the bulk of a facility's clinical and patient care workforce.

Trained and practiced at patient assessment and prioritizing care, hospital RNs also liaise regularly with physicians, support services, and ancillary staff, making them uniquely adept at caring for patients and negotiating the hospital system, however compromised it may be in a disaster.

Registered nurses comprise a very diverse profession and practice in vastly different settings throughout various medical facilities. The education, skill level, and clinical experience among nurses also vary significantly.

Thus, defining the already diverse "role of nursing" is difficult, except in very general terms—even among hospital nurses—in the inherently unpredictable setting of a disaster response.

Areas of responsibility

Nursing roles and areas of responsibility are defined to some degree by hospital disaster plans, which vary from facility to facility and should be accessible and familiar to and rehearsed by all staff. No guidebook or chart can prepare staff or account for all variables or all contingencies in a disaster. Flexibility is essential.

Most hospital RNs will fall into a specific area of responsibility based on skill set.

Triage (emergency RNs)

The RN is part of most hospitals' triage team, ideally paired with an experienced physician and two ancillary staff members.

RNs must be familiar with disaster triage:
- Perform triage based not only on patient acuity and potential survivability of condition but also on available resources—e.g., supplies, blood, personnel, and access to definitive care—rationing to do the most good for the greatest number

Triage nurses may be required to provide life- and limb-saving interventions not frequently practiced in the non-disaster setting.

Triage may occur outside the facility:
- At the scene of the disaster
- Decontamination area
- Ambulance staging area

RNs must be prepared to work in inclement weather, with limited staff and supply resources, and under potentially hazardous conditions in which long hours may be required.

The triage area supervisor is typically an RN, facilitating the flow of supplies and personnel to the triage area and patients to appropriate physical locations based on category.

Emergency department (ED)/immediate care RNs

- Assist with and provide life-saving interventions, potentially surgical interventions under less than ideal conditions
- ED charge or supervising nurse ensures efficient flow of patients to definitive care areas

Definitive care

Provision of this care involves operating room (OR) nurses and intensive care unit (ICU) RNs, post-anesthesia care (PACU) RNs, and RNs normally working on "step-down" level units.
- ICU capability may overlap the post-anesthesia area and overflow into areas usually populated by less critically injured patients
- ICU care may have to be provided in an austere environment. Limited equipment availability may force staff to improvise or do without altogether and may affect the level of care that can be provided
- ICU staffing may have to be augmented by RNs with limited intensive-care experience, placing ICU RNs in the role of care provider in addition to supervisor and instructor to those unaccustomed to caring for the critical or postsurgical patient

The impact on RNs in these areas may not be immediate but may become overwhelming based on volume and acuity.

Floor/clinic nurses

RNs could be called to assist with casualties in the "immediate" care area—usually the ED or other areas, especially in the initial phase of a disaster response.
- Nurses may be tasked to common areas, such as gymnasiums, to set up and care for "delayed" category patients in contingency wards.
- Minimally injured "walking wounded" may require nothing more than first aid or minor care by nurses.
- Large numbers of psychiatric casualties, also categorized as "minimal," may require care by RNs—even those not specialized in psychiatric care.
- RNs may be assigned to expectant casualties to provide comfort care and pain management.
- In the event of a disease outbreak, hospital nurses may also fulfill community tasks to provide immunizations, health screenings, etc.

Administrative/supervisory positions

RNs normally in administrative roles may be required to provide patient care, and their administrative duties fulfilled by nonproviders.

Nurses as liaisons

As providers involved most directly in bedside patient care, nurses in all roles will be involved with assisting not only patients but also family members' needs, including the following:
- Access to clergy, social services, etc.
- Access to telephones, sources of information
- Referral to relief organizations or other resources

Disaster-specific nursing response

Disaster size (in terms of number of casualties and degree of damage to infrastructure) and type (natural vs. man-made), as well as the nature of casualties generated by a disaster, will dictate the type of response.

RN roles are assigned on the basis of patient population and need. Actual disaster responses may be prolonged given the nature of the disaster. In a pandemic, victims may present over a period of weeks.

Additional staffing will likely be required, not just in the initial phase of the disaster but in the coming weeks to months, to provide care not only for the primarily injured but also for subacute illness in an increased long-term regular volume of patients.

It is important to consider the impact of stress-induced secondary complaints, or illness or injury related to environmental sequelae of a disaster: exposure, food and water contamination, lack of sanitation, mold, or vermin or insect infestation.

Varying types of disasters will dictate nursing roles.

Natural disasters
- These may affect the infrastructure of the facility. In-coming patients may need to triaged to alternate facilities or evacuation provided for inpatients.
- Roadways may be affected, delaying rescue arrival on scene, patient arrival to facilities from a disaster, and staff arrival to the hospital.

Biological/pandemic
- Influx of patients may last for days to months.
- Patients requiring isolation may increase the strain of facility resources and space.
- Nurses need to be diligent in the use of personal protective equipment (PPE).
- RNs in primary care roles may be first to recognize disease or symptom trends heralding outbreaks.

Chemical/nuclear
- A decontamination station needs to be set up at a distance sufficient (given prevailing winds and weather conditions) to prevent contamination of the medical facility.
- Ensure that all staff are appropriately protected from the hazardous material prior to caring for contaminated patients.
- Staff members need to be conscious of the added strain of sustained working in protective equipment.
- There will be a probable increase in the number of expectant patients.
- Radiological casualties are initially triaged no differently than conventional casualties. Casualties themselves do not become radioactive and are relatively easy to decontaminate.

Facility capability and nursing staffing

Surge capacity
- Caring for casualties while maintaining usual standards of care.
- Capacity often determined by nursing staffing availability.

Overflow capacity
- Standards of care must be compromised to provide the greatest good to the greatest number.
- Actual physical capacity of the facility may be the limiting factor.
- Staffing ratios will not be maintained, and clinicians may be mandated to remain on duty for extended periods.

Physical capacity may be limited by internal disasters
Loss of structural integrity or fire, flood, or contamination may affect capacity.
- This necessitates unconventional use of intact parts of the facility or alternate facilities as defined by the hospital's internal disaster plan or as improvised in the face of unforeseen circumstances.
- Alternate sites, such as gymnasiums, schools, hangars, office buildings, and other large shelters, may be set up as ad hoc treatment facilities.
- Equipment customary for the treatment and care of ill and injured patients may be unavailable. RNs and providers must rely on ingenuity and critical thinking skills to provide the best care possible.

Training

RNs must be familiar with their facility's disaster plan and their expected role in it and take advantage of training in responding to specific types of disasters. RNs must also participate in facility disaster drills.

As casualties mount, usual nurse-to-patient ratios may no longer be practical, and RNs may be asked to perform duties beyond their usual role.

Nurses who do not practice in critical care settings but who may be expected to do so in a disaster have a professional responsibility to familiarize and educate themselves (and should be supported by if not required to participate in such training by their employer) with "basic and essential disaster medical knowledge." This includes usual and customary skills to provide basic care to critical care patients such as respiratory failure and ventilator management, recognition and treatment of shock, sedation and pain management, and physiological monitoring.

This training should include the following elements:

Regular disaster plan drills
- Hospital or region-wide involvement
- The Joint Commission mandates two drills per year. These drills are often underutilized as training opportunities, involving only some components of the disaster response, or run as a tabletop-only exercise
- Random and unannounced drills provide more realistic training.
- Training should include setup of decontamination area, if applicable.
- Specific and general disaster situations
- Specific to geographical area

Individual training for nurses
- Review specific facility and ward standard operating procedures and update them as needed
- Disaster triage specific training
  - IDME: Immediate, Delayed, Minimal, Expectant. This is different from conventional triage, in which the most severely ill and wounded are given highest priority
- Ongoing training for identification and treatment of disease, as well as in chemical, radiological, and nuclear disasters
- All nurses need to be fitted for and understand proper application of all available PPE that they may need to use in a response
- Equipment training
- Basic emergency and critical care training for all nurses expected to respond in a disaster
- Review of policies for reporting of diseases and disease trends
- Online training available at http://www.fema.gov and other Web sites

Summary

Nursing is a major part of disaster response in a medical facility. Nursing roles in a disaster are extensive but difficult to define, as responsibilities vary according to type of disaster, skill set of RN, and the facility's capability. Some nurses are better prepared than others for response and, like all clinicians, require training and realistic practice.

Suggested reading

Gebbie KM, Qureshi, K (2002). Emergency and disaster preparedness: core competencies for nurses: what every nurse should but may not know. *Am J Nurs* 102 (1):46–51.

Mitani S, Kuboyama K, Shirakawa T (2003). Nursing in sudden-onset disasters: factors and information that affect participation. *Prehosp Disast Med* 18(4):359–366.

Part 3

Pre-Disaster Considerations

Disaster length: an overview

Kelly R. Klein

Ashika Jain

Henry H. Truong

Cindy Baseluos

Overview

What is a disaster? The definition of a disaster depends on one's perspective. The World Health Organization (WHO) defines a disaster as any occurrence that causes damage, ecological disruption, loss of human life, or deterioration of health and health services on a scale sufficient to warrant an extraordinary response from outside the affected community or area.

Volatile political situations can result in humanitarian disasters, which have been termed "complex emergencies."

A medical disaster exists in a hospital when the number of patients presenting in a given time frame exceeds the emergency department's ability to provide minimal care without external assistance.

Put simply, a disaster will be present on any level if the death, human suffering, and societal disruption are such that the existing available resources of the affected population are not enough.

In the developed world, a community affected by a disaster expects that the established public health and health care systems will continue to provide services. The degree of human suffering will be amplified if the existing health care infrastructures are not prepared to meet these expectations.

It is therefore imperative that the medical and public health care community be prepared to deal with the immediate medical conditions created by the event. Additionally, they must continue to provide health care for patients with day-to-day emergencies, chronic medical conditions, and other special needs.

All disasters, whether short term, long term, or extended term, have the following timeline in common:
- *Inciting point:* the time when the disaster starts (train collision, power failure, earthquake, infectious disease outbreak)
- *Chaos:* the period immediately following the incident until order begins to return (cellular phone systems overwhelmed and limited communication available about the event)
- *Structure:* when a framework of assistance and repair is established (electricity is being restored, potable water is available, health-care facilities if closed, begin to reopen)
- *End:* when day-to-day life has returned to normality, infrastructure is restored, and outside assistance is no longer necessary. This is a variable point that is highly dependent on the individual, community and government perspective (children have returned to school, curfew is lifted, local health care has returned to pre-event normal)

In its initial stage, the chaos phase of the disaster is managed by the community itself: local EMS, emergency management, and citizens. Those who are already in the area are best positioned to carry out search and rescue, provide medical first aid, and conduct rapid needs assessments.

As communication networks are often temporarily interrupted and it takes time to organize a response from outside the immediate area, outside assistance will arrive too late to impact this critical window of intervention—often arriving 96 hours after the event has begun. That is why robust coordination efforts between public and private stakeholders are essential and preplanned integration of local faith-based and community-based organizations are essential for an immediate response and should be strongly encouraged in disaster planning efforts.

Given the initial media coverage, there is often an abundance of well-meaning independent medical professionals who want to assist, as seen during Hurricane Katrina and the Asian tsunami. Unless specifically requested by the affected community, "self-deployed" medical teams should be discouraged, as they generally lack the infrastructure to function independently and be self-sufficient.

This is particularly relevant in international disaster situations where the outside medical personnel arrive days after the immediate emergency medical needs have been handled by the local health-care systems. Additionally, these non-native groups are a resource burden, as they do not speak the local language or understand the local customs, and they require food and shelter when they arrive.

If the disaster warrants outside assistance, state and regional assistance will ideally arrive within 24 hours. If federal assistance is requested, a presidential disaster declaration of an emergency will generally provide further aid within 72–96 hours.

New federal directives and the Joint Commission (TJC) are now requiring hospitals to be able to manage a disaster situation independently for a period of 96 hours.

Examples of federal assistance include Disaster Management Assistance Teams (DMAT), the Federal Emergency Management Agency (FEMA), Urban Search and Rescue (USAR), the military, and private-sector resources such as the American Red Cross.

National Incident Management System (NIMS)

Post-9/11, the U.S. government developed and mandated the implementation of NIMS. Although most emergencies are handled on a daily basis by a single, local jurisdiction that has its own command structure, NIMS was developed to provide a system that would help emergency mangers and responders from different jurisdictions and disciplines work together more effectively in disasters and in large geographic emergency situations.

Incident Command System (ICS)

In the 1970s, after a series of wildfires in California, a need was identified for an emergency management system that would allow firefighters from different jurisdictions to work together. The ICS was developed after that event, and since 9/11 it is mandated for any organization receiving federal funds, including hospitals and private industries.

The ICS organizational chart can be tailored according to the changing needs of the event. It is important to realize that not all of these positions are necessary and, depending on the event size, and one person can have multiple roles.

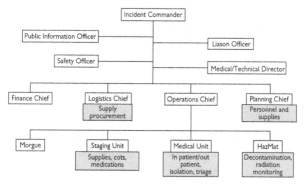

Figure 21.1 Example of Hospital Incident Command System (HICS).

Emergency management

Once a disaster has struck, an effective response involves *assessment, implementation,* and *continuous evaluation.* While the need may not be apparent in the immediate chaos of a disaster, a *needs assessment* is a crucial management tool, which effects decision-making, planning and control of an organized response.

The fluidity of these situations requires ongoing surveillance and monitoring as well as evaluation of disaster response to rapidly adapt to changing conditions.

There are four phases of management for disasters and emergencies: mitigation, preparation, response, and recovery.

- *Mitigation* focuses on long-term measures for reducing or eliminating risk. This phase of a disaster is most often overlooked
  - *Examples:* placing generators on the higher floors of hospitals in a flood zone, robust building codes in hurricane- or earthquake-prone areas, redundant computer network servers, smoke detectors, or sprinkler systems
- *Preparation* involves advance planning for a disaster response
  - *Examples:* stored water and food for 96 hours for all employees and patients, hurricane area evacuation plans, child and elder care for hospital employees who must remain at work
- *Response* involves actions taken by health-care providers, rescuers, and agencies
  - *Examples:* search-and-rescue teams, efforts to get communication and computer systems working, evacuation
- *Recovery* constitutes the actions resulting in a return to a normal way of functioning. This process begins immediately after the event has occurred and lasts until normality is restored
  - *Examples:* providing dialysis for renal-failure patients, keeping pharmacies open for medication refills, returning community members to their homes

Many hospitals, public health systems, and businesses have emergency management committees. These committees address the four phases of emergency and disaster planning at their facility.

Emergency management is also an integral part of TJC inspection requirements for hospitals. An effective and proactive committee in the hospital setting should be made up of a cross section of the hospital departments, including physicians and nurses, as well as support from other departments, including environmental services and housekeeping, social work, infectious disease, medicine, safety, physical plant operations, communications, purchasing, finance, patient transport, ambulance, and dietary.

Emergency management committees should meet on a monthly basis and prepare plans, create an IC template, procure funding for projects, and make recommendations to the administration regarding mitigation, preparedness, response and recovery. During an actual disaster event, the emergency management committee traditionally would not be in charge but would be part of the advisory team, if needed.

Evacuation

Evacuation, although a term used frequently during disaster planning, is a very complex undertaking. The decision to evacuate is resource and monetary dependent.

Research indicates that once a decision is made to evacuate, a considerable amount of time may elapse before people in the affected area hear, absorb, and decide to respond to the instructions. Crucial evacuation resources include transport, traffic flow management, and safe destinations.

Hospital evacuations require preplanning and generally a day or more to execute. Ongoing clear communication with the affected population through trusted sources is necessary to facilitate the evacuation and for the eventual return home.

If a prolonged period of displacement is expected, temporary shelters should be the last option. All efforts should be made to relocate displaced people in homes of relatives or friends.

Return to a normal routine and secure living environment is a critical step in the mental health recovery of disaster survivors.

Special-needs populations

While disasters may occur randomly, they do not randomly affect the population. Vulnerable members of society face increased risk from a given hazard.

For example, people of lower socioeconomic status may not have the financial means to evacuate when a hurricane threatens. Children and pregnant women may be more vulnerable from the effects of radiation. Those who are at the extremes of age, who are disabled or developmentally delayed, or who suffer from chronic medical or psychological conditions will face increased risks in disaster situations.

This vulnerable subset of the general population will require increased attention to routine medical care, shelter, nutrition, communication networks, and mental health needs.

Disasters are becoming more common. Some factors contributing to this phenomenon include the following:

- Increases in population density and mobility
- Climate changes and erosion of environmental barriers
- Economic inequity, global interconnectedness
- Threats of emerging infections

While no one can predict exactly where and when a disaster will strike, steps can be taken to minimize damage and to foster an effective response and recovery.

Disasters can affect local communities or widespread regions, lasting days to decades. They may require the single response of a particular hospital or a complex multinational response that includes multiple organizations and countries.

Familiarity with the priority actions and resources available for a short-term, long-term, or extended-term disaster is critical for effective disaster management on all levels and improved coordination among responders.

Suggested readings

Federal Emergency Management Agency. Emergency support function annexes. Retrieved December 21, 2008, from http://www.fema.gov/emergency/nrf/

Federal Emergency Management Agency. National Emergency Management System (NIMS). Retrieved October 24, 2008, from http://www.fema.gov/pdf/erergency/nims_doc_full.pdf

Federal Emergency Management Agency. Overview of Stafford Act support to states. Retrieved December 21, 2008, from http://www.fema.gov/emergency/nrf/

Ginter PM, Duncan WJ, Abdolrasulnia M (2007). Hospital strategic preparedness planning: the new imperative. *Prehosp Disaster Med* 22(6):529–536

Noji EK, Kelen GD (2004). Disaster preparedness. In Tintinalli J, Kelen G, Stapczunski J, eds. *Emergency Medicine: A Comprehensive Guide*, 6th ed. New York: McGraw-Hill, pp. 27–35.

Pan American Health Organization (1993). *Mitigation of Disasters in Health Facilities: Evaluation and Reduction of Physical and Functional Vulnerability. Volume II: Administrative Issues.* Washington, DC: Pan American Health Organization.

The Joint Commission (2009). *History Tracking Report: 2009 to 2008 Requirements*, Oakbrook Terrace, IL: The Joint Commission.

Sorensen JH, Vogt BM, Mileti DS (1987). *Evacuation: An Assessment of Planning and Research* (report prepared for U.S. Federal Emergency Management Agency, RR-9).

World Health Organization. Risks, emergencies, and disasters, p. 91. Retrieved December 11, 2006, from http://www.wpro.who.int/internet/files/pub/297/part1_1.6.pdf

World Health Organization and Pan-American Health Organization (2003). *Hospitals in Disasters: Handle with Care.* Report of a meeting held in San Salvador, El Salvador, 8–10 July 2003.

Chapter 22

Short-term events

Kelly R. Klein

Ashika Jain

Introduction

Short-term disasters are finite and not long-lived. Short-term disasters can last from only a few hours to up to a few weeks.

Examples
- Power outages
- Snow and ice storms
- Computer failure
- Mass gatherings
- Pipe explosion
- Plane crash

The following discussion lists priority actions for health-care providers and emergency management personnel to consider during short-term disasters. This list is not exhaustive and may not be applicable for all situations.

Short-term disaster mitigation

Most health-care systems have disaster mitigation infrastructures. These are standing orders or resources already in place to prevent a problem should a short-term disaster occur.

An example would be putting in a redundant server system for a computer system so that if one goes down, the other one would take over without service interruption.

Short-term disaster preparedness

- Decontamination plans; these are a Joint Commission (TJC) requirement
- Updated contact numbers for all essential personnel
- 96 hours of supplies in hospital (TJC requirement)
  - Pharmaceuticals and antidotes
  - Generator fuel
  - Food, water, and basic needs for hospital staff, family, and patients
- Evacuation plan

Short-term disaster response

Implementation of Incident Command System (ICS)

Decontamination

Best-practice recommendations suggest that the hospital be able to decontaminate ambulatory and nonambulatory patients within 3 hours of the incident occurring, with a minimum expectation of 100 people.

Triage

A valid triage system should be based on four factors: patient's medical condition, available equipment, training of the responders or health-care providers available, and transportation capabilities.

Assessment

• Even in an expected short-term disaster, someone should be tasked with identifying available resources and expected vulnerability
• A method of rapidly identifying available inpatient and critical care beds should be in place (i.e., surge capacity)
• Collaboration with other area hospitals should be used to establish regional resources and ability to transfer patients if the need arises

Communication

• Traditional communication may not always be functioning in an acute response phase. Be flexible and creative
• Timely, regular briefings for health care workers should be implemented. It is imperative to keep health care workers informed of the developing situation
• A public information officer (PIO) should be utilized early for the media to prevent confusing and inappropriate information going to the public

Protection of health care and emergency response workers

• Health care and emergency response workers may be directly threatened in certain disaster situations
• Securing a disaster scene for safe triage and search and rescue should be a priority, prior to sending in large numbers of health care and emergency care workers
• Enhanced hospital security should be addressed early in a disaster situation

Short-term disaster recovery

Post-disaster evaluation
- Debriefing with hospital and ancillary staff
- Recommendations for future mitigation and preparedness

Psychological trauma
Even in limited-duration events, the resulting psychological effects may last for long periods and may require ongoing evaluation and treatment.

Suggested readings
Rosenthal MS, Klein K, Cowling K, Grzybowski M, Dunne R (2005). Disaster modeling: medication resources required for disaster team response. *Prehosp Disaster Med* 20(5):309–315.

The Joint Commission (2009). *History Tracking Report: 2009 to 2008 Requirements*, Oakbrook Terrace, IL: The Joint Commission.

U.S. Department of Labor Occupational Safety and Health Administration (2005, July). OSHA best practices for hospital based first receivers or victims from mass casualty incidents involving the release of hazardous substances. Retrieved December 21, 2008, from http://www.osha.gov/dts/osta/bestpractices/firstreceivers_hospital.html

Chapter 23

Long-term events

Kelly R. Klein

Henry Truong

Introduction

A long-term disaster can have lasting effects that may be felt for months or years. This type of disaster requires both state and federal assistance during the response and recovery phase.

Examples
- Hurricane or typhoon
- Large earthquake
- Economic down turn
- Epidemics
- Terrorist act
- Drought
- Forest fires

The following discussion lists priority actions for health-care providers and emergency management personnel to consider during long-term disasters. This list is not exhaustive and may not be applicable for all situations.

Long-term disaster mitigation

For the vast majority of new health facilities, the incorporation of comprehensive disaster protection from earthquake and weather events into designs adds only 4% to the initial building cost.

Long-term disaster preparedness

Memorandums of understanding (MOU) should be in place prior to any large-scale event with surrounding hospitals, EMS providers, and supply vendors to help with surge, evacuation, and equipment needs.
- Pharmaceutical needs readily available or stockpiled
- Prophylaxis for staff and their families
- Medical supplies to meet the needs of a displaced population

The New Emergency Health Kit, used by the World Health Organization (WHO), was created to meet the primary health needs of a displaced population of 10,000 for 3 months.

Long-term disaster response

Needs assessment

Even if brief, it is essential to initially identify to what extent people can help themselves, what the population is doing now, and what the unmet immediate needs are. This process should be repeated regularly.

- Data points include people and area affected, numbers of people displaced, water and sanitation needs, food and nutrition needs, shelter needs, and health services.
- Any outside assessment team must be self-sufficient in food, water, shelter, medical supplies, transport, and communications.
- Assessment references include the following:
  - Rapid Health Assessment Protocols for Emergencies (WHO)
  - Handbook for Emergencies (UNHCR)
  - Assisting in Emergencies (UNICEF)
  - Humanitarian Charter and Minimum Standards of Disaster Response (SPHERE)
  - Refugee Health (MSF)
  - Rapid Health Assessment of Refugee or Displaced Populations (Epicentre)
  - Famine-Affected, Refugee, and Displaced Populations: Recommendations for Public Health Issues (CDC)
  - War and Public Health (ICRC)

Strategic national stockpile (pharmaceuticals, ventilators and medical supplies)

DMAT (medical teams), VMAT (veterinarians), DMORT (morticians, dentists, and forensic specialists), FEMA (needs assessment, disaster relief)

National Guard

Red Cross

The Red Cross plays a valuable role in providing essential items of shelter, clothing, and basic health care.

Other personnel

Other personnel who might be called to service or already available include the following:

- Local volunteers who are members of the community will be the most valuable and generally the first to respond locally.
- Faith- and community-based organizations provide a focal point of trusted information for the population and should be clearly integrated into any communication strategy.
- If concerned personnel are coming into a disaster area to help, they should be prepared to provide for all of their own basic needs, including food, water, and shelter, and not rely on the local infrastructure to support them.
- Mental health workers should be prepared to refer anyone who appears psychotic or is having suicidal ideation. Many health-care and

emergency-care workers may acutely require mental health counseling depending on the nature of the event.

Donations
- Large numbers of nonessential items create a burden for the affected area.
- Be careful regarding what is asked for from the general public.
- Inappropriate drug donations can take huge amounts of time and money to dispose of properly.
- All items brought into a disaster area should be based on the requests of the population and a valid needs assessment.

Long-term disaster recovery

Economic
- Individual and family grants
- Public assistance for relocation or rebuilding
- Hazard mitigation grants

Return to normal routine and functioning
- This is a key step in recovery.
- If victims are unable to immediately return to their home or job, it is important to actively involve them in the reconstruction efforts so they do not feel helpless.
- Providing a structured education for children will help them to establish a normal routine, which is important for mental health recovery.

Psychological trauma
- Psychological trauma may persist for years after a disaster.
- Patients who exhibit symptoms of psychological trauma should be appropriately referred.

Infectious disease

New disease epidemics are rare in disaster settings, but like the novel H1N1 pandemic, it can be disastrous for health-care systems.

During natural disasters, when disease outbreaks do occur, they are either endemic to the area or have been brought into the area by refugees or via zoonotic vectors.

The most important measures to prevent massive infectious disease outbreaks during a disaster include ensuring adequate water and sanitation, necessary vaccinations, avoiding overcrowding, and public health surveillance.

The dead

There is often the false belief during a disaster that large numbers of dead bodies are an epidemic hazard. In only a few special cases, such as cholera or hemorrhagic fevers, are recently dead bodies known to pose a health risk to those still living in the area.

Proper identification and burial of the bodies, while adhering to traditional cultural norms, is important for the psychosocial recovery of disaster victims. Prior to burial or cremation, legal documentation and forensics are often necessary.

In the U.S. disaster response system, the Disaster Mortuary Operational Response Teams (DMORT) may be deployed by the federal government to support local resources in the event of mass fatalities. DMORTs bring with them forensic experts, dentists for identification, embalming capability, and sophisticated data-collecting systems.

Suggested readings

Noji E (2005). Public health in the aftermath of disaster. *BMJ* 330:79–100.

Pan-American Health Organization and the World Health Organization (2003). *Protecting New Health Facilities from Disasters: Guidelines for the Promotion of Disaster Mitigation*, Washington, DC: PAHO/WHO.

The Sphere Project. (2004). *Humanitarian Charter and Minimum Standards in Disaster Response*. Oxford: Oxfam Publishing.

World Health Organization (1998). *The New Emergency Health Kit 98*. Retrieved September 25, 2008, from http://www.who.int/medicinedocs/pdf/whozip31e/whozip31e.pdf

Extended events

Kelly R. Klein

Cindy Baseluos

Introduction

Extended-term disasters are large scale and affect nations and communities for decades, if not generations. They can result mass population displacements and complex humanitarian emergencies.

Examples
- Exxon Valdez oil spill
- Rwandan genocide
- Famine
- Chernobyl
- War

This following discussion lists priority actions to consider during extended-term disasters. This list is not exhaustive and may not be applicable for all situations.

Extended-term disaster mitigation

- Safe farming practices and topsoil retention
- Peace agreements and efforts to create stable economic and political situations
- Not building in disaster-prone environments

Extended-term disaster preparedness

- Early warning systems for storms and earthquakes and tsunami in high-risk areas
- Disease and famine surveillance
- Regional agreements for assistance during emergencies
- Collaborative cross-border agreements to respond to infectious disease risks
- Stockpiling of food, fuel, and vaccines
- Training of appropriate personnel
- Watch groups
  - Physicians for Human Rights
  - WHO, UNICEF

Extended-term disaster response

- Provision of basic minimum needs (see WHO Sphere)
  - Clean water, sanitation, and shelter
  - Food rations
  - Treatment of micronutrient deficiencies (vitamin A administration)
- Health
  - Vaccinations
    - Measles
  - Malaria
    - Vector control and treatment
  - Provision of medications for chronic medical conditions
  - Reproductive health
  - Mental health
  - The New Emergency Health Kit (WHO)
- Family-tracing programs

Extended-term disaster recovery

- Return to a normal routine is a critical aspect of recovery for the affected population
- Participation of the affected communities in the recovery effort is important for them to regain control of their lives
- Post-traumatic stress disorder (PTSD) can be expected in vulnerable people years after the disaster
  - Children may have behavioral problems or difficulty in school, or may be withdrawn
  - Increase in substance abuse
  - Increase in divorce rates
  - Increase in domestic violence
  - Increase in suicides
- Population resettlement
  - Returning displaced populations to their homes is preferred over resettlement
  - Shelters should be a last resort, and only as a temporary situation
  - Any shelter situation must provide for the safety of the inhabitants and be culturally appropriate

Suggested readings

Button BV (1995). "What you don't know can't hurt you": the right to know and the Shetland Island oil spill. *Hum Ecol* 23:241–257.

The Sphere Project (2004). *Humanitarian Charter and Minimum Standards in Disaster Response.* Oxford: Oxfam Publishing.

Chapter 25

Hazard vulnerability analysis

Dinah Cannefax

Introduction

A *hazard* is a source of potential danger or cause of adverse events. A *hazard vulnerability analysis* (HVA) is an assessment of potential hazards that considers probability, risk or level of impact, and preparedness.

HVA tools vary from lengthy descriptive documents to succinct tables with quantifiable rating systems. Regardless of the type, the intent of the tool is to guide an organization or community in prioritizing their mitigation and planning efforts based on their hazards.

Probability

Whether it is a man-made event, such as a terrorist attack, train wreck, utility failure, or a natural event, such as a tornado or hurricane, disasters are not predictable with any degree of accuracy. However, several steps can be taken to assist the team in estimating the probability of each hazard.

- From the local jurisdiction (e.g. city, county, state), ask to review the current HVA for the community. This will provide insight as to how their emergency management professionals determined probability.
- Complete a literature search on local disasters.
- Review weather histories (i.e., number of tornado and/or flood warnings).
- Review geographic reports to look for flood plains and fault lines.
- Review area business by type (e.g., chemical plant, mass transit hubs).
- Identify venues where large numbers of people gather and how frequently (e.g., stadiums, malls).
- Internal disaster or utility failure reports.

One area often overlooked when an organization is working on their HVA is vulnerability due to technology. A simple transformer on a hospital campus can cause serious implications for patient-care activity. With many providers implementing an electronic health record, which is dependent on multiple business systems, a single electric or network failure can hinder patient care.

It is important to understand that the probability of man-made events grows exponentially as technological advances are made.

Establishing the probability of an occurrence is part objective and may be statistical if data are available. Even so, the determination of probability for each hazard is considered highly subjective.

Risk or level of impact

Risk is the potential impact that any given hazard may have on the organization. Risk should be analyzed to include a variety of factors specific to the organization completing the HVA.

For example, a hospital has several critical factors (as defined by The Joint Commission in 2008) that can be listed as the following:

- Communications
- Supply and equipment
- Safety and security
- Staffing
- Utility and plant operations
- Clinical and support services

For example, in analyzing the impact of a flood in the community that does not affect the hospital campus, the safety of those on campus may not be a problem. However, supply and staffing resources may be reduced significantly if transportation is hindered by high water and road closures in the community surrounding the hospital campus.

Level of preparedness

In order for any organization to analyze the level of disaster preparedness, one must consider how well the organization is prepared internally and how well the community is prepared. Of the three categories analyzed for each hazard, preparedness is the most objective.

It is critical that the group rate their program honestly. Failure to do so may result in a false sense of security and wrongfully direct resources to less threatening hazards.

When determining the level of preparedness for the organization or for the community, the following are indicators to be considered:

- The current status of emergency response plans
- Whether their response plans consider sustainability in critical areas such as utilities and supplies
- The frequency and level of staff training completed
- How often and how thoroughly the organization conducts practice exercises of its response plans

The level of preparedness between the organization and the community at large is often very different. For this reason, the internal level of preparedness should be analyzed and/or rated separately from the external or community level of preparedness.

For example, a small hospital may be unable to support a large decontamination team for chemical hazards because of lack of staffing and of funds for equipment maintenance. Their local fire department, on the other hand, may have a well-equipped hazardous materials team.

Steps to completing an HVA

The following list outlines the general steps to completing an HVA for an organization:

- Assemble a multidisciplinary team from your organization to assist in an HVA brainstorming session.
- List all possible hazards, regardless of their likelihood or impact.
- Consider grouping the hazards into typical categories such as man-made threats and natural events. This is a popular technique, but not required.
- Assess your completed list to be sure that only hazards are listed and not outcomes. This is a common mistake in developing an HVA and will cause confusion when ranking probability, impact, and preparedness.
- Discuss the probability of each hazard.
- Discuss how each hazard would impact key areas within the organization (i.e., staffing, supplies, etc.).
- Discuss how each hazard would impact the infrastructure of the supporting community (e.g., transportation, utilities).
- Discuss how well the organization and supporting community are prepared to respond to each hazard.
- Review the data gathered for each hazard and prioritize the list. Determine which hazards threaten the organization most.
- List mitigation, planning, response, and recovery activities needed to reduce the risk of each hazard at the top of the prioritized list.

Conclusions

To summarize, every organization will assume certain levels of risk inherent to employing staff and providing services. Analyzing individual hazards that threaten the organization will initiate a process of identifying the areas on which the organization may want to concentrate their mitigation and planning efforts.

HVAs should be done on a facility and a regional level and should be reviewed regularly for possible changes.

An example of a regional HVA is given in Table 25.1.

Table 25.1 Sample hospital hazard vulnerability analysis (HVA)

Event	Probability	Internal Impact of Critical Areas						External Impact		Level of Preparedness		Rank of Risk
	Likelihood this will occur	Internal Communications	Supply and Equipment	Safety and Security	Staffing for Care and Command	Utility and Plant Operations	Clinical and Support Services	Potential for Pt Influx (MCI)	Business Interruption	Internal	External	Relative Threat
Roman = Natural	0 = N/A	0 = N/A						0 = N/A		0 = N/A		
Bold = Technical	1 = Low	1 = Low						1 = Low		1 = High		
Italic = Man Made	2 = Moderate	2 = Moderate						2 = Moderate		2 = Moderate		
	3 = High	3 = High						3 = High		3 = Low or none		
Tornado	3	3	2	2	3	3	3	2	3	1	1	26
Epidemic/Pandemic	2	1	3	2	3	2	3	3	3	2	2	26
Info Systems Failure	2	3	2	2	3	3	3	1	3	2	1	25
Terrorist (CBRNE)	1	2	1	3	2	3	3	2	3	3	2	25

											Total
Electrical Failure	2	2	2	2	2	3	2	1	3	2	23
Bomb Detonation	1	2	2	1	3	3	1	3	3	1	23
Chemical, External	1	1	2	2	3	2	2	3	2	2	23
Generator Failure	1	3	2	3	3	3	0	3	1	1	23
Severe Thunderstorm	3	2	2	2	3	2	1	1	2	2	22
Telecom Failure	3	3	2	2	3	2	0	2	2	1	22
Ice Storm/ Blizzard	2	2	2	2	3	2	2	2	1	2	22
Radiologic, External	1	1	3	2	2	3	2	2	3	2	22

Table 25.1 (Contd.)

Event	Probability		Internal Impact of Critical Areas					External Impact		Level of Preparedness		Rank of Risk
	Likelihood this will occur	Internal Communications	Supply and Equipment	Safety and Security	Staffing for Care and Command	Utility and Plant Operations	Clinical and Support Services	Potential for Pt Influx (MCI)	Business Interruption	Internal	External	Relative Threat
Water Failure	1	0	2	2	1	3	3	1	3	3	3	22
Fire, Internal	1	2	2	2	1	3	2	1	3	2	2	21
Construction/ Demolition	2	3	1	3	1	3	3	1	1	1	1	20
Civil Disturbance	1	1	2	3	2	1	2	2	2	3	1	20
Fuel Shortage	1	1	3	1	2	3	3	0	2	2	2	20
Sewer Failure	1	0	3	1	1	3	3	1	3	2	2	20
HVAC Failure	3	2	1	2	2	3	3	0	1	1	1	19
Medical Gas Failure	2	0	3	3	1	3	3	0	1	2	1	19
Hurricane	1	2	2	1	1	3	2	1	1	2	2	18
Natural Gas Failure	2	0	1	0	0	3	3	0	2	3	3	17
Transport/ Mass Transit	1	1	1	2	2	1	2	2	1	2	2	17

Hazmat, Internal	2	0	0	3	2	3	2	0	0	2	2	16
Extreme Heat	3	1	1	1	1	3	1	1	1	1	1	15
Area Flooding	2	1	1	1	1	2	1	1	1	2	2	15
Earthquake	1	1	1	1	1	1	1	1	1	3	3	15
Flood, Internal	2	2	1	2	2	2	2	0	0	1	1	14
Steam Failure	2	0	2	0	0	3	3	0	0	2	2	14
Hostage Situation	1	1	0	3	2	0	1	0	1	3	1	13
Infant Abduction	1	0	0	3	2	0	1	0	1	2	1	11
Medical Vacuum Failure	1	0	0	0	0	3	3	0	1	1	0	9
Drought	2	0	1	0	0	2	0	1	0	1	1	8
Wild Fire	2	0	0	0	0	0	0	1	0	2	2	7

Suggested readings

Kaiser-Permanente Hazard Vulnerability Analysis Tool. Retrieved January 20, 2011, from http://www.calhospitalprepare.org/category/content-area/planning-topics/healthcare-emergency-management/hazard-vulnerability-analysisLast

McIsaac J (2006). *Hospital Preparation for Bioterror—A Medical and Biomedical Systems Approach*. St. Louis: Elsevier Academic Press.

Noiji EK, Sivertson KT (1987). Injury prevention in natural disasters. A theoretical framework *Disasters* 11(4):290–296,

Drills and evaluation

Brenda O'Connell Driggers

The telephone rings

You are in your hospital's emergency department at 2:00 on Sunday morning when the phones begin to ring, one after another. Emergency Medical Services dispatch is calling, along with other EMS services giving you the heads-up that a disaster has occurred at the local airport.

A commercial aircraft has crashed, and public safety personnel on the scene estimate greater than 75 patients with traumatic injuries and burns, many contaminated with aviation fuel. Estimates of the number of deaths are unreliable but are growing.

We all dread this scenario and hope it never happens. With the proper training and participation in disaster exercises, individuals and organizations can be better prepared to mount a measured response and provide the best possible care for disaster victims, with minimum stress and confusion.

Introduction

All hospitals must be prepared to accommodate a response to a broad spectrum of disasters:
- Natural disasters (flood, earthquake, hurricane, etc.)
- Man-made accidental disasters (air crash, building collapse, etc.)
- Terrorism incidents
- Large-scale natural disease outbreaks

The scale of catastrophic incidents is also a factor:
- Limited casualty
- Mass casualty incident (MCI)
- Super MCI
- Mass casualty/mass fatalities
- Mass fatalities incident

Plans for appropriate response should be
- Clearly written (to a sixth- to eighth-grade reading level)
- Disseminated to all responder partners
- Tested via drills and exercises
- Revised regularly (at least annually)

In addition, there are four phases in any disaster, all of which could be tested in the course of an exercise:
- Mitigation (efforts to reduce the severity of an incident)
- Preparedness (identify resources that might be used)
- Response (activating the plan and operating under it)
- Recovery (resuming "normal" operations)

The federal government requires hospitals to develop disaster plans and conduct exercises using these plans. Exercises and drills not only test assigned resources and personnel but also will provide insight into a system's strengths and weaknesses, providing insight to remedy the weaknesses and build on strengths. One cannot rely on disaster plans to function properly if they are written but never tested.

In order to conduct any exercise, some basic questions have to be addressed:
- What are the objectives of the exercise? (Must begin with objectives)
- What will be tested during the exercise?
- What agencies will be involved?
- Will tabletop or functional exercise be used?
- How long will the exercise take?
- Who will be involved in the planning?
- Who will be asked to conduct an evaluation?

There are numerous examples available to help develop a good exercise. The Homeland Security Exercise and Evaluation Program (HSEEP) is a good example. This information can be found at https://hseep.dhs.gov. Not only does it provide all of the tools to prepare a successful exercise, it also provides exercise evaluation guides (EEGs) that cover the target capabilities list (TCL).

With theses guides, FEMA has done most of the structural work to prepare an exercise—all that remains is to choose a scenario. Assuming the opening scenario in the first paragraph is the premise for a drill, what should the objectives be? Possibilities include the following:

- To implement and test the Hospital Emergency Incident Command System (HEICS) and response time involved
- To test the decontamination team call-back tree and response time
- To stress capabilities of the current decontamination team members
- Is the communication system capable of handling this size disaster?
- To implement the complete external disaster plan

Objectives should be realistic. If an exercise is created from a current disaster plan, it should include actual exposure to risks that exist in the community. It would be pointless to train, for example, for an earthquake response in an area of the country that doesn't experience earthquakes.

The scope of the exercise should be reasonable so that results of the exercise can be realistically evaluated. Any deficiencies that are revealed by the exercise will need to be corrected.

Objectives will also serve as the components of the disaster response that will be evaluated. One way to select realistic objectives is to conduct a vulnerability assessment. Factors that could help define a potential impact on the hospital and community should be identified:

- What are the normal environmental exposures (tornados, snowstorms, floods, etc.)?
- What man-made hazards are present (nuclear power stations, chemical plants, large commercial airports, etc.)?
- What internal failures could enter the scenario (power failure, fire)?
- What is the probability or consequence value for each factor (high or low probability and high or low consequence)?

Who gets to play?

Once the scenario and objectives have been decided, a decision should be made regarding which agencies and organizations will be involved. During the planning phase, it is important to always involve at least one outside agency to help test the hospital's internal functions.

In the example scenario given, several agencies could offer such assistance, including local fire departments, EMS agencies, airport officials, and COBRA teams. Involvement of these stakeholders is helpful to meet all the planned objectives.

Exercise design

When planning an exercise, there are four types of exercises to consider:
- Drills—single procedure or area
- Tabletop—group discussion
- Functional—some resources are deployed with simulated events
- Full-scale—all resources are deployed

Drills are normally a single procedure or activity with limited involvement in order to test a portion of a facility's disaster plans (e.g., conduct fire drills or communication drills).

Tabletop exercises involve a group of people gathered at a table discussing disaster plans and procedures based on a scripted scenario. The event provides a good environment for problem solving, and it usually involves little or no stress.

There is no use of equipment, no resources are used, and it is very cost-effective. Normally, tabletop exercises last between 3 and 6 hours.

Functional exercises involve simulated events with some resources deployed. This type of exercise can be very realistic without deployment of large numbers of personnel and with minimal deployment of supplies and equipment. The emergency operations center (EOC) is usually activated during a functional exercise.

This is the most popular type of exercise for realistic-event scenarios. Functional exercises can last for several hours or may run all day.

Full-scale exercises involve full deployment of resources, are conducted in real time, involve multiple agencies, and are usually multijurisdictional. The level of support and organization needed to conduct a full-scale exercise is greater than that for any other type and is more costly to everyone involved.

Normally, this type of exercise is used to evaluate disaster plans in communities and counties and to evaluate interagency participation.

Hospitals and other health-care providers should choose specific goals and plan exercises and drills designed to satisfy these goals.

Goals and objectives

Depending on the needs of the community and the success or failure of previous drills and exercises, specific goals should be identified for each exercise planned. Components can include the following:

- Communications (both technical and human)
- Effectiveness of warning and notification systems
- Response times
- Asset availability
- Authorities, roles, and responsibilities
- Personnel readiness
- Logistical support
- Special-needs populations
- Resupply and staff relief functionality
- Agency interoperability
- Contaminants and decontamination efforts
- Media and public relations
- Legal impediments and liabilities
- Availability of state and federal support
- Others as dictated by local needs

The selection of components to be tested should be intentionally limited and clearly defined. Specific objectives should be articulated for each element in the exercise.

For example, if a notification system is being tested, the effectiveness of that system is under examination, not the ability of the notified agencies to respond quickly in large numbers.

Objectives for testing can include the following:

- Effectiveness (did the plan work at all?)
- Efficiency (how well it worked, and the yardstick for grading)
- Intentionality (did it work as planned, or via improvisation?)
- Endurance (how long before performance gaps appeared?)
- Impediments (intentionally injecting limits and challenges)

Exercises may have fixed-length time frames, but there should always be flexibility to end an exercise early if warranted or to extend the exercise to test component durability.

All exercises, particularly when evaluating new or untested plans, should be carried out until a major element fails. Exercises that don't induce failure haven't really tested the system.

Evaluators and evaluation tools

Evaluation exercises are crucial in order to meet objectives and test the effectiveness of disaster plans. The Homeland Security Exercise and Evaluation Program (HSEEP) at https://hseep.gov has excellent information on exercises, including exercise evaluation and improvement planning.

During an exercise, the evaluators can use Homeland Security's exercise evaluation guides (EEGs) to document whether tasks and activities have been performed, and whether the policies and procedures for the disaster were accurate and enabled staff to complete their functions. EEGs will help define whether objectives have been met.

In the best-case scenarios, outside evaluators should be used to give an unbiased opinion.

Staging the drill or exercise

Extensive planning is critical before an actual drill. The following are some key points that FEMA has provided on the HSEEP Web site (https://hseep. dhs.gov) to remember during the staging process:

- Keep the events of the exercise as quiet as possible prior to the event. In order to test the system, it has to be as realistic as possible.
- All participants should arrive early (2–3 hours early) to handle any logistical or administrative issues.
- Controllers are exercise participants who plan and direct exercise play. They give information and data to players and may initiate certain player actions. They report to a senior controller.
- Evaluators observe and record the actions of the players but do not interfere with the exercise flow. They should arrive early and should understand the expectations of evaluating the exercise.
- Players perform tasks that demonstrate the capabilities being assessed during the exercise.
- Actors are volunteer players who simulate specific roles during the exercise. Actors may also serve as evaluators acting on behalf of an agency or organization that is not playing in the exercise.
- The exercise site should be set up at least 1 day prior to the event.
- Brief everyone prior to the start of the event, making sure that everyone understands their role and what the objective is.
- Always put safety first! The number one priority is to have a safe and successful exercise.

After-action review and report

After the exercise has ended, it is very important to conduct a critique and review. Remember that the entire reason to conduct an exercise is to see what works and what does not. Immediately following the completion of all activities (usually announced by the senior controller), all evaluators and controllers must report all key activities to the senior controller. This is termed "debriefing" or wrap-up activities.

A "hot wash" provides players with an opportunity to provide immediate feedback while everything is still fresh and they can provide accurate answers. The hot wash also allows evaluators and controllers to capture information and make notes for the after-action report (AAR).

This is also an opportunity to report on how well the exercise played out, identify any issues, problems, or concerns, and offer comments and observations on any areas that need improvement. It is very beneficial to provide players with a preprinted feedback form, which is also used to generate an AAR. All forms and reports can be found on the HSEEP Web site.

Participant attendance lists should be collected. These lists will be included with the AAR and other exercise information.

The purpose of collecting and analyzing the data generated by exercise participants is to make changes that lead to improvement in the response process. In both the short and long term, this analysis should become the basis for the following:

- Existing disaster response plan modification
- Development of new training and exercise scenarios
- Multi-year development plans for
  - Purchasing new or additional equipment
  - Specialized training and certification for staff
  - Establishment of new facilities
  - Revision and integration of support plans

Traditionally, many AARs focus on the successful aspects of the exercise and downplay the negatives. The result is an unrealistic view of the readiness of the community to manage in a disaster.

It is vital that an atmosphere of openness and scrupulous attention to all of the results, both positive and negative, be fostered prior to, during, and after the conducting of the exercise.

Suggested readings

Federal Emergency Management Agency Homeland Security Exercise and Evaluation Program (HSEEP) home page. https://hseep.dhs.gov/pages/1001_HSEEP7.aspx

Federal Emergency Management Agency Homeland Security Exercise and Evaluation Program (HSEEP) Exercise Evaluation Guides. https://hseep.dhs.gov/pages/1002_EEGLi.aspx

McGowan DE, Jervis JA, Revere M (2004). *Mass Casualty Management*. San Clemente, CA: Law Tech.

Milsten A (2002, April). Hospital disaster exercises: a blueprint for success disaster medicine 11.2, American College of Emergency Physicians. http://www.acep.org/ACEPmembership.aspx?id=38412

Saruwatari M (2008, October 22) Hospital exercises, straight from the EM's mouth. Homeland 1 online.

Part 4

Fundamental Principles of Disaster Management

Communications

Constance J. Doyle

Introduction

Communications in disaster situations is important to allow maximum efficiency and facilitation of safety of responders and patient care on a real-time basis. Communications must be redundant, interoperable, and readily available resources to pass important information between all responders to a disaster, including public health, Emergency Operations Centers (EOC), Medical Coordination Centers (MCC), field operations, and patient care areas, whether they are in the field or in definitive medical facilities. Resources include hardware, software, information, human operators, and design of systems. In disasters, communications systems that can handle ordinary traffic become overloaded, and failures occur. Failures also occur because human operators do not communicate with all agencies involved, do not understand information needs of agencies, and often the information is not timely. In addition, where infrastructure damage occurs, ordinary systems may not be available, and alternate systems must be available. A larger number of agencies may be involved in communication when a disaster occurs. Many agencies have different communication systems that serve their routine needs, but they need to be interoperable with other agencies in times of community crises.

Efficient medical communications systems will facilitate patient care and transfer of care as well as patient tracking. These systems will allow communications with all responders, including hospitals, in a disaster. Medical communications systems should also serve the public and the media, and they should assist in public safety and the safety of responders. Surveillance systems for hazards and forensic reasons and for review of care and after-action review will be important to evaluate areas for improvement in care and for review and planning purposes.

- Surge Capacity

Graded response capability to add additional capacity and resources as needed in times of high patient volume and when community disasters occur. Scaleable event systems can add additional capacity for mass casualty care and movement of casualties.

Communications systems must be:
- Scalable.
- Interoperable.
- Redundant.

The system will need to address:
- Hardware and equipment needs.
- Equipment software and programming.
- Communication between and among response partners.
- Information management.
- Costs to acquire and maintain systems.
- Costs of training.
- Costs of pre-event planning and drills.
- Information Planning and Operations Planning will need to provide analysis of information.
- Decision making based on field information.
- Information resources to field providers (Haz-Mat information, patient-care information).

- Pre-event messages.
- Who needs to communicate and to whom?
- What is the message?

Common messaging for multiple groups
- What equipment that would best accomplish the goal.
- What equipment will serve in a back-up capacity if original equipment is unavailable or overloaded.
- Medical information planning and response.
- Pre-event communications:
  - Ordinary systems:
    — Land-line telephone.
    — Call Banks:
      – Reverse 911.
      – 211 systems.
      – Call banks with prerecorded message.
    — Cellular phone systems.
    — Text messaging.
    — PDA (Personal Digital Assistant).
    — Paging systems.
    — Satellite telephone.
    — Internet systems:
      – Data.
      – E-mail.
      – Twitter.
      – Internet phone systems.
    — Broadcast/Blast Fax.
    — Health-Alert Networks.
    — HEAR (Hospital Emergency Administrative Radio) radio network.
    — EMS radios.
    — Police, Fire and First responder (EMS) common communications systems and pathways.
    — 800 MHz Systems for ordinary EMS and other responders.
    — Hospital 800 MHz systems.
    — GPS and automatic crash system notification.
    — Patient tracking systems.
  - Post-event disaster systems/back-up systems:
    - All above and expanded use of
      — HEAR radio network.
      — EMS radios.
      — 800 MHz systems including special-event channels.
      — Encryption in high-security events.
      — Satellite systems.
      — Portable radio systems.
      — RACES (Radio Amateur Communications Emergency Services)—Ham Radio systems.
      — FRS (Family Radio Systems) radios—walkie talkies.
      — PBX telephone systems—Plug-in boxed systems with multiple receivers per line.
      — Microwave systems.

    — 800 MHz Systems for ordinary EMS and other responders.
    — Wireless priority systems (WPS)—Allows cellular users who are authorized, to get next available cell.
    — Government Emergency Telephone Systems (GETS), preauthorized card number dialed into central government telephone line.
    — Patient tracking systems.

- Systems design:
  - System requirements will depend on locality and types of information that must be communicated.
  - Voice.
  - Data.
  - Operations information including medical information.
  - Public warning and information.
- Interoperability:
  - Preplanned systems that allow common channels on radios, back-up systems if radios are overloaded, or planned systems that allow diverse responders and agencies to communicate during a crisis. These preplanned systems such as 800 MHz systems can be preprogrammed with talk groups and event channels that will be available to groups of responders. Some channels can be encrypted for high security communications.
  - Frequency incompatibility between agencies has been a problem for many disasters and other solutions such as black-box technology, which can serve as interface to connect cellular phones and radio systems with other systems to provide interoperability. Some Emergency Operations Centers and Mobile Command Centers as well as dispatching centers may have this capability.
  - Agencies that need to communicate with each other in an emergency need to preplan for both ordinary communication needs as well as expanded communications with multiple partners.
  - Costs include planning, additional operators, hardware, software updates, maintenance, and drills to keep operators familiar with communications systems.

Information management

Field, interhospital and intrahospital information needs will be different. Field information on types of patients, exposures, or contamination, and resource needs will need to be communicated to incident command and other responders. Numbers of patients and distribution to hospitals will be important information to provide to hospitals. Hospitals and Emergency Departments (ED) will want to know what numbers and severity of patients are estimated, how casualties will be distributed, and to how many hospitals, and whether contamination or exposure is suspected. (up to 80% of casualties can arrive outside of EMS). Hospitals and EDs will base their ramp-up and resource allocation based on this information. EOCs and Medical Coordination Centers will also need access to the same information to coordinate community-wide responses. Distant resources will need to be officially obtained through established plans. Intrahospital information will allow communication between the hospital emergency command center (HEOC) and the Emergency Department or receiving center for incoming patients. Additional patient information requiring HEOC coordination is required in order to move patients within the hospital as well as to open all available beds and ramp up personnel and other resources. Generally the HEOC will coordinate between other hospitals, the local emergency operation center (EOC), and the mobile command center (MCC).

- Who will be doing communication?
- Who is the intended audience?
- What information will need to be communicated?
- What is the priority of the information?
- How will the information be communicated?
  - Are there special audiences for whom accommodation will need to be made (such as hearing impaired or language barriers)?
- What organizations or partners will need to communicate?
- Will a joint information center (JIC) be responsible for a common message?
- What media will carry the message?
- What type of equipment will be used for what types of information: voice, data, patient information?
- Paramount in importance is determining what redundant equipment is needed in the event of primary communications equipment failure.

Additional information planning issues

Pre-incident familiarity with primary modes of communications.
- Regular use of equipment.
- Periodic testing of surge equipment for disaster communication including battery checks.
- Periodic drills to test function and communications.
- How information Coordination and Stratification will be managed: What needs to be communicated and how and in what order and by whom.
- Coordination of information to and from various agencies with different goals.
- Joint Information Center (JIC) coordination and response to the JIC.
- Lead agency coordination.
- Media responses.
- Resources for additional information.

Disaster situation assessment needs

Plan of response.
- Call-up of immediate response personnel.
- Prioritization of needs.
- Warnings:
  - To whom?
  - What message?
  - Pre-incident preparedness messages.
- Resources assessment to determine what is needed.
- Call-up/out of additional resources and vendors.
- What communications equipment will be needed in the field if additional resources are needed?
- How will patient care needs and tracking be communicated?
- Casualty distribution:
  - Emergency department and hospital-bed availability.
  - Patient transport and coordination.
  - Casualty transport systems.
  - Field medical-care needs if hospital capacity is exceeded.
- Standard and uniform terminology.

Medical coordination and resource coordination through coordinating emergency operations centers, public health, medical coordination centers.
- Call-up and demobilization of disaster communications should be clear.

Medical operations

- EMS coordination in field.
- Field to hospital.
- Hospital to hospital.
- Intrahospital communications.
- Medical coordination/operations center.
- Public-health communications.
- State medical communications.
- Alternate care sites.
- Joint information about healthcare.

Equipment and frequencies for medical operations

- Telephone land lines
  - Can be overloaded or disrupted in natural disasters.
  - Narrow Band width.
  - Voice only
  - DSL and coaxial cable.
  - Fiber-optic cable.
  - Carries voice and capable of large amount of data including video and interactive communications.
- Cellular phone.
  - Towers and base stations can be disrupted in emergencies.
  - Easily overloaded.
- RTL—Radio telephone link.
  - Can link hospital telephone and EMS radios.
  - Can be overloaded. Single call at a time.
- Radio frequencies.
  - Low frequency 30–300 KHz.
  - Medium Frequency MF 300–3000 KHz.
  - High Frequency 3–30 MHz.
  - Super High Frequency 3–30 GHz.
  - Extremely High Frequency 30–300 GHz.
  - UHF TV 450–470.
- Broadcast TV.
  - Antennas and dishes can be disrupted in natural disasters.
- AM/FM radio.
  - May have battery or generator back-up.
  - Vulnerable to station antenna damage in natural disasters.
- EMS radios-bands assigned by FCC (Federal Communications Commission).
- VHF (Very High Frequency): 30–300 MHz Both low band and high band.
  - Low band.
    — Long distances—reflected by upper atmosphere.
    — Weather interference.

- — Other electrical equipment-pagers, business communications, wireless microphones.
- — Don't penetrate buildings well.
- — Dead areas.
- — Interference from far away radio traffic.
- — Voice only, no data.
- — One person talks in sequence.
- — Line of horizon.
- High band.
  - 150–174 MHz.
  - Line of sight.
  - Need repeaters.
  - Don't penetrate buildings/dense terrain well.
  - Voice only.
  - One person talks in sequence.
  - Repeaters may be needed.
- UHF (Ultra High Frequency) 300–3000 MHz.
  - Line of sight.
  - Will penetrate buildings.
  - Limited in rugged terrain.
  - Voice and telemetry.
  - Specific medical channels.
  - Higher frequencies >2,500 telemedicine.
- 800 MHz 806–902 MHz.
  - Technically UHF, but unique programmable talk groups.
  - Computer-programmed radios with assigned frequencies.
  - Additional special-events channels.
  - Separate talk groups for medical/hospitals.
  - Special-events groups can include responders to a specific event.
- Satellite.
  - Fixed systems transmitters and receivers.
    - — Can relay information from distant points locally.
    - — Interface with telephone and other communications.
  - GEO (Geosynchronous Earth Orbit).
    - — Few satellites can cover the globe.
    - — Voice and data, Internet, broadband.
    - — Voice and low-speed data to mobile receivers.
  - LEO (Low Earth Orbit).
    - — Multiple satellites to cover globe.
    - — Can be accessed by hand-held receivers.
    - — Voice, position, data, Internet, and fax.
    - — Telephone interface.
  - Need satellite transmitters and receivers.
    - — May be fixed receivers or mobile antennae.
    - — Multiple types of data: voice, Internet, messaging systems.
    - — Fixed transmitters and receivers and antennas can be disabled in natural disasters.
- Telemedicine.

Various Internet systems allow remote diagnosis and monitoring and with rule-based logic and remote consultation for remote areas and for disaster operations where additional expertise and monitoring is needed. Internet-based systems based on various types of land lines. Cable and dish networks will require infrastructure integrity and electricity.

- PDA (Personal Digital Assistant).
  - Information systems.
  - Portable.
  - Some with Internet capability and can download information.
  - E-mail, fax, voice, and camera capabilities.
- Additional law enforcement and military frequencies.
- Ham radio frequencies-RACES Radio.

Limitations of communications systems

Jamming of frequencies by high-volume traffic.
- Limitations of radio traffic.
- Scanners that can monitor sensitive and patient information.
- Tone activated receivers need to be heard.
- Designated emergency calling frequencies.
- HEAR (Hospital Emergency Administrative Radio) network often overloaded in disasters.
- Frequency-sharing agreements.
  - Mutual agreement to share frequency for joint operations.
  - 800 MHz special-event/special-ops channels.
- Radio and other equipment caches.
  - Designated responsibility for testing, battery charging or swap, battery chargers, repeaters.
  - Deployment plan.

Conclusion

Communications failures are system failures. Normal systems may be overloaded. Each agency is usually autonomous and often used to making and executing decisions in real time without cooperation. Incident Management Systems (ICS) help, but in real time, chaos may fail to change to a more cooperative mode. Some failures occur because no one agency has an overview of what has been communicated and that all who need to know have been included. Preplanned communications and familiarity with routine and scaled-up operations are vital, but drills cannot completely simulate real situations. Multi-agency responses will need common communications channels and know National Incident Management Systems (NIMS). Roles of other agencies that respond, their needs, and what resources they can provide to the matrix of communication must be recognized.

Suggested readings

Auf der Heide, E. *Disaster Response* 2000. Chapter 5 Inter-Agency Communications. http://orgmail2.coe-dmha.org/dr/flash.htm downloaded 9/22/2008.

Disaster Response: Principles of Preparation and Coordination: Chapter 5 Inter-Agency Communications: http://orgmail2.coe-dmha.org/dr/DisasterResponse.nsf/section/05?

Disaster Communications Part 1 Global: Disaster relief Communications Foundation: www.reliefweb.int/library/dc1/dcc1.html

Disaster communications *Guidebook/Preparedness and Public Education*. Missouri Department of Mental Health. www.dmh.mo.gov/diroffice/disaster/disaster.htm

Garshnek, V and Burkle, FM (2007). Communication and information technology tools for disaster response and medical assistance. In *Disaster Medicine*. 2nd ed. Wolters Kluwer/Lippincott Williams and Wilkins, Philadelphia.

Landesman, LY (2005). *Disaster Communications in Public Health Management of Disasters.* Washington D.C.: American Public Health Association.

Region 2 South Communication Plan. (2008). www.2south.org contact information

State of Minnesota. (2007) *EMS Radio Ccommunications Plan. A Radio Planning Guide for Minnesota EMS and Hospitals.*

Suter, RE and Martinez, R (2006). Chapter 9: Communications. In Brennann, JA and Krohmer, JA (eds) *Principles of EMS Systems*, 3rd ed. Sudbury, MA: American College of Emergency Physicians, Jones and Bartlett Publishers.

Twitter: mobile and Internet access to activities, locations and brief message http://twitter.com

Washtenaw L (2008). County Medical Control Authority (Michigan) Communications Policy 1-31.

Wahhtenaw, L (2008). County Medical Control Authority (Michigan) Mass Casualty Protocol 1-06.

Wood, M. Disaster Communications. http://www.reliefweb.int/library/dc1/dcc1.htm. (Accessed 9/22/2008).

Decontamination

James J. Augustine

Introduction

Decontamination is the process to remove from a victim as much of a hazardous substance as possible, in a timely manner, to prevent injury or death. Decontamination can take a variety of forms, and use a variety of substances to remove or neutralize. The timeliness and effectiveness of the decontamination process is guided by the clinical condition of the patient, which must be factored into decisions by rescuers. Decontamination may be assisted by first responders, by EMS providers, by hospital emergency department personnel, or by a combination of those individuals. Decontamination is a "one shot" opportunity for rescuers - if timely and effective removal of hazardous materials does not occur it may have life-ending or life-long implications for the victim. Contamination of multiple patients can occur in natural or man-made circumstances, and requires a larger scale operation to address all patient needs.

History

Decontamination principles were developed following wartime use of asphyxiants and blister agents in the ground battles of World War I. Military principles of decontamination used strong cleaning agents and neutralizers for these chemicals. Civilian utilization of decontamination processes developed in the cold war period after World War II, and radioactive contamination was used as the planning scenario. The process used firm brushes, cold water, corn starch, and tincture of green soap as the cleaning materials.

Experiences with patients contaminated in industrial mishaps brought about the development of scientific principles of wet decontamination for a wide variety of chemical agents. Multiple casualty incidents in Bhopal, India and Tokyo, Japan led to the development of mass decontamination plans. Biologic incident management has developed after exposures in the anthrax attacks of 2001 and the SARS outbreak of 2003.

Overview

Decontamination is the process of removing or neutralizing hazardous materials to save the victim's life, limbs, lungs, or eyes. Many chemical exposures are threats to health and must be removed immediately, since human injury is a result of both concentration and time of exposure. For example, an industrial acid sprayed in the eye must be irrigated out immediately, or irreversible damage to the cornea will blind the victim. A victim left to lay on clothing soaked in gasoline will evolve a full thickness skin injury within 60 minutes if it is not removed.

Rescuers are asked to prevent the spread of the material to avoid exposure of other civilians or health care personnel, or damage to the environment. "Keep it in the HOT ZONE." However, governmental agencies have written guidelines that specify that victim decontamination and lifesaving efforts take priority.

Methods of decontamination

- Dry decontamination is utilized for biologic and radiologic exposures. This form of decontamination requires the victim or rescuers to remove clothing, wash hands and face, and place the victim in uncontaminated clothing.
- Emergent eye decontamination is the most common, and uses appropriate quantities of clean water until the victim reports relief of symptoms.
- Wet decontamination uses clean water, soap, and friction to remove contaminants on the skin, hair, and other external surfaces.
- Internal decontamination is removing or neutralizing a hazardous material that has already been ingested or inhaled.
- Mass decontamination is wet decontamination for large numbers of victims.
- Technical decontamination is the operation used by hazardous-material responders prior to suit removal from entrants in Chemical Protective Clothing. This is usually a planned event, and will be considered as soon as Chemical Protective Clothing is donned.

Decontamination—protecting the rescuer

- Structure Firefighting Gear protects for 15–30 minutes, depending on the material. Some hazardous materials, like organophosphates in oil, may contaminate the rescuers gear and require it to be destroyed. Airway protection for the rescuer (breathing apparatus) is needed if exposure was to vaporous material (nerve gases), but less protection for the rescuer is needed when victim's clothes are removed. When in doubt, protect the rescuers.

- Dry decontamination is utilized for most biologic and radiologic exposures. This form of decontamination requires the victim or rescuers to remove clothing, wash hands and face, and place clothes in an uncontaminated container. This process is facilitated by the development of dry decontamination materials in a pack, with preprinted instructions. In situations of mass exposure to biologic substances, this process is the most timely for preventing bad outcomes or spread of the agent. A description of a dry decontamination pack is attached.

- Biological agents almost always are managed with dry decontamination. Do it as soon as the contamination is recognized, and contain the dirty clothing. Typically biological contamination does not have the same time urgency as chemical contamination. Consider input from medical control physicians or the public health officials.

- Emergent eye decontamination is the most commonly performed type of decontamination, because hazardous material exposures to the eyes occur routinely, often in relation to law enforcement activities. This form of decontamination uses appropriate quantities of clean water until the victim reports relief of symptoms. Some commercial devices have been developed to assist in large volume irrigation, and some providers improvise by using a nasal oxygen cannula to deliver water or saline to the orbital areas. Eye devices should never be inserted in the eyes when a severe chemical exposure has occurred, because the device may rub against damaged tissue and worsen the injury.

- Wet decontamination uses clean water, soap, and friction to remove contaminants on the skin, hair, and other external surfaces. Remove outer clothing. 80% of contaminants will remain on outer clothing. Use warm water to clean any areas the victim knows has been exposed. Soap and water and friction work best. Use of a soft cloth or sponge will remove substances more quickly from the skin, hair and nails. Do not use firm brushes. Use only the friction you would want used on you if you had a burn on your skin, and someone was scrubbing it. Do not rinse victims with cold water, unless it is absolutely lifesaving. Nothing worse than a victim who is hypothermic and ill from chemical contamination. In cold weather decontamination must be done with warm water, and in a sheltered environment.

A skilled rescuer must decide for each patient what the priorities are for best outcome of the patient, balancing the needs of immediate medical care with the need for decontamination. A decision grid to assist in decision making for contaminated hazmat patients is shown in Table 28.1.

- If victims are symptomatic from a chemical exposure, there is no need to wait on soap, or set-up of the containment system. It is not necessary to contain the runoff in a lifesaving mode. It is appropriate to contain runoff when doing planned decontamination, like technical decontamination. Once clothing is off, the exposure risk to rescue personnel is from chemical in the victim's airway, lungs, or stomach. It should be recognized that patients from chemical blast incidents, from intentional ingestions, or from falling into chemical tanks may have large and dangerous quantities of chemical in airway, lungs, or stomach. Transport in an EMS vehicle will pose a risk to EMS personnel if the victim is expelling chemicals from one or more of those sources.

- For a few chemicals, and for radioactive materials, the effectiveness of decontamination operations can be evaluated using detection and monitoring devices. In most circumstances, only the victim's symptoms will guide the rescuer about when the danger has past. When in doubt, strip clothing off the victim and perform decontamination until the chemical is visibly gone or the patient is cleared of all symptoms.

- Regarding the length and quantity of decontamination, there are a few guides. Chemicals typically collect in clothing, shoes, and personal materials. Significant risk exposure will be reduced by removing from the victim the worst contaminated material, the clothing and shoes, to make the victim completely naked. When using and collecting the runoff, prior study has found that the vast majority of a hazardous material will be removed from a human with about 8 gallons of water for a contaminated extremity, and about 25 gallons for a whole body contamination.

- EMS personnel should always contact the receiving hospital as soon as possible. They must be informed prior to your arrival. Be prepared to advise them of the following:
  - The victim's medical complaint and the way the exposure occurred
  - Name of the chemical.
  - Extent of contamination.
  - The type and extent of decontamination performed at the scene.
  - Acknowledge that EMS will stay outside the ED until their personnel direct entry into the facility.

- Mass decontamination is wet decontamination for large numbers of victims. It may be facilitated by large hoses, open shower areas, or prepared areas at worksites or outside hospitals. It follows the principles of wet decontamination. Victims in a mass decontamination scenario that are not ambulatory will require assistance from rescuers.

- Technical decontamination is the operation used by hazardous material responders prior to suit removal from entrants in Chemical Protective Clothing. This is often a planned event, is not so time critical, and must be considered as soon as Chemical Protective Clothing is donned. This process may use special solutions to decontaminate pieces of equipment.

Table 28.1 Decision Making for Contaminated Hazmat Patients

	Critical Ill, Trauma, Burn	Moderate Ill, Trauma, Burn	Extremity Burn or Trauma
Heavily contaminated Highly toxic	II	III	III
Heavily contaminated Low toxicity	I	II	II
Low-level contamination Highly toxic substance	II	III	III
Low-level contamination Low toxicity	I	I	II
Chemical in eyes	Decontaminate thoroughly		

Regardless of where the decontamination takes place, rescuers may wish to develop and distribute a Uniform Information Release Sheet, to standardize information given to victims. A sample of these information forms is attached.

Medical decision making for contaminated hazmat patients

Decontamination and treatment decisions are made after determining the degree of contamination and assessing the victim's illness, trauma, and burn status, as shown in Table 28.1.

• Priority III decontaminate first!
Decontamination the highest priority. Chemical contamination of the body with associated minor burn, trauma, or illness. Priority is complete and thorough decontamination ASAP.

• Priority II mixed problems
Medical care needs are balanced with priority to decontaminate. Victims with significant illness, trauma, or burns who have not been decontaminated and have a dangerous level of contamination. Risk continues from ongoing exposure to hazardous material and from associated medical problems. Manage airway, breathing, shock, and threats to life simultaneous with decontamination.

• Priority I medical care first!
Medical care needs outweigh immediate decontamination, and victim should be grossly decontaminated only as priority to transport serious or critical illness, trauma, or burn and still contaminated. Decontaminate to make the victim as safe as possible while addressing life threats.

Process for development and use of decontamination packs

Rescuers must be prepared to decontaminate patients with suspected or confirmed exposure to radioactive, biological, or chemical hazards. Any person who is able to will prefer to clean themselves, whether in a shower, sink, or tub. There are several methods for decontamination that are safe and effective. What all of them share in common is the final point in the process—a group of individuals who have been stripped of their clothing (and often, their dignity) awaiting emergency evaluation and care. Regardless of the method of decontamination employed, these individuals must be dressed in something, have their clothing and valuables placed in an airtight bag that can stay with them, and know what to do with their potentially contaminated belongings.

Dry decontamination incident management includes these elements:

- Greet patient and conduct the initial interview outside the ED (prevents contamination of any part of the ED).
- Do not bring any materials (like an envelope) into the building.
- If the patient and his/her clothing are potentially contaminated, remove the clothing outside, place it in a bag with the patient's name on it, leave it outside, and ask the patient to wash his/her hands and face.
- Place the patient in a gown and escort him or her into the ED for assessment.
- Provide medical triage, then appropriate patient evaluation and treatment.

A **Decontamination Pack** should include the following contents:

- A printed plastic bag with a cinch tie at the top. On one side instructions should be printed on how to use of the decontamination pack. The other side should contain a blank space with a surface that can be written on.
- A large pair of nonsterile hospital gloves should be attached to the outside of the bag.
- The bag should contain the following contents:
- An instruction sheet on how to properly dispose of belongings.
- A small clear plastic bag marked VALUABLES, with a writing surface for the victim's name. This bag should be able to be sealed; 10 inch Zip-Lock type bag would be ideal.
- A marking pen for writing the victim's name on the bags.
- Postdecontamination clothing for the person—inexpensive, lightweight cloth coveralls of a standard color would be ideal (like old hospital scrubs). Ideally, the color of these clothes will be distinct, so victims will not be mistaken for emergency workers (bleach the old hospital scrubs or dye them).
- Foot coverings (booties).
- A personal mask to cover the victim's nose and mouth.
- 2 wet-wipe napkins.
- Another dry soft wipe to clean glasses or hearing aids.
- An identification bracelet.
- Instructions for proper disposal of clothing.
- A second pair of nonsterile gloves (placed inside the bag).

- Using this pack and its instructions will facilitate rapid cleaning of large numbers of people. Each of the decontamination packs would be self-contained, and with minimal instruction by the emergency staff, allow the victims to be uniformly cleaned, masked, carrying a bag of valuables including their identification documents, and placing a bag of (potentially) dirty belongings in a central collecting area. After the victims have been appropriately assessed and any care provided, the emergency staff should have determined whether it is safe to return the bag of belongings. The only additional items that victims might need at the end of the incident are follow-up instructions and any prescriptions (these instructions are listed in Table 28.2),.

Table 28.2 Sample Uniform Information Release Sheet

HAZARDOUS SUBSTANCE EXPOSURE INSTRUCTIONS

You have been evaluated in the Emergency Department following an exposure to a hazardous substance.

To the best of our knowledge, the material you were exposed to was_____

The usual reactions to this substance can include:

You have been treated or checked for any severe problems, but occasionally a problem can develop hours to days later. We ask that you call your family doctor, company medical facility, or return to the Emergency Department if any of the following symptoms occur:

You have a severe headache, chest pain, or abdominal pain.

You feel short of breath.

You pass out or have a seizure.

You develop a severe rash.

You pass blood in vomit or bowel movement.

If we are informed by authorities of other problems related to your exposure, we will contact you at the phone number or address you have given us. Please call 911 or return to the Emergency Department if you develop any problem you think is serious.

Decontamination of a hazmat contaminated patient

Identify product, life threat, and route of exposure. Determine need for and type of decontamination.

- Control access, and take the appropriate precautions for decon personnel (suits, SCBA, etc.).
  - Do not enter hazardous environment unless adequately protected!
- Set up a minimum two-stage decontamination process that is upwind and uphill from the contaminated area.
  - First stage is having the victim completely disrobed, and use a water rinse.
  - Second stage is soap and water scrub and rinse.
  - Third and fourth stage decontamination may be needed, depending on product.
  - Use warm, clean water if possible.
- Evaluate ABC's, stabilize spine (if trauma suspected), establish patent airway and breathing.
  - Rescuers in Level A suits (fully encapsulated) will not be physically able to do anything other than drag victims.
- Move victim away from contact with hazardous material to a cleaner area, or to Decon Area.
  - If not breathing, use oxygen and bag valve mask (BVM). Consider triage to Black.
  - If victims are ambulatory, direct them to leave the Hot Zone, to assist others with evacuation, and to decontaminate themselves under the direction of the Decon Officer.
- Remove clothing.
  - Isolate/control the airway with an oxygen mask over the patient's mouth and nose, or by endotracheal intubation.
  - Strip the victims of clothing and jewelry and double-bag the items.
  - Clothing contaminated with dust should be removed dry with care taken to minimize any dust becoming airborne.
  - Dust should be brushed off the face prior to fitting the mask or respirator.
  - Brush off or vacuum clean any solid particle contaminants.
- Flush the entire body with plain water for 2–5 minutes.
  - If chemical unknown or uncertain, obtain a predecon swab for later chemical analysis.
  - Flush exposed eyes and other body surfaces with copious amounts of water for 2–5 minutes.
  - Use low pressure water flush, and try not to splash the material around!
  - Follow with soap and/or shampoo scrub, followed by additional water flushing.
  - Clean under nails with scrub brush or plastic nail cleaner.
  - Hazmat victims are at high risk for hypothermia if washed with cool water.

- If extreme weather conditions, consider appropriating nearby facility. Almost any facility will be less expensive to decontaminate than a hospital, and both patients and emergency workers are at less risk if patient is decontaminated early.
- Most contaminants can be removed by using 8 gallons of water and a soft scrub on each extremity or small area of contamination. Save this amount of runoff.
- For whole body decontamination, it is necessary to use about 25 gallons of water and soft scrub. Save this volume of runoff.
- A victim who has been involved in an explosion or near-drowning can have large volumes of chemicals in the airway, lungs, and/or stomach. Save all suction material, emesis, urine, and tissue that may be contaminated.
- Contaminated wounds (lacerations, abrasions, and punctures) have a very high priority:
  - Secure a drape around the wound. Irrigate or flush with warm normal saline for 5 minutes, while gently scrubbing the wound.
  - If contamination persists, consider surgical debridement. Save all tissue.
  - After open wounds are decontaminated, cover with Saran Wrap or self adherent occlusive dressing and proceed with complete decontamination of other areas.
- Contaminated nares and mouth:
  - Turn head to side or down as the patient's condition permits.
  - Rinse with large amounts of water and use suction if needed.
  - Prevent water from entering the stomach.
  - If a blast occurred, or if the mouth is contaminated, expect that contaminated material is in the stomach. Insert NG tube if trained. Suction and save gastric contents.
- Contaminated eyes:
  - Remove contact lenses. Numb the eye if possible.
  - Rinse eyes thoroughly at least 1,000 cc normal saline or water each eye, or for 15 minutes.
- Contaminated intact skin:
  - Gently wash with soap and water using a scrub sponge for 3 minutes.
  - Dawn detergent is an appropriate soap for almost all compounds.
  - If contamination persists, wash with mildly abrasive soap.
  - Monitor and repeat as needed.
  - Do not irritate the skin with harsh rubbing or with hot water!
- Contaminated hair:
  - Shampoo hair with mild soap for 5 minutes and rinse at least 5 minutes.
  - If contamination persists, clip hair off. DO NOT SHAVE AREA!
- When collecting the contaminant:
  - Save the life first.
  - Collect the worst contaminated material—the clothing.
  - Collect one small container (about 8 gallons) for a contaminated extremity.
  - Collect about 25 gallons for a whole-body contamination.

- Removal of patient from decontamination area:
  - Noncontaminated personnel should bring a clean stretcher into the decon area.
  - Clean personnel should transfer the patient to the clean stretcher. Make sure not to pull contaminated fluid (including that used for decon) onto the clean cart.
  - Wrap the clean patient in a sheet and, if appropriate, collect a postdecon swab specimen in the clean area.
- Technical decontamination for rescuers performing patient care when patients are in protective gear:
  - When rescue personnel are ready to exit from the Hot Zone, each member must proceed to technical decontamination.
  - One person in the contaminated area assists others in disrobing and cleaning, taking the discarded garments as others remove them, and placing them in barrels.
  - Remove tape from sleeves.
  - Remove outer gloves first, turning them inside-out as they are pulled off.
  - Remove mask.
  - Remove gown, turning it inside-out. Avoid shaking it. Remove one foot, and step over into clean area. Remove other foot and bring foot into clean area.
  - While leaning into containment area, remove inner gloves and discard.
  - Shower and change into clean clothes. If personnel sustain contamination of personal clothing, it will be necessary to discard personal clothing inside the decon area.
  - If personnel sustain body contamination, use the same procedure as for contaminated patients.

Overseeing a decontamination process: instructions for ED staff

Patients identified by Fire Department, EMS, hazardous material, or law enforcement personnel as being a potential victim of an exposure incident or highly infectious disease should be greeted outside the ED. These patients should be managed outside the ED until it is safe to bring them inside the building. A physician or public health official should dictate which decontamination process will be utilized for contaminated or exposed individuals.

- At the hospital it is appropriate to designate a Hospital Safety Officer.
  - Confirm with Incident Command. Safety Officer's role is to protect the hospital facility and staff.
  - Confirm which ED physician will be directing patient care and the need for decontamination.
  - Direct Security to establish a perimeter around the area of contamination and patient care.
  - Until incident is complete, oversee all operations to ensure safety of hospital facility and staff.
- The hospital and emergency department staff should have preparedness training that addresses these priorities.
  - This is infrequent and different than normal patient processing.
  - Protect hospital staff from harm.
  - Allow the patient to be moved quickly to "regular" care.
  - Simplify all the necessary paperwork.
  - Have someone who knows what they are doing clean up the mess, usually a contractor.
  - Use a Public Information Officer to make appropriate interactions with the media.
- Wet Decontamination:

Wet decontamination is needed for chemical contamination, either in the prehospital setting, or upon arrival to the ED. Ideally, wet decontamination should be done with warm, clean water and some form of soap. Dawn detergent is an ideal cleaner for a wide range of contamination substances. At the end of the shower, the patient(s) should use towels to dry off, and then dress in appropriate patient clothing and foot coverings.

Emergency personnel should realize that any person who is physically able to decontaminate him or herself will want to do so. Individuals who are well enough to comply with directions should be handed a decontamination pack and directed to a cleaning shower. Once there, the patient should disrobe, go into the shower, wash, dry, and then put on their new clothing, foot coverings and mask. Towels provided to dry off will need to be collected.

Other items that may be needed to facilitate complete wet decontamination include:
- Eye flush.
- Contact lens cases.
- Topical anesthetic agent (Proparacaine).

- Sanitary napkins and belts.
- Bags appropriate for contaminated trash.
- Containers for wet towels, if they can be laundered.

If patients have any open wounds (including burns), they will need Saran Wrap or an occlusive dressing (OpSite™ or Tegaderm™) to cover the wounds once they are decontaminated. Victims and rescuers should be instructed to clean the wounds first, then cover them with an occlusive dressing to allow complete decontamination of surrounding tissues.

● Dry Decontamination:

Although exposure to chemical agents often requires "wet" decontamination, many incidents may be safely managed using the "dry" technique. This includes exposures to most infectious agents. The key process for decontaminating these patients is removal of clothing, the cleaning of hands, and placing a mask on the patient's nose and mouth to limit the droplet spread of infectious or dangerous agents from one individual to another. This should be accomplished before the victims are brought into the building. A decontamination pack will be utilized.

If the number of victims is not too great to preclude privacy, each patient should be given a private area and asked to disrobe. Trash containers should be provided for dirty items, including gloves, clothing that people don't want or can't keep, and items used for cleaning. Once disrobed, patients should put on the temporary clothing that is in the bag and place their old, contaminated clothing and personal effects in the bag. Make sure that patients write their name on clothing and valuables' bags.

Other items that may be needed to facilitate complete dry decontamination include:

- Eye flush.
- Contact lens cases.
- Topical anesthetic agent (Proparacaine).
- Sanitary napkins and belts.
- Bags appropriate for contaminated trash.

Emergency personnel will need to determine whether the bags of contaminated clothing and belongings can be returned to the owners. The bags should be kept outside the building, so that no contaminated materials will be introduced into the hospital. The bags should be secured so that no one will misplace or steal the items. All valuable bags should be kept with the patients. When a clear determination can be made about the exposure of the victims and the potential hazard of their belongings, then the bags can be returned to the victims as they leave the ED or they can be turned over to the appropriate authorities for safe disposal. This process of disposal is why valuables must be removed and kept with the victims, in a sealed bag.

The community should approach exposure incidents in a consistent manner. Depending on the nature of exposures, most situations will be managed by dry decontamination using the process and the materials provided in the decontamination pack. The process we have described, and the use of these packs, will facilitate the rapid decontamination and re-clothing of large numbers of victims. Preparing hundreds of these packs, which have an indefinite shelf life, and distributing them to public safety agencies, represents a cost-efficient method for communities to prepare for mass casualty incidents of a chemical, biological, or nuclear nature.

Some hospitals and communities may find it necessary and beneficial to personalize the decontamination packs. If so, the packs can be adapted to include multilingual instructions, different sizes of clothing, and pediatric and infant-care items.

Essential concepts

- Decontamination Best Practices include approaches to patients contaminated with
  - Radioactive material (not irradiated).
  - Chemical materials.
  - Biological agents.
  - Mixed contamination.
  - Unknown contaminant.
- Various modes of decontamination can occur in the prehospital or hospital locations:
  - Dry decontamination is utilized for biologic and radiologic exposures.
  - Emergent eye decontamination.
  - Wet decontamination uses clean water, soap, and friction to remove contaminants.
  - Internal decontamination involves removing or neutralizing material that has already been ingested or inhaled.
  - Mass decontamination is wet decontamination for large numbers of victims.
  - Technical decontamination is used by hazardous material responders in chemical protective clothing.
- Hospital Processes:
  - Hospitals must be prepared for walk-in patient(s).
  - EMS notification and reception can facilitate set-up of the ED.
  - "Protect the house" by not allowing hazardous materials or contaminated patients into the building.
  - Protect the EMS and ED staff.
  - Incorporate a Hospital Safety Officer.
  - Internal incidents within the walls of the hospital from hospital processes requires processes for containment and cleanup.
  - Document Best Practices with the use of worksheets.
  - Report, law enforcement interaction, and evidence preservation.
- Priority dentification for Patient Management:
  - Matching clinical care needs with priority for decontamination.
  - Decision Diagrams and Algorithms for Patient Management will improve consistency and serve as educational tools.
  - Decision documents and training should stress the priorities for decontamination versus medical treatment and evaluation.
  - Evidence preservation may need to occur in terrorist or criminal events.
- Organizing the Decontamination Priorities, from the Customer's Perspective.
- We can define needs for the various persons in a hazardous-material event by establishing a customer-service priority list.

Patient Customer Service Priorities:
  - "Don't make me wait."
  - "Save my life and limbs."
  - "Don't hurt me anymore. Don't make me cold."

- "Explain what you are doing."
- "Get me through the decontamination quickly and into 'regular' care."
- "Find out what contaminated me, how much, and what the risk is."
- "Explain to me what, if anything, I need to do next"
- "Talk to my boss."
- "Confidentiality, please."

Suggested readings

In Preparing for Decontamination Operations

Agency for Toxic Substance and Disease Registry(2000). Patient management. In *Managing Hazardous Materials Incidents*. Vol. 2. Retrieved from http://www.atsdr.cdc.gov/mhmi-v2-3.pdf.

Augustine JJ (2006). Burn baby burn. *Managing Victims of Unexpected Hazardous Material Incidents*, 35(3): 34–36.

Barbera JA, Macintyre AG, DeAtley CA (October 2001). Chemically Contaminated Patient Annex (CCPA), Hospital Emergency Operations Planning Guide. *OEP/USPH*.

Hick JL, D. Hanfling D, Burstein JL, Markham J, Macintyre AG, and Barbera JA (2003). Protective equipment for healthcare facility decontamination personnel: Regulations, risks, and recommendations. *Annals of Emergency Medicine* 42(3): 370–380.

Horton DK, Berkowitz Z, and Kaye WE (2003). Secondary contamination of ED personnel from hazardous materials events, 1995–2001. *American Journal of Emergency Medicine* 21: 199–204.

Koenig K (2003). Strip and shower: The duck and cover for the 21st entury. *Annals of Emergency Medicine*. 42(3): 391–394.

Lehmann J (2002). Considerations for selecting personal protective equipment for hazardous materials decontamination. *Disaster Manag Response*: 21-25.

Macintyre AG, et al. (2000). Weapons of mass destruction events with contaminated casualties. *JAMA*: 242–249.

MMWR. (2001). Nosocomial poisoning associated with emergency department treatment of organophosphate toxicity – Georgia, 2000. *Morbidity and Mortality Weekly*, 49(51): 1156–1158.

NIOSH. (2003). NIOSH pocket guide to chemical hazards and other databases (online edition). Cincinnati, OH: National Institute for Occupational Safety and Health (NIOSH), Department of Health and Human Services (DHHS) http://www.cdc.gov/niosh/npg/npg.html (Accessed November 11, 2008).

Nozaki H, Hori SO, Shinozawa Y, et al. (1995). Secondary exposure of medical staff to Sarin vapor in the emergency room. *Intensive Care Med* 21:1032–1035.

U.S. EPA. (2000). First responders' environmental liability due to mass decontamination runoff (EPA 550-F-00.009). U.S. Environmental Protection Agency, Office of Solid Waste and Emergency Response .

http://yosemite.epa.gov/oswer/Ceppoweb.nsf/vwResourcesByFilename/onepage.pdf/$File/onepag e.pdf

Vogt BM and JH Sorrensen. (2002). How clean is safe? Improving the effectiveness of decontamination of structures and people following chemical and biological incidents – Final Report (ORNL/TM-2002/178).Prepared by Oakridge National Laboratory for the U.S. Department of Energy http://emc.ornl.gov/EMCWeb/EMC/PDF/How_Clean_is_Safe.pdf (Accessed September 2004).

In Responding to Contamination Incidents

Agency for Toxic Substance and Disease Registry (ATSDR) www.atsdr.cdc.gov

Centers for Disease Control and Prevention (CDC) www.bt.cdc.gov

CHEMTREC, American Chemistry Council Emergency HAZARDOUS MATERIAL Information 1300 Wilson Blvd. Arlington, VA 22209 (703)741-5000 Web page: www.americanchemistry.com

Cleanup of Clandestine Methamphetamine Labs Guidance Document. Colorado Department of Public Health and Environment. Hazardous Materials and Waste Management Division. July 2003. http://www.cdphe.state.co.us/hm/methlab.pdf

Environmental Protection Agency (EPA) – www.epa.gov

The National Response Center, Chemical/HAZARDOUS MATERIAL Spills National Response Center c/o United States Coast Guard (G-OPF)-Room 2611 2100 2nd Street, S.W. Washington, DC 20593-0001 (202) 267-2675 or (800) 424-8802 Web page: www.nrc.uscg.mil/index.html

Evacuation

Peter Kemetzhofer

Eric S. Weinstein

Indications through a hazard vulnerability assessment

One of the most important objectives of a county emergency manager, in partnership with the Local Emergency Preparedness Committee (LEPC), is the completion of the county Hazard Vulnerability Assessment (HVA). This systemic evaluation of the probable risks of natural and man-made disasters and subsequent consequences guides the mitigation, preparation, response, and recovery efforts of county emergency management.

Initial steps or actions

Once the most likely natural and man-made incidents are determined:
- Multidisciplinary agencies (Table 29.1) establish evacuation planning.
- Develop table-top and live exercises with critical review leading to plan revision.
- Delineate specifics of evacuation based on the time period that the community has to begin the evacuation.

Sudden or unpredictable natural disasters like an earthquake or volcano will have no advance warning, requiring evacuation planning to be paramount to prepare the community to know what to gather quickly and how to follow evacuation directions based on a variety of measures such as public media (radio, television), road signage, and traffic routing. Similarly, sudden man-made incidents like an industrial explosion, a transportation crash, or an act of terrorism, with release of hazardous materials, disruption of essential public services such as water, sewer, electricity, or natural gas will also have no advance warning (Table 29.2).

Natural disasters may occur with minimal notice (determined by surveillance) such as a flash-flood or wildfire. A community at risk for a radiologic or industrial release will be able to draw from their safety plans to facilitate an orderly, rapid evacuation through previously established community-alerting mechanisms like sirens, the Emergency Broadcast System, radio, television, pagers, cell phones, and reverse 911 systems.

Table 29.1 Evacuation Committee

Lead Agency: Municipal, county or state government emergency management that will issue the evacuation order as defined by state or local statute
Chief Participating Agencies: Law enforcement, fire/rescue, department of transportation, Health and Human Services (or similar), public works from the same government authority issuing the evacuation
Other Representatives from: the LEPC; large business, factories, industry or other population-dense structures; chemical creation and storage sites; health-care facilities, nursing homes, assisted-living facilities, homes for the mentally ill, substance abusers, or other chronic-care facilities; schools, adult and child care, colleges; lodging industry; gasoline, food and beverage dealers; bus, rail, water craft, airline companies; print, radio, Internet, television, cellular phone, pager, and other communication companies

Table 29.2 Evacuation materials

Money, ATM cards, credit cards, bank statements, jewelry and other valuables

Legal documents, marriage certificates, deeds, titles, diplomas, licenses, certificates

Insurance papers, business documents, and other pertinent items to establish ownership

Medication, durable medical goods, supplies, medical records, and any other important documents to continue medical and mental-health care

Food, water, clothes, bedding or sleeping bags, items to occupy time like books or board games; similar to the preparation for a hurricane or other disaster planning to stay in your home for 72–96 hours with little to no essential public services

Communication plans to alert family, friends and co-workers of the evacuation, destination, and re-entry

Cell phones, chargers, and other electronics essential for communication and maintenance of business operations

Family heirlooms and irreplaceable mementos that permit a safe and effective long, tedious evacuation journey

Hurricanes, flooding, and wildfires may require a vast regional population to move great distances. Frequently, advance notification is possible with establishment of best routes for a staged evacuation. An epidemic, civil unrest, or long-term disruption of essential public services due to numerous causes may require a large population or a portion of a region or regions to evacuate for a longer time frame. Advance preparation may be possible to establish safe routes of evacuation and establishment of resources for the evacuated population.

Authority

Office of the chief executive

The legal basis for an evacuation of (an entire or portions of) a municipality, city, county or state lies in the office of chief executive of the specific governmental agency determined by the statute governing that office.

Proclamation for voluntary or mandatory evacuation

This authority will issue a proclamation for voluntary or mandatory evacuation in specific language. The emergency management plan will designate a lead agency for evacuation.

Essential information in proclamation

Provide additional assurances for the safety of material possessions of the evacuated population (i.e., measures to prevent looting).

- Identify what services (law, fire, EMS, sanitation, etc.) and essential services (water, sewer, electricity, natural gas, etc.) will not be available.
- Detail in clear and concise language the risks of remaining:
  - "You stay at your own risk."
  - "Expect no city services."
  - "There will be no water or electricity."
  - "No one will be available to rescue you."
- Some proclamations may detail civil and criminal charges brought against any person or persons who disobey the mandatory evacuation to include those found guilty of looting.

The safety of rescue personnel is paramount and exceeds the risk of rescue. This information should be repeated during public education efforts and during the process announcing the incident evacuation. Memories of those who did not leave when ordered ahead of Hurricane Katrina (Coastal Louisiana and Mississippi 2005) and Hurricane Ike (Galveston Texas, 2008) may prompt naysayers to leave accordingly.

Specifics

ESF Annexes

The evacuation responsibilities of each lead agency is defined in an annex (Table 29.3) to the state, county and municipal (city) emergency management plan. These Emergency Support Functions (ESFs) may have a different number, specific to each jurisdiction's plan, but they have the same format beginning with an introduction stating the clear rationale to create and maintain a written plan for the design, notification, and implementation of the timely and orderly movement of an affected population. All-hazards emergency management is fulfilled when the mission of this ESF extends evacuation traffic management to any incident threatening public

Table 29.3 Sample Evacuation or Traffic-Management Emergency Support Function Annex to Jurisdiction Emergency Management Plan

Primary Lead Agency:

Support Agencies:

Terms and Definitions:

Referenced ESFs:

I. Introduction

    a. Rationale for evacuation and traffic management

    b. Specific hazards for this jurisdiction

    c. Selection of agencies

II. Mission statement

III. Concept of operations, (may require references to other ESFs)

    a. Lead agency's role

    b. Jurisdiction's traffic-management strategy

    c. Coordination among local jurisdictions

    d. Coordination with state emergency management

    e. Specific civilian evacuation routes: no notice, short notice, advance notice

    f. Primary/alternate inspection routes

    g. Primary/alternate lifeline routes

    h. Traffic control points

    i. Provisions for special jurisdiction or local jurisdiction sites: nuclear, military, airport, harbor, rail, major industry, or other sites

    j. Provisions for specific natural or man-made incidents

    k. Intera-gency evacuation communication

    l. Re-entry process and procedures

    m. Public information

TABLE 29.3 (*Contd.*)

IV. Responsibilities
a. Preparedness
b. Mitigation
c. Response
d. Recovery
e. Review
f. Reporting
V. Administration and logistics
a. Situation reports
b. Logistics
c. Financial
d. Information exchange
e. Other
VI. Annex review and maintenance
VII. Coordinating instructions
VIII. Signatures of jurisdiction authority and lead agency chief administrator

safety, such as an ice storm, wildfire, wind storm, or major transportation crash, which requires re-routing of the normal traffic flow. The Concept of Operations will be specific for each threat as determined by the HVA, with the peculiar factors relating to the area's geographic, topographic, or population density. These specifics may require additional ESF annexes or inclusion in other ESF annexes.

State emergency management division

States use a traffic-demand-forecasting-spreadsheet model, which uses demographic information extracted from evacuation areas and then calculates the number of people to be evacuated, depending on time of day, day of the month, month of the year, due to tourists, colleges, and other population-dependent factors. This is converted from people to vehicle volume, assuming no public transportation, which may or may not be feasible, depending on the incident and evacuation proclamation advance notice. This is then assigned to the expected evacuation route from that specific evacuation zone for that specific incident to calculate the time needed for the evacuation. Estimates of projected time of each evacuation should be communicated to the evacuees, promoting patience and setting realistic expectations to give citizens the confidence to leave as instructed and to follow evacuation procedures and destination objectives.

Traffic control points

Traffic Control Points (TCPs), adapted from military checkpoints, are established to reduce if not eliminate choke points or bottlenecks created by mass movement of traffic against normal traffic patterns.

- Lane reversal (traffic moving in all lanes in one direction).
- Contra-flow (three of four lanes are in the direction of the evacuation and one lane remains in the original direction).

Locations of TCPs

TCPs are located at key intersections approaching major transportation routes like interstate, state, and county highways. Key components of an evacuation are the re-routing of traffic, which may require the closing of on- and off-ramps. TCPs will be located to restrict potential movement in a manner that may reduce the effectiveness of the designed evacuation, like closing back-road traffic routes on local roads.

Computer modeling, table-top, and live exercises and effective after-action review of actual evacuations have been shown to be consistently helpful in the refinement and maintenance of the TCPs and thus the design of specific evacuation routes for general and specific incidents.

Staffing of TCPs

Physical staffing of each TCP may be from municipal (city), county, or state agencies or contracted private firms. The signage of a TCP may be permanent or may be placed in a temporary fashion, aided by various electronic devices already in place for other traffic messages. Design of barriers that are common across the country establishing high occupancy vehicle interstate and state highway lanes have been effectively adapted to aid the closure of on- and off-ramps as well as assisting new traffic flow. In an effort to expedite an evacuation, tolls may be suspended for the period of the evacuation, either stated in the evacuation proclamation or in existing legislation or regulation that apply during a disaster or emergency.

Communications

Intra-agency communication has proven to be a consistent area of improvement during an evacuation, with the myriad public and private agencies involved, at times during inclement weather or other austere environmental conditions. Evacuation ESFs communication plans are promulgated by preexisting radio channels only for evacuations or previously purchased stored communication equipment.

Re-entry of evacuated populations

Re-entry or the return of an evacuated population remains the primary challenge of an evacuation. The authority that issues the evacuation proclamation also has to issue a proclamation that ends the emergency and directs re-entry. Local emergency managers have significantly more input into the re-entry process that is not as well defined within an ESF annex or other plans due to the unknown effects of the incident to infrastructure, critical essential services, and supply lines delivering food and other supplies. Time will be required to remove hazards, not only along main transportation interstate, state, and local roads, but also airports, railroads, subways, and waterways. Only crews on the ground can assess downed electrical wires, leaking natural gas, and contaminated water delivery while engineers assess structural competency. Days if not weeks may be required to repair even temporary measures to establish sufficient services for the evacuated population to return, even if for a few hours a day to calm fears regarding their property. High-rise buildings, large-scale industrial livestock waste, and other dams, chemical storage facilities, nuclear and other power plants, and other potentially damaged infrastructure must be assessed.

Incremental or phased re-entry identification cards, papers, or stickers, specific for the incident can be issued at TCPs or other designated locations to disaster rescue and recovery personnel via their agency or organization as issued by the incident-management team. Evacuated citizens or those from outside the area with financial, property, or personal concerns in the affected area have to be considered with re-entry. Some jurisdictions have established plans, either contained in a re-entry ESF or other means to issue official cards or paperwork that can be displayed in returning vehicles or furnished upon request at a TCP. Others have issued yearly stickers that owners place on a vehicle window in a specific location that can easily be seen at a TCP. State issued identification such as a business license, driver's license, or property-tax receipt have also been used to permit re-entry. Regardless of proof of identification or purpose to return, all concerned must be aware, from those manning TCPs to those wishing to return, not only in any official proclamations, communications, or situation reports, but also in standard media like television, radio, Internet, and newspapers of specific risks and availability of essential public services and medical care.

The affected population from the city, county or state, or even multiple states will have to evacuate to an area determined to be safe from the incident. This may be in areas in other parts of the state or other states requiring long-term planning to assure specific assets are in place to handle the surge of people. States may have to work within the parameters of the Emergency Management Assistance Compact to assure that their citizens are provided the best chance of weathering the incident until they can return home. The evacuation proclamation will outline areas safe to evacuate to, even naming specific towns. The planning process will consider destinations for specific evacuation scenarios and invite representatives from these distant emergency-management agencies to assist the establishment of appropriate destinations.

Emergency-management public information has the opportunity to follow the successful education that families have incorporated into their own emergency preparedness with maintenance of a three-day supply of essential supplies, food, and water if faced with an incident of limited access to resupply as well as essential public services. This duty may be tasked to a representative in the specific county emergency-management office, or additional duties to the PIO from the authority's office that issued the evacuation proclamation, or the PIO from law enforcement, EMS or fire. Regardless, this responsibility commences with the advent of the committee or group that maintains plans, exercises, mitigation efforts, the evacuation response, re-entry, and review. This PIO should be at the table to best communicate the evacuation process, through a consistent voice.

Special considerations

- MOUs with portable latrines, food and beverage, and gasoline distributers are important aspects of an evacuation ESF. Locations for deployment include current rest areas, truck weigh stations, public buildings, and service areas easily accessed from evacuation (and then re-entry) routes as well as private properties that can be identified and contracted via an MOU. Current private establishments dispensing food, beverages, and gasoline will be challenged to meet the demand in an evacuation (and re-entry), with their supply lines stretched if not eliminated due to demand placed on their suppliers as well as limited access due to the incident itself. Public fuel depots and gasoline stations created specifically for a specific evacuation should be considered, especially in rural or frontier areas where there are limited commercial stations. Price gouging is the scourge of any disaster; specific states, counties, and municipalities (cities) have passed laws prohibiting price gouging with parameters set to guide proprietors as well as firm penalties if found guilty.

- Lodging will begin to fill with the threat of an imminent hurricane or other advance notice incident, and once a voluntary proclamation has been issued it may be too late to phone ahead or book a room via the Internet. In the event of a sudden, no-notice evacuation, proprietors may not have the time to gear up for the sudden surge of business. Therefore, state emergency-management agencies may consider advance targeting of commercial lodging, establishment of evacuation-specific shelters in concert with the EMAC and other interagency agreements and using the Federal Emergency Management Agency (FEMA) to solidify shelter plans for large-population evacuations. County emergency-management agencies in locations with increased risk of evacuation have varied in their approach to educate at-risk populations with campaigns to add an evacuation destination in family-disaster planning.

- Community residents that rely on public transportation cannot evacuate easily. School buses and private sector transportation companies, buses, trains, water craft, and airlines can be contracted through MOUs for evacuation. Once these companies have been identified, the process for a citizen to gain access to the transportation asset can be defined to include a muster point, or a place where they can get on the bus or transport. This may be a public location, like a current bus stop, school, or large parking lot associated with a stadium or other building. There may be plans to gather at one location to then be taken to another where the actual transport may be located. This information can be arranged, communicated, and even tested via computer, table-top, or live exercise. Citizens should understand what they can bring on a limited scale. Tracking systems utilizing bar codes will facilitate family communication during the evacuation and sheltering process. With a registration process, a potential evacuee can receive advance education, providing the emergency-management agency valuable information to aid in the planning process, as well as information to guide future exercises. County emergency managers can utilize religious gatherings, local newspapers, direct mailings, physicians' offices, and other common paths to gain attention to the evacuation process for potential shut-ins and those without a means to evacuate. The destinations of these evacuees can be predetermined to facilitate family communication, as well as arrange for medical and other chronic care.

- Dialysis, chemotherapy, IV infusion therapy, hospice, and home health patients should have evacuation planning via their health- care provider. Some states even incorporate the planning process into health-care regulations, with requirements to file patient evacuation plans with state officials. Not only is the specific evacuation means defined, the destination and recipient health-care provider is identified with their ability to acquire current medical records, their latest medical and other therapy, and means to communicate with the patients' primary care or other physician during the evacuation and sheltering period. The goal is to not burden the destination health-care facilities, unless otherwise arranged, with the creation of special-medical-needs shelters.

- Durable medical equipment suppliers are also required in some states to similarly create, maintain, and furnish evacuation and sheltering plans for their patients to satisfy requirements for continued funding of their patients during standard operations. Nursing- home, assisted-living, in-patient mental-health, and other similar facilities in some states are required to furnish evacuation plans, to include how they plan to notify families, physically transfer the patients to safe accommodations or special-medical-needs shelters previously determined to maintain care while evacuated and how they plan to return the patient to the originating facility. Prisons exist under separate ESFs, depending on the circumstances including no-notice, sudden incidents. Adult and child daycare, public and private schools, including colleges, should develop evacuation plans as part of any orientation process for each student or client, to best facilitate a timely and orderly evacuation, with minimal distress for all concerned with the full evacuation process discussed, including the notification of an evacuation, the means of actual transportation, destination, shelter facility, and how to alert families about the evacuation and return of the evacuees to their families. Emergency managers want to avoid families descending on an evacuation area, searching for their loved ones, when their goal is for a timely and safe evacuation. Bar codes can be utilized and planned far in advance to aid tracking and communication.

- Evacuating with pets can be a challenge. Keeping the pet in the car during the long commute, to finding lodgings that permit pets, and to maintain pets during the evacuation period can be difficult. Just as the family has to plan their evacuation process, route, destination, and re-entry, they have to plan for their animals, including any medication, special food, or other accommodations that they require. Simply leaving the animal(s) at home with what an owner may believe to be sufficient food and water is not acceptable and should be communicated to animal owners via county emergency management

along with all other evacuation education and planning, specifically targeting animal owners through their veterinarians and pet stores.
- The key to an evacuation is patience. Communities must
  - Gather all constituents to develop plans.
  - Establish community and constituent education programs.
  - Create viable computer, table-top and live exercises.
  - Reinforce that the necessary evacuation will be boring, lengthy, and an adventure.

Proper planning, setting realistic expectations through consistent and recurrent family, neighborhood, and work communication will set the tone for a successful evacuation.

Suggested readings

Drabek T (2010). *The Human Side of Disaster*. New York: CRC Press.
Riad JK, Frank H, Norris R, Ruback B (May 1999). Predicting evacuation in two major disasters: Risk perception, social influence, and access to resources." *Journal of Applied Social Psychology* 29(5): 918–934.

Chapter 30

Force health protection

Richard Schwartz

Gerald Beltrab

Overview

This chapter describes the protection of forces responding to a disaster. This is a complex and involved process that has was initially developed by the military as part of the unit-deployment process. Although force health protection has it roots in the military, the fundamental concepts are just as applicable to civilian disaster-response operations. These fundamental concepts are based on the promotion and maintenance of a fit and healthy responding force, prevention of illness and injury to the responders, protection from potential hazards to health and well-being of those providing aid, rendering medical care to the sick and injured, and configuration as well as maintenance of an infrastructure that supports these activities. The underlying strategy integrates prevention and clinical activities implemented to protect the forces rendering aid.

Due to recent historical disaster events, both man-made and natural, there has been a dynamic modification to the manner in which response teams have addressed their mission. This has been influenced by continuous budgetary and personnel constraints leading to the deployment of a smaller force to support these missions. In preparation for potential disasters, the paradigm has changed from one of clearly defined threats to one of potential threats and what medical means are required to mitigate these threats. This process of evaluating the potential medical threats is commonly referred to as medical- threat assessment.

Force health protection addresses methods of prevention of casualties during all phases of deployment, including before, concurrent, and after the disaster. This occurs through:

- Services that accentuate fitness, readiness, and prevention.
- Observation and vigilance of threats as well as forces rendering care.
- Cognizance by both leaders and individuals of medical hazards prior to affecting force functioning.
- Medical occupational support of the force during deployment.

In addition to prevention, force health protection addresses the medical care and treatment of disaster casualties. The care rendered in the field is critical in casualty management. It can prevent morbidity and mortality. Additionally, timely and efficient removal of casualties to definitive care also directly impacts patient morbidity and mortality. Uninterrupted care from injury location to final-care location greatly improves patient outcome. By modifying previous paradigms from acute care to prevention, in addition to the effective implementation of newer medical technologies, casualty outcomes have greatly improved.

History

Force health protection has rapidly evolved over the last few decades. Prior to the 1980s, it simply focused on mission accomplishment. The primary force health protection goal was maintenance of health until the force returned home when the illnesses and injuries would be managed. After Desert Shield and Desert Storm, it was recognized that force health protection capabilities had been exceeded by the needs of the forces.

In particular, concern was raised after Desert Storm about the Gulf-War syndrome, with many citizens, politicians, and soldiers inquiring about environmental risks to the forces participating in this conflict. This led to greater emphasis being placed on force health protection and modification of the existing paradigm to address concerns and new threats.

Deployment and environmental surveillance became integral to force health protection. The equipment and process of relaying the information from surveillance to implementation has improved tremendously and continues to improve. For example, air and water sampling equipment is not only becoming smaller and easier to deploy, it is now possible to monitor potential and newly identified hazards. With real-time force data becoming a reality, the integration of this force health data renders greater protection to deployed personnel.

Just prior to 2000, the importance of force health protection was recognized by the U.S. Army, and it was given voting capabilities in the Army System Acquisition Review Council as well as the Cost Review Board. This allows for input into the weapons systems acquisition process to address the force health protection needs and concerns.

The role of force health protection has only recently been recognized. Its role has enlarged and become integrated into mission planning and implementation. As new potential threats are identified, this role will only continue to expand.

Essential concepts

There are three key concepts relative to force health protection:
• A healthy and fit force.
• Prevention and protection of the deployed force.
• Medical care and rehabilitation.

Each of these concepts, when integrated in their entirety, ensures the health and well being of the deployed force as well as the casualties relying upon their care.
• Fit and Healthy Force.

A force that is at optimal health and fitness ensures maximal opportunity for success of the mission for which it is deployed. This maxim is a requisite for force health protection.

Physical fitness allows the deployed assets to function optimally in their mission. All persons who may be deployed should be encouraged to maintain their physical fitness. Health promotion type programs, occupational-health programs, and managed-health-care programs should also be emphasized to maintain assets at peak health. This ensures peak physical performance and maximum protection from disease, illness, and injury. Should an injury or illness occur, this helps force members to quickly and readily recover.

To maximize physical fitness, cardiovascular health, skeletal muscle strength and endurance, flexibility, dexterity, and body composition need to be addressed. Implementation of an evidenced based or scientifically based physical fitness program oriented to the mission is important to meet this goal. This may be difficult to enforce in a volunteer disaster response team such as a Disaster Medical Assistance Team (DMAT). Inclusion of physical fitness activities in training sessions or incentives may help motivate individuals to meet or exceed fitness standards. Time should be allocated to nondeployed and deployed personnel to continue fitness training. Equipment and facilities should be readily available to encourage

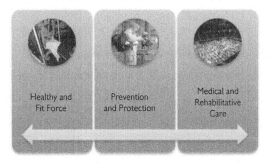

Figure 30.1 Spectrum of force health protection.

maintenance of fitness. Planned fitness and health assessments should be performed regularly to continuously monitor physical readiness of the operational force. Deployment, medical readiness, and self-assessments should also be used to track readiness of deployable personnel.

The caloric intake by deployed individuals is important to optimize physical performance, health, and morale. It should be tailored to meet individual needs relating to physical activity, nutritional needs, and preference. Predeployment activities should allow for logistics related to preparatory staff, food preparation, supplies, and sanitation. Healthy eating habits should be promoted and reinforced during predeployment and deployment.

Utilization of technology can aid with obtaining and monitoring personnel consumption in addition to body composition measures. This allows for education and modification of dietary intake in combination with estimated daily caloric expenditure.

Water is critical in maintaining hydration and peak efficiency during deployment, especially in warm environments. It is estimated that the body can survive 30 days without food, but only 4–10 days without water during a time of inactivity. Water represents about 45%–70% of an individual's weight and is essential in maintenance of normal cellular function as well as thermal regulation. There is an inherent water requirement that varies from individual to individual. In all cases, water requirements increase with activity. This is due to increased water loss from the skin, respiratory system, and GI tract. Personnel will usually not feel thirsty until dehydrated by about 1.5 liters. During replacement, the average person can only absorb approximately 1–1.5 liters of water in the gastrointestinal tract.

The Wet Globe Temperature Index is a measure that takes into consideration temperature, humidity, wind, and direct sunlight. This is a commonly utilized tool to guide activity of deployed forces. Heat index based on the wet globe temperature index is divided into 5 distinct categories. Each category has recommendations for water intake and activity. See Table 30.1.

Table 30.1 Heat Category/Wet Globe Index Chart

Heat Category	Wet Globe Index	Activity	Hydration Requirements
1	78–81.9F	Continuous	Minimum ½ quart per hour
2	82–84.9F	40 minutes activity followed by 20 minutes rest	Minimum ½ quart per hour
3	85–87.9F	30 minutes activity followed by 30 minutes rest	Minimum 1 quart per hour
4	88–89.9	20 minutes activity followed by 40 minutes rest	Minimum of 1.5 quarts per hour
5	> 90F	10 minutes of activity followed by 50 minutes rest	Minimum of 2 quarts per hour

Source: Medical College of Georgia Tactical Operator Care Course handbook May 2008

The effects of heat stress should be recognized by deployed personnel. Knowledge of the various forms of heat illness is essential.

- One form of heat illness is heat cramps. It manifests as uncomfortable muscle spasms. The spasms usually occur after exertion and significant intake of water. Its etiology is believed to be from salt deficiency and treatment consists of oral replenishment of electrolytes. In mild cases this can be done by a mixture of an electrolyte solution (e.g., Gatorade™) mixed in a 1:1 fashion with water. With more severe symptoms, intravenous normal saline or lactated ringers can be utilized.
- Another form of heat illness is heat edema. This can be recognized by the swelling of the hands and feet. Heat edema is believed to be due to vasodilation and pooling of interstitial fluid in the dependent extremities. It can be treated by simply elevating the affected extremity.
- An additional form of heat illness is heat syncope. This is loss of consciousness caused by both peripheral vasodilation and dehydration. This resolves by placing the casualty in a supine position and providing oral rehydration.
- Another form of heat illness is heat exhaustion. This is a syndrome associated with hypovolemia secondary to heat stress. It can be described as either the water-depletion type or salt-depletion type. The water-depletion type is due to insufficient fluid intake. Individuals working in a hot environment usually only drink enough fluid to replace about two-thirds of their net water loss, leading to a voluntary dehydration and hypovolemia. Older individuals or those with limited access to water are also predisposed to dehydration and hypovolemia. The salt-depletion type typically occurs over a longer period of time. It develops when large volumes of fluid loss are replaced by water with insufficient salt. It typically presents with hyponatremia, hypochloremia, diminished urinary sodium and chloride with a normal body temperature. With either type of heat exhaustion management consists of moving the person from the warm environment to a cooler one. An oral electrolyte solution can be given in mild cases to help with the hypovolemia and any electrolyte depletion. Similar to the treatment used for heat cramps, the ideal oral solution is a mixture is a 1:1 fashion of water with an electrolyte solution (e.g., Gatorade). However, in more severe cases intravenous fluids can be given.
- The most severe form of heat illness is heat stroke and is a medical emergency. This can present with an increase in temperature, central-nervous-system alteration (e.g., delirium, convulsions, coma), dry or wet skin, rapid respiratory rate, hypotension, nausea, vomiting, and diarrhea. The management of this ailment is rapid cooling. The affected individual should be taken from the hot environment and moved to a cooler environment. Clothing should be removed. Cooling can be performed by any of the following methods: cold or ice water immersion, cool spray and fanning, or ice packs to the axillae, neck, and groin. Care should be taken to try to avoid shivering by either administration of benzodiazepines or massage. Approximately 1-2 liters of intravenous fluids should also be administered as part of the

treatment. Patients with heat stroke should be evacuated to medical facilities for further care.

Of particular concern during deployment is the potential for enteritis or diarrheal illness. This can cause significant discomfort, dehydration, and may be a harbinger of more serious illness. To minimize the risk, individuals should be counseled and educated on the risks of drinking water that has not been purified. Ice cubes prepared without purification should also be avoided. Foods that are prepared with unpurified water and that are uncooked should be avoided. Foods that necessitate refrigeration for storage should constantly be maintained at temperatures below 7.2°C (45°F), except during preparatory and serving activities. Heated foods should be cooked to adequate temperature (Table 30.2) then maintained at temperatures greater than 60°C (140°F) to minimize the risk of food illness. Education concerning proper hand-washing during food preparation and prior to eating is also helpful in staving off enteritis.

Potable water is a key element in maintenance of health. There are many methods for making water useable in the field.

- Boiling water is very effective at destroying enteric pathogens, but has no effect on sediments or toxins.
- Distillation is very effective at destroying pathogens, removing sediments, and removing toxins. Its limitation is its bad taste and the removal of electrolytes.
- Reverse osmosis filtration is extremely effective in removing pathogens, sediment, and toxins. However, it requires special equipment.
- Simple filtration is fairly effective, but is limited by the size of the filter. The more fine the filter, the more effective it is in removing pathogens and sediment. This method also requires frequent changing of the filter to avoid tears of the filter.
- Halogenation is another method used to make water more useable. Its limitation is in the residual taste of the water and its limited ability to affect pathogens such as protozoans and helminthes.
- Field sanitation is critical in preventing illness during deployment. There are several device types available for removal of human waste. At a bivouac, a chemical toilet is most often utilized. If that is not

Table 30.2 Cooking temperatures for safe food

Product	Minimum Internal Temp
Poultry	165°F for 15 seconds
Pork	145°F for 15 seconds
Ground Meat	155°F for 15 seconds
Roasts (Beef or Pork)	145°F for 3 minutes
Beef Steaks, Veal and Lamb	145°F for 15 seconds
Fish	145°F for 15 seconds

Source: East Jefferson General Hospital

available, a burn out latrine can be used. When mobile in the field, individual collection bags are utilized. It is mandatory that local, state, national, and host-nation regulations be followed regarding human waste disposal.

- The location of the latrine in the field is important in minimizing its impact to health and field operations. Ideally, it should be placed at least 100 meters from food operations. If possible, it should also be placed downhill and downwind from food operations, work areas, and living areas. It must also be placed at least 30 meters or more from water sources such as wells, springs, and streams. The latrine should be constructed or setup as soon as personnel move into the area. Cleaning of the facility should occur daily with personnel assigned to spraying insecticide as required. Hand washing is mandatory after latrine use.

- Dental health is another component of a fit and healthy deployable force. The pain and discomfort of poor dentition can greatly affect an individual's ability to concentrate on the mission. Pre-deployment education and preventative care is essential. During deployment reinforcing dental as well as oral care will minimize dental-care issues during deployment.

- Mental well-being also contributes to asset effectiveness. This component of health includes behavioral, emotive, spiritual, social, and intellectual. It helps define how an individual will respond to stressors. Ultimately, this entails identifying persons at greatest risk, developing programs to aid with self-management skills and behavioral skills, utilizing community and force resources, emphasizing primary prevention instead of acute care, and changing negative perceptions of individuals receiving mental health care. This gives personnel stronger coping skills and healthy relationships at work and at home, allowing the individual to better focus on the force mission. Training in conflict as well as anger management, stress, and performance, substance abuse including alcohol, identification of suicide risk factors, and family communication furthers this goal by giving the individual the tools to better deal with deployment and home stressors.

- Prevention

The best manner to maintain the force at peak readiness is through prevention of disease and injury. This mandates that team commanders and members adopt a philosophy that stresses safety, preventative medicine resources and tools, and modification of behaviors that are unnecessarily risky.

Maximizing the goal of prevention requires:

- Identification of threats to health that could jeopardize the force mission including a predeployment threat assessment.
- Surveillance of disease and injury; transmittal of surveillance data to decision makers and commanders.
- Utilization of technology emphasizing immunizations, fitness, prophylaxis, screening tools, systems integration for medical intelligence.
- Utilization reduction or cessation of alcohol, tobacco, and drugs inclusive of over the counter medicines and supplements.

As part of any mission predeployment preparation, a threat assessment should be conducted, which includes identification of local diseases, injuries, plants, animals, and arthropods. The plan for the mitigation of the threats is dependent upon the medical threat assessment. The identification for each of these and their potential threat for each geographical location is beyond the scope of this section. There are several reliable Internet sites that are continuously updated to provide medical threat assessments. See Box 30.1.

There are secure sites available for conducting threat assessment, which require a government or military e-mail address. See Box 30.2.

There are also several classified sites requiring a justification, clearance, and access to a computer terminal rated for secret clearance and higher. Specific disease entities should be identified during the predeployment threat assessment, allowing for immunization and medicinal prophylaxis as well as customization of drug inventory.

The predeployment medical threat assessment should also include environmental and occupational hazards; potential chemical, biologic, and radiological hazards; heat and cold hazards; and other stressors. Infectious disease monitoring and management must be performed, especially in the following areas when there are large groups of people together in one area: waste and sewage disposal, immunizations and chemoprophylaxis, water quality, personal protection (e.g., hand washing, sharing of food, gloves when working with patients, insect repellant, and net surround sleeping area where appropriate), and food quality as well as food sanitation (e.g., cooking food well).

Box 30.1 Resources for medical threat assessments
- Center for Disease Control at http://www.cdc.gov/ (specifically http://wwwn.cdc.gov/travel/default.aspx)
- World Health Organization at http://www.who.int/en/ (specifically http://www.who.int/ith/en/index.html)
- Department of State http://travel.state.gov (specifically http://travel.state.gov/travel/travel_1744.html)
- U.S. Department of Health & Human Services at http://www.hhs.gov/
- U.S. Department of Defense Global Emerging Infections Surveillance and Response System at http://www.geis.fhp.osd.mil/
- U.S. Army Center for Health Promotion and Preventive Medicine at http://chppm-www.apgea.army.mil/
- Armed Forces Health Surveillance Center at http://afhsc.army.mil/index.asp.

Box 30.2 Secure resources for conducting a threat assessment
- Armed Forces Medical Intelligence Center at http://www.afmic.detrick.army.mil
- Law Enforcement Online at http://www.leo.gov.

Based on this medical threat assessment, steps should be taken to minimize the risk of arthropod/insect exposure. Insect repellent is one means to address this. N,N-diethyl-M-Toluamide (DEET) is an insect repellent that can be applied to all exposed skin in a light, even coating. It should be re-applied after 8–12 hours or if insect bites start occurring. It should not be applied to eyes, lips, or damaged skin. Clothing should also have repellent applied to discourage insect/arthropod exposure. Permethrin can be applied to clothing, bed nets, ground cloths, and tent liners. It will remain active even after repeated washings. Permethrin should not be applied directly to the skin, underwear, or hat, and it should only be applied in a well-ventilated area or outdoors.

Bed netting should be utilized when sleeping if indicated by the medical threat assessment. It should be tucked under sleeping pad or sleeping bag to prevent any openings. Bed netting should be inspected daily for any rents; if there are any holes they should be repaired.

Spiders, scorpions, and centipedes should be removed from tents and building to reduce the risk of bites and stings. Clothing and footwear should be shaken to dislodge any spiders, scorpions, or centipedes. Clothing should also be worn with the shirt sleeves rolled down and pants bloused in footwear. Shirts should also be buttoned to the neck and wrist. Scented soaps, shampoo, conditioners, cologne, perfume, aftershave, and scented deodorant should be avoided as they attract arthropods.

Malaria chemoprophylaxis, if applicable, must be addressed as part of the medical threat assessment because it is estimated that one million people die worldwide each year from malaria, and there is no vaccine against this mosquito borne illness. Antimalarials taken before, during, and after exposure to an environment where malaria exists minimize the risk of contracting malaria. Prevention or suppression of symptoms caused by this parasite is the concept behind chemoprophylaxis. If there is antimalarial medication resistance, the chemoprophylaxis should be adjusted accordingly. See Table 30.3.

Protection from the sun is also critical in both maintaining peak mission readiness and personnel comfort. Ultraviolet (UV) radiation causes damage and discomfort to both the skin and eyes. Clothing prevents the UV rays from damaging the epithelial cells. Any exposed skin can be protected

Table 30.3 Malaria chemoprophylaxis

Chloroquine Phosphate	Malaria risk areas: Mexico, Haiti, Dominican Republic and some areas in Central America, Middle East, and Eastern Europe
Doxycycline Hyclate	Extensive chloroquine resistance (e.g., Africa, Southeast Asia)
Mefloquine	Extensive chloroquine resistance (e.g., Africa, Southeast Asia)
Atovaquone Proguanil	Extensive chloroquine resistance

Source: U.S. Pharmacist

by use of sunscreen and lip balm with a minimum sun protection factor of 15. The eyes can be protected with UV protection eyewear and should be used with any sun exposure.

While deployed, constant surveillance for chemical, biologic, and radiological contamination should be performed on each team member based on the threat assessment. This may be as simple as monitoring the health of deployed personnel and looking for trends.

After deployment, surveillance of all deployed individuals should be performed, monitoring again for biologic, chemical, and radiological changes. Long-term measure may also be employed for those who may experience chronic conditions related to environmental exposures during deployment. This surveillance should be guided by the medical threat assessment.

* Occupational prevention is critical in minimizing potentially preventable casualties by affecting the research and development lifecycle; implementing prevention measures; development of techniques aiding in individual adaptation to altitude, climate, and assorted environmental stressors; and promulgation of doctrine and processes to support individuals and their mission performance.

* Force health protection prevention includes identification of individuals at greatest physical risk of injury. These assets include people who are involved in high-risk activities (e.g., diving, sport with high rate of physical contact, etc.), those who regularly perform new activities (e.g., new food preparation with new cutting instruments, utilization of new medical equipment, etc.), and those who have preexisting conditions predisposing them to injury (e.g., illness, past injury, poor physical fitness, etc). Additional training or other activities to mitigate these risks help to reduce the risks to these individuals. If poor baseline physical fitness is a risk for a person, a gradually challenging fitness regimen may be implemented. Rest should regularly be scheduled and sleep maximized as the mission permits.

At times during deployments, sleep cycles may need to be adjusted to coincide with work shifts, time zones, or continuous operations. Under medical supervision, certain medications are available to aid with sleep. Some of the more commonly utilized medications include zolpidem tartrate, zolpidem tartrate extended release, zaleplon, and eszopiclone. Typically, these medicines are taken at a predetermined time prior to start of desired sleep. They each have different effects on the individual using them. Utilization during training permits determination of side effects, optimal use, and best timing of use for each individual. Effects on cognition and physical performance can be better understood during training to minimize the risk to personnel during deployment.

Other medications can be used to reduce the need for sleep or postpone sleep in a stressful or hazardous environment and have been successfully utilized for shift workers. The most commonly used medication for this purpose is modafinil. This medication should only be considered in extraordinary conditions, with the authorization of the deployment commander, and under medical supervision. If this medication is to be utilized during deployment, it should also be used during training to understand the side effects, optimal use, and best timing for use for each individual. This medicine also has effects on behavior and physical performance.

Those at greatest risk for becoming mental-health casualties are those with a poor support system, use psychoactive medicines, have a disciplinary history, and have a history of family problems. Prevention in this arena incorporates family support services, stress debriefings related to critical incidents, counseling (both voluntary and command referred), implementation of rest and relaxation policies incorporating individual preferences, and support from family and friends through phone, letters, and internet.

Force health protection prevention relating to chemical, biological, radiological, and nuclear injuries is becoming more and more important as criminal and terror elements contemplate their use to further the goals of terrorizing the public at large. These types of weapons are utilized to terrorize the public out of proportion to the threat that they actually pose. Prevention starts with intelligence and neutralization of these threats to prevent development and deployment of these types of weapons. Surveillance includes environmental detection capabilities. The earlier a threat is detected, the earlier steps can be implemented to contain the threat. Additionally, decontamination, immunization, and chemoprophylaxis can be utilized as threats are identified.

- Medical Management and Rehabilitative Care

Care provided to casualties of a disaster or to responders of a disaster mandates prompt care in the field with immediate extraction to a site of definitive care as quickly as possible. Technology permitting clinical information to be relayed prior to casualty arrival as well with arrival must be integrated with the patient's medical record.

The initial response for a victim of trauma is critical in reduction of morbidity and mortality. Stabilization or attempts at stabilization are of the utmost importance in giving the casualty the best possible outcome. First responders who are extremely familiar with rendering aid rapidly are very useful when deployed among the rapid and mobile forces in austere and hostile environments. They are most efficient at initial management of casualties at potential chemical, biological, or radiological threat locations compared to other resources. In general, the first responder's primary goal is immediate medical care as well as stabilization of the injured. Additionally, as a secondary function, they may provide treatment for common acute minor illnesses and injuries.

Medical management has a role in prevention. Typically, first responders monitor the effectiveness of prevention strategies for individuals and groups. They also provide information to unit commanders about mandatory prevention strategies. They identify threats that may be mitigated, for example utilization of new technologies or techniques for identification of chemical, biological, radiological, and other environmental threats.

Conclusion

Force health protection is a vital component for personnel deployed for disaster support. Planning and preparing for force health protection begins long before the deployment and has components that extend into the post-deployment period. Adequate planning, preparation, and implementation of force health protection will assist commanders in successful mission accomplishment.

Suggested readings

Embrey EP (February 13, 2007). Force health protection. ASMUS. Available at: http://www.amsus.org/sm/presentations/Feb07-B.ppt (Accessed 09/01/2008).

Reimers K (2008). Nutritional factors in health and performance. In: Baechie TR and Earle RW eds. *Essentials of Strength and Conditioning*. Champaign, IL: Human Kinetics, pp. 217–218.

Environmental Emergencies: Tactical Operator Care 1 Course (TOC 1) by the Medical College of Georgia. May 2008.

Salvator V (2006). Heat illness. In: Marx JA, Hockberger RS, and Walls RA, eds. *Rosen's Emergency Medicine Concepts and Clinical Practice*. Philadelphia, PA: Mosby, pp. 2258–2265.

U.S. Army. *Army Field Manual 21-10* (2000). Washington, D.C.: HQ Dept of the Army. http://www.brooksidepress.org/Products/OperationalMedicine/DATA/operationalmed/Manuals/fm2110.pdf (Accessed 09/01/2008).

U.S. Department of Defense. Force health protection. Available at: http://deploymentlink.osd.mil/pdfs/fhpcapstone2004.pdf (Accessed 09/01/2008).

U.S. Government Accountability Office. Defense health care. Available at: http://www.gao.gov/new.items/d05120.pdf (Accessed 09/01/2008).

Young SE and Pierluisi GJ (2008). Operational performance and preventive medicine. In Schwartz RB, McManus JG, and Swienton RE, eds. *Tactical Emergency Medicine*. Philadelphia, PA: Lippincott Williams & Wilkins, pp. 133–134.

Incident command system

William Mastrianni

Introduction

The Incident Command System (ICS) was established in the 1970s in response to catastrophic wildfires at California's rural-urban interface, where there was widespread property damage and loss of life. Analysis of the outcomes indicated that rather than inadequate resources, lack of adequate incident management was the single largest contributing factor.

ICS is a standardized management tool that:

- Meets the demands of large or small incidents and is scalable during the incident.
- Can be used for emergency and non-emergency (preplanned) incidents.
- Provides a common operational structure for a wide variety of organizations and jurisdictions.
- Is applicable across a variety of disciplines, bringing them together to meet common goals and objectives.

Features of an incident command system

An incident command system is normally structured into five main functional areas:

- Command.
- Operations.
- Planning.
- Logistics.
- Administration.
- Finance.

Regardless of structure, any incident command system should have the following features:

- Common terminology.
  - Allows responder communication with clarity and common understanding.
- Modular organization.
  - Incident management is developed from command down, based on the size and complexity of the incident. Functions are activated or deactivated as the incident requires (scalable).
- Management by objectives.
  - Common goals are established for the incident, which lead to the development of strategies and tactics for each objective.
- Incident Action Plan.
  - Development of the Incident Action Plan (IAP) provides a means of communicating the incident objectives in a coherent manner, and elucidates both operational and support activities.
- Chain of command and unity of command.
  - Chain of command is the orderly lines of authority within the ranks of an incident management system. Unity of command requires that every individual have a single designated supervisor to whom they report at the incident.
- Joint or unified command.
  - In any incident involving multiple agencies, multiple geographic jurisdictions, or multiple agencies from multiple jurisdictions, unified command allows agencies to work together without loss of individual authority, legal responsibility, or accountability.
- Designated incident locations and facilities.
  - Depending on the type and complexity of the incident, a variety of incident locations and facilities may be established. These include establishment of control zones, mass casualty triage and treatment areas, decontamination corridors, command posts, responder rehabilitation sites, and any others that the incident dictates.
- Resource management.
  - Incident resources must be requested, dispatched, tracked, recovered, and accounted for. This also includes any necessary processes for reimbursement as may be appropriate. Resources include personnel, vehicles and equipment, expendable supplies,

and such facilities as may be necessary for the successful completion of the incident.

- Information and intelligence management.
- The incident-management system must have an orderly process for collection, recording, and dissemination of incident related information and intelligence. Integrated communications.
  - The development and use of a common communications plan will facilitate incident completion and enhance responder safety.
- Transfer of command.
  - Command should be established by the initial arriving responder, and it should be transferred as appropriate. Such transfer should be done face-to-face, with a briefing that ensures all appropriate information on the status of the incident is communicated for continued safe and effective operations.
- Accountability.

Effective accountability is paramount to responder safety at all levels of response. Included in effective accountability are the following principles:

- Check in. All arriving responders must check in to receive an assignment and to account for their presence at the incident.
- Unity of command. Each individual involved in the incident will report to only one supervisor.
- Span of control. Effective span of control is essential to both accountability and overall incident management. Supervisors must be able to manage and account for their assigned personnel. The span of control should range from three to seven subordinates for anyone with incident-management supervisory responsibility.

Resource tracking

Incident resources must be tracked from the point of ordering, through dispatch, to arrival at the incident, and then throughout deployment until they are recovered and returned to service.

Deployment

Personnel and equipment should respond only when requested, or dispatched by the appropriate incident authority. Resources not requested should be denied entry. Law enforcement may be necessary to enforce perimeters. The term *freelancing* is used to describe individuals or teams of responders who arrive at an incident without being properly requested, and should not be allowed.

Application of incident command to disaster management

Unlike an isolated incident, a disaster (defined as an incident that cannot be managed with mobilization of all readily available resources) is very unlikely to be managed solely from the incident site by a single response agency. Widespread geographic impact limits the ability to manage the incident from the scene. Each agency involved will have its own incident commander, and incident management system. This is a setting that requires unified command (UC). All necessary disciplines (fire, rescue, law enforcement, health and medical, public works, etc.) must work cooperatively to achieve their common goals. Command personnel assigned to a unified command post must have the authority to speak for their parent agencies with minimal need for consultation with other agency leadership. Each of the five main functional areas, or sections (command, operations, planning, logistics, administration and finance) should have representatives of each discipline. At the command level, each major jurisdiction involved should also be represented. Each functional section will have an assigned section chief, with each major discipline supplying deputy chiefs as necessary.

The modular nature of the ICS structure lends itself to expansion from a single incident location to a widespread or complex disaster scenario. This will require the establishment of a facility capable of supporting this expanded management structure, commonly termed an Emergency Operations Center (EOC) or, with multiple jurisdictions involved, a Joint Operations Center (JOC). Depending upon the particular scenario this may be in the proximity of the incident, but must be in a secure location, with infrastructure to support the disaster response operations.

In a widespread or complex incident, the IC/UC will have a support staff, commonly referred to as the command staff. This includes a safety officer, a public information officer, and a liaison officer. Each of these positions may require one or more assistants, from each discipline and/or jurisdiction involved. Depending on the phase of the incident, the spokesperson for each officer position may vary between individual assistants as appropriate.

- The Public Information Officer (PIO) is responsible for interfacing with the media and the general public, or with other agencies that have a need for information. Generally, only one PIO is assigned, but assistants from each discipline may be necessary to provide appropriate specific information. Any incident specific information released must be approved by the IC/UC. The establishment of a Joint Information Center (JIC) adjacent to the EOC or JOC may be particularly helpful when there are significant numbers of media needing updated information on an extended operation.
- The Safety Officer (SO) is responsible for establishment of the incident safety plan, and monitoring incident operations to advise the IC/UC of any incident specific safety concerns. Although the overall responsibility for incident and responder safety rests with the IC/UC and each supervisor, the SO is responsible for identifying any known hazards and putting in place a system for hazard identification and

mitigation. In a UC situation, there will be a single SO responsible for overall safety issues, and to coordinate with Assistant Safety Officers from other jurisdictions, functional agencies, and other governmental entities and nongovernmental organizations (NGOs) that may be involved. The SO has the emergency authority to stop an operation to mitigate a safety hazard or unsafe act.

- The Liaison Officer (LNO) is responsible for being the point of contact for other governmental agencies, NGOs, and/or private entities that may be assisting or cooperating with the resolution of the incident or disaster. Assistants from agencies involved in incident management under unified command may be assigned to the LNO to facilitate this coordination.

General staff

Each of the four remaining sections (operations, planning, logistics, and administration/finance) are referred to as the general staff and they report to the IC/UC. A section chief, with Deputy Chiefs assigned from each functional area or jurisdiction as necessary or appropriate, manages each section. The general staff is responsible for carrying out the goals and objectives as established by the IC/UC. Sections may be further subdivided into functional branches or units, and/or geographic divisions.

Operations section

The operations section is responsible for managing all tactical operations necessary at an incident to reduce or eliminate immediate hazards, save lives, and protect property and the environment, establish situational control, and restore normal operations. The need to expand the operations section is dictated by the number of tactical resources involved, and the variety of functional disciplines engaged. In order to maintain appropriate span of control, operations may be divided into a number of branches, divisions, and/or groups. Branches may be functional, such as a hazardous materials branch or represent a large geographic area in a widespread disaster scenario.

Under the operations section there may be a law enforcement branch, a medical branch, an air operations branch, and so on, all headed by an appropriate branch director. An incident or disaster may be further divided into physical or smaller geographic divisions (i.e. north division, river division, etc.) to maintain optimum safe operational span of control.

The operations section chief (OPS chief) is responsible to the IC/UC for direct management of all incident-related operational activities. The OPS chief will establish the specific tactical objectives for each operational period to meet or work toward meeting the established goals. In a multidisciplinary operation, there will usually be deputy OPS chiefs from each discipline to direct their part of the overall operation under the OPS chief. This maintains both span of control and unity of command at large or complex operations.

Planning section

The planning section is responsible for the collection, organization, and evaluation of incident-specific information and dissemination of this information to the IC/UC and incident-management personnel. The planning section is also responsible for preparation of incident status and situation reports, maintaining the status of incident resources, documentation of the incident action plan (IAP) based on guidance from the IC/UC, with information gathered from both the operations and logistics sections. The planning section chief (plans chief) reports to the IC/UC.

The planning section may be broken down into a variety of units, such as the resources unit, situation unit, demobilization unit, and documentation unit, each with it's own unit leader. Also assigned to the planning section may be a number of technical experts such as scientific support, epidemiologists, weather analysts, structural engineers, and other specialized expertise as may be needed to assist in evaluating the current and ongoing situation, evaluating data being collected, developing planning options, and forecasting resource requirements for further ongoing operations.

Logistics section

The logistics section is responsible for all support elements required to ensure effective and efficient incident management. This includes, but is not limited to, such things as facilities, equipment and equipment maintenance, fuel, personnel, supplies, food services, communications support, responder medical care and rehabilitation, transportation, and the distribution of necessary resources. The logistics section is also responsible for the establishment of staging areas for incoming equipment and supplies, and maintains the needed inventory of resources to support incident operations.

Within the logistics section, a variety of subsections, or units can be established as incident needs require. A medical unit can be established to oversee the medical needs of responders. This unit may be collocated with the rehabilitation unit. When resources from multiple agencies and/or jurisdictions are involved, a communications unit should be established to ensure that a common communications plan allows for information dissemination. A ground support unit may be necessary to handle fuel and maintenance issues that arise, ensuring that vehicles and equipment remain in service as needed.

Finance and administration section

The finance and administration section is activated when the scope or complexity of the incident requires financial accounting and administrative support. Although not all incidents will require establishing this section, accounting for personnel, equipment, supplies, and other essentials is easily overlooked and often difficult to reconstruct retrospectively. In the scenario of a widespread or complex disaster, tracking of resources assigned to the incident(s) will quickly overwhelm the command staff.

A procurement unit might be established to process resource orders identified by the resource unit in the planning section and approved by the incident commander as part of the incident action plan. As personnel and equipment are checked in to staging, their arrival may be communicated to a time unit who will track their time on scene. The demobilization unit will also notify the time unit when the incident commander releases those resources. This information then allows the compensation and claims unit to process the appropriate payroll information. This unit would also be responsible for the documentation necessary for any claims, such as responder injuries, that might arise in the course of the response. If necessary, a cost unit can be established to maintain a running tally of the overall cost associated with the resolution of an ongoing incident. This is sometimes referred to as the burn rate, and assists the command staff in making cost/benefit analysis and decisions concerning various strategic goals.

Summary

It is likely that a disaster scenario could involve multiple separate incidents of varying duration, geographic scope, and complexity. An incident management system is utilized to maximize efficient and effective management of a wide variety of emergency response incidents. The structure of the system can be as simple or complex as the incidents demand. The system can grow as the complexity of the incident response increases, adding additional functions as needed. As the incident comes under control and moves toward resolution, the incident management system can be contracted, combining units divisions and sections as appropriate.

A widespread or complex disaster, potentially comprising many individual incidents, spanning a large geographic area or spanning an extended period of time will require an elevated level of coordination. An emergency operations center can be established at the level necessary to coordinate competing demands for resources. The same principles of organization that apply to management of a single incident can be utilized to manage these multiple demands for resources.

Suggested readings

ICS 200 – *Incident Command System for Single Resources and Initial Action Incidents.* Emergency Management Institute, Federal Emergency Management Agency, United States Department of Homeland Security

ICS 300 – *Intermediate Incident Command for Expanding Incidents.* Emergency Management Institute, Federal Emergency Management Agency, United States Department of Homeland Security

ICS 400 – *Incident Command for Command and General Staff – Complex Incidents.* Emergency Management Institute, Federal Emergency Management Agency, United States Department of Homeland Security

Incident Command System for Emergency Medical Services. National Fire Academy, United States Fire Administration, Federal Emergency Management Agency, United States Department of Homeland Security

Integrated Emergency Management Course (IEMC). Emergency Management Institute, Federal Emergency Management Agency, United States Department of Homeland Security

ISC 100 – *Introduction to Incident Command System.* Emergency Management Institute, Federal Emergency Management Agency, United States Department of Homeland Security

Chapter 32

Mass sheltering

Michelle Daniel

Christopher Daniel

Introduction

- Disasters occur in many forms. Although each disaster is unique, they often have one critical element in common: large numbers of people may be forced to leave their homes. Shelter is critical to survival, and mass sheltering may be necessary to meet the basic needs of a population until it is safe to return home. There may be only a handful of families who need shelter or there may be hundreds of thousands of internally displaced persons or refugees seeking accommodation.
- Sheltering options in developed and developing nations vary significantly, as do the governing bodies, resources, and health concerns in each country.
- Most mass-care shelters in developed nations are intended to operate only for a limited time—days to weeks.
- Large-scale shelters or camps in developing nations often remain in place for extended time periods.
- While in operation, mass shelters must meet a multitude of human needs, both physical and psychological.

The best emergency shelters are established before the people arrive and have public health measures built into their design.

Agencies involved in mass sheltering

The primary disaster response agencies responsible for mass care operations in the United States are federal, state, and local governments, who generally use the American Red Cross and its subsidiaries to coordinate sheltering. Deployment of medical personnel in a mass sheltering scenario would fall under Emergency Support Functions #6 and 8 (refer to Chapter 33 through a primary agency such as the Federal Emergency Management Agency (FEMA,) or a state Department of Health.

Outside the United States, the major actors in mass-sheltering scenarios include national governments, agencies of the United Nations (UN), such as the Office for the Coordination of Humanitarian Assistance (OCHA), and the office of the United Nations High Commissioner for Refugees (UNHCR,) as well as other multilaterals like the International Committee of the Red Cross (ICRC) Medical personnel are often deployed as part of a nongovernmental organization (NGO) operating under the UN cluster system for coordination of sectoral responses to large-scale emergencies.

Facility and site selection considerations

Mass sheltering in the United States and other developed areas most commonly occurs within large public buildings, such as schools or halls, that have been designated in advance as appropriate sites. In less well-developed areas, or following the destruction of preplanned sites, shelters may need to be erected where none existed previously in the form of temporary camps. Several factors must be taken into consideration when choosing a shelter site:

- The site must be secure and should be located a safe distance from external threats (natural, man-made, and disease vector.)
- Adequate space must be available. The layout should take into consideration privacy, clustering according to family and community norms, as well as separate accommodation for single men, women, children, and special-needs victims.
- Proximity to an adequate supply of clean water is critical.
- Sanitation and solid waste services must be in place or easily implemented (i.e., pit latrines.) The toilets should be located a maximum of 50 meters from the dwelling. Ensure users are consulted regarding toilet design such that it is culturally appropriate.
- If a preexisting structure is to be used, it must be structurally sound. A professional assessment may be needed if the structure itself may have been affected by the disaster.
- Essential services should be accessible from the site (schools, child-care, places of worship, recreational facilities, and health care).
- Transportation, land, and market access are important for continuation or development of livelihood opportunities.
- A sufficient number of easily accessible emergency exits must be present.
- Heating, cooling, and ventilation should be considered. Needs vary by climate.
- Provisions for pets and livestock may be needed.
- Care should be given to minimize the long-term impact of the shelter on the environment. Existing plants and trees should be left in place when possible to reduce soil erosion.

Table 32.1 Minimum standards for use in shelter planning

Water (survival needs)	2.5–3 L per day (adjust for climate) per person
Water (basic hygiene)	2–6 L per day per person
Water (cooking)	3–6 L per day per person
Total basic water needs	7.5–15 L per day per person
Max users per water source	250 per tap with flow 7.5 L/min
	400 per open well with flow 12.5 L/min
	500 per hand-pump with flow 16.6 L/min
Covered floor space	3.5 m² per person
Total space	45 m² per person
Toilet/latrines	1 per 20 persons (ideal) 1 per 50 (max in acute phase)

Shelter registration

Upon arrival at the shelter, every individual should be registered. Preprinted shelter registration cards should be used if available. A shelter registration card should contain the following information:
- Name (including maiden name if applicable,) age, date of birth.
- Name of family members traveling with you.
- Predisaster address, planned post-disaster address.
- Date arrived in shelter, date departed.
- Health problems, allergies to medications, special needs.

Registration cards should be made in duplicate. One copy should be retained by the shelter occupant, and the other copy by the shelter manager. Shelter rosters may then be generated. A copy of this roster should be forwarded to coordinating agencies to assist in distribution of food and nonfood items (NFIs), and to assist in location of missing persons.

Food

Ensuring that shelter occupants have access to enough food, water, and other nonfood items to meet their basic needs is a critical role of mass shelters.

Food may be secured from readily available stockpiles used for government sponsored or other existing food aid programs. Food rations may come in dry or wet form, and may be prepared en mass or by individual families. In a shelter environment, where persons are displaced and have no access to any food at all, the distributed rations should meet a resident's total daily nutritional requirements. A generic basic ration should contain 2100 kcal (for complex adjustments, refer to Table 32.2) In disaster situations where residents are able to obtain some food by their own means, they should be encouraged to do so, so as not to foster dependency. The rations should then be planned to make up the difference between their nutritional requirements and what people can provide.

Food in disaster-affected areas must be properly stored and handled to prevent outbreaks of food borne illnesses. Persons affected by disasters are already at high risk of malnutrition, and the food they consume must be safe. Food-related disease outbreaks have been known to kill as many persons as the disaster itself. Inadequate washing, improper food handling, and incomplete cooking of food before consumption are the primary causes of food-borne disease. Shelf stable rations such as meals ready to eat (MREs) are the safest food items as they do not require cooking or handling. They are also particularly useful when there is a

Table 32.2 Nutritional recommended daily allowances (RDA)*

Age/Sex	Energy (kcal/d)	protein(g/d)	Fat (g/d)
Child 1–3 yrs	1300	16	45–58
Child 4–6 yrs	1800	24	40
Child 7–10 yrs	2000	28	45
♀ 11–50 yrs	2200	47	45–50
♀ 51+ yrs	1900	50	36–42
♂ 11–14 yrs	2500	45	50–56
♂ 15–18 yrs	3000	59	57–67
♂ 19–50	2900	60	55–65
♂ 51+	1900	63	36–42
Pregnant ♀	+ 300	+13	+6–7
Lactating ♀	+500	+18	+10–11

Source: Subcommittee on the Tenth Edition of the Recommended Dietary Allowances, Food and Nutrition Board, Commission on Life Sciences, National Research Council. *Recommended Dietary Allowances*, 10th ed.. Washington, DC: National Academy Press, 1989.

shortage of cooking fuel. Things to consider in food preparation and storage include:

- Food should be stored away from walls, and off the floor. Adequate food cover and ventilation is important. Food should be stored in sealed containers, and spills should be promptly cleaned to prevent attraction of pests, especially rats.
- Water should be boiled or otherwise treated before being consumed or used to make food.
- Any food suspected of being contaminated or spoiled should not be used.
- Food handlers should be trained in personal hygiene and hand-washing. Food handlers should not be suffering from any illness. Specifically, people with diarrhea, vomiting, jaundice, fever, sore throat, visible skin lesions, or discharge from the eyes, ears, or nose, should not handle food.
- Food should be thoroughly washed. Raw food (especially meat) preparation areas should be separate.
- Careful consideration should be given to refrigeration capacity, and food should never be allowed to sit out for prolonged periods.

As soon as families have reestablished their capacity to cook for themselves, food will most likely be distributed in the form of dry rations. People should be shown how to prepare the foods. They must also be instructed in cooking safety (open flames, hand hygiene, safe food handling, and adequate cooking / reheating techniques.)

Nonfood items (NFIs)

When populations are displaced following a disaster, loss of personal property ensues. People flee with few possessions and will require several basic nonfood items (NFIs) for survival. NFIs are typically supplied to shelter staff in kits or in bulk for distribution based on the number of shelter residents. NFI needs vary according to culture and context and should correspond to the needs of the population and climate. Items to consider include:

- Tarps, tents, plastic sheeting.
- Blankets, sleeping mats, impregnated mosquito nets.
- Soap (250 g per person per month) personal hygiene supplies (i.e. toothbrush, toothpaste, feminine products) towels, cloth diapers, laundry detergent.
- Jerry cans to collect drinking water.
- Clothing or material to make clothing and shoes.
- Cooking supplies (pots, plates, utensils, cups, stove / fuel).

Disease control and prevention

People who present to a shelter may be sick when they arrive. Primitive living conditions increase disease transmission via three major mechanisms: fecal-oral, respiratory droplet, and vector-borne spread. Public health measures are needed in mass-sheltering scenarios to help prevent the spread of disease. Basic measures include:

- Instructing residents on hand hygiene (posters, education sessions, megaphone announcements,) particularly in regard to toileting and food preparation.
- Ensuring an adequate supply of cleaning / disinfecting products and enlisting volunteers to assist in cleaning.
- Providing medical waste receptacles (sharps containers, red bags).
- Ensuring pest control (insect, rodent).
- Screening new arrivals for illness and malnutrition.
- Implementing disease and malnutrition surveillance within the shelter. Focusing future public-health efforts on the findings.

Mass shelters generally do not provide more than basic first-aid medical services. Arrangements should be made to transfer individuals who are acutely ill to appropriate medical facilities.

Specific health considerations

The five leading causes of death among internally displaced persons and refugees during complex humanitarian emergencies in developing nations are:

- Diarrhea/dehydration.
- Measles.
- Malaria.
- Acute respiratory infections.
- Malnutrition (which contributes to death from first four).

Diarrhea and dehydration are best prevented by ensuring an adequate supply of potable drinking water, good hand hygiene, and food handling practices, and good waste/sanitation systems. Children's feces tend to have the highest content of infectious agents, and proper diaper cleaning/feces disposal in designated areas is paramount. Fly control is also important. Flies land on feces and then land on food items. Shelter occupants should be educated on keeping their food covered and pesticide spraying may be indicated. An adequate supply of oral rehydration solution (ORS) should be on hand in shelters. Shelter staff should be trained in the proper administration of ORS.

Measles is spread by droplet transmission of the Rubeola virus. It is highly contagious. 90 percent of people sharing a living space with an index case will contract the virus. Extensive experience in humanitarian emergencies in developing countries has shown measles vaccination to be effective at saving lives. Measles vaccination should be part of the emergency relief effort following disasters in populations where measles vaccination rates are low. Mass shelters should be targeted for vaccination campaigns. All children ages 6 mo–5 yrs should be vaccinated. Where malnutrition rates are high, it may be prudent to extend vaccination to children ages 6–14 yrs. Any child immunized between 6 and 9 months of age should be re-immunized at 9 months. If insufficient vaccine is available, priority should be given to the malnourished and very young.

Vitamin A deficiency enhances the virulence of measles, and increases morbidity and mortality associated with the illness. Vitamin A supplementation (100,000 IU po for children < 12 months, 200,000 IU po for children > 12 months) can be administered simultaneous to measles vaccine in the same target population. Surveillance of camp populations for cases of measles is important. Symptoms include fever, cough, coryza, conjunctivitis, a generalized erythematous rash, and Koplik spots. Vaccines for other illnesses (diphtheria, pertussis, tetanus, TB, polio, meningitis, yellow fever, typhoid, etc.) are generally not indicated in the acute setting except in special circumstances.

Malaria cases may occur in greater numbers following disasters involving flooding. Malaria is a chronic threat in endemic regions and whenever possible, camps should be located away from mosquito habitats. Spraying with pesticides within camps may provide marginal benefits. Use of mosquito netting should be encouraged. Chemoprophylaxis is rarely feasible in the emergency setting, but should be considered during epidemics in immune naive groups and targeted populations (i.e., malnourished

Table 32.3 Micronutrient deficiency diseases

Micronutrient	Disease	Symptoms
Iron/B12	Anemia	Pallor, fatigue, weakness, dyspnea
Iodine	Hypothyroidism	Goiter, mental retardation
Vitamin A	Blindness Immune deficiency	Decreased night vision, frequent infections
Thiamine (B1)	Beriberi (wet/dry)	Cardiac dysfunction / CHF or neurologic disease
Niacin (B3)	Pellagra	Diarrhea, dermatitis, dementia
Vitamin C	Scurvy	Anemia, skin hemorrhages, gingivitis
Vitamin D	Rickets/ Osteomalacia	Impeded growth, long bone deformities, bone fragility

children.) Prompt identification and treatment of symptomatic individuals is important. Fever in an endemic area should be considered malaria until proven otherwise.

Acute respiratory infections may spread rapidly within mass shelters. Helping victims stay dry and warm helps prevent susceptibility to respiratory infections. Potential for outbreaks exist. During influenza season, consideration may be given to vaccination of shelter occupants. Tuberculosis is another common respiratory ailment among individuals in shelters. Cohorting of these individuals may be desirable to help reduce spread.

Providing for basic food needs as described in the previous section is important for preventing protein-energy malnutrition. Attention to micronutrients is also important. Outbreaks of scurvy, beriberi, and pellagra have been reported in internally displaced person camps. Screening of new arrivals for malnutrition using weight for height or arm circumference standards is important. Malnourished individuals should be targeted to receive additional rations. The formula for determining adequate caloric intake is: kcal/kg = (RDA for age x ideal weight) / actual weight. Periodic screening within the shelter or camp for malnutrition and micronutrient deficiencies is prudent. Breastfeeding should be encouraged.

Suggested readings

Famine-Affected, Refugee, and Displaced Populations: Recommendations for Public Health Issues. (1992). *CDC, MMWR, 41:* RR-13.
The Sphere Project Handbook: Chapter 4: Minimum standards in shelter, settlement, and Non-Food Items. http://www.sphereproject.org
Toole, MJ and Waldman, RJ (1993). Refugees and displaced persons: War, hunger, and public health. *JAMA 270* (5), Aug 4: , 600–605.
Toole, MJ and Waldman, RJ (1997). The public health aspects of complex humanitarian emergencies and refugee situations. *Annu. Rev. Public Health,* 18:283–312.
UNHCR Global Annual Health Report 2007. http://www.unhcr.org/48ee02984.pdf

The National Response Framework

Robert Gouglet

James Geiling

Introduction

The federal government has identified 15 "threats or hazards of national significance with high consequence" for national planning scenarios to help develop national preparedness standards. The challenge for any hospital or community that experiences a devastating disaster is that all support to the affected people and institutions begins with local response efforts, that is, all disasters are initially local events. With rare exceptions (terrorism), the response is stepwise, from local to substate regional to state to federal.

Any federal response to a disaster will be limited, both in time and in scope. Although the federal government can provide enormous resources (including the military) to respond to emergency events, these are most useful in undertaking a massive and prolonged response for a large-scale event such as Hurricane Katrina. Federal resources, conversely, cannot provide a rapid response to smaller events, and they are limited in scope in a way that makes them less suitable to respond to a nationwide event such as pandemic flu. It is unfair for us, then, to assume that the federal government will bail us out of any significant event that affects our community. It is our obligation as citizens, local planners, and state representatives to ensure that we are able to respond to the best of our abilities quickly and efficiently, beginning within our own communities.

Contrasting our past experiences in hurricane Katrina with our recent experiences in hurricanes Gustav and Ike, we learned that a well-coordinated and planned, multiagency, multijurisdictional response with all key partners is the only possible way to minimize illness, deaths, and suffering. It is essential for the federal government to work with all state and local partners to aid this country during catastrophic emergencies. By effectively coordinating responses, from local to substate to state to federal levels, only then can we say that we have done the most good for the most people in our nation with the resources available at the time of the incident. Coordination can lead to improved rather than delayed response, as shown in Figure 33.1.

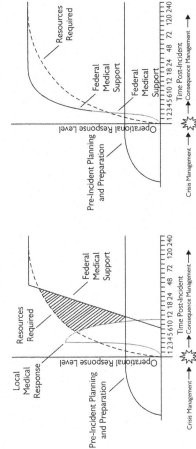

Figure 33.1 What happens when National Response Plan is delayed by lack of surge capacity for casualties or evacuation. Reprinted with permission from Rosen JM, Grigg EB, McKnight MF, et al. Transforming Medicine for Biodefense and Healthcare Delivery. *IEEE Engineering in Medicine and Biology Magazine* 2004; 23(1): 89 – 101. © 2004 IEEE. Reprinted, with permission, from *IEEE Engineering in Medicine and Biology Magazine.*

History of disaster response in the United States

In 1964, a large earthquake in Alaska caused major damage, and local resources were unable to meet the emergency response needs. Following this disaster, federal emergency management officials discussed what, in the future, should be the federal government's responsibility and ability to respond to such a disaster. This led to the enactment of the Disaster Relief Act of 1974, which described the procedure that state governors should follow to seek federal help in the event of any disaster. Later, in 1979, the Federal Emergency Management Agency (FEMA) was created; initially FEMA's role was to respond to Cold War needs, but in 1989, its scope was broadened to respond to any general disaster. Currently, the main law governing federal disaster response is the Robert T. Stafford Disaster Relief and Emergency Assistance Act (the Stafford Act), enacted in 1988. This law provides "an orderly and continuing means of assistance by the federal government to state and local governments in carrying out their responsibilities to alleviate the suffering and damage that result from such disasters"

Current response structure: Where do you call for help?

Calling 911 is currently the best way to ask for aid and to generate all levels of response in the event of an emergency. The agencies that may become involved at every level are described below.

Local and substate support

As a result of the Stafford act, response efforts to all disasters begin at the local level. Communities may develop Local Emergency Planning Committees (LEPCs), multiagency groups (hospitals, emergency management services, public works, law enforcement, fire and rescue, Red Cross, etc.) that oversee community response efforts. Other community resources or town/community emergency management agencies may augment these local committees. A variety of volunteer organizations may also be available to support community efforts; their participation, including their capabilities and limitations, must be integrated into any community disaster plan. The goal of these groups is to facilitate a multi-disciplined approach to the four phases of a disaster: mitigation, preparation, response, and recovery.

When community or city resources have been exhausted, state assets may need to be integrated in to the response effort. Initially, substate regions or counties may have capabilities to coordinate, re-allocate, or repurpose community assets in order to maximize the response at a local level. These regions may have additional assets of their own such as public health entities. New Hampshire, for example, has developed 19 all-hazards health regions with their own support for Neighborhood Health Clinics (NEHCs), for low-acuity patients; Points of Distribution (PODs), to distribute medications or vaccines; and Acute Care Centers (ACCs), to provide low levels of care for patients who require a bed.

Federal support may actually be available at the local or regional level in the form of the Department of Homeland Security's Medical Reserve Corps (MRC) or Community Emergency Response Teams (CERTs). These are medical and multidimensional teams, coordinated and trained with federal support under FEMA, but entirely designed to function independently at the local level to support community response efforts. DHS/FEMA also sponsors 124 Metropolitan Medical Response System (MMRS) programs to assist highly populated jurisdictions to develop plans, conduct training and exercises, and acquire pharmaceuticals and personal protective equipment, to achieve the enhanced capability necessary to respond to a mass casualty event caused by a WMD terrorist act. The MMRS system provides quick support to local jurisdictions until substantial additional support arrives. Finally, additional federal assets that might be available for local or statewide support include Department of Defense bases or medical treatment facilities as well as Veterans Affairs hospitals or clinics.

State support

After local, regional and substate emergency response systems have been activated, state resources are the next in line to respond to a local or statewide disaster. Each state may have its own organizational structure for its medical emergency management agency, but all states share commonalities of a defined Emergency Operations Center (EOC) designed to coordinate the state's resources of law enforcement, fire departments, hazardous material (HAZMAT) teams and public utilities. . Medical coordination varies with each state, but often includes the state's hospital association. States also have at their disposal the National Guard, whose organization includes the recently developed Weapons of Mass Destruction Civil Support Teams (WMD-CSTs), which are highly-resourced 22-person teams of active-duty guard members who respond to local events within 90 minutes at the direction of the state's Adjutant General and Governor.

When states are unable to provide support within their boundaries, they may be able to seek help from adjoining states through mutual-aid agreements without having to ask the federal government for assistance. Legislated in 1996 as Public Law 104-321, the Emergency Management Assistance Compact (EMAC) is a mutual aid agreement and partnership between states that exists because of the common threat from a variety of disasters; it is a legal mechanism and not an organization. Requests for EMAC assistance are legally binding contracts, permitting states to both ask for assistance, and provide available resources with a minimal amount of "bureaucratic wrangling." Table 33.1 shows local, substate, and state levels of support.

National support

Once local capabilities and state assets have been exhausted, a governor may ask for help from the federal government via the Stafford act. Although the federal government has many assets to support local and state efforts, federal resources take time to mobilize, and they have limited ability to respond to widespread and prolonged events, especially a pandemic. Some assets, from Department of Defense (DOD) for example, may not even be available due to other concurrent obligations and missions. The federal government, realizing its limitations, has made significant progress in working with its key partners in developing its disaster support plan for the nation. Disaster support from the national level has changed over the past several years, morphing from the Federal Response Plan to the National Response Plan to its current National Response Framework released in January 2008. The distinction between *federal* and *national* response is important; *federal* refers to the federal government only, whereas *national* means how we respond as a nation with all our resources, government and civilian, from local through state and federal governments. The current guidelines focus on a national response; a comprehensive, national, all-hazards approach to domestic incident response rather than isolating the plan to just the federal government's response effort.

The National Response Framework (NRF)

The National Response Framework is a guide that details how the United States conducts all-hazards response,,from the smallest incident to the largest catastrophe. This document establishes a comprehensive, national approach to domestic incident response. The framework identifies the key response principles, as well as the roles and structures that organize

Table 33.1 Examples of local, substate and state resources to complement federal aid

LOCAL	SUBSTATE (regions and counties)	STATE
Local Emergency Planning Committees (LEPC)	Neighborhood Health Clinics (NEHCs) for care of moderately ill patients	Emergency Operations Center (EOC)
Multiagency groups (hospitals, emergency management services, public works, law enforcement, fire and rescue, Red Cross, etc	Points of Distribution (PODs) for vaccinations and medicines	State's Hospital Association
Town/community emergency preparedness agencies	Acute Care Centers (ACCs) for patients requiring beds	Weapons of Mass Destruction Civil Support Teams (WMD-CSTs),
Volunteer groups	Federal Resources acting at the substate level:	Mutual Aid Agreements with other states (inter state aid)
	(1) Department of Homeland Security's Medical Reserve Corps (MRC) or Community Emergency Response Teams (CERTs): medical and multi-dimensional teams, coordinated by FEMA	(1) the Emergency Management Assistance Compact (EMAC)
	(2) Metropolitan Medical Response Systems	
	(3) DoD Bases or Medical facilities and VA hospitals and clinics.	

national response. It outlines how communities, states, the federal government, and private sector and nongovernmental partners apply these principles for a coordinated, effective national response. It describes special circumstances in which the federal government exercises a larger role, and lays the groundwork for first responders, decision makers and supporting entities to provide a unified national response.

The National Response Framework is designed to:

• Be scalable, flexible and adaptable.
• Always be in effect.
• Articulate clear roles and responsibilities among local, state, and federal officials.

The NRF is multidimensional: it contains the Emergency Support Function Annexes and Support Annexes, a total of 23 individual documents that describe operations, procedures, and structures for achieving response directives for all partners in fulfilling their roles under the NRF, including needed medical support and transportation, communications and other essential functions. See Table 33.2 below.

The outline of the NRF is shown in Figure 33.2.

Table 33.2 The 15 Essential Support Functions in the National Response Framework, their missions, and their coordinating agencies for emergency support.

Essential Support Function	Scope/Mission	Coordinating Federal Agency
ESF #1 - Transportation	• Aviation/airspace management and control Transportation safety • Restoration/recovery of transportation infrastructure • Movement restrictions • Damage and impact assessment	Department of Transportation (DOT)
ESF #2 - Communications	Coordination with telecommunications and information technology industries • Restoration and repair of telecommunications infrastructure • Protection, restoration, and sustainment of national cyber and IT resources • Oversight of communications within the federal incident management and response structures	Department of Homeland Security/National Communications System (DHS/NCS)
ESF #3 – Public Works and Engineering	• Infrastructure protection and emergency repair • Infrastructure restoration • Engineering services and construction management • Emergency contracting support for life-saving and life-sustaining services	Department of Defense/U.S. Army Corps of Engineers (DOD/USACE)

Table 33.2 (*Contd.*)

Essential Support Function	Scope/Mission	Coordinating Federal Agency
ESF #4 – Firefighting	• Coordination of federal firefighting activities • Support to wildland, rural, and urban firefighting operations	U.S. Department of Agriculture/Forest Service (USDA/FS)
ESF #5 – Emergency Management	• Coordination of incident management and response • Issuance of mission assignments • Resource and human capital • Incident action planning • Financial management	Dept of Homeland Security Federal Emergency Management Agency (DHS/FEMA)
ESF #6 – Mass Care, Emergency Assistance, Housing, and Human Services	• Mass care • Emergency assistance • Disaster housing • Human services	DHS/FEMA
ESF #7 – Logistics Management and Resource Support	• Comprehensive, national incident logistics planning, management, and sustainment capability • Resource support (facility space, office equipment and supplies, contracting services, etc.)	DHS/FEMA and General Services Administration (GSA)
ESF #8 – Public Health and Medical Services	• Public health • Medical • Mental health services • Mass fatality management	Health and Human Services (HHS)
ESF #9 – Search and Rescue	• Life-saving assistance • Search and rescue operations	DHS/FEMA
ESF #10 – Oil and Hazardous Materials Response	• Oil and hazardous materials (chemical, biological, radiological, etc.) response • Environmental short- and long-term cleanup	Environmental Protection Agency (EPA)

Table 33.2 (Contd.)

Essential Support Function	Scope/Mission	Coordinating Federal Agency
ESF #11 – Agriculture and Natural Resources	• Nutrition assistance • Animal and plant disease and pest response • Food safety and security • Natural and cultural resources and historic properties' protec-tion and restoration • Safety and well-being of house-hold pets	U.S. Department of Agriculture (USDA)
ESF #12 – Energy	• Energy infrastructure assessment, repair, restoration • Energy industry utilities coordina-tion • Energy forecast	U.S. Department of Energy (DOE)
ESF #13 – Public Safety and Security	• Facility and resource security • Security planning; technical re-source assistance • Public safety and security support • Support to access, traffic, and crowd control	Department of Justice (DOJ)
ESF #14 – Long-Term Community Recovery	Social and economic community impact assessment • Long-term community recovery assistance to States, local governments, and private sector • Analysis and review of mitigation program • Implementation	DHS/FEMA
ESF #15 – External Affairs	• Emergency public information and protective action guidance • Media and community relations • Congressional and international affairs • Tribal and insular affairs	DHS

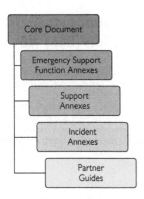

Figure 33.2 Sections of the National Response Framework.

Specific national medical support: Emergency Support Function (ESF) #8

Although medical leaders and providers must be aware of the multiple support capabilities outlined in the NRF, most will want to be thoroughly appraised of the specific medical assets within ESF 8, Public Health and Medical Services. ESF #8 also covers behavioral health needs, including mental health and substance abuse assistance for both incident victims and response workers; support for individuals who need additional medical response assistance; and support for veterinary and/or animal health issues. ESF #8 provides supplemental assistance to state, tribal, and local governments in the following core functional areas:

- Assessment of public health/medical needs.
- Health surveillance.
- Medical care personnel.
- Health/medical/veterinary equipment and supplies.
- Patient evacuation.
- Patient care.
- Safety and security of drugs, biologics, and medical devices.
- Blood and blood products.
- Food safety and security.
- Agriculture safety and security.
- All-hazard public health and medical consultation, technical assistance, and support.
- Behavioral health care.
- Public health and medical information.
- Vector control.
- Potable water/wastewater and solid waste disposal.
- Mass fatality management, victim identification, and decontaminating remains.
- Veterinary medical support.

The National Incident Management System (NIMS) and its relationship to NRF

NIMS integrates existing best practices into a consistent, nationwide, systematic approach to incident management that is applicable at all levels of government, nongovernmental organizations (NGOs), the private sector, and across functional disciplines in an all-hazards context. Five major components make up the NIMS approach:

- Preparedness.
- Communications and Information Management.
- Resource Management.
- Command and Management.
- Ongoing Management and Maintenance.

NIMS provides the template for the management of incidents, regardless of cause, size, location, or complexity. The National Response Framework is an all-hazards plan that builds upon the NIMS. The NRF provides the structure and mechanisms for national-level policy and operational direction for incident management to ensure timely and effective federal support to state, tribal, and local related activities. The NRF is applicable to all federal departments and agencies that participate in operations requiring a coordinated federal response.

Summary

The NRF is a functional guide to mobilizing the nation's capabilities to support a local disaster. Obtaining such support requires detailed planning at the local and state levels prior to seeking any help from the federal government, whose assets, though substantial, may take time to arrive, or may be committed elsewhere.

Local medical providers, therefore, must actively engage in disaster preparedness to mitigate the effects of any disaster on patients, staff, facilities, and their communities. In order to achieve optimal disaster preparedness, it is important to conduct a hazard vulnerability analysis (HVA) in order to prioritize planning efforts. No individual or organization operates in a vacuum, so providers must understand the organizational diagram of the facility, community, and state in order to effectively manage a response effort. Most follow the basic principles of the Incident Command System (ICS) under current National Incident Management System (NIMS) guidelines. Finally, although risks, capabilities and organization are important, no plan works without periodic, realistic training. Effective training ensures that local providers can best prepare to care for their patients, peers, and facilities until state or national resources arrive after a disaster event.

Key documents

National Response Framework (NRF): Delineates our Nation's response doctrine, responsibilities, and structures.

- National Incident Management System (NIMS): Establishes a systematic approach for managing incidents nationwide.
- ESF, Support, and Incident Annexes: Provide concept of operations, procedures, and structures for achieving response objectives.
- National Strategy for Homeland Security: Reflects the National Preparedness Guidelines, which include the National Planning Scenarios.
- Response Partner Guides: Provide a ready reference of key roles and actions for local, tribal, State, Federal, and private-sector response partners.

Suggested readings

Compilation of Laws and Basic Authorities, Robert T. Stafford Disaster Relief and Emergency Assistance Act, http://149.168.212.15/mitigation/Library/Stafford.pdf

http://www.FEMA.gov/NRF

http://www.ngb.army.mil/features/HomelandDefense/cst/factsheet.html

http://www.medicalreservecorps.gov/

http://www.citizencorps.gov/cert/

http://www.fema.gov/mmrs/

http://dms.dartmouth.edu/necep/projects/mmrs/

http://www.emacweb.org/

http://www.fema.gov/pdf/emergency/nrf/about_nrf.pdf

http://www.fema.gov/emergency/nims/

Pediatric concerns

Daniel B. Fagbuyi
Lou E. Romig

Introduction

Over the past decade, terrorism and natural disaster events have enabled society to begin to appreciate the necessity of disaster preparedness. Today, even with society's heightened awareness and lessons learned from previous disasters, the unique vulnerabilities and special needs of the pediatric population remain unaddressed in disaster plans at all levels of organizational emergency management.

Resources compiled by experts in the field of disaster medicine are available through the American Academy of Pediatrics (AAP), American College of Emergency Physicians (ACEP), Emergency Medical Services for Children (EMSC), Centers for Disease Control and Prevention (CDC), and many other organizations (Box 34.1).

Disaster characteristics

Disasters generally outstrip or overwhelm local resources and may or may not involve large numbers of victims. Some disasters occur without warning, whereas others are slow in onset and afford the opportunity to prepare for and mobilize resources prior to the incident. Disasters have a physical and psychological impact on people, especially children. Such psychological reactions are very pronounced in children regardless of proximity to the incident. For this reason, terrorists have targeted and continue to target children (e.g., schools, parks, sporting events).

Box 34.1 Internet resources for medical professionals and family disaster education and planning

FEMA Publications Library
http://www.fema.gov/library/prepandprev.shtm

FEMA for Kids
http://www.fema.gov/kids/index.htm

American Academy of Pediatrics (AAP)
http://www.aap.org/disasters/about.cfm

American Red Cross Community Disaster Education Materials
http://www.redcross.org/pubs/dspubs/cde.html

US Search and Rescue Taskforce
Family Disaster Planning
http://www.ussartf.org/family_disaster_planning.htm

National Disaster Education Coalition
Talking about Disaster: Family Disaster Plan
http://www.nfpa.org/Education/TalkingAboutDisaster/DisasterPlan/DisasterPlan.asp

Children are unique

Children differ from adults developmentally, anatomically, physiologically, immunologically, and psychologically. The various differences must be accounted for during disaster planning, triage, assessment, diagnosis, management, and disposition. Failure to address the pediatric differences in all areas of disaster preparation and management, either by omission or commission, may result in increased pediatric morbidity, mortality, or both.

Developmental

- Depending on the age, children are unable to localize pain or verbalize their symptoms.
- Children possess limited motor skills to flee from danger or incident site.
- Children have limited cognitive ability to identify a threat.
- Rely on parents/caregivers for food, clothing, and shelter.
- Unable to fully communicate their wants and needs.

Anatomical considerations

- Airway. The pediatric airway can be more difficult to secure and maintain. Children have large tongues compared to their oropharynx. The larynx is more anterior, and the narrowest portion of the airway is the cricoid ring. The short trachea and small lung volume place children at risk for airway compromise secondary to right mainstem bronchus intubation and pneumothorax from barotrauma.
- Children are shorter than adults and vulnerable to toxicity from agents that accumulate on the ground close to their breathing zone.
- Children have limited blood volume and fluid reserves compared to adults and are at risk for hypovolemic shock from blood loss or excessive vomiting and diarrhea. Depending on the age, estimated circulating blood volume in young children ranges from 70 to 90 ml/kg.
- Small body mass enables a greater amount of force to be transmitted per unit of body area with resultant multiple organ injury.
- Children have a more pliable skeleton that is not completely calcified, putting them at risk for underlying serious internal organ injuries.
- The head is the largest, heaviest part of a child's body and particularly vulnerable to injury in most traumatic mechanisms. The relatively thin skull offers little protection to the brain, and the weaker neck muscles may fail to stabilize the head and brain when subjected to outside force. The developing brain is vulnerable to shearing forces and the effects of toxins crossing the blood-brain barrier.
- Age-dependent anatomic radiographic differences make interpretation of x-ray films, especially cervical spine films, difficult to interpret. Injury to the pediatric cervical spine usually involves the upper cervical vertebra and ligaments.
- Body-surface area and skin keratinization differences in children place them at risk for hypothermia, severe burns, dehydration, and rapid systemic effects from toxin absorption.

Physiological considerations

- Cardiovascular collapse in the pediatric population is usually from respiratory compromise, whereas it is of cardiac origin in the adult. Careful attention to airway and respiratory status are paramount in the pediatric population. Remember the ABCs (Airway, Breathing, and Circulation).
- Children have higher minute ventilation than adults. This increased respiratory exchange allows for exposure to higher toxin doses (e.g., aerosolized nerve, chemical, or biological agents) over the same period of time. Children will often become symptomatic more rapidly.
- Children vigorously compensate for hypovolemia by increasing their heart rate and peripheral vascular resistance. Changes in blood pressure occur late in the sequence of shock. Providers not accustomed to caring for children may miss the earliest indicators of shock (tachycardia, altered skin perfusion and mental status changes). Failure to institute adequate fluid resuscitation in the pre-shock child may lead to rapid deterioration and a poor outcome.
- Fluid resuscitation and medication administration in children are based on weight in kilograms (kg). Moreover, it is difficult for providers with limited pediatric experience to estimate a child's weight without the use of some quick reference tool (e.g., Broselow™ Pediatric Emergency Tape).
- Careful attention must be paid to the type of fluid prepared for hydration (bolus) in children as hypotonic fluids can result in hyponatremia and seizures. Isotonic fluid is recommended.
- Pediatric vital signs vary with age. Health care providers should be able to rapidly interpret the vitals as normal or abnormal.

Immunological considerations

- Children are at increased risk for infection due to an immature immune system.
- Children are susceptible to many infectious agents. Certain agents, especially the biologicals, pose a significant threat to the pediatric population. Moreover, children have less herd immunity from rare agents or those that have been eradicated (e.g., smallpox).

Psychological considerations

- Psychological responses of children vary based on their stage of development, which encompasses age and cognition.
- Infants do not understand a disaster; their needs are primarily food, comfort, and a familiar caretaker.
- Toddlers and preschoolers understand to some extent and may react by mirroring the reactions of parents/family. In addition, some may exhibit regressive behaviors, muteness, tics, clinging, decreased appetite, and vomiting. Children at this stage also may reenact events through play.
- School age children understand and seem to have the most marked reactions including fear, anxiety, poor school performance, sleep problems, and sibling hostility in addition to somatic complaints including abdominal pain, vomiting, headache, constipation.

- Adolescents are fully cognizant of the causes and consequences of a disaster. Some, especially boys, feel invulnerable. Depression, suicide, risk-taking behaviors, and aggression may result.
- A child's personality, proximity to the event, experience of personal loss, and preexisting risk factors including prior exposure to traumatic event or disaster, dysfunctional family or background psychological illness place children at risk and may determine their psychological response and resiliency.

Children and families—pragmatic considerations

Emergency Medical Services (EMS), emergency departments (ED), hospitals, and clinics should consider the various unique needs of the pediatric patient well in advance of a disaster. Some of the areas of consideration include:

Equipment

- The availability of pediatric resuscitation equipment in sufficient quantities and sizes to handle large numbers of infants and children is of paramount importance, especially during a disaster.
- Neonatal and pediatric size-specific equipment likely to be required in a disaster includes endotracheal tubes and other airway devices, oxygen masks, bag-valve-mask devices, intravenous catheters, intraosseous devices, and equipment for spinal and fracture stabilization.
- Prior organization of pediatric equipment into size ranges, such as that promoted by the Broselow™ Tape's color-coding principles, is highly recommended for improved patient safety and provider confidence.

Triage

- Mass casualty or Multicasualty Incident (MCI) triage must be put into play when medical needs greatly outstrip the immediately available medical resources. Contrary to customary daily ED or EMS triage, MCI triage must seek to balance relatively scarce resources with overwhelming demands. The focus changes from doing the best for each patient to doing the best possible job for the greatest number of patients. Patients with grave injuries may not be treated because the resources they require may be better used to salvage a greater number of patients with lesser injuries. Children are not exempt from this process. The additional stress of having to make potential treat/not treat decisions about pediatric victims makes MCI triage even more psychologically difficult for those attempting to perform the task.
- MCI triage is probably best initiated using objective guidelines that can be easily and consistently used by providers in a chaotic and stressful environment. Such objective guidelines must address both adult and pediatric patients.
- A number of objective MCI triage tools are in used in the field and Emergency Departments around the world. Several tools specifically address pediatric needs (JumpSTART11, the Smart Tape™, the Sacco Triage Method™). Unfortunately, no existing MCI triage tool has been validated by clinical research on patients in MCI settings.
- The JumpSTART Pediatric MCI Triage© tool (Figure 34.1) is the method most commonly used by EMS agencies and Emergency Departments in the United States. It is the pediatric corollary to START (Simple Triage And Rapid Treatment) Triage™, the most commonly used adult tool. Both prioritize patients physiologically through a rapid assessment of the ability to ambulate, presence/

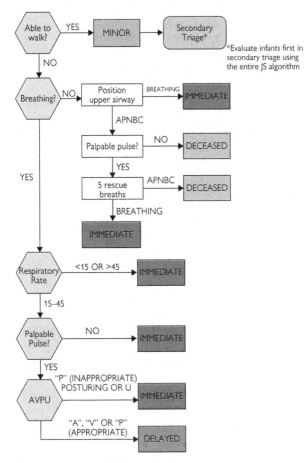

Figure 34.1 The JumpSTART pediatric MCI triage tool

absence of respirations, respiratory rate, perfusion, and mental status. Both are primary triage tools only, used for the initial gross sorting of victims. Further triage must take place as assessment and treatment resources become available.

• Field MCI triage must be accompanied by plans and systems for determining transport priorities of patients and should consider the most effective utilization of transport modalities and fixed medical facilities. In larger incidents, pediatric tertiary care resources should be utilized primarily for the most critical children, even if it means children with lesser injuries may need to be cared for initially at facilities less accustomed to caring for pediatric patients. Plans must acknowledge the fact that adults will refuse to be separated from their children and compromises in transport destinations may need to be made.

Decontamination

- In some types of disasters, victims require decontamination (decon) as a part of initial treatment and to avoid contaminating responders and care providers. Decontaminating children poses several unique problems:
  - Lack of ability to follow instructions to decontaminate themselves, thereby increasing the number of personnel needed to assist victims with the procedure.
  - Unaccompanied children require personnel-intensive direct supervision.
  - Families may not cooperate with instructions if it means separating family members.
  - Risk of hypothermia during and after the decon process.
  - Need for pediatric-appropriate postdecon garb.
  - Psychological consequences of the decon process.
- Available resources for planning for pediatric decontamination include "The Decontamination of Children," Agency for Healthcare Research and Quality (AHRQ)/Children's Hospital of Boston. DVD available from AHRQ.

Resuscitation and technical needs

- Intubation and intravenous access are not easy in the pediatric patient, especially those who present in shock. Technical skills need to be constantly refined.
- Alternative pediatric resuscitation equipment must be available and should include oro/nasopharyngeal and supraglottic airways and intraosseous access devices.
- In some types of chemical exposure, antidotes may need to be given by intramuscular (IM) injection due to time and other resource constraints. Although some pediatric autoinjectors are available, some antidotes will have to be administered using multi-dose vials and standard IM injection techniques.
- Pediatric patients requiring intensive resources for field and/or ED resuscitation attempts may be triaged as expectant in larger incidents and receive only comfort care when those resources are available. In a true disaster, patients in cardiac arrest are offered no treatment, regardless of their age.

Treatment

- Pediatric dosages are weight based. Pediatric-appropriate medications should be available.
- Terrorism-specific pediatric antidotes should be readily available, preferably with easy access to informational resources detailing

pediatric dosing and medication administration. One such resource is the Broselow™ Pediatric Antidotes for Chemical Warfare Tape which uses the same length-based color-coded approach as the Broselow™ Pediatric Emergency Tape.
- For disasters that require personal-protective equipment (PPE):
  - Provider dexterity may be compromised with reduced ability to successfully perform procedures.
  - Providers become dehydrated, experience heat-related illness, or both.

Reunification

- Children may be at day care, school, home, or in transit when a disaster strikes. Family, school, and community disaster plans should be clear, concise, and interwoven. Inevitably, there will be some children not reunited with their families. It is paramount that childcare centers, schools, community youth centers, and shelters, ensure a safe environment and keep in contact with local police and emergency responders while making every effort to contact guardians.

The aftermath

- Children are at increased risk for injuries after disasters as a result of:
  - Lack of adult supervision; preoccupation with recovery efforts.
  - Environmental hazards from collapsed structures, remodeling equipment, open chemical containers, sharp objects, and debris.
  - Unsecured firearms and other weapons used to protect personal property and interdict looting.
  - The use of open flames for light, heat, and cooking increases the risk of fire and burn injuries.
  - Motor-vehicle-related trauma may increase due to nonfunctioning traffic lights and intersection signage.
  - Child abuse and associated domestic-partner abuse in a stressful environment.
  - Lack of available supervisory resources such as day care and school.
- Children are at increased risk for illnesses and injuries after disasters.
  - Viral illnesses like Influenza, Rotavirus, Norovirus, Respiratory syncytial virus (RSV) spread rapidly in shelters or group homes.
  - Poor sanitary conditions after a disaster can increase the risk and spread of infectious diseases such as gastroenteritis.
  - Contaminated food or water can result in epidemic outbreaks of infectious diseases. Epidemics of cholera and typhoid, seen commonly in developing-country disasters, have not been seen postdisaster in the United States.
  - Postdisaster weather and the lack of usual environmental control may lead to hypo or hyperthermia, sunburn, and exposure to other environmental threats such as insects.
  - The unsafe use of alternative heating, cooking, and power generation sources can result in carbon monoxide exposure.
  - Environmental contaminants or stress can exacerbate asthma in children.

- Medication for chronic illnesses may be used up, forgotten, or destroyed in a disaster with resultant disease exacerbations.
- Stress in children can manifest as somatic complaints like headache, abdominal pain, appetite changes, vomiting, and chest pain.
- Children are at increased risk for psychological/behavioral problems.
  - Monitoring children for signs of mental illness after a disaster should be a part of recovery planning by families, school systems, social service agencies, primary-care providers, and mental-health professionals.
  - Most children have enough mental and emotional flexibility to adapt; they benefit from their ability to express their feelings freely, and they have fewer worries than adults who are trying to put their lives back together.
  - Children can suffer from acute and chronic emotional distress and mental illness after disasters. Many studies have shown that children may experience a variety of psychological sequelae, including posttraumatic stress disorder, even if they were not directly involved in the disaster themselves
  - In the immediate postdisaster stage, it is important to re-establish a sense of order and routine and to assure children that they are safe.
  - Expect regressive behaviors; children may wet the bed or cling to their parents instead of showing their usual independent spirit.
  - Rapid mood changes, interrupted sleep, and nightmares may occur.
  - It is important to explain a disaster to children in words they can understand, not to lie about loved ones or acquaintances that might have been injured or killed, and to encourage children to express their feelings through talk, play, or art.
  - Adults should express their own concerns and feelings in front of their children but shouldn't subject them to extreme emotional displays.
  - Children should be shown images of the disaster so they have an authentic picture of what happened, but this should be done in an environment that permits guided discussion.
  - Children should not watch television news clips that repeatedly display disturbing images or footage that graphically portray injury and death.
  - Children who exhibit signs of ongoing stress and depression, such as headaches, chronic abdominal pain, recurrent nightmares, changes in sleep patterns, deterioration in behavior or school performance, personality changes, drug abuse, or suicidal ideation should undergo full medical and psychological evaluation.
- Health-care dilemmas encountered by children and families.
  - Families may not have the ability to seek medical care for their ill or injured child in a timely manner.
  - Families may have lost their means of transportation or the transportation and road system may be disrupted so badly by damage or disaster relief traffic that a trip outside the area for medical care might take an entire day.

- Basic survival needs such as food, water, ice and other supplies may take precedence over seeking medical attention.
- Local medical treatment facilities may be nonoperational.
- Wound care is compromised in austere environments where water for bathing is in short supply and every-other-day wound checks are next to impossible.
- Compliance with medical follow-up depends on the availability of scarce resources. For instance, an asthmatic who needs frequent nebulizer treatments may have to be separated from loved ones so as to have access to a generator every few hours to comply with treatment recommendations.
- Pharmacies may not be open in the affected area; families may have to rely on being mobile to drop off and pick up prescriptions.
- Altered Emergency Department care
  - Emergency and primary care practitioners may need to change their usual prescribing patterns to accommodate family needs (e.g., 90-day prescriptions for chronic conditions).
  - Emergency and primary-care practitioners may have to admit children who would ordinarily be discharged with close outpatient follow-up.
  - Supplies for injury, illness prevention, and health maintenance may be distributed by hospitals to patient families and visitors.
  - Targeted patient and family education efforts should be increased in an environment in which access to care is restricted.
  - Disseminating safety and health tips, as well as the locations of temporary medical facilities and pharmacies in the local area to patients and their family members.

Special populations

The emergency medical services task force for children describes children with special health-care needs as "those who have or are at increased risk for a chronic physical, developmental, behavioral, or emotional condition and who also require health and related services of a type or amount beyond that required by children generally."

- Most are technology assisted children (vagal-nerve stimulator, cerebral-spinal-fluid shunt, gastrostomy-tube, tracheostomy-tube, etc).
- Consist of children with a broad spectrum of disease entities.
- ~15 million children in the United States.
- Most have unique health-care needs that may consist of medications and supportive health-care equipment (e.g., insulin, home ventilator).
- Extremely dependent on their parents, home-health-care providers, school teachers, school nurses, and primary-care provider.
- It is important not to separate the caregiver and child as they are very cognizant of what is normal for the child and able to provide the child's needs. Separation may result in a high-risk situation, converting a stable patient to unstable.
- The AAP and ACEP developed Emergency Information Forms (EIFs) to provide critical patient information to care providers when evaluating special-needs patients. It contains information about medications, allergies, settings for special medical equipment, patient's normal vital signs, diagnoses, child's and parent's languages, parent and physician contact phone numbers.
- Some examples include children with bronchopulmonary dysplasia (BPD), cyanotic heart disease (CHD), cerebral palsy (CP), hydrocephalus, spina bifida, cancer, HIV/AIDS, genetic disorders, and so on.

Pregnant women and the fetus

- Premature labor and delivery can emanate from the stress of a disaster or infection in utero.
- Radiation exposure in utero increases the child's risk for cancer.
- Fallout from nuclear and radiation settles on grazing grass and secondarily contaminates sources of nutrition.

Considerations for children with special health-care needs

- Families with children or other loved ones with special health-care needs must plan very carefully to meet those needs either with the assistance of a hospital or shelter or on their own.
- Extra equipment and supplies should be stocked and inventoried regularly, especially at the beginning of a disaster season.
- When sheltering in place during an anticipated event, arrangements should be made to have extra oxygen, batteries, replacement parts, medications, consumables, biohazard disposal equipment, generators and fuel delivered well in advance, with plans for automatic restocking as soon as possible after the event.

- Plans should include bug-out criteria, sets of circumstances under which the family absolutely must evacuate in order to assure their own safety and adequate medical care.
- Families evacuating from their homes must identify in advance where they will go.
- Some hospitals open their doors to shelter special-needs patients under the care of a few family members but cannot shelter entire families
- Some shelters depend on families to provide all equipment, supplies, and patient care, whereas others provide some level of skilled medical assistance and supplies.
- Third-party payers may also have protocols providing for special needs patients in disasters.
- Hospitals and emergency management agencies may have registries not only for special needs patients but also for those who are frail or might need assistance with evacuation. These registries often provide additional educational materials and preparedness checklists.

Role of the pediatric health-care provider

- Participate in community (especially school and day care), local (including hospital associations and pediatrician offices), state or federal-level efforts to establish response plans.
- Assist in developing protocols for offices and medical treatment facilities.
- Accept key role of identifying sentinel cases of illness.
- Educate colleagues and trainees on pediatric disaster management issues and medical response.
- Provide anticipatory guidance to families.
- Depending on type of disaster he/she may be tasked to:
  - Identify a bioterrorism event.
  - Identify specific agent/organism.
  - Prevent secondary cases.
  - Initiate appropriate therapy.
  - Prophylaxis when appropriate.
  - Communication with proper authorities.
  - Disseminate appropriate information to the public.

Liability during disasters (individual volunteerism)

- Be part of an organized program. Don't go solo.
- Most malpractice coverage is limited to the provider's scope of practice and practice setting.
- Good Samaritan statute varies among states. Check with your state.
- To be covered during a disaster, it is recommended to practice under the umbrella of an official disaster agency.

Summary

Children are at increased risk for injury and illness both during and after disasters. However, with the exception of the more sudden, violent types of disasters, most injuries and illnesses are in keeping with typical childhood patterns. Emergency and primary care providers in the postdisaster setting must be prepared to adjust their normal practices to conform to the constraints placed upon patients and their families because of the disaster. Mental-health issues have been frequently identified in pediatric disaster victims and may affect children and their families far beyond the time when physical injuries have healed. All child advocates must be aware of these potential problems and learn how to incorporate childhood mental-health surveillance and interventions into their ongoing disaster plans.

Table 34.1 Post-disaster Emergency Department constraints and altered decision patterns

Constraint	Altered Decision Patterns
Lack of electricity at home	• Prescribe metered dose inhalers with spacer chambers for inhaled medications • Provide a few power outlets or pressurized oxygen/room air tanks or outlets for use by families for aerosol treatments with their own medications (without undergoing the entire ED routine) • For younger children, prescribe chewable tablets and liquid medication preparations that do not require refrigeration. Consider non-chewable tablets and use of a pill cutter. • Lower admission threshold for children who require treatment with hard-wired electrical equipment.
Unavoidable environmental exposure	• Distribute sunscreen, sunburn care products, insect repellent, umbrellas, hats, disposable fans, chemical cold or hot packs. • Advise family of ongoing risks and the possible need to send the child away from the area. • Distribute safety literature about preventive measures and what to look for in cases of environmental illness.
Infectious diseases	• Consider parenteral antibiotic treatment as starter dose • Consider acceptable shorter course of antibiotics and increased dosing interval to improve compliance. • Consider need for isolation. Decrease admission threshold if child and family are living in a shelter environment and can't make alternative arrangements. • Demonstrate a child's ability to take and keep down fluids before discharge with gastroenteritis. Liberalize IV and/or formal oral rehydration practices and antiemetic administration. • Distribute oral rehydration solution, diapers, diaper wipes, alcohol-based hand cleansing solutions. • Distribute educational literature regarding measures to prevent spread of disease.
Poor follow-up/ decreased access to care	• Learn what temporary medical facilities have been set up in the affected area and ask patients to follow-up there if possible. Send a note with patient describing what care is needed. • Specifically instruct families as to what complications absolutely require further medical evaluation. • Distribute wound care supplies. • Instruct families in suture removal procedures • Confirm alternate contact methods (leaving message with relative, etc) for children discharged with test results pending, especially cultures. • Confirm actual current address (shelter, relative's house) as well as usual address. • Decrease admission decision thresholds for any condition that might require frequent follow-up or pose a risk of sudden deterioration.

Future directions

- There is need for formal curricula that focus on pediatric implications of bioterrorism and disaster.
- Enormous gaps exist in the understanding of how weapons of terror and the varied disasters affect children medically and psychologically.
- Research on antidotes or preventive agents for terror attacks are nonexistent.
- Participating in disaster drills/efforts, being informed and educated on disaster topics, and reviewing lessons learned from various disasters are first steps in preparedness.

Suggested readings

Aghababian R, ed. (2008). *Pediatric Disaster Life Support (PDLS©)*, 2nd ed. Worcester, MA: University of Massachussetts.

Curtis T, Miller BC, Berry EH (2000 Sept). Changes in reports and incidence of child abuse following natural disasters. *Child Abuse Negl. 24*(9):1151–1162.

Committee on Pediatric Emergency Medicine. American Academy of Pediatrics (1999 Oct). Emergency preparedness for children with special health care needs. *Pediatrics. 104*(4):e53.

Foltin G, Tunik M, Treiber M, et al. (2008). *Pediatric Prehospital Disaster Preparedness Resource*. New York: Center for Pediatric Emergency Medicine.

Hagan JF, Jr. (2005 Sept). Psychosocial implications of disaster or terrorism on children: a guide for the pediatrician. *Pediatrics. 116*(3):787–795.

Markenson D, Redl,ner I (2004). Pediatric terrorism preparedness national guidelines and recommendations: Findings of an evidenced-based consensus process. *Biosecur Bioterror, 2*(4):301–319.

Markenson D, Reynolds S (2006 Feb) The pediatrician and disaster preparedness. *Pediatrics, 117*(2):e340–362.

Pfefferbaum B, Gurwitch RH, McDonald NB, et al. (2000 Mar) Posttraumatic stress among young children after the death of a friend or acquaintance in a terrorist bombing. *Psychiatr Serv. 51*(3):386–388.

Pfefferbaum B, Nixon SJ, Tucker PM, et al. (1999 Nov)Posttraumatic stress responses in bereaved children after the Oklahoma City bombing. *J Am Acad Child Adolesc Psychiatry. 38*(11):1372–1379.

Pfefferbaum B, Seale TW, McDonald NB, et al. (2000 Winter). Posttraumatic stress two years after the Oklahoma City bombing in youths geographically distant from the explosion. *Psychiatry. 63*(4):358–370.

Romig LE (2002 Jul) Pediatric triage. A system to JumpSTART your triage of young patients at MCIs. *JEMS. 27*(7):52–58, 60–53.

Schonfeld DJ (2002 Jul). In times of crisis, what's a pediatrician to do? *Pediatrics.110*(1 Pt 1):165.

Schonfeld DJ (2002 Aug). Almost one year later: looking back and looking ahead. *J Dev Behav Pediatr. 23*(4):292–294.

Smith M. (2001 Mar). Get smart: jumpSTART! *Emerg Med Serv. 30*(5):46–48, 50.

Yule W, Bolton D, Udwin O, Boyle S, O'Ryan D, Nurrish J. (2000 May). The long-term psychological effects of a disaster experienced in adolescence: I: The incidence and course of PTSD. *J Child Psychol Psychiatry.41*(4):503–511.

Personal protective equipment

Liudvikas Jagminas

Introduction

Personal protective equipment (PPE) refers to garments, respiratory equipment, and other barrier materials used to protect first responders and medical personnel from exposure to chemical, biological, or nuclear hazards. Personal protective equipment is used during the primary decontamination of casualties at the scene, as well as by hospital personnel during the secondary decontamination process, and during the initial medical evaluation and stabilization.

Decontamination is defined as the reduction or removal of chemical, biological, or nuclear agents so they are no longer hazards. Agents may be removed by physical means or be neutralized chemically (detoxification). Decontamination of the skin is the primary concern, but decontamination of other systems must also be done when necessary. To ensure appropriate and timely patient care as well as optimal response, emergency personnel must understand decontamination procedures and the proper use of personal protective equipment.

Assessment, decontamination, and initial treatment of patients

Primary goals for emergency personnel in a hazardous materials incident:
- Establishment of decontamination zones; hot, warm, & cold zones (see Figure 35.1).
- Cessation of patient exposure.
- Patient stabilization.
- Containment of the hazard to prevent further contamination.
- Patient treatment without jeopardizing emergency personnel safety.

Although not all chemicals pose a hazard for secondary contamination, until the risk is known, prevention of exposure is best accomplished by removing the patient from the incident area and then decontaminating the patient. The essential requirements for any decontamination process include:
- Safe area to keep a patient while undergoing decontamination.
- Method for washing contaminants off a patient.
- Means of containing the rinsate.
- PPE (see Table 35.1) for personnel who are treating the patient.
- Disposable or cleanable medical equipment to treat the patient.

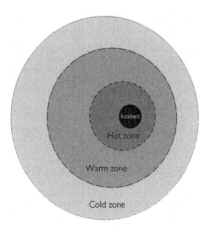

Figure 35.1 Decontamination zones.

Table 35.1 Personal protective equipment

	Description	Advantages	Disadvantages
Level A	Completely encapsulated suit and self-contained breathing apparatus (SCBA)	Highest level of protection available for both contact and inhaled threat High level of protection adequate for unknown environment entry, supplied air ensemble with increased mobility and dexterity	Expense and training requirements restrict use to hazardous materials response teams, lack of mobility, heat and other physical stresses, limited air supply time
Level B	Encapsulating suit or junctions/seams sealed, supplied air respirator or SCBA	High level of protection adequate for unknown environment entry, supplied air together with increased mobility and dexterity	Dependence on air line or limited air supply time; heat and physical stresses; expense and training significant; fit testing required
Level C	Splash suit and air-purifying respirator	Significantly increased mobility, decreased physical stress, extended operation time with high levels of protection against certain agents; no fit testing required for blood-type	Not adequate for some high concentration environments or less than atmospheric oxygen environments or high levels of splash contamination; expense and training minimal
Level D	Work clothes, including standard precautions for healthcare workers (e.g., gloves, splash protection)	Increased mobility, decreased physical stresses, extended operation time	Offers no protection against chemical or other agents; expense and training minimal

Establishment of decontamination zones

Hot zone
- Immediately dangerous to life or health.
- Level A personal protective equipment with self-contained breathing apparatus or supplied air respirator is required for first responders or other personnel.

Warm zone
- Uncontaminated environment into which contaminated victims, first responders, and equipment are brought.
- Adjacent to and upwind from the hot zone.
- Level C PPE is generally sufficient unless there is heavy contamination with liquid or powder.
- Vapor or aerosol exposure leaves no or minimal contaminant on victims, and material inhaled into the lungs is not exhaled to contaminate others.
- Victims exposed to biological aerosols pose little risk.

Cold zone
- Completely uncontaminated.
- Victims exposed to certain biological warfare agents may develop disease that can be transmitted to others. This situation poses a risk of secondary spread to medical personnel. The type of PPE required depends on the route of transmission of these infectious diseases.

Limitations of PPE

More protective levels of PPE are more difficult to use. Associated with potential limitations including:
- Time to don the suit and equipment: Level A PPE takes the longest.
- Impaired dexterity leading to difficulty in performing some life-saving interventions.
- Impaired mobility, especially with the use of a simple air-purifying respirator (SAR) because the wearer must retrace his or her steps along the supplied airline to exit hot zone.
- Impaired communication: Wearing a face piece or mask commonly results in poor speech intelligibility.
- Impaired vision: Face pieces may also limit the wearer's visual field.
- Heat stress: Encapsulation and moisture-impermeable materials lead to heat stress.
- Increased weight: Level A with SCBA is the heaviest PPE.
- Psychological stress: Encapsulation increases the psychological stress to wearers and patients.
- Limited duration of use: Wearing level A PPE for longer than 30 minutes is difficult.

Choice of PPE

- Whenever possible, select the level of PPE based on the known properties of the hazard. If the type of hazard is unknown, assume a worst-case exposure and use the highest level of adequate PPE.
- The primary consideration in selecting appropriate PPE is whether it will be worn in the hot zone (exclusion zone or contaminated area) or in the warm zone (contamination reduction zone or area where decontamination of patients takes place).

Known biological-warfare-agent hazards

- Personnel handling victims contaminated with bioterror (BT) agents require level C PPE and a powered air purifying respirator (PAPR) with a high-efficiency particulate air (HEPA) filter.
- When victims are contaminated with a known liquid or powder, Level D and PAPR with a HEPA filter are required until decontamination is complete.

Known chemical-warfare-agent hazards

- Personnel handling victims contaminated with chemical warfare agents require respiratory and skin protection.
- Level C PPE with PAPR and chemical cartridge is required until decontamination is complete.

Known radiation hazards

- No PPE is required if victims are exposed to external radiation and are not contaminated with a radiation-emitting source.
- All victims should be surveyed with a Geiger-Müller (G-M) counter.
- If contaminated externally with radioactive material (on their skin, hair, wounds, clothes), use level D PPE (for example, waterproof barrier materials, such as surgical gown, mask, gloves, leg, and/or shoe coverings; universal precautions) until decontamination is complete. Double layers of gloves and frequent changes of the outer layer help reduce the spread of radioactive material.
- Handle radioactive materials with tongs whenever possible.
- Lead aprons are cumbersome and do not protect against gamma or neutron radiation.
- Health-care workers should wear radiological dosimeters while working in a contaminated environment.
- When dealing with victims who are internally contaminated with radioactive material, wear latex gloves when handling body fluids (urine, feces, wound drainage).

Unknown hazards (Biological, Chemical, or Both)

- Level C PPE with PAPR (with organic vapor cartridge and HEPA filter) provides adequate protection until decontamination is complete.
- No single ensemble of PPE can protect emergency care personnel against all hazards.

Respiratory Droplet/Airborne Particles

- PAPR with HEPA filter provides the greatest degree of respiratory protection against biological-associated disease spread by respiratory droplet (such as smallpox or pneumonic plague) or airborne particles (possibly smallpox) when treating victims with obvious disease.
- Disposable HEPA filter masks also work.
- Medical personnel should wear latex gloves while handling the skin of people with smallpox, since smallpox may potentially be transmitted by contact with pox lesions that have not yet crusted over.

Blood or Body Fluid

- Level D PPE (standard precautions) is generally protective while in contact with victims who have contracted biological-associated disease spread by blood or body-fluid contact (hemorrhagic fever from Ebola, for example).
- Higher levels of protection may be necessary, however, if such victims have coughing or extensive bleeding.

Respirators

- Level C protection is the recommended minimum level of protection.
- If there is no information at all, then Level B protection is recommended.
- Powered air-purifying respirators are recommended over simple air-purifying respirators.
- Canisters should provide HEPA filtration and protection against organic vapor and acid gases at a minimum.
- FR57 canisters provide NIOSH-approved protection against organic vapors, acid gases, ammonia, methylamine, chlorine dioxide, HF, and formaldehyde; they are also effective in military testing against nerve agents, mustard, riot-control agents, cyanide, and acid-gas-related agents.

Suits

- If the threat is unknown, level B protection is suggested.
- An average person will take an XL suit at the smallest since flexibility of garments are minimal, and tearing is a concern if too small a suit is worn.
- Duct tape (or chemically resistant tape) can be used to reinforce the zipper front and crotch of the suit as additional protection.
- Tyvek SL™ offers moderate general protection against a majority of chemical agents, including nerve agents and mustard, but resistance to many organic agents is limited. This is probably a reasonable minimum level of protection for the healthcare decontamination setting.
- Tychem F™ offers improved protection against chemical and other BT agents.
- Tychem BR™ offers even a higher level of protection.
- For more information, visit http://personalprotection.dupont.com/ protectiveapparel/products/ applications.html

Booties
- Abrasion resistance booties are generally suggested since tearing of suit booties may go unnoticed.
- In the warm or cold zone, butyl rubber booties that can be pulled over shoes are sufficient protection.
- Junctions between the suit and booties should be taped with duct tape careful not to leave an opening.

Gloves
- Heavy butyl over gloves and thinner nitrile inner gloves offer protection against a broad range of agents, and are inexpensive.
- Cuffs should be long enough to reach at least 2 inches above the sleeve cuff.
- Silvershield™ inner gloves may also be used and provide additional protection against prolonged contact with halogenated hydrocarbons.
- Junction between gloves and suit should be sealed with duct tape.

Radiologic
- Standard suits block alpha and beta particles.
- Neither the suits nor radiology lead aprons are effective against gamma radiation.
- Inhaled radioactive dusts are generally well-controlled by a HEPA level filter.
- Decontamination personnel should have radiation badges or radiation pagers immediately available to their personnel as well as having G-M counters.

Critical Incident Stress Management

Situations involving large numbers of ill or injured individuals and situations that risk harm to the responder(s) are sources of critical incident stress. To minimize the occurrence of acute or long-term psychological consequences in response personnel, stress debriefing sessions should be held shortly after the incident. Acute stress reactions recognized during and after the incident should be immediately addressed by qualified peer debriefers or other mental-health professionals.

Suggested readings

Burgess JL, Kirk M, Borron SW, Cisek J (1999, Aug). Emergency department hazardous materials protocol for contaminated patients. *Ann Emerg Med 34*(2):205–212. [Medline].

Levitin HW, Siegelson HJ (1996, May). Hazardous materials. Disaster medical planning and response. *Emerg Med Clin North Am 14*(2):327–348. [Medline].

Macintyre AG, Christopher GW, Eitzen E Jr, et al. (2000, Jan). Weapons of mass destruction events with contaminated casualties: effective planning for health care facilities. *JAMA 283*(2):242–249. [Medline].

Occupational Safety and Health Administration. OSHA best practices for hospital-based first receivers of victims from mass casualty incidents involving the release of hazardous substances. OSHA. Available at www.osha.gov/dts/osta/bestpractices/ firstreceivers_hospital.pdf.

Stopford BM, Jevitt L, Ledgerwood M. Development of models for emergency preparedness: Personal protective equipment, decontamination, isolation/quarantine, and laboratory capacity. US Department of Health and Human Services. Available at http://www.ahrq.gov/research/devmodels/devmodels.pdf.

Wetter DC, Daniell WE, Treser CD (2001). Healthcare facility preparedness for victims of chemical or biological terrorism. *Am J Public Health 91*:710–716.

Chapter 36

Regional mass care

Anthony J. Tomassoni

Introduction

Regional mass care system stressors range in scope from daily emergency department overcrowding to catastrophic natural and manmade disasters. Disaster response requires leadership and coordination of resources in excess of those available in single organizations or localities—a regional approach. Regional systems must be ordered, resourced, and practiced while incorporating flexibility, creativity, and timely response. Pragmatic movement toward regionalization of disaster planning and response continues among legislators, grantors, public and private organizations, and individuals. Improved communication, planning, stockpiling, coordination of human and material resources, reduction of duplicative efforts, and economy of scale are a few benefits of regional planning.

Preparedness for disasters is a target goal never to be reached. Events that define disasters outstrip the resources available to address them. All incidents should be managed at the lowest organizational and jurisdictional level possible, though they may span numerous organizations and jurisdictions.

Multijurisdictional regions require a coordinating framework. States and regions must plan toward interfaces with national architecture to effectively integrate federal and out-of-state resources.

- National Response Framework (NRF).
- National Incident Management System (NIMS).
- National Response Coordination Center.
- Regional Response Coordination Center.
- Interagency Incident Management Group.
- Joint Field Office.
- Principal Federal Official.

Regions are the fundamental units of preparedness. Base the coordinated planning and response efforts on regional hazard-vulnerability analysis, capability and capacity assessments, and asset inventories to optimize resource allocation. Regional architecture should facilitate receipt and allocation of internal and external resources to minimize the cost of disasters in human and economic terms, facilitate recovery, study the results of interventions, and mitigate the effects of future disasters.

Despite improvements in preparedness across the nation, substantial improvements remain to be made. Municipalities and health-care organizations have reason to remain uneasy regarding current levels of preparedness. Coordinated integration of health-care delivery networks into the fabric of regional response remains incomplete; renewed focus on regional coordination of resources will bear dividends.

History

- The U.S. approach to emergency preparedness and response has traditionally relied upon localities. Governance is addressed at local, state, and federal levels, therefore, regional, multijurisdictional approaches to policy have been challenging.
- State and federal support systems had limited capacity to share in-depth expertise with individual localities before disasters.
- In some locations, public regional councils of governments and regional planning organizations have historically coordinated transportation and/or environmental planning. Some have coordinated recruitment, training, and operations of public safety personnel.
- Special needs intensified regional planning and response efforts. Past regional efforts to respond to hazardous-materials incidents (due to the Hazardous Waste Operations and Emergency Response Standard [HAZWOPER]) are an example.
- In 1997, the Metropolitan Medical Response System (MMRS) program began distributing funds to metropolitan areas to enhance capabilities to manage mass casualty incidents. The list of eligible areas has expanded and includes a rural tri-state model (Northern New England).
- MMRS addresses mass-casualty preparedness and response; provides structure for medical incident management; enhances mutual aid, regional collaboration, and capabilities; includes hospitals; and provides framework for funding from the Department of Homeland Security (DHS) and the U.S. Department of Health and Human Services (HHS).
- The events of 9/11/2001 heightened awareness of limited regional coordination and interoperability. Resulting homeland-security policy is a relatively new field.
- Subsequent expenditures of federal-preparedness funds highlight the magnitude of resources needed to prepare the nation and generate a focus on evolving regional-preparedness efforts. Examples include the State Homeland Security Grant Program, several programs from HHS, and the Urban Areas Security Initiative (UASI).
- Overhaul of federal and state response plans and incident management systems reinforced the need for regionalization of preparedness efforts. This resulted in facilitation of bidirectional information and resource flow.
- Federal funding catalyzed the trend toward regional planning. Awareness of the NRF, NIMS, wider understanding of the ICS, widespread implementation of the Hospital Incident Command System (HICS), and business continuity planning facilitated stronger regional collaboration.
- Subsequent large-scale natural disasters provided tests and feedback for system modifications in progress further highlighting the inherent advantages of regional ESF-8 planning, especially at the state/federal interface.
- Health-care organizations and providers, businesses, chambers of commerce, civic organizations and citizens are embracing larger, more

active roles in regional preparedness efforts and business continuity planning.

- Taken as a whole, these events have made regional and national programs dependent on regional resource coordination.

FEMA and HHS have regionalized operations, bringing federal resources closer to the site of disasters and improving the success of federal disaster response efforts. Although distinct from regional mutual-aid efforts in the traditional sense, this less-centralized structure has improved communications and coordination with affected localities.

Some current federal first-provider grant programs are intended, in part, to foster regional coordination and cooperation. Much more remains to be done. Regional coordination and cooperation maximize the effectiveness of scarce preparedness funds, eliminate duplication of effort, and build effective preparedness and response networks by combining and targeting federal, state, local, and private assets. Mutual-aid agreements, regional coordination plans, and interstate compacts such as the Emergency Management Assistance Compact (EMAC) facilitate regional coordination and reduce legal risk.

Scenario-based planning vs. all-hazards approach

In the recent past, an all-hazards approach to preparedness has often been advocated. Although the all-hazards approach is a useful starting place for building the backbone of disaster plans, filling gaps common to many scenarios, the merits of this approach have some limits. Scenario-specific gaps will remain. Scenarios to guide planning are available, and planning should proceed in priority order according to regional Hazard Vulnerability Assessment (HVA). Regional scenario-specific planning represents a next step in the evolution of disaster planning.

Size and boundaries for a region

Numerous determinants for optimal definition of a region exist. These vary by region. Some factors include service and administrative areas (EMS; trauma distribution; public health; hospital/hospital system; borough, city, county, or other governmental and nongovernmental divisions). These factors are further influenced by economic and social factors, population density, service availability (or lack thereof), law, natural and man-made geographic boundaries, travel patterns, infrastructure, and public perceptions of service quality and convenience available from competing suppliers. Regions defined by any of these single factors are seldom congruent and often independent of administrative areas (borough, city, county, etc.). In metropolitan areas, a "region" may consist of part or all of a city, whereas in rural areas a "region" may be better defined as part of a state (even considering interstate collaboration for some purposes). In defining regions, it is important to consider surge capacity and capabilities available/needed to respond to high impact and high probability disasters that may affect a prospective region as lines are considered. Planners may employ fundamentals of hazard vulnerability analysis, emergency management/business continuity using internal functions and governmentally defined Emergency Support Functions (ESFs) as starting points for their checklist.

Care must be exercised in comparing details of emergency planning among actual or prospective regions. The process is not straightforward, depending on population density, variable supplies of assets, travel patterns, utilization rates per capita for supplies and services, and other variables that must be controlled or normalized for accuracy.

Regional coordinating constructs

A regional coordinating entity may be designed to facilitate planning and response. In an established example of emergency response regionalization familiar to many hospitals, a hospital would be designated by the Local Emergency Planning Committee (LEPC) to receive patients contaminated with hazardous materials. That hospital would be obliged to have an emergency response plan, appropriate decontamination facilities, equipment (including personal protective equipment), and trained personnel as established under the Superfund Amendments and Reauthorization Act of 1986 (SARA) and the subsequent Occupational Safety and Health Administration (OSHA) HAZWOPER standard effective in 1990. Emergency-response drills are used to evaluate hazardous waste operations and emergency response standard (HAZWOPER) compliance. Of note, the Joint Commission requires accredited hospitals to implement their emergency response plan in a planned drill or in response to a real event twice yearly. The dual requirements may be fulfilled by properly configured combined drills to minimize costs and effort.

Trauma systems are also familiar examples of regional coordination. A well-developed trauma system illustrates many of the attributes of a regional coordination system for disaster preparedness and response. For example, the planning areas of Maine's three Regional Resource Centers for Public Health Emergency Preparedness were designed in collaboration with public health and hospital leaders to share geographic and social determinants of the state's trauma and hospital delivery network systems. Together they maintain practiced response patterns, equalize allocation of resources and populations served, facilitate contracts, and foster acceptance of the model.

Organizations sharing capabilities build regional plans and responses

Participation by diverse stakeholders/organizations/jurisdictions in regional forums provides opportunities to formulate regional problems and priorities, and to agree on potential solutions and resource allocation. Where collaboration is not well established, regulatory or financial inducements or incentives may lead stakeholders to engage in regional planning. Some federal grant programs require collaborative action or strategic planning on a regional scale; some allow flexibility to collaborate in ways optimized for regional circumstances.

Planning and resourcing processes must include **all partners,** and not solely those with whom relationships are established or alliances are convenient. These processes require individuals and organizations to champion relationship and planning development. Impartial consultants serve important functions when they guide, coordinate, facilitate and evaluate planning and training. However, paper plans constructed by consultants for an organization or a region defeat the purpose of planning; paper plans that reside on a shelf are neither understood nor implementable at the time of a disaster. The value of the knowledge gained, plans made and resourced, and interpersonal relationships developed through the planning process is inestimable.

It is incumbent on each organization within a region to understand the ways in which that organization will depend on others, and to prepare in advance for other-organization expectations in return. It is essential for partners to understand the limits of preparations and expected operations for each organization within a region and for all to understand the process and point of contact required to trigger the flow of regional resources, mutual aid, contracted assets, and state and federal assets when needed. Stakeholders may include, but are not limited to, the following:

- Interstate, state, county, tribal and local agencies and organizations.
- Hospitals (including VA hospitals), extended-care facilities, home-health agencies, urgent-care facilities, clinics, and their associations.
- Public health at each level, including public-health laboratory representatives and health educators.
- Public safety including emergency medical services, law enforcement, fire, HazMat and environmental representatives.
- Established mutual-aid partners.
- Emergency-management-agency representatives at each level.
- Homeland-security representatives.
- Primary-care and medical-specialty associations (emergency medicine, toxicology, infectious disease, pediatrics, geriatrics, psychiatry, trauma-advisory committees, etc.)
- Metropolitan Medical Response System representatives
- Disaster Medical Assistance Team (DMAT), Urban Search and Rescue (US&R) and Medical Reserve Corps (MRC) representatives.
- Public and private critical infrastructure owners and operators.
- Citizen Corps Council.
- National Guard/WMD-Civil Support Team representatives.

- Federal Bureau of Investigation/Joint Terrorist Task Force.
- Regional Poison Center.
- American Red Cross chapter representatives.
- Representatives from contiguous regions.

An extensive and cataloged portable contact database is a powerful tool for planners and responders. Coupled with effective and redundant communications devices, shared training, and exercises, it can turn the tide for a response.

Challenges to collaborations

Despite the apparent benefits of collaboration, challenges persist. Organizations or jurisdictions may cite loss of local control, jobs, or independence as barriers to collaboration. Lack of local or regional history of collaboration may be (at least in part) overcome by necessity, through the need to satisfy grant requirements, regulation or prescription, or even via partnerships built during emergent response. Few organizations have personnel in excess of those needed for routine operations to engage in preparedness planning.

Interorganizational competition for scarce resources may also prove problematic, particularly in difficult economic times or when a potential partner is perceived as resource rich. In the health-care arena, resource allocation to high-probability events may eclipse disaster preparedness needs (perceived as low-probability, high- consequence events). Competition for market share, labor issues, the need to focus on employee protection and concerns regarding liability also may provide challenges to collaboration in some settings.

Smaller localities have traditionally relied on mutual-aid agreements with similar neighbors, but they may be reluctant to enter agreements with large metropolitan areas for fear of losing rights to separate funding. Conversely, large metropolitan areas may be reluctant to enter agreements with surrounding localities because they often run at or near capacity on a daily basis and may be concerned about being overwhelmed in the event of a disaster.

Interagency differences of opinion about the merits of an all-hazards planning approach versus scenario-based approaches may place obstacles in the path to regional coordination and response. The frequent lack of sufficient interoperable communications equipment, protective items, and training heighten competition for funds. Shifting program-funding levels and lack of ongoing funds for maintenance or continued operations of emergency services, created with limited-time funds, raise serious questions among stakeholders about the sustainability of their efforts.

Processes in planning and response

For regions to engage in the emergency management cycle (mitigation, preparedness, disaster, response, recovery), provision must be made for stakeholders to engage in coordinated, concurrent processes of assessment, planning, education, organization (including command and control), budgeting, staffing, reporting, and reassessment to occur throughout the phases. The importance of developing relationships and interpersonal ties through these processes cannot be overemphasized. Familiarity and trust formed during planning and joint actions facilitate the flow of resources and operations during disasters and improve outcomes. Many case studies highlight the benefits of regional resource coordination and the value of the planning process even for the unexpected, including Maine's response to a covert chemical threat observed by the Centers for Disease Control and Prevention (CDC).

Community level planning and coordination

Decentralized positive action based on prior planning is the eventual goal of the disaster-planning process. It is not unusual for planners to underestimate the frequency and impact of disasters and to overestimate assets and response capacity/capabilities when planning. It is essential to tie plans to resources that exist under regional context and control even while planning for state and federal assistance, because all disasters begin locally (with "shock waves" that extend outward from the center of the disaster). Planners must anticipate actual behavior patterns learned from past disasters, avoiding false perceptions. When a region commits a specific resource to a particular job or purpose, the facts must be shared with planning partners to avoid conflicting allocations (example: multiple agencies planning for exclusive use of a meeting facility). In particular, volunteer staff may be overestimated because many potential volunteers may have accountability in public-service jobs or to multiple volunteer agencies.

True preparedness efforts must encompass all partners required to plan for and respond to the full spectrum of potential disasters that may befall a community. Allocation of scarce resources needed for mitigation and preparedness efforts must be based on formal hazard- vulnerability analysis, including likely worst-case scenarios. As first receivers and centers of community support, health-care organizations must be a focal point of preparation and response to disasters. Both the scope and magnitude of issues to be addressed in the creation of preparedness for any individual organization highlight that organization's dependence on other responding and supporting organizations within the region.

Although many names and structures have been given to organizations designed to foster collaboration, planning, and response, their functions and goals remain similar. Regional Resource Centers (e.g., Maine) or Centers of Excellence (e.g., Connecticut) for public-health emergency preparedness are, in effect, coordinating centers that bring together partners to facilitate regional planning for public health and health-care emergency planning and response. Such centers may be designed to accommodate any selected regional needs for coordination of efforts and resources, command and control, networking, regional standardization, and interoperability.

Coordination of resource utilization

Given an existing level of preparedness at a moment in time, one measure of success in response to a disaster occurring at that moment depends on the coordinated deployment of regional resources and effective recruitment of outside resources. In order to coordinate the expenditure of available resources within a region to the best and highest purposes during a disaster a collaborative approach must be set up in advance. Resources should be organized under a system that considers staffing, space for operations, and supplies for each responding entity, with contingency plans to cover the loss or evacuation of critical functions within the region. The pivotal tool is a shared and frequently exercised communications plan in which all partners understand the most appropriate initial information exchange that will enhance partners' awareness of challenges faced and trigger the optimal flow of resources.

Topic areas to consider for inclusion in a regional collaboration

Consider setting up work groups or task forces to address the planning needs of your region. Add other topics to reflect needs in your region.

- Regional hazard-vulnerability analysis and casualty prediction.
- Communications plan and redundant communications and IT networks.
- Interoperability.
- Risk communications and population warnings.
- Public health.
- Public safety.
- Emergency medical services.
- Health-care planning and response.
- Pediatric planning and response.
- Behavioral health planning and response.
- Occupational medicine planning and response.
- Ethical issues/allocation of scarce resources.
- Stockpile planning and management.
- Credentialing.
- Citizen corps/ESAR-VHP planning/volunteer and donation management.
- Training and exercises.
- Communicable-disease modeling and implications for staffing and service loads at the regional level.
- Triage planning.
- Planning for alternate health-care sites.
- Shelters.
- Evacuation planning.
- Mutual-aid planning and response.
- NIMS/ICS implementation and exercises.
- Incident management.
- Legal and legislative issues.
- Regional governance structure and continuity.
- Regional response planning and coordination.
- Regional response teams (HazMat, etc.).
- Informatics/cyber security.
- Critical infrastructure protection and business continuity.

Regional command and control

Regional command and control authority over operations should be planned and exercised in advance of an incident. The Incident Command System (ICS) should be followed, with clear lines of communication in place to initiate disaster-response mechanisms on-site and among partner organizations in order to trigger the appropriate cascade of resources. Lines of communication between the incident-site and health-care responders and receivers must be clear, with callers prepared to convey essential information such as the hazard(s) faced, number and type of victims, provisions for triage, and appropriate distribution of casualties among health-care facilities to optimize salvage. Clear specification of the agency/party responsible for this information transfer is essential to avoid system failure due to lack of notification and sufficient information to optimize response. Health-care facilities should have in place a dedicated link/liaison to the ICS structure to assure timely and accurate bidirectional flow of information. Additionally, both responders and receivers may expect to manage unexpected outside agency assistance and volunteers.

Upon forming or altering your regional planning and coordinating body, collaboratively designate and equip a robust regional Emergency Operations Center. Those who will occupy seats in the center during a disaster must drill in the center frequently enough to use the tools and communications devices available fluidly.

Practical considerations and steps to regional preparedness

- Focus proactively on regional planning for large-scale disasters, response-gap analysis, and gap closure; plan for concurrent emergencies.
- Triage available resources to close gaps in priority order according to HVA and highest yield in lives/property affected.
- Plan for the loss of infrastructure, including hospitals, which may be victims or targets themselves; plan for evacuation of health-care facilities and forward movement of patients from surges or evacuations.
- The strategic planning process is familiar to hospitals and other organizations; use it as a technique to engage organizations in regional efforts and to build relationships.
- Little surge capacity (and capability) exists in health-care organizations today; the creation of additional capacity and capability requires regional modeling, drilling, and exercising of mass casualty event plans.
- Gaps will remain despite preparations; plan to close high-priority gaps as resources are made available.
- Creative thinking and unconventional resource utilization can serve to close gaps, even when disasters strike in advance of preparations.
- Form one or more regional collaborative/regional resource centers to facilitate multiagency coordination regional training, drills, exercises, responses, and mitigation.
- Plan together to respond together; train as you will respond to real events and respond as you were trained.
- Ensure that organizations and collaboratives do not plan in isolation; include the needs of vulnerable populations.
- Update plans regularly; include principles of joint planning and response.
- Establish contracts (MOUs, MOAs, mutual-aid agreements) for facilities, goods, personnel, and services needed to avoid multiple claims on the same resource during a disaster.
- Practice joint training among responders/receivers within regions and in neighboring regions; assure clear lines of communication.
- Select interoperable communications, lifesaving and protective equipment; plan for alternate means of clear, high-volume communications.
- Strengthen critical regional infrastructure (e.g., hospitals, water supplies, etc.); provide for augmented security.
- Teach household preparedness and self-sufficiency to critical infrastructure staff and the public to cover the first 96 hours of an emergency.
- Develop and apply improved decision-analysis tools; test them in advance of major disasters.
- Prepare for the integration of regional and national resources in local contexts; consider resources such as DMAT, MMRS, medical strike teams, DMORT, and the strategic national stockpile, among others.

- Inventory pharmaceuticals and supplies that may be needed in the first hours of a disaster response before federal assets can reach the region; base purchases on regional HVA and immediacy of need.
- Agents that are expensive or infrequently used and that may be needed immediately following a disaster may lend themselves to regional stockpiling.
- Consider stockpiling supplies of those items needed emergently or urgently to protect responders, to save lives, and to stabilize victims: examples may include PPE, antidotes to chemical or radiological agents, trauma supplies, ventilators, antibiotics, antivirals, and more.
- Work with regional experts and state/federal officials to consider shelf-life extension for inventory that cannot be replaced.
- If vendor-managed inventory is used in lieu of stockpiling, assure that the correct inventory will be delivered in a relevant time frame upon demand; clarify details of payment and product specifications in advance.
- Locate regional assets where they will be accessible for transport throughout the region 24/7/365; consider potential obstacles to transport that may arise (floods, rail disasters, bridge outings, etc.).
- Plan for Temporary Medical Operations and Staging Areas (TMOSA) and/or Search and Rescue Base of Operations (SARBOO) areas where need may arise.
- Complete waste-and-debris management plans and related contracts.
- Complete regional emergency transportations plans and related contracts.
- Plan for critical-asset shortages that cannot be remedied; consider ethical and legal ramifications of altered standards of care; educate providers about potential need for altered standards and palliative care.
- Anticipate the need for public-risk communications messages; script likely messages in advance for adaptation at the time of a public health emergency; drill Joint Information Center (JIC) operations with partners.
- Use real events and responses as learning opportunities; refine avenues for command, control, and coordination.
- Use the tools and communications pathways you will use during disaster as frequently as possible in exercises or daily operations (e.g.,. triage tags, diversion plans); update public and professional emergency notification systems including the Health Alert Network.
- Share effective after-action review and mitigation processes in response to drills, exercises, and real events.
- Regional collaboratives and compacts continue to evolve as increasingly effective tools for coordinating preparedness and response despite the modest resources available to most regions.
- Become familiar with regional, state, and federal assets, tools, and procedures before a disaster strikes.

Conclusion

Regional planning for disasters is not complete until all partners' needs have been addressed, plans are fully developed, resourced, drilled, exercised, and revised until no links remain untested and resources are adequate for all predictable disaster scenarios that may befall the region.

Suggested readings

American Hospital Association. Model hospital mutual aid memorandum of understanding. Accessed at http://www.aha.org/aha/content/2002/pdf/ModelHospitalMou.pdf.

Federal Emergency Management Agency. (2004, August). *Are you ready? An In-depth guide to citizen preparedness.* Jessup, MD.

Auf der Heide E. (1989). Disaster response: Principles of preparation and coordination. Accessed at http://orgmail2.coe-dmha.org/dr/flash.htm.

Chaffee MW, Oster NS. (2006). The role of hospitals in disaster. In Ciottone G ed., *Disaster Medicine*, pp. 34–42. Elsevier, PA.

Clements B, Evans RG. (2004, January–February). Bioterrorism preparedness coordination: An ataxic saga continues. *Public Health Rep 119*(1): 16–18.

Dart RC, Borron SW, Caravati EM, Cobaugh DJ, et al. (2009, September). Expert consensus guidelines for stocking of antidotes in hospitals that provide emergency care. *Ann Emerg Med 54*(3):386–394.

Dart RC, Stark Y, Fulton B, et al. (1996). Insufficient stocking of poisoning antidotes in hospital emergency departments. *JAMA 276*:1508–1510.

Department of Homeland Security, FEMA Center for Domestic Preparedness, Anniston, AL website and multi-disciplinary course list at https://cdp.dhs.gov/.

Hick JL, Hanfling D, Burstein JL, et al. (2004, September). Health care facility and community strategies for patient care surge capacity. *Ann Emerg Med 44*(3): 253–261.

Hick JL (2005)Trauma systems and emergency preparedness: the hand bone's connected to the arm bone. *Acad Emerg Med 12*(9):875–878.

Joint Commission on Accreditation of Healthcare Organizations. (2007). Comprehensive accreditation manual for hospitals. Oakbrook Terrace, IL: Joint Commission on Accreditation of Healthcare Organizations.

Koh HK, Elqura LJ, Judge CM, et al. (2008, April). Regionalization of local public health systems in the era of preparedness. *Annu Rev Public Health 21*;29:205–218.

Olson D, Leitheiser A, Atchison C, et al. (2005). Public health and terrorism preparedness: Cross-border issues. *Public Health Rep 120*(1): 76–83.

Phillips SJ, Knebel A, eds. (2007, February). Mass medical care with scarce resources: A community planning guide. AHRQ Publication No. 07-0001. Agency for Healthcare Research and Quality, Rockville, MD. http://www.ahrq.gov/research/mce/.

Pinkowski J ed. (2008). *Disaster Management Handbook.* CRC Press, Taylor and Francis Group. Boca Raton, Fl.

Robinson R, McEntire DA, Weber RT. (2003).Texas homeland defense preparedness. The Century Foundation's homeland security project working group on federalism challenges. A Century Foundation Report, New York,. http://www.tcf.org/Publications/HomelandSecurity/robinson.pdf.

Root ED, Allpress JL, Cajka JC, Lambert SB, Savitz LA, Bernard SL. (2007). Emergency Preparedness Atlas: U.S.Nursing Home and Hospital Facilities. Prepared by RTI International under contract no. 290-00-0018. AHRQ Pub. No. 07-0029-2. Rockville, MD: Agency for Healthcare Research and Quality.

Rubinson L, Hick JL, Hanfling DG, et al. (2007). Definitive care for the critically ill during a disaster: a framework for optimizing critical care surge capacity: from a Task Force for Mass Critical Care summit meeting, January 26–27, Chicago, IL. Chest. 2008 May;133(5 Suppl):18S–31S.

Skolfield S, Lambert D, et al. (1997). Inadequate regional supplies of antidotes and medications for poisoning emergencies. *Clin Tox 35*(5).

Tomassoni AJ, Simone K, Watson W. (2004). Lessons learned from response to a covert chemical threat. *Clin Tox 42*(5).

Tomassoni AJ, Simone K. (2004). Development and use of a decentralized antidote stockpile in a rural state. *Clin Tox 42*(5).

Tomassoni AJ, et al. (2007). Analytical emergencies arising from atypical exposures: creative problem solving. *Clin Tox 45*(6): 629.

U.S. Department of Labor, Occupational Safety and Health Administration. Guidance on Preparing Workplaces for an Influenza Pandemic. OSHA 3327-02N 2007. www.osha.gov.

U.S. Department of Labor, Occupational Safety and Health Administration. (1997). Hospitals and community emergency response – What you need to know. Emergency Response Safety Series, OSHA 3152. http://www.osha.gov/SLTC/emergencypreparedness/general.html.

U.S. Department of Labor, Occupational Safety and Health Administration. (2005). OSHA best practices for hospital-based first receivers of victims from mass casualty incidents involving the release of hazardous substances. OSHA 3249-08N. http://www.osha.gov/dts/osta/bestpractices/html/hospital_firstreceivers.html

U.S. Department of Labor, Occupational Safety and Health Administration. (2007). Pandemic influenza preparedness and response guidance for healthcare workers and healthcare employers. OSHA 3328-05. http://www.osha.gov/Publications/3328-05-2007-English.html.

U.S. Government Accountability Office. (2004, September). Response to the chairman, committee on government reform, House of Representatives,. Homeland security: Effective regional coordination can enhance emergency preparedness.; 441 G Street NW, Room LM; Washington, D.C. 20548. To order by Voice: (202) 512-6000 TDD: (202) 512-2537 Fax: (202) 512-6061 www.gao.gov

Wineman NV, Braun BI, Barbera JA, et al. (2007). Assessing the integration of health center and community emergency preparedness and response planning. *Disaster Med Public Health Prep* 1(2):96–105.

The Preparedness Report - Archives 2004 to present

Yale New Haven Center for Emergency Preparedness and Disaster Response. 1 Church Street, 5th Floor; New Haven, CT 06510. (203) 688-3224. E-mail center@ynhh.org

http://www.ynhhs.org/emergency/commu/archives.html

American Red Cross National Headquarters

2025 E Street, NW

Washington, DC 20006

Phone: (202) 303-4498

www.redcross.org/pubs/dspubs/cde.html

Centers for Disease Control and Prevention

1600 Clifton Rd, Atlanta, GA 30333, U.S.A

Public Inquiries: (404) 639-3534 / (800) 311-3435

www.cdc.gov

Citizen Corps http://www.citizencorps.gov/

National Weather Service

1325 East West Highway

Silver Spring, MD 20910

www.nws.noaa.gov/education.html

U.S. Geological Survey Information Services

P.O. Box 25286

Denver, CO 80225

1 (888) 275-8747

www.usgs.gov

Provider mental health

Irving "Jake" Jacoby

Introduction

Mental-health considerations for disaster-response providers are an integral part of the disaster response. The responder who is most capable of dealing with the mental-health issues that arise during disaster responses is the responder who considers these issues for each phase of the disaster cycle.

Preparedness phase

Responders should be physically fit and have adequate training, immunizations, and appropriately fitted personal protective equipment (PPE) prior to any deployment. Hard hats, respirators, particulate masks, steel-toed footgear, and uniforms appropriate for anticipated missions and conditions are all essential in assuring the responders that their well-being is anticipated and being considered. Lists of items anticipated to be useful or necessary can help the responder be prepared for loss of utilities, power, communications, and standard sanitary supplies. Training responders to recognize that certain emotional and physical responses are normally expected during and following disasters can prepare them for dealing with such feelings and symptoms both in themselves and their colleagues during a deployment response. The resilient disaster responder is a prepared one.

Response phase

A significant need for disaster responders in the field is the ability to communicate with family members and loved ones. Knowing what is going on at home will allow responders to remain focused on their jobs and not distracted by personal concerns.

Monitoring responder well-being and facilitating responder safety are essential disaster-site functions. Disaster mental-health workers should be tasked to monitor team member responders for signs and symptoms of fatigue, depression, and critical-incident stress. Individual responders are often overlooked during a response. Box 37.1 lists characteristics of posttraumatic stress disorder (PTSD), and Box 37.2 lists clinical signs and symptoms that may be indicators of PTSD.

Enforcing work shifts to assure responders are getting adequate rest should be a priority for managers and team leaders. Proper diet, limiting junk-food consumption, and assuring adequate oral fluid intake to avoid hypotensive episodes, fainting, and heat-stress illness are essential to both physical and mental well-being. Use of a buddy system to have pairs of team members look out for each other can assist in monitoring personnel, may lead to early detection of critical incident stress, and forestall more serious issues.

At times, responders may also be victims, particularly when responding to incidents in their own community. Working while other family members have lost utilities, a home, or have become homeless can be distracting to a responder and can increase stress. Additional fears, such as exposure to corpses, infectious-disease agents, toxins, radiological agents, contaminated air or water, terrorism threats, or the occurrence of aftershocks during an earthquake response will add to incident stress levels,

---

Box 37.1 Aspects of Posttraumatic Stress Disorder

- Intrusive recollections of the trauma.
- Physiologic arousal.
- Numbing, withdrawal and avoidance.

Box 37.2 Signs and Symptoms of Possible Posttraumatic Stress Disorder

- Flashbacks.
- Memory disturbances.
- Traumatic dreams.
- Self-medication, especially alcohol.
- Anger, irritability, hostility.
- Withdrawal, persistent depression.
- Dazed or numb appearance.
- Panic attacks.
- Phobia formation.

particularly if the response system or agency is not providing adequate personnel protection. Other events that may trigger critical incident stress include the death of another provider in the line of duty, deaths or significant events involving children, or suicide of an emergency worker.

Recovery phase

Critical Incident Stress Management (CISM) programs are designed to prevent the development of dysfunctional and potentially disabling PTSDs. The medical literature has a growing number of attempted controlled trials and reports to assess whether Critical Incident Stress Debriefings (CISD) are successful. The complex nature of the process, superimposed on the complex personalities of providers and the variability in individual experiences, even during the same incident, has suggested the need for continued reporting of cases and other disaster data in addition to improved study design in future events.

Specifically, CISD refers to a 7-phase structured group meeting, usually within 10 days of the end of the deployment or crisis. It is designed to mitigate acute symptoms, assess the need for follow-up, and provide psychological closure to the event. Responders who have completed CISD and are identified as lacking closure, are referred for one-on-one psychological assessment, counseling or support, and other clinical interventions upon return home. The debriefings that are held are part of the continuum of CISM, and are not in themselves a replacement for longer-term interventions that some responders may need. Providers of such debriefings must undergo adequate and specific training. They may also benefit from accompanying other debriefers to gain some experience prior to taking on the task on their own.

Disasters can significantly impact the family members of responders. A disaster-responder's family may be exposed to the stress of often staying past the end of a shift, safety fears, and uncertainty about degree of involvement when incidents are broadcast by the media, disruption of family activities by response-related events, and interference of job-related emotional events with those of the family. Other stressors on families include dealing with symptoms being experienced by the responder to critical incidents and the impact of the stress that such interactions might have on children within the home. Symptoms of PTSD were reported in 50 percent of wives of firefighters involved in the response to the Oklahoma City Federal building bombing. Although the area of CISM has been developing and evolving in the last two decades, few programs address the CISD issues in family members. These programs should be of greater concern to planners, employers, EMS directors, and disaster managers.

CISD sessions should be a planned part of the demobilization plan under the Incident Command System for agencies and hospitals. Social workers, psychologists, and hospital psychiatry departments need to take a greater role in becoming involved in providing these services to community organizations and agencies.

Mitigation phase

Once an event has occurred, the postevent assessment, whether it be called a hotwash, an after-action meeting, or a critique, should include consideration of the following:

- Was an area designated for responders to rest and relax away from the patient flow (rehabilitation area)?
- Was a mechanism in place and were personnel assigned to detect signs of critical-incident stress in employee responders and providers?
- Was a procedure in place that enabled taking an individual off-line for a time period for rest and recuperation in a nonthreatening fashion?
- Was a group CISD session scheduled for employees? Their families? Is there a mechanism for referral if further psychological interventions are indicated?
- Were systems in place to address possible employee needs to maintain the workforce, such as child care for employee's children, special needs sheltering for dependent adults, and calling family members to assure their safety?
- Were the PPE and tools provided adequate for the hazards that had to be dealt with?
- Were emotional and safety concerns on the part of employee responders and their families anticipated such that standard, accurate answers were planned to be available for common concerns and questions? If not, were they produced in a timely fashion?

Negative responses to these items should be taken through appropriate channels and incorporated into the planning phase of the next disaster cycle. This will serve to mitigate them in future disaster events.

Suggested readings

Everly Jr. GS, Flannery Jr RB, Mitchell JT. (1999). Critical incident stress management (CISM): A review of the literature. *Aggression and Violent Behav* 5 (1): 23–40.

Everly Jr. GS, Lating JM, Mitchell JT. Innovations in group crisis intervention. In: Roberts AR, ed. *Crisis Intervention Handbook: Assessment, Treatment and Research*, 3rd ed, pp. 221–245. New York: Oxford University Press.

Mitchell JT, Everly GS (1997). Critical incident stress debriefing: An operations manual for CISD, defusing and other group crisis intervention services, 3rd ed. Ellicott City, MD: Chevron Publishing Corp.

Regehr C (2005). Crisis support for families of emergency responders. In: Roberts AR (Ed.), *Crisis Intervention Handbook: Assessment, Treatment and Research*, 3rd ed, pp. 246–261. New York: Oxford University Press..

Disaster triage

Carl H. Schultz

Alexis Lieser

Introduction

- Triage is the process of prioritizing patients for care after a mass casualty event, treating as many as possible with the limited resources available.
- The goal is to do the most good for the most people.
- Triage does not always direct care to those most critically injured but to those most likely to survive with emergent aid.
- Most current triage methods are based on limited evidence. With one exception, the performance of these systems has not been adequately evaluated in real disaster events.

Overview

Algorithms developed for triage of civilian populations after a natural disaster, bioterrorism attack, or other mass-casualty event can be classified broadly as primary or secondary triage systems.

- Primary triage systems are designed to assess patients in the field in order to determine who should be evaluated for further medical care and in what order. These systems rank victims by acuity.
- Secondary triage is designed to designate which patients will receive care, in what order, and whether initial care will be at medical facilities or in the field if there is a significant delay in transportation.

These systems incorporate not just acuity but also potential for survival with treatment. Secondary triage instruments will frequently recommend withholding care for patients with mild conditions and those critically ill with little chance of survival.

Brief history

- The word triage comes from the French word *trier*, meaning "to sort."
- Credit for initially developing the concept of triage is usually given to Napoleon's surgeon-in-chief Dominique Jean Larrey in the late seventeenth century.
- Multiple civilian triage systems exist today. The creation of these instruments mirrors the development of emergency medical systems in the early 1970s.
- Most current triage systems were developed by consensus with limited evidence supporting the various decision elements.
- Multiple countries have adopted related but unique triage systems (France, United Kingdom, Australia, United States).

Primary triage systems

Among the primary triage instruments, START is the most commonly used in the United States. JumpSTART was developed to include assessment of pediatric patients. CareFlight is used in parts of Australia, and some evidence exists that it is more specific for critical injury and faster to administer when applied to trauma patients. Triage Sieve is primarily used in the United Kingdom and is the accepted method for the North Atlantic Treaty Organization (NATO). Sacco Triage Method (STM) is a computer-based system that is the only empirically derived method. Except for STM, primary triage tools separate patients in four categories.

General primary triage categories

Black – decreased or expectant
- Dead or not expected to survive due to severity of illness or injury.

Red – immediate
- Life-threatening injury or illness requiring immediate intervention.

Yellow – delayed
- Significant by not immediately life threatening conditions.

Green – ambulatory
- Minor injuries.

Simple Triage And Rapid Treatment (START)
- Patient assessment within 60 seconds.
- Utilizes only two interventions during the triage process: direct pressure for bleeding and basic airway-opening maneuvers.

Red – any of the following
Nonambulatory patients with:
- Respirations > 30 breaths/min.
- No palpable radial pulse.
- Not able to follow commands.

Yellow
- Nonambulatory who do not meet black or red criteria.

Green
- Able to walk to a designated safe area for further assessment.

Black
- Not breathing despite one attempt to open the airway.
- Recent data from an actual disaster (train collision) suggest START has an acceptable level of undertriage (red sensitivity of 100% and green specificity of 90%) but moderate amounts of overtriage.

JumpSTART
- Modified version of START to assess children ages 1–8.
- Normal respiratory rate 15–40.
- Mental status measured by AVPU scale (Alert, responds to Voice, responds to Pain, Unresponsive).

CareFlight
- Similar to START method.
- Respiratory rate not evaluated.
- Assessment of mental status done prior to assessment of circulation.

Triage sieve
- Similar to START method.
- Does not measure level of consciousness.
- Includes heart rate >120 beats/minute and respiratory rate <10 or >29 as criteria for the immediate (red) category.
- Decreased sensitivity and specificity when compared with START or CareFlight triage.

Sacco Triage Method (STM)
- Computer-based system designed to estimate patient's chances of deterioration accounting for physiologic parameters and available resources.
- Sacco score calculated based on patient's respiratory rate, heart rate, and best motor response. Requires use of computer for calculations.
- Patients divided into three groups:
  - Group 1 - probability of survival <35 percent, high rate of deterioration.
  - Group 2 – probability of survival 49–85 percent, may deteriorate rapidly.
  - Group 3 – probability of survival >90 percent, slow deterioration.
- Includes incident command software to determine optimal EMS transportation strategy and alert hospitals of the number, severity, and scheduled arrival of patients. Software is proprietary and system may be expensive to implement

Secondary triage systems

Secondary triage instruments were developed to help health-care providers further prioritize victims for treatment with severely limited resources. Due to the nature of mass-casualty events, the treatment of patients may be significantly delayed either at the receiving hospital or in the field. Patients often have evolving injuries and will continue to deteriorate. Therefore, reassessment is often necessary using these instruments. Victims are assessed using secondary triage tools in the order of acuity assigned by primary triage.

Secondary Assessment of Victim Endpoint (SAVE)

- Main goal of SAVE triage is to estimate probability of survival and prioritize treatment of those who qualify for care.
- Treatment prioritized for those whose likelihood of survival is >50 percent, given available resources.
- Uses existing tools such as Glasgow Coma Score, limb-salvage score, and burn-survivability data to estimate probability of survival.
- Also will identify those who will not receive care.

Triage sort

- Secondary system for Triage Sieve.
- Uses Revised Trauma Score (Glasgow Coma Scale, blood pressure, respiratory rate).
- Patients within the initial immediate (red) category further divided into immediate, urgent, and delayed categories. Then yellow and green patients assessed.
- Only ranks patients by order of acuity. Does not consider probability of survival before assigning treatment.
- Does not weigh components of revised trauma score but treats all three components equally. This is less accurate.

Controversial issues

- In evaluating the accuracy of triage systems, objective measurement of outcomes currently uses two systems. One is based on the numerical injury severity scores (ISS), identifying immediate patients as having an ISS of 16 or greater. The other system identifies patient acuity using a resource utilization model. It remains unclear which of these approaches will become the standard.
- Data supporting the selected respiratory rates in various triage systems is lacking. Recent evidence suggests that rates of 30 for adults and 45 for children older than 2 may be excessive.

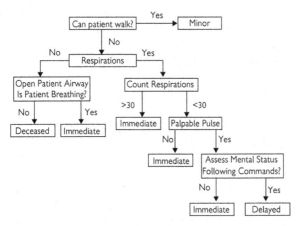

Figure 38.1 Modified START algorithm.

Table 38.1 Triage physiological parameters

	Ability to Walk	Ability to Breathe	Perfusion	Follows Commands	Motor Response
START	X	Respirations	Radial pulse	X	
Care Flight	X	Yes/No	Radial pulse	X	
Triage Sieve	X	Respirations	Cap refill		
STM		X	X		X

Suggested readings

Websites

- Critical Trauma and Illness Foundation START background
  - www.citmt.org/start/background.htm
- PowerPoint presentation on triage
  - http://www.emergencymed.co.za/powerpoint/5_7_06triage.ppt
- Newport Beach Fire Department START Triage FAQs
  - www.start-triage.com/START_TRIAGE.htm

Literature

- Al-Salamah MA, McDowell I, Stiell IG, Wells GA, Perry J, Al-Sultan M, Nesbitt L (2004). Initial emergency department trauma scores from the OPALS study: The case for the motor score in blunt trauma. *Acad Emerg Med* 11: 834–843.
- Baumann MR, Strout TD. (2005). Evaluation of the emergency severity index (3rd edition), Triage algorithm in pediatric patients. *Acad Emerg Med* 12: 219–224.
- Benson M, Koenig KL, Schultz CH. (1996). Disaster triage: START then SAVE. A new method of dynamic triage for victims of a catastrophic earhtquake. *Prehospital and Disaster Medicine*; 11(2): 117–124.
- Garner A, Lee A, Harrison K, Schultz CH. (2001). Comparative analysis of multiple-casualty incident triage algorithms. Ann Emerg Med 38(5): 541–548.
- Jenkins J, McCarthy M, Sauer L, Green B, Stuart S, Thomas T, Hsu, E. (2008). Mass-casualty triage: Time for evidence based approach. *Prehospital and Disaster Medicine* 23(1): 3–8.
- Kahn CA, Schultz CH, Miller KT, Anderson CL. (2009). Does START triage work? An outcomes assessment after a disaster. *Ann Emerg Med* 54: 424–430.
- Sacco WJ, Navin DM, Fiedler KE, Waddell II RK, Long WB, Buckman Jr RF. (2005).Precise formulation and evidence-based application of resource-constrained triage. *Acad Emerg Med*;12: 759–770.
- Tanabe P, et al. (2005). Refining emergency severity index triage criteria. *Acad Emerg Med* 12: 497–501.

Vulnerable populations

Alexander Wielaard

Andrew Milsten

Definitions

To be "vulnerable" in disaster-medicine terminology means having particular risk for physical or emotional damage due to a disastrous event. The damage is any loss of health, including disability, illness, or death. A "population" is any group of inhabitants occupying or making up an area or sharing a common characteristic.

Combining these two ideas, it follows that a "vulnerable population" is any group of people that share some common characteristic (medical or not) rendering them particularly susceptible to loss of health due to a disaster.

In disaster medicine, there is no official consensus regarding the definition of who should be considered vulnerable.

Why define them?

- Identifying at-risk individuals enables their special needs to be better addressed during predisaster planning in hopes of preventing illness and injury.
- A targeted emergency medical response based on a community's vulnerabilities can more effectively deliver appropriate medical care to those who need it most.
- More efficient allocation of emergency medical resources benefits all members of a population affected by a disaster.

Many factors contribute to an individual's ability to handle the challenges created by the stress of a disaster. This chapter will highlight common medical considerations; however, any complete discussion of health-care delivery should note the interaction between social, economic, cultural, and political factors.

Examples

Visually impaired
- Corrective lenses to legal blindness.

Problems
- Loss or damage to corrective lenses (contact lenses, eyeglasses).
- Loss or damage to assistive devices (walking sticks, canes).
- Care and well-being of service animals.
- ↓ access to transportation (e.g., unable to drive).
- Navigating unfamiliar routes.

Solutions
- Emergency supply of assistive devices.
- Verbally communicate written instructions.
- Tactile and Braille lettering, localizing tones.
- Braille mobile phones and two-way communicators.
- Service animals are NOT house pets.

Hearing impaired
- Hard of hearing to deafness.

Problems
- Loss or damage to hearing aids.
- Hearing aids ↑ volume of sound, not clarity.
- Understanding speech by some hearing-impaired individuals.
- Power outages → ↓nonverbal communication.
- Literacy levels may vary.

Solutions
- Simple written communications (5th grade level).
- Centrally located signs (symbols, illustrations).
- Captioning of televised alerts and updates.
- Basic nonverbal communication (pen and paper).
- Sign-language interpreters.

Mobility impaired
- ↓ independent mobility.
- Crutches, canes, walkers, or wheelchairs.

Problems
- Loss or damage to assistive devices.
- Environmental factors (debris, flooding, stairs) → ↓mobility.
- ↑risk for falls.
- ↓mobility → ↓ ability to evacuate

Solutions
- Wheelchair accessibility (vehicles, shelters, stair-descent devices).
- Fall precautions.
- Availability of medical assistive equipment.
- Physical assistance when necessary (1 and 2 person carries).

Cognitive impairment
- Mental retardation.
- Learning disabilities, dyslexia.
- Dementia and Alzheimer's disease.

Problems
- Variable levels of understanding, communication.

Solutions
- Early identification and screening.
- Simple, clear instructions.
- Varied, redundant modes of communication (written, verbal, pictorial).
- Specialized aid workers, emergency personnel.

Language barriers
Problems
- Illiteracy spectrum.
- Non-native language speakers.

Solutions
- Simple written communication (5th grade level).
- Universal signage and symbols.
- Foreign-language translators.

Psychiatric illness
- Schizophrenia, Depression, Anxiety, PTSD.

Problems
- Interrupted medical therapy.
- ↑ circumstantial stress.
- ↓ social support (therapists, family, friends)
- Schizophrenia may ↑paranoia toward government, aid workers.
- PTSD → flashbacks of previous disasters (ex. Hurricane-endemic areas).

Solutions
- Expect ↑ after a disaster
- ↑ availability of counselors, therapists, support groups.
- Aggressive antidepressants, anxiolytics, mood stabilization.

Chemically dependent
- Physiologic dependency: ethanol, opiates.

Problems
- Interrupted supply (alcohol, opiates) → withdrawal.
- EtOH withdrawal → DTs, seizures.
- Opiate withdrawal → GI disturbances, diaphoresis, generalized pain.
- Illegal activity → ↑reluctance to seek aid.
- ↑co-morbid mood disorders.

Solutions
- Access to aggressive medical Rx for withdrawal (EtOH).
- Substance abuse counseling.
- Rx of mood disorders.

Acute medical conditions

When a disaster strikes, patients in the acute phase of an illness may be ill-equipped to care for themselves due to the challenges of the event as well as the consequence of their acute illness.

- ↓ familiarity with medical situation.
- ↑acute functional limitation.

Examples

- Recently postoperative patients (wound care, pain).
- Orthopedic injuries (crutches, fixators, splints).
- Ongoing outpatient rehabilitation needs → delayed recovery.
- *Contagious illnesses need to be identified early for appropriate infection control (influenza, tuberculosis, Neisseria meningitis, etc).*

Chronic medical conditions

Examples

- End-stage renal disease → need for ongoing dialysis.
- Chronic lung disease →oxygen supply.
- Asthma →inhaler/MDI need.
- Cancer patients →chemotherapy, neutropenic infection control.
- HIV→antiretroviral medications.
- IDDM→ insulin, glucometer, test strips, regular meals.
- Ostomy patients →ostomy care supplies.
- Morbid Obesity →mobility and access limitations.
- Example: 1999 – Hurricane Floyd struck the North Carolina coastline →flooding and closure of 21 outpatient dialysis and chemotherapy centers. Patients had to be routed to additional facilities, some many miles away

Elderly and nursing home residents

Problems

- ↑risk for injury   ↑recovery time.
- ↑chronic medical conditions (polypharmacy, lost medical records).
- ↑ socioeconomic limitations (fixed income, social isolation).
- ↑visual, hearing impairments.
- ↓mobility (↓balance, strength, exercise tolerance).
- ↓transportation options.
- *Functional capacity in and out of home is NOT equal.*
- Dementia, Alzheimer's, Parkinsonism →cognitive, functional limitations.
- Nursing homes →↑↑ functional needs.

Nursing homes face significant challenges as they balance the risks and benefits associated with emergency evacuations. Residents often require relocation into living arrangements with very specialized equipment and staff, possibly for an extended duration.

- *Elderly receive a ↓ amount of appropriate aid.*
  - Counseling and social resources offered.
  - Financial and housing assistance most needed.
- Falsely assumed to be financially secure.
- Reality: underinsured, ↓creditworthiness, ↓ reserve.

Solutions

- Redundant, appropriate communication.
- Priorities are housing and financial aid.
- ↑outreach programs to *offer* help, rather than meet requests.
- Strengthen and employ specific elderly service organizations.
- Anticipate ↑ need for medical access.

Homeless and shelter-dependent

Problems

- Socially marginalized.
- Poor/delicate support systems.
- ↓use of mass communication.
- ↓mobility restrictions.
- ↑ isolation.
- ↑psychiatric comorbidities.
- ↑chronic medical conditions.
- *Domestic violence victims residing in specialized shelters need a continued source of safe and supportive housing.*

Solutions

- Coordination with existing local agencies and community support resources.

Legal offenders

Examples

- Prison inmates.
- Ex-convicts.
- Offenders "at large."

Problems

- Evacuation of incarcerated populations →large-scale operations.
- Fear of arrest/persecution →↓ evacuation, ↓acceptance of aid.

Solutions

- Facilitate a nonjudgmental emergency response.
- Ensure the security of ALL people involved.

Transients and tourists

Problems

- Isolated, high-risk areas   mountains, beaches, historical structures.
- Unfamiliar environment.
- Separation from usual support networks.
- Language problems.
- ↓knowledge of local emergency procedures.
- ↓personal reserves → ↓food, water, and clothing.

Solutions

- Predisaster planning with travel agencies, resorts, and embassies.
- Targeted emergency communications.
- Repatriation insurance.

Pregnant and lactating women
* ↓mobility.
* Milk/formula → storage/supply.
* Dietary needs.

Chemically and environmentally sensitive
* ↑environmental exposures.
* Bites and stings→ epi-pens!
* Dust, mold, and pollen.
* Food →allergies, vegetarians, Kosher needs.
* Detergents, soaps, and perfumes.
* Latex.

Group sheltering and mass distribution of aid supplies requires consideration of these factors. If possible, these individuals should bring personal supplies with them upon evacuation. When possible, emergency rations should be fragrance, dye, and irritant-free.

Disaster planning issues

* Considering special-needs characteristics can identify commonly overlooked areas during design of emergency response systems.
* In certain communities, a significant majority of the whole population might be identified as vulnerable using these criteria, rendering the definition meaningless as it pertains to efficient resource allocation.

2005 Hurricanes Katrina and Rita

* Special-needs groups consisted of greater than 50 percent of the U.S. Gulf Coast population.
* raditional definitions of *vulnerable populations* during emergency planning contributed to imprecision in the disaster response.
* To address the issues, new concepts in disaster management advocate for a paradigm shift toward a more applicable definition of vulnerable populations.

C-MIST

- Categories of *functional* vulnerability (again not mutually exclusive).
  - **Communication** – limitations involving receipt of or effective response to information.
  - **Medical** – acute or chronic medical conditions that impair adaptability to a disaster (including control of contagious illnesses).
  - **Independence** – a disability to maintain basic functional independence during all phases of a disaster.
  - **Supervision** – related to a circumstantial decrease in social support on which individuals normally rely.
  - **Transportation** – impaired mobility needed for effective response to emergency situations.
- C-MIST attempts to ↓complexity of traditional vulnerability.
- ↑flexibility for varied populations and events.
- ↑the efficacy of disaster responses.
- Not prospectively validated.

Suggested readings

Aldrich N, Benson W. (2008, January). Disaster preparedness and the chronic disease needs of vulnerable older adults. *Preventing Chronic Disease 5*(1).

California Governor's Office of Emergency Services (2000 May). Meeting the needs of vulnerable people in times of disaster: A guide for emergency managers.

CDC Health Aging Program. Accessed at www.cdc.gov/aging/pdf/disaster_planning_goal.pdf.

Fernandez LS, Byard D, Lin CC, Benson S, Barbera JA (2002). Frail elderly as disaster victims: Emergency management strategies. *Prehosp Disaster Med 17*(2):67–74.

Lubit, Roy MD, PhD (2005). After the tsunami - Human rights of vulnerable populations.. Acute treatment of disaster survivors. Berkely, CA: Human Rights Center Univ. California at Berkeley Accessed at , www.emedicine.com/med/topic3540.htm

Public health workbook to define, locate and reach special, vulnerable and at risk populations in an emergency. Accessed at www.bt.cdc.gov/workbook/pdf/ph_workbook_draft.pdf

Vulnerable Population Links and Resources List. Accessed at http://www.preparenow.org/pop.html/

The White House. (2006). The federal response to hurricane Katrina: Lessons learned. Washington DC. Accessed at http://www.whitehouse.gov/reports/katrina-lessonslearned.pdf.

World Bank Disability and Development Team. Report of the online forum on disabled and other vulnerable people in natural disasters.

Part 5

Special Considerations in Disaster Management

Research in disaster and triage settings

COL John McManus

Introduction

Investigators must be familiar with and adhere to all legal and ethical obligations prior to conducting any type of research. Researchers in both the civilian sector and military-related tactical environments have an ethical obligation to allow potential participants to have input into actions that affect them.

Basic ethical principles established by the 1979 Belmont Report:

- Beneficence.
- Justice.
- Respect for persons (autonomy).

Examples of controversial research investigations conducted prior to the Belmont Report:

- The Continental Army's use of compulsory variolation (exposure of uninfected individuals to matter from smallpox lesions).
- The use of an experimental cholera vaccine on nonconsenting prisoners located in the American-occupied Philippines during the Spanish-American War, resulting in 13 deaths.
- The infamous Tuskegee Syphilis Study in which subjects were denied treatment and were misled after being diagnosed with secondary syphilis.
- Nazi war experiments such as sterilization of men and women without their permission or knowledge by use of radiation, injection of an irritating solution, or surgical procedures.

Although these and other past military-sponsored research practices engendered distrust toward Federal medical institutions, these events have become some of the most influential in shaping public perceptions of research and fostering the government's role in human subjects' protection. Indeed, at the conclusion of World War II, the Nuremberg Medical Trial became "the most important historical forum for questioning the permissible limits of human experimentation."

The Nuremberg Code and research ethics

The Nuremburg Code was the first international standard for the conduct of research on human subjects and was affirmed in 1954 in the United States when the Army Surgeon General's Office issued a memorandum for human subject protection during research, becoming one of the first official documents to guide the conduct of human experimentation by military researchers.

Currently, there exist stringent regulations that must be followed to conduct research on soldiers and civilians on the battlefield and in tactical situations. This chapter serves as an introduction and brief overview of some of the terms and regulations that concern the conduct of research in the tactical environment; many of these principles are also directly applicable to research conducted in disaster environments. Prior to beginning any type of research, the authors recommend seeking guidance from local authorities that govern the conduct of all animal and human research.

Definition of human subjects research

Federal regulations define *research* as:

> A systematic investigation, including research development, testing, and evaluation, designed to develop or contribute to generalizable knowledge.
> or
> Human subjects research is any research or clinical investigation involving human subjects.

Research includes studies that involve patient interviews, follow-up contact of patients to determine the effectiveness of a program or a treatment, chart review, analysis of computer-stored clinical and administrative data, and mailed questionnaires. Additionally, randomized trials of experimental drugs, devices, and procedures must be reviewed and approved by the Institutional Review Boards (IRB) because there is contribution to generalizable knowledge.

Federal regulations governing human subjects research:
- Department of Health and Human Services (HHS) regulations 45 CFR Part 46.
- FDA regulations 21 CFR Part 50 and 56.

What is a human subject?
HHS regulations define a human subject as a living individual about whom an investigator conducting research obtains:
- Data through intervention or interaction with the individual or
- Identifiable private information.

Federal law requires review of research involving human subjects. The laws and regulations regarding research on human subjects have specific requirements for IRB and study administrators. To ensure no ethical or legal violations occur during the conduct of research, the authors recommend that all human-subject research and all other activities, that, in part, involve human-subject research, regardless of sponsorship, must be reviewed and approved by an IRB prior to initiation.

Institutional Review Board
An IRB is charged with protecting the rights and welfare of people involved in research and reviews plans for research involving human and animal subjects. Institutions that accept research funding from the federal government must have an IRB to review all research involving human subjects (even if a given research project does not involve federal funds). The Food and Drug Administration (FDA) and the Office of Protection from Research Risks (part of the National Institutes of Health) set the guidelines and regulations governing human-subject research and IRBs.

An IRB is a committee usually within a university or other organization consisting of at least five members of varying backgrounds.

An IRB must have members with the following affiliations:
• At least one scientist member.
• At least one member whose primary concerns are nonscientific.
• Additionally, there must be one member who is not otherwise affiliated with the institution (a community representative).

The IRB reviews the proposals before a project is submitted to a funding agency to determine if the research project follows the ethical principles and federal regulations for the protection of human subjects. The IRB has the authority to approve, disapprove, or require modifications of these projects.

Rules and regulations for conducting military research

The foundation for the Department of Defense (DOD) rules and regulations governing the conduct of human-subject research is primarily based on the regulations that govern all federally funded research. DOD regulations apply whether research is conducted on the battlefield, in a foreign theater of operations or within medical treatment facilities in the United States.

In 1974, the Department of Health and Human Services (DHHS) drafted the 45 Code of Federal Regulations (CFR) Part 46, Protection of Human Subjects, which governed human research protection. This policy was revised to include specific protections for pregnant women and fetuses (Subpart B), prisoners (Subpart C), and children (Subpart D). It was finally adopted by 17 other federal agencies to include the Department of Defense in 1991 and became known as "The Common Rule."

The Common Rule incorporates the Belmont principles of beneficence, justice, and respect, and it requires that an Institutional Review Board approve all human-subject research before implementation of the study.

In 1972, prior to the establishment of 45 CFR § 46, Congress inserted into appropriation bills the 10 U.S.C. § 980 requirement for the DOD entitled "Limitations on Use of Humans as Experimental Subjects." This code required the process of informed consent to be obtained in advance for all DOD funded research. 10 USC § 980 states:

> Funds appropriated by the DOD may not be used for research involving a human being as an experimental subject unless 1) the informed consent of the subject is obtained in advance; or 2) in the case of research intended to be beneficial to the subject, the informed consent of the subject or a legal representative of the subject is obtained in advance.

Informed consent and the waiver process

Amended three times by 1985, the most current version of USC 980 was amended to allow for an exceptional waiver by the Secretary of Defense of the advance informed consent process if a research project would:
1. Directly benefit subjects.
2. Advance the development of a medical product necessary to the military.
3. Be carried out per all laws and regulations including those pertinent to the Food and Drug Administration (FDA).

This change allowed the conduct of specific emergency research to be carried out under the provisions of the Emergency Research Consent Waiver, 61 Federal Register 51531–51533. Legal interpretation of 10 USC § 980 stipulates that, for cases in which surrogate consent must be obtained, the IRB must determine if the research is intended to benefit all subjects. This interpretation has limited DOD participation in placebo-controlled studies or those that involve a standard-of-care arm, for which surrogate consent is required and participants may not receive any direct benefit.

Human-subject research by DOD agencies is also impacted by FDA regulations that govern investigational drugs and devices. The 21 CFR §56 governs the function and responsibilities of the IRB reviewing and approving human studies, including those involving investigational drugs, while 21 CFR §50 specifically addresses the requirements and elements of the informed consent process. DOD Directive 6200.2, "Use of Investigational New Drugs for Force Health Protection," establishes policy and assigns responsibility for compliance for the use of investigational new drugs for force health protection and designates the Secretary of the Army as the DOD executive agent.

Likewise, there are more specific regulations and directives that govern DOD research that delineate unique issues to the DOD than the more general Office of Human Research Protections regulations.

- 32 CFR § 219, "Protection of Human Subjects" is the DOD version of the Common Rule.
- DOD Directive 3216.2, "Protection of Human Subjects and Adherence to Ethical Standards in DOD-Supported Research" was updated in December 2002 and provides updated changes from other federal regulations.
- DOD Directive 6000.8, "Funding and Administration of Clinical Investigation Programs," updates DOD policy and responsibilities regarding the administration and funding of clinical investigation programs in military medical and dental treatment facilities and the Uniformed Services University of the Health Sciences.

Within each branch of the military, there are more service-specific regulations that govern different types of human-subject research. Army Regulation 70–25, "Use of Volunteers as Subjects of Research," also governs the conduct of research within the Army Medical Research and Materiel Command (MRMC). This provides more specific restrictions on the recruitment, consent, and payment of volunteers to which the investigator must adhere during the conduct of the study. The conduct of research at any U.S. Army medical treatment facility is specifically governed by Army Regulation 40–38, "Clinical Investigation Program" that adheres to DOD, FDA, and OHRP federal regulations.

Tactical research considerations

As with combat research, there are several regulations and rules that apply to research conducted in the civilian environment. These regulations can be obtained on the HHS web site at: http://www.hhs.gov/ohrp/ However, one topic worthy of discussion is research conducted on prisoners and detainees. The current military policy is that no research shall be conducted in the combat zone on detainees.

However, in the civilian sector, certain types of research can be done on prisoners if the rules and regulations are followed and one obtains IRB approval. According to 45 CFR 46.303(c) a prisoner means any individual involuntarily confined or detained in a penal institution, including individuals detained in other facilities that provide alternatives to criminal prosecution or incarceration, and individuals detained pending arraignment, trial, or sentencing. Finally, all research involving colleagues, victims, and medical personnel also requires IRB approval.

Challenges to conducting research in disaster or tactical settings

Research on the battlefield (whether its basic design is social, behavioral, or biomedical) and in civilian tactical or disaster situations presents a challenge to the entire research community and research process. The aim of medical care is to treat the wounded and either return them to duty or evacuate the severely injured to definitive care. Given the primary focus of tactical operations upon mission accomplishment, coincidental human-subject research by necessity is relegated to a subordinate role. Thus, development and implementation of either prospective studies requiring informed consent or retrospective studies of existing data requires a very clear, well-defined protocol that can be conducted during the deployment time period but without compromise to the tactical mission. Concurrently, ethical considerations of conducting such research on the battlefield must be considered, to include the rights of research subjects, which are complicated by the traditional commander-subordinate role.

Clinical researchers desiring to conduct research in this setting must first develop an appropriate protocol, with the *a priori* conclusion that such research could not be replicated in a satisfactory manner in a domestic setting. Once such a protocol has been developed and its methodological and ethical validity confirmed by peer review, formal approval should then be sought from the commanders of the units to be impacted by the proposed research, and subsequently from the command element of the theater of operations to be studied. This command approval ensures that the proposed research can be conducted in a tactical environment without jeopardizing the mission and at the same time ensuring the integrity of the study.

Ensuring that the rights and welfare of subjects are protected, no matter where the study is conducted, is still the responsibility of an IRB. All services currently have an IRB that performs external review for combat research. Soldier-subjects should be afforded the same research protection as all other civilian research volunteers. Prospective research involving informed consent can only be done when the Soldier-subject is able to provide his or her own written informed consent. The prohibition of 10 USC 980 with its intent-to-benefit clause does not allow surrogate consent as an alternative to research on the battlefield. Due to the similar high level of vulnerability of populations affected by war and disaster, many of these same principles are also applicable to research conducted in disaster and humanitarian-relief operations.

Soldiers and victims of disaster as a vulnerable population

The performance of patient-oriented clinical research by the U.S. military requires investigators to also look at some of the ethical implications and the ability for soldiers or victims of disaster to give informed consent. Because of the structure of the military environment, soldiers, in some circumstances, may be considered a vulnerable population.

> In clinical research a **vulnerable population** is one that is unable to give informed consent or is susceptible to coercion.

The very nature and location of the soldier in combat (e.g., battlefield) contributes to a sense of vulnerability and may also be a source of unintended coercion. Furthermore, any subject in a study involving traumatic injury may have an impaired capacity to consent, also raising questions of validity of consent procedures. In a similar vein, victims of disaster are, by nature, vulnerable and potentially susceptible to coercion.

At the best of times, during a combat or disaster situation, can informed consent be truly obtained? The mere stress of battle or a soldier's eagerness to please may not actually represent the ability of an individual to make a fair, informed decision. However, one could argue that the same concept applies to most trauma patients who are asked to participate in research. Are these patients any less vulnerable than soldiers?

Furthermore, because soldiers are told to obey all lawful orders from officers, they may feel compelled to obey "requests" from senior officials conducting research. To assure protection of the rights and welfare of the military research subjects, the IRB may sometimes require an ombudsman to be present during the informed- consent process.

However, the ability of soldiers and their surrogate (legal representative) to refuse some medical interventions is restricted. For example, vaccinations that have been proven to be safe and effective are generally required for soldiers. This regulation may be misinterpreted by soldiers and/or surrogates, resulting in confusion between a mandatory procedure (e.g., vaccinations) and medical research. The army has revised the regulations covering medical subjects to prevent unintended coercion. Army regulation 40–38 states that soldier's commanders or supervisors may not be in the room during the consent process.

Ensuring informed consent

Informed-consent research can be performed in an ethically legitimate fashion on today's battlefield and in disaster scenarios if investigators can ensure subjects are protected. Despite some controversy, the DOD and its investigators have an ethical responsibility for protecting its service members. Following the aforementioned policies and procedures as well as using appropriate research ethics will allow military and civilian investigators to ensure human subject protection.

Conclusions

- Research investigators in both the civilian sector and military-related tactical environments hold an ethical obligation to allow potential participants' input into actions that affect them.
- Currently, there exist stringent regulations that must be followed to conduct research on soldiers and civilians on the battlefield and in tactical situations.
- The conduct of all research in the tactical setting should undergo review by an Institutional Review Board.
- Development and implementation of either prospective studies requiring informed consent or retrospective studies of existing data requires a very clear, well-defined protocol that can be conducted during the deployment time period but without compromise to the tactical mission.
- Military and tactical colleagues should be viewed as members of a vulnerable population and afforded the same protection as other vulnerable populations, including minors, prisoners, or the economically disadvantaged.

The conduct of military and tactical medical research has and will serve as an important contribution to both the civilian and military medical communities. Tactical research, when performed properly, is rewarding and aids in reducing morbidity and mortality. The lessons of Vietnam and the development of trauma systems, the "golden-hour," hemorrhage control products, and air medical services provide additional reminders of the mutual benefits gained by military and civilian tactical research. The role of medical research in the tactical setting continues to be diverse, conflicting, and disquieting at times, yet it remains a pioneering and crucial part of modern medicine and national defense.

Suggested readings

Annas GJ, Grodin MA (1992). The Nazi doctors and the Nuremberg code: Human rights in human experimentation. Oxford, England: Oxford University Press.

Army Regulation 70–25. (1990, December). Use of volunteers as subjects of research, Department of the Army, Washington, D.C.

Army Regulation 40–38. (1989, September). Clinical investigation program. Headquarters, Department of the Army, Washington, D.C.

Chernin E. (1989). Richard Pearson Strong and the iatrogenic plague disaster in Bilibid Prison, Manila, 1906. *Rev Infect Dis.* 11(6): 996–1004.

Department of Defense Directive 6200.2. (2000, August) Use of investigational new drugs for force health protection.

Department of Defense Directive 3216.2 (2002, March). Protection of human subjects and adherence to ethical standards in DOD-supported research.

Department of Defense Directive 6000.8. (1999, November). Funding and administration of clinical investigation programs.

National Commission for the Protection for Human Subjects of Biomedical, Behavioral Research (1979). The Belmont report: Ethical principles and guidelines for the protection of human subjects of research. DHEW Publications No. (OS) 78–0012. Washington, DC, US Government Printing Office.

Pape TL, Jaffe NO, Savage T, Collins E, Warden D (2004). Unresolved legal and ethical issues in research of adults with severe traumatic brain injury: Analysis of ongoing protocol. *Journal of Rehabilitation Research Development* 41(2): 155–174.

U.S.C. Title 10 – Armed Forces, Subtitle A – General Military Law, Part II – Personnel, Chapter 49 – Miscellaneous Prohibitions and Penalties §980. "Limitation on use of humans as experimental subjects."

White RM (2006). The Tuskegee study of untreated syphilis revisited. *Lancet Infect Dis* 6(2): 62–63.

Disaster training and education

John L. Foggle

Introduction

Although disaster training and education in the United States predated this millennium, it was not until after the September 11, 2001 terrorist attacks and the 2005 Hurricane Katrina disaster that training courses were rapidly developed and steps were taken to improve disaster management. The biggest challenges for disaster education are the heterogeneity of disasters (e.g., management of a infectious disease disaster such as H1N1 influenza differs dramatically from an environmental disaster or radiological mass casualty incident), and the various medical and nonmedical target audiences that need education and training. The all-hazards approach lumps together disasters involving contaminated victims and those involved in a natural disaster. Each disaster is unique and entirely unpredictable, so disaster training will always be incomplete. Moreover, mock disaster scenarios and simulation exercises are far from real-world conditions. The goal of disaster education and training should focus on core competencies, learned routines, teamwork, and communication. These components are pertinent and transferable to any type of disaster. There are legal, ethical, and psychological issues that also must be addressed as part of any training program.

There are additional issues:
- Disaster-management courses and training are not typically included in medical-school curricula or in residency training programs.
- Even when disaster education does exist, it is often institution or residency-specific and not readily transportable to other disciplines.
- Disaster courses are neither evidence based nor standardized.
- There are no scientific studies that show that disaster-management training courses affect patient outcomes.
- Published data on disasters and disaster training is limited.
- The chaotic nature and environment of almost any disaster limits the ability to design and run prospective, controlled, and objective studies while maintaining accepted ethical standards.

There are a series of key competencies that span across all medical disciplines and all institutions that are pertinent for both medical and nonmedical personnel, including:
- Command.
- Coordination.
- Communication.
- Decontamination.
- Law and risk management.
- Medical management.
- Psychological-stress reaction.
- Response.
- Triage.

Disaster training is a critical component for achieving an effective and coordinated disaster response. Fundamental knowledge and skills are required to function independently while being part of a team. This chapter will review the current state of disaster education, define opportunities for acquiring disaster training, and explore future needs in disaster education.

Disaster-training mandates

- Association of American Medical Colleges (2003): recommended that bioterrorism education be included in each of the four years of all medical-school programs in the United States.
- The Joint Commission: requires that any accredited organization that provides emergency services must have an Emergency Operations Plan (EOP) that addresses both external and internal disasters so that patient care can be continued effectively in the event of emergency situations. The EOP should be general and allow for specific responses to the types of disasters likely to be encountered by the organization, based on an evaluation of incident probability/frequency specific to the organization. In addition, any such organization must provide at least one annual, community-wide, disaster drill that includes an influx from outside the organization of volunteer or simulated patients. Enough "victims" should be used for the mass-casualty exercise to adequately test the system, with the number of victims necessary to test the organization's resources and reactions under stress.
- Pandemic and All-Hazards Preparedness Act, (December 2006): calls "to improve the Nation's public health and medical preparedness and response capabilities for emergencies, whether deliberate, accidental, or natural."
- Homeland Security Presidential Directive 21, HSPD-21, (October 2007): calls for a national strategy for disaster medical education, training, and preparedness in public-health fields.

Existing training programs

- United States Army Medical Research Institute: Offers computer-based training, as well as multiday courses for uniformed personnel and civilian employees, such as Hospital Management of Chemical, Biological, Radiological/Nuclear, and Explosive Incidents (CBRNE).
- Combat Trauma Patient Simulation (CTPS) program: Designed primarily for military purposes and has been used to assess and analyze combat casualties and other types of manmade disasters in massive simulation field exercises. Care of trauma patients from medics to first aid stations to receiving hospitals are part of the drills.
- United States Department of Health and Human Services: provides an Emergency Preparedness Toolkit for states and offers courses and numerous educational materials regarding disaster management.
- Team STEPPS (Team Strategies and Tools to Enhance Performance and Patient Safety): A teamwork system designed for health- care professionals that focuses on patient safety, improved communication, and teamwork skills that was developed by the United States Department of Defense's (DOD's) Patient Safety Program in collaboration with the Agency for Healthcare Research and Quality. Although it does not focus directly on disaster training, it teaches skills and methodology applicable to disaster training. It has been used for disaster-response-team training for field teams.
- MedTeams: like TeamSTEPPS, is focused on teamwork, communication, and patient safety. The MedTeams System, developed by Dynamics Research Corporation, is based on well-documented and tested human factors and Crew Resource Management (CRM), principles that were originally designed for aviation crews in military settings. MedTeams has been used to assess teamwork skills, communication, and different aspects of hospital emergency plans and disaster preparedness
- American Medical Association (AMA) in 2003, along with a group of leading academic medical institutions and the National Disaster Life Support Foundation (NDLSF), developed a nationally standardized all-hazards series of education programs for medical and nonmedical personnel. These programs have been taught in the United States as part of the National Disaster Life Support (NDLS), and abroad as part of International Disaster Life Support (IDLS). The goal was to standardize emergency response training, and the NDLS and ILDS are the most widely taught disaster training courses in the world.

The NDLS DISASTER training focuses on each part of its paradigm, including:
- Detection.
- Incident command.
- Scene security and safety.
- Hazards assessment.
- Support.
- Triage and treatment.
- Evacuation.
- Recovery.

Federal Emergency Management Agency (FEMA) programs

- Center for Domestic Preparedness (CDP) offers courses for healthcare and emergency response personnel in Chemical, Biological, Radiological, Nuclear, and Explosive (CBRNE) incident response, toxic-agent training, and health-care response for mass casualty incidents, Radiological Emergency Preparedness (REP) program courses, ield-force operations, and the National Incident Management System (NIMS).
- Community Emergency Response Team (CERT) program focuses on civilian volunteers and trains them to be better prepared to respond to emergency situations in their communities.
- FEMA Emergency Management Institute (EMI) Independent Study Program offers self-paced courses designed for people who have emergency-management responsibilities as well as to the general public. The Program offers courses that support the nine mission areas identified by the National Preparedness Goal: Incident Management, Operational Planning, Disaster Logistics, Emergency Communications, Service to Disaster Victims, Continuity Programs, Public-Disaster Communications, Integrated Preparedness, and Hazard Mitigation.
- National Training and Education Division (NTED) courses are taught in a classroom, at a training facility, as mobile training usually taught by FEMA-funded instructors at any location, or via self-paced online training.

Free training options

- American College of Emergency Physicians (ACEP): offers a disaster curriculum with topics such as: "Bombings: Injury Patterns and Care."
- American Red Cross (ARC): offers introductory online (as well as in-person) disaster-training courses and modules.
- Federal Emergency Management Agency (FEMA): offers self-paced, web-based, emergency management courses that cover a range of disasters.
- Salvation Army offers National Disaster Training Program (NDTP) and Critical Incident Stress Management courses, available online and with classes at Salvation Army locations around the United States.
- The National Center for Disaster Preparedness (NCDP) at Columbia University offers online courses and webinars through its School of Public Health, with topics such as "Geospatial Intelligence, Social Data, and the Future of Public Health Preparedness and Response"
- Centers for Disease Control and Prevention (CDC): offers an array of mostly online courses that can be downloaded for free (in either English or Spanish).

Training modalities and medical simulation

There are several different disaster-training options, especially field drills, which are the principal form of applied mass-casualty training used around the world. The benefit of simulated field drills is that the educators can focus on specific strengths and weaknesses in the exercises (such as team-work and communication) without focusing on specific medical aspects unless it is warranted. Such drills usually utilize either moulaged stand-ardized patients or simulation-based high fidelity life-sized, programmable manikins. Although both can interactively communicate, the manikins can be used for training interventional procedures and resuscitations. The use of multiple manikins in a disaster drill can also enhance learning in a mass casualty incident.

Medical simulation

Many academic medical centers routinely utilize medical simulation in dis-aster education. In addition, Laerdal Medical and METI, two leading design-ers, programmers, and manufacturers of high-fidelity simulation manikins, have programmed terrorism scenarios to meet training challenges, ranging from first responders to the military to hospital personnel.

Standardized patients

Pros:
• Can simulate any type of hazard.
• Can target any level of medical training or experience.
• Size of the exercise is limitless.
• Relatively inexpensive.
• Excellent for triage, communication, teamwork, and incident command.

Cons:
• Requires many "volunteers."
• Cannot do any medical interventions or true resuscitations.

High-fidelity simulation

Pros:
• Can focus on critical medical management and intervention in disaster scenarios.
• Any type of intervention or resuscitation is theoretically possible.
• Can ensure a reproducible curriculum for all trainees.

Cons:
• Labor and time intensive in programming the manikins.
• Expensive technology.

Other training modalities include tabletop exercises, such as those designed and offered by FEMA, and virtual reality triage training. A table-top exercise is a method of team-based problem solving that can be used to prepare for disasters. There is no simulated drill. Instead, participants gather to talk through the event and possible solutions as the disaster unfolds, and ultimately facilitates a discussion of how an organization would plan, protect, respond, and recover from a disaster.

Virtual reality triage training and other computer-based exercises facilitate teamwork, role responsibilities, and enable exposure to uncommon scenarios and situations where rapid coordinated response is critical for success. Virtual reality allows immersive, repetitive practice that can also be used as an assessment tool. In addition, scenarios can easily be modified to focus on any type of disaster, and training can be customized to focus on specific skill sets and lessons to be learned. Lastly, refresher courses and periodic re-training are facilitated by using this evolving technology. Two important issues with virtual reality are its enormous start-up costs and lack of standardization.

Future challenges

- Designing appropriate disaster training to a diverse group of individuals across multiple medical disciplines.
- Determining how often to teach refresher courses, as one-time training only provides passing familiarity with disaster terms and concepts that will decay over time.
- Promoting disaster management research and publishing peer-reviewed articles that focus on disaster education and training.
- Analyzing the existing courses, such as NDLS and annual training drills mandated by the Joint Commission to determine whether they can be used as a reasonable national standard.
- Creating tools to assess disaster education courses and establish best practices in training that can then be disseminated to create a standardized approach.
- Developing a set of disaster core competencies that can span across health specialties, levels of medical training, and professions.

Suggested readings

Hsu EB, et al. (2006). Healthcare worker competencies for disaster training. *BMC Med Educ 19*: 1–9.

Kobayashi L, et al. (2003). Disaster medicine education: The potential role of high fidelity medical simulation in mass casualty incident training. *Med Health RI 86*(7): 196–200.

Pfenninger, EG, et al. (2010). Medical student disaster medicine education: The development of an educational resource. *Int J Emerg Med 3*: 9–20.

Scott LA, et al. (2010). Disaster 101: A novel approach to disaster medicine training for health professionals. *J Emerg Med 39*(2): 220–226.

Subbarao I, et al. (2008). A consensus-based educational framework and competency set for the discipline of disaster medicine and public health preparedness. *Disaster Med and Pub H Preparedness 2*(1): 57–68.

Williams J, et al. (2008). The effectiveness of disaster training for health care workers: A systematic review. *Ann Emerg Med 52*(3): 211–222.

Chapter 42

Medical ethics in disasters

Wayne Smith
Lee Wallis

Ethical principles

Ethics can be defined as the study of standards of conduct and moral judgement, or a system or code of morals (concepts of right and wrong). Medical ethics has been based on four principles:

- *Beneficence*—to do the best for the patient so as to optimise outcome
- *Nonmaleficence*—to do no harm
- *Autonomy*—medical staff need to respect the informed decisions of patients as pertaining to their own medical care
- *Justice*—ensure that medical resources are equally distributed among all.

A disaster situation presents the medical fraternity with many ethical considerations and dilemmas which may seem to be in direct conflict with the principles of medical ethics. This arises due to an acute imbalance between the medical needs of the victims and the medical services required to provide care to these victims.

Despite this, the overarching principle remains for the health-care practitioner to adhere to the ethical code as stated in the Hippocratic Oath, which obligates the medical professional to assist in the relief of human suffering and alleviation of pain. Careful consideration is required when applying these principles in the context of a disaster.

Some ethical considerations are listed in the sections following. They do not represent a complete list but rather some of the more common issues that may face the health-care practitioner in a disaster situation:

Duty to care

The American Medical Association in a 2004 policy document states that "Because of their commitment to care for the sick and injured, individual physicians have an obligation to provide urgent medical care during disasters. This ethical consideration holds even in the face of greater than usual risk to their own safety, health or life."

Triage

The principle of justice requires that care and medical resources must be distributed equally. Triage is the tool to achieve this, and must be performed fairly without any consideration to race, age, gender, or creed. The aim of triage is to do the most for the greatest number of patients. It is unethical for a medical professional to persist at attempting to save the life of one individual at the expense of many others that may benefit from the scarce resources. Likewise patients who were not direct victims of the disaster, but were being treated by the same limited medical resources when the disaster struck, would now also need to be triaged alongside the actual victims.

In some cases, the expectant triage code may be evoked. This occurs in situations in which the resources required are totally inadequate for the number of patients to be treated. Those that are triaged as expectant are suffering from injuries so severe that survival is unlikely. These patients should receive palliative care and not be abandoned. However, the level of care given to expectant patients is at a level that will not compromise the care given to patients with a greater chance of survival. The expectant triage code is unlikely to be used in civilian incidents, and is more often used in the military environment. Palliative care in the disaster setting is also discussed in Chapter 50.

Media

The media has a responsibility to advise the world of the developments in a disaster. In this way, world attention and subsequent support can be directed by prudent media coverage. Medical professionals should be aware of the important role the media may play, but need to ensure that patient dignity and confidentiality are maintained. Photographs of patients should not be taken without their express permission.

Humanitarian assistance

In a complex emergency, humanitarian assistance may prolong the conflict. Often, one or the other of the warring factions confiscates the assistance to supply its own fighters. Although this may prolong the conflict, the withholding of humanitarian assistance is unethical because it may subject other complex disaster victims to unbearable suffering.

Disaster research

In the acute phase of a disaster, research is inappropriate if researchers only record information without providing assistance to disaster victims. It is at this stage that the number of victims is most likely to outnumber the amount of assistance readily available, and it would be unethical for the researchers not to provide assistance. Research conducted in the latter phases of a prolonged incident may be more acceptable, provided the results of such studies are seen to possibly improve the outcome of future similar events.

Informed consent

Most codes of medical ethics require that informed consent is obtained before providing medical care. In a disaster situation, the ethical requirement shifts to the ability to provide the best for the most number of patients. In such a situation, it may not be possible to obtain informed consent.

Sustainability

If long-term medication is started and/or long-term treatment is commenced, can it be sustained once the response agencies withdraw? Another ethical question that may arise is, When is it appropriate for medical professionals to withdraw?

Armed conflict

The World Medical Association (WMA) advises that the medical ethics in time of armed conflict should be identical to medical ethics in time of peace. The primary obligation of the medical professional is performing their professional duty, and have their conscience as the supreme guide.

Disaster situations require that ethical decision-making is structured to ensure that the issue of collective ethics is added to the individual ethics practiced on a daily basis by the medical fraternity.

To manage these ethical dilemmas the practitioner must ensure that ethical principles are given due consideration during the planning phase of disaster preparedness. The ethical codes for disaster response should also be dealt with in a transparent and inclusive manner to ensure that all disaster providers are able to accept and apply them in the face of a disaster.

Suggested readings

Lin JY, Anderson-Shaw L (2009). Rationing of resources : Ethical issues in disasters and epidemic situations.. *Prehospital Disast Med* 24(3):215–221.

Ruderman C, Shawn TC, Bensimon CM et al. (2006). On panademics and the duty to care: Whose duty? Who cares? *BMC Medical Ethics* 7: 5.

World Medical Association. (1994, September). Statement on medical ethics in the event of disasters - Adopted by the 46th General Assembly. Stockholm, Sweden.

Politics and disasters

John T. Carlo

Hurricanes, earthquakes, and the like are acts of God. The extent of the damage they cause often depends on the politics and economics of man.

Marvin Olasky (2006) *The Politics of Disaster: Katrina,*
Big Government and a New Strategy for Future Crises.
Nashville: Thomas Nelson

Disasters and elected officials

Major disasters have the impact of pulling the nation together, encouraging a centralization of authority, and mobilizing governmental action. The perceived success or failure by an elected official in his/her response to a disaster will often be the determinant of their political future. Because of this, elected officials must understand the organization of emergency management, but perhaps more importantly, convey a solid image of leadership to their constituents during a disaster event.

Elected officials' responsibilities

- Respond to the needs of their constituents and direct the public as to what steps they can take to promote their safety.
- Convey how the government is responding and what steps are being undertaken to aid in the recovery.
- Leverage public-private relationships to improve responding capability.

Elected officials and the medical responder

Disasters often afford medical responders a unique opportunity to be directly engaged with elected and senior governmental officials where they would have not have been engaged otherwise. Such interactions can be beneficial in opening opportunities to obtain necessary response elements, or they can be a time-consuming and anxiety-provoking event.

Since most medical responders likely do not have prior experience with meeting elected officials, it is important to understand that elected officials' visitations are often part of the process of the response and recovery and not an all-encompassing element. These interactions can be opportunities to convey concerns, but it is important for the responder to understand the role of an elected official during a disaster response. Further, it is important for medical responders not to go outside their role or knowledge base during these interactions and only discuss problems that are directly associated with their operational activities.

Medical responders should be aware of any policies and procedures set forth by the institutions that they are either working for or represent prior to engagement with elected officials. Most hospitals have public information or public affairs offices that are responsible for coordinating meetings with elected officials and guests.

As such, it is important to obtain approval by these departments prior to meeting with the elected officials. These offices are often helpful to the medical responder by providing speaking points and scripted information that both convey need but also avoid any negative images of the institution and its representatives.

When operating under the Incident Command System (ICS), elected officials' visits should be facilitated through the ICS Command Staff. The Incident Commander should be aware of any visit by an elected or senior government official. Typically, the liaison officer should facilitate engagements with elected officials. The liaison officer should be the point of contact and be responsible for directing meetings with medical responders. The Public Information Officer (PIO) will likely also be involved as often as elected officials often will have media representatives with them.

Characteristics of elected officials

Although current perception is that elected officials are categorically dishonest or incompetent, most studies have shown exactly the opposite. Many elected officials studied by psychologists exhibit exceptional skills in transformational leadership style. They can inspire motivation and achieve an improved performance of those working toward common goals. Often, elected officials have a background of being a successful business owner or a successful career in the legal profession. They often have proficient interpersonal skills and are empathic individuals who can drive change through leadership. Because of this, a responding elected official can be extremely helpful during a crisis.

Keys to successful engagement of an elected official during a disaster response

- Do not speak about issues beyond your control. If you are a responding medical provider, speak only about what you are seeing in your patients, for example. The elected official is there to gather first-hand information, so it's best to provide only that and not extraneous information.
- Speak to an elected official in an understandable and empathic language like you would to a patient, but be careful to not be condescending. Many elected officials have experience in the healthcare industry and have a basic understanding of medical problems.
- Have in your mind a short list of engagement goals. Many leaders will feel compelled to contribute, and if they ask, giving them actionable items will enable the elected official to feel involved and add to the benefit of bringing them into the response.

Disasters and socioeconomics

Although the effect of a disaster may be felt by all members of the community, the impact is almost never equally experienced across the entire population. The economically disadvantaged, those who live in poverty and near-poverty tend to have the least resilience and the least amount of resources available in order to recover.

In industrialized nations, disasters often result in large losses of capital, however, the number of fatalities are often much lower than the numbers observed in impoverished nations. The management of individuals who are in poverty is a politically charged issue, because these individuals are frequently the focus of the media. The overall response to the disaster is likely to be measured by how well those who are least able to take care of themselves are taken care of by the overall disaster response.

Shelter use

Determination of whether individuals will require public shelter depends mainly on the evacuees' economic status rather than the actual characteristics of the event or official notifications. Recent experience with hurricane disasters along the Gulf Coast demonstrated that most of the population who utilized public-assistance shelters were from lower socioeconomic backgrounds. Individuals exhibited disproportionately higher rates of untreated, chronic medical conditions and mental-health disorders, including substance abuse, than the general population. Lower socioeconomic groups tend to have higher rates of distrust in government.

Table 43.1 Examples of disasters in which the poor were disproportionately affected in the United States

Disaster	Demographic Effected	Source
1900 Honolulu's Chinatown Fire	5,000 homes of poor immigrant neighborhoods were burned as a result of actions to control the plague epidemic	Mohr, James. 2005. *Plague and Fire: Battling Black Death in the 1900 Burning of Honolulu's Chinatown.* New York: Oxford University Press
1918 Spanish Influenza Pandemic	Poorer households were more likely to have cases and secondary cases	Jordan, E. 1927. *Epidemic Influenza: A survey.* Chicago, IL: American Medical Association.
Chicago heat wave 1995	Nearly all of the 700 deaths were elderly low-income individuals	Klinenburg, E. 2002. *Heat Wave: A social autopsy of disaster in Chicago.* Chicago, IL: University of Chicago Press.
Hurricane Katrina, New Orleans 2005	Most remaining residents were poor	Olasky, M. 2006. *The Politics of Disaster: Katrina, Big Government and a New Strategy for Future Crises.* Nashville, TN: Thomas Nelson.

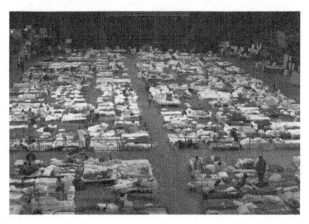

Figure 43.1 Taken from Reunion Arena, Dallas, Texas during the Hurricane Katrina Evacuation, 2005.

Public Response to Disasters

Compliance

An important factor for a successful response to a disaster is how well the public responds. Often this response is gauged by how well the public complies with official recommendations. Studies have demonstrated that response compliance depends on:

- How citizens assess the risk to themselves and their loved ones.
- What resources they have available.
- How well the official response appears organized.
- What other consequences could be anticipated (looting, separation from family members, abandonment of pets, etc.).

Studies have shown that the public will generally follow official advice during a disaster. The media clearly plays an important role in informing the public concerning the disaster. Recently, newscasts were a primary source of information for evacuees to gain further information during the Hurricane Katrina disaster.

Recent work by federal, state, and local public-health agencies has been directed toward improving crisis communication and utilizing the media as a major tool of information dissemination. Guidelines have been produced by the Centers for Disease Control and Prevention (CDC) that can be used by medical responders to facilitate communication with the media and generate important messages to the public. Remember, that although the public perceives physicians as medical experts, coordinating a single message by an official spokesperson carries the highest likelihood of achieving a coordinated public response to a disaster.

Crime

Criminal activity following a disaster remains a concern. Visual depictions of looting and violent crime in the media can reinforce the fear that public panic and disorganization systematically follows any disaster. However, it has also been shown that disasters afford the opportunity for the demonstration of altruistic behavior, which can cause a reduction of violence and crime compared to normal levels. This is also observed with the increase in donations by the public to charitable organizations during disasters.

Reports have shown that rates of domestic violence and child abuse increase immediately postdisaster. This may be the result of associated stress, feelings of helplessness, and frustrations over losses incurred. VanLandingham in 2007 demonstrated a significant increase in the murder rate for the City of New Orleans in the two years following hurricane Katrina. Suicide rates have also shown to increase after disasters, again as a result of the increased feelings of hopelessness and frustration experienced by disaster victims. Looting and theft often follow natural disasters. Responding to criminal activity is an important component of assuring the public to return to normal status. Officials must be responsive to media reports of criminal activity and assure the public that restored infrastructure offers them protection and safety. Adequate protective services must be in place not only for citizens but also for responders.

Suggested readings

Centers for Disease Control and Prevention. (2002). Crisis and emergency risk communication. Available at http://emergency.cdc.gov/cerc/pdf/CERC-SEPT02.pdf

Dombroski M, Fischhoff B, Fischbeck P (2006). Predicting emergency evacuation and sheltering behavior: A structured analytical approach. *Risk Analysis 26*(6): 1675–1690.

Sylves Richard T, Waugh, Jr. William L eds. (1996). *Disaster Management in the U.S. and Canada.* Springfield, IL: Charles C. Thomas.

VanLandingham Mark. Murder rates in New Orleans, 2004–2006. (2007). *American Journal of Public Health 97*(9): 1614–1616.

Rural approaches

Evan Avraham Alpert

Kobi Peleg

Introduction

Although government agencies often focus disaster resources on urban areas, it is important to remember the potential for rural disasters. The first documented case of bioterrorism in the United States occurred in rural Oregon in 1984 when the Rajneeshee religious cult intentionally poisoned the local salad bars with Salmonella typhimurium in an attempt to sicken the local population. In 2005, hurricane Katrina, although frequently depicted in the media for its devastation of New Orleans, also affected large rural areas of the southern United States. In May 2007 a level EF-5 tornado destroyed 95 percent of the rural community of Greensburg, Kansas.

Although many injury patterns and treatment will be the same as in urban disasters, this chapter will highlight some of the unique issues affecting rural disasters.

Facts

- Approximately 50–60 million Americans live in rural areas.
- There are 2,200 rural hospitals.
- Rural areas account for 20 percent of the U.S. population but only 11% of its physicians.
- 80 percent of U.S. land is classified as rural.

Types of rural hospitals

- Not for profit.
- For profit.
- Large referral centers.
- Small isolated hospitals.
- Critical-access hospitals (15 or fewer acute-care beds; keep inpatients an average of less than 4 days; 35 miles from another hospital, or are designated so by the state).

Potential for rural disasters

- Proximity to military bases.
- Proximity to dams.
- Proximity to industrial plants .
- Proximity to nuclear plants.
- Proximity to natural gas pipelines.
- Proximity to hazardous material manufacturers.
- Areas that employ migrant or international workers may be at risk for infectious disease.
- May damage the agricultural industry that then becomes a public-health threat.

EMS issues

- Fewer resources.
- Less system-wide capacity.
- Increased reliance on volunteers.
- Longer response times.
- Longer transport time to and from the hospital.
- Longer time to centralize enough EMS and health-care teams.
- In a recent survey, only 3 percent of rural EMS systems felt that they could effectively handle 25 patients simultaneously.
- Better prepared for Hazmat events than biological or infectious disease events or terrorist attacks.
- Helicopter is often best means of transportation.
- Treatment according to prehospital trauma life support (PHTLS).
- Often forced to "stay and play" (e.g., invasive procedures such as intubations, chest tubes, and central lines will be placed in the field).

Hospital issues

- Fewer available critical resources such as CT, MRI, operating rooms, ICU beds, and so forth.
- Less available space and equipment for surge capacity.
- Less available funding for capital improvements for up to date facilities and equipment.
- Lack of enough single-air-return systems for isolation.
- Disaster event in an urban area could lead to an exodus to a rural area.
- If a disaster event occurred during tourism peaks in certain rural areas, it could easily overwhelm the system.
- Inability to divert patients as they are likely the only hospital in the region.
- Less disaster funding to areas with a smaller population.

Personnel issues

- Limited number of health-care providers.
- Often not enough personnel to fill all the positions in the Incident Command System, especially for more than one shift.
- Less specialist coverage including trauma surgeons and ICU specialists.
- Often need to develop plans to rely on retired or volunteer health-care providers.
- More difficult to spare personnel for training as limited number of staff.
- Often less continuing medical education sources than in urban areas.
- Physicians in rural areas are often overworked and have less time for CME issues.
- Primary care providers will also have to manage the mental-health issues of a disaster.

Improving the system

- Regional collaboration among hospitals.
- Telemedicine.
- Procedures for emergency credentialing of volunteers.
- Maintain an all-hazards approach to disaster preparedness.
- Improving interagency communication.
- Increasing involvement in regional planning.

Suggested readings

Chesser, et al. (2006). Preparedness needs assessment in a rural state: Themes derived from public focus groups. *Biosecurity and Bioterrorism: Biodefense Strategy, Practice and Science* 4(4): 376–383.

Chang, et al. (2001, July–September). A comparison of rural and urban emergency medical system (EMS) personnel: A Texas study. *Prehospital and Disaster Medicine* 6(3):117–123.

Clawson A, Brooks Robert G (2003). Protecting rural communities from terrorism: A statewide, community-based model. *The Journal of Rural Health* 19(1): 7–10.

Edwards, et al. (2008). Promoting regional disaster preparedness among rural hospitals. *The Journal of Rural Health* 24(3): 321–325.

Furbee P, et al. (2006). Realities of rural emergency medical services disaster preparedness. *Prehospital and Disaster Medicine* 21(2): 64–70.

LeBosquet III Thomas P, Marcozzi David. (2006). Medical care in remote areas. In Ciattone, Gregory R, ed. *Disaster medicine*, 3rd ed., pp. 274–277. St. Louis, MO: Mosby.

Ricketts, Thomas (2000). The changing nature of rural health care. *Annu. Rev. Public Health* 21: 639–657.

Rosenthal, Thomas. (2003). Rural bioterrorism: Are we exempt? *The Journal of Rural Health* 19(1): 5–6.

Van Fleet-Green, et al. Identifying the Gaps Between Biodefense Researchers, Public Health, and Clinical Practice in a Rural Community," *The Journal of Rural Health*.

Urban approaches

Evan Avraham Alpert

Kobi Peleg

Introduction

From the earthquake in San Francisco in 1906, the World Trade Center bombing in 2001, to the devastation of New Orleans by hurricane Katrina in 2005, the United States has had to prepare for and deal with disasters in its urban areas. Increasing urbanization over the last several decades with its corresponding increased population density can lead to a higher number of casualties than in a rural area. Large population centers in seismically active areas, flood plains, or tornado zones can lead to large numbers of injured victims. This can occur through structural collapse of multistory buildings, which can lead to large numbers of entrapped victims with many suffering from blunt trauma. Fires can ignite, dams can be damaged, causing secondary flooding, and hazardous materials can be released. The close living quarters of urban populations can facilitate the spread of disease. On the other hand, the increased resources such as medical personnel and health-care facilities can provide for more rapid triage and treatment. This chapter will explore various issues in urban disaster management.

History of urban disaster relief in the United States

- 1803: New Hampshire asks for funding for assistance after fires
- 1905: Red Cross receives Congressional mandate to provide disaster relief in the United States.
- 1906: Earthquake hits San Francisco.
- 1941: President Roosevelt creates Office of Civilian Defense (OCD), which created air-raid procedures and black-out drills to be carried out by volunteers.
- 1950: Civil Defense Act under President Harry Truman created the Federal Civil Defense Administration (FCDA), which created shelter, evacuation, and training programs for state and local governments.
- 1974: Robert T. Stafford Disaster Relief and Emergency Assistance Act unified federal funding of civil defense and disaster assistance programs.
- 1979: Federal Emergency Management Agency (FEMA) established by President Carter to be the executive branch coordinator for disaster response.
- 1989: FEMA established the National Urban Search and Rescue Response System.
- 1991: FEMA developed the Federal Response Plan (now National Response Plan) sponsoring 25 urban search and rescue forces.
- 2001: World Trade Center attack. FEMA focuses on National Preparedness and coordinates its activities with the newly formed Department of Homeland Security.
- 2005: Hurricane Katrina resulted in over 1,800 deaths and widespread criticism of implementation of government disaster relief.
- 2006: President Bush signs Post-Katrina Emergency Reform Act, reorganizing FEMA.

Urban search and rescue

- Urban search and rescue: involves the location, extrication, and stabilization of victims from confined spaces.
- Multihazard discipline involving all types of disasters.
- If required nationally, FEMA will deploy 3 closest task forces within 6 hours. Additional deployments if needed.
- 28 national task forces.
- Task force: 62 positions.
- At the ready: 130 trained people, 4 canines, equipment.
- Self sufficient for first 72 hours.
- Incident support team helps with logistics, electronics, and coordination.
- Medical team:
  - 6 people.
  - 2 medical team managers: EM physicians with prehospital experience.
  - 4 medical team specialists: level of paramedic.
  - Adequate supplies for 10 critical, 15 moderate, 25 minor patients.
- Responsibility:
  - Take care of rescuers.
  - Take care of victims directly encountered.
  - Taker care of others as needed.
  - Evacuation triage: triage to transfer to medical facilities.

Some of the issues that EMS and FEMA task-force members will face in urban disasters will be rescuing victims entrapped in confined spaces, as well as treating crush syndrome.

Confined-space medicine

- Medicine practiced in areas with limited access and ventilation, usually due to structural collapse.
- Rescuer safety first.
- Types of collapse:
  - Pancake collapse: all of the floors fall on top of each other.
  - Lean-to collapse: floor, wall or beam collapses but still supported by a remaining wall.
  - V-collapse: floor or roof collapses into a lower level in the shape of a V.
  - Cantilever collapse: outer wall is destroyed leaving the roof and upper floors dangling.
- Need to be careful for secondary collapse.
- Medical team uniform: helmet, dust mask, ear plugs, safety glasses, latex gloves under leather gloves, steel -toe boots, coveralls.
- Golden day: 24–48 hrs after the event.
- No golden hour: If victims can't be reached, they will die.
- Patients who will die in 4 to 24 hrs will do so from either shock or airway issues.
- Patients who will die in >24 hrs will do so from sepsis or multi- organ failure.
- Medical team is responsible for patient.
- Rescue team performs the extrication.
- May need to deal with minor canine problems.

Table 45.1 Common injuries seen in victims trapped in collapsed structures

Fractures
Multiple trauma
Closed head injury
Hypothermia
Dehydration
Crush injury/crush syndrome
Hazmat issues
Laceration and punctures especially from wood structures
Dust inhalation such as from adobe and brick

Crush injury and crush syndrome

Crush injury
Direct injury to the limb or organ by compressive forces.

Crush syndrome
Systemic effects of the crush injury.
- Includes rhabdomyolysis, renal failure, sepsis, ARDS, DIC, bleeding, arrhythmias, electrolyte imbalance.
- After trauma, most frequent cause of death from earthquakes.
- After recent earthquakes many victims developed renal failure requiring dialysis but there was no organized effort to help them.
- Pathophysiology: impaired kidney perfusion, intratubular obstruction by myoglobin and uric acid.
- Treatment: early fluid resuscitation, best within 6 hrs, even while victim is under the rubble.
- While under rubble, administer saline 1 L/hr= 10–15cc/kg/hr
- After removal, can change to hypotonic saline adding 50meq sodium bicarbonate to every second or third liter to maintain urinary pH over 6.5. This prevents deposition of myoglobin and uric acid in the tubules.
- If urine output (UO) is greater than 20cc/hr then 50cc of 20% mannitol per liter of fluid at 1–2gm/kg/day for total 120gm (5gm per hr/24 hrs)
- Once hospitalized, want urine output to be greater than 300cc/hr. Therefore, may need to up to 12 L per day which would mean 4–6L of intravenous fluids includes sodium bicarbonate.
- Electrolyte abnormalities:
  - *Hypocalcemia*: only treat if symptomatic because victim can later develop hypercalcemia.
  - Calcium gluconate 10%/10cc or calcium chloride 10%/5cc over 2 minutes.
  - *Hyperkalemia*: monitor and treat as needed based on level and EKG changes
    1. Calcium as above.
    2. Albuterol, nebulized.
    3. Sodium bicarbonate 1 meq/kg slow IV.
    4. Regular insulin 5–10 U IV.
    5. D50 1–2 ampules IV bolus.
    6. Kayexylate 25–50g with sorbitol PO or kaexylate in retention enema.
    7. May require dialysis.
- Blood products as needed.
- Monitor for 5 Ps of compartment syndrome: pain, parasthesias, paralysis, pallor, pulselessness.
- Fasciotomy usually if pressure is greater than 40.

Box 45.1 FEMA Task-Force Equipment Cache for the Medical Section

- Antibiotics/Antifungals
- Patient Comfort Medications
- Pain Medications
- Sedatives/Anesthetics/Paralytics
- Steroids
- Intravenous Fluids/Volume
- Immunizations/Immune Globulin
- Canine Treatment
- Basic Airway Equipment
- Advanced Airway Equipment
- Eye Care Supplies
- Intravenous Access/Administration
- Patient Assessment Care/General
- Patient immobilization/extrication

Source: Department of Homeland Security, Federal Emergency Management Agency. National Urban Search and Rescue Response System Task Force Equipment Cache List, August 2003.

Emergency medical services response

- May be overwhelmed because of multiple casualties.
- May have greater ability to respond due to greater number of ambulances in proximity to the incident.
- Short distance and duration from scene to hospital = greater ambulance availability, meaning the ambulance can respond multiple times to bring in casualties.
- Scoop & Run- protect the airway and control bleeding; often preferred in urban-disaster setting due to proximity to medical centers.
- May have the ability to divert less injured patients to other hospitals.

Emergency department response

- Verify via EMS the nature and extent of the disaster.
- Activate the hospital emergency plan.
- All potentially hospitalized patients should be admitted and workups continued on the wards.
- Inpatients who can be discharged should be as soon as possible.
- The resuscitation area should be readied.
- Set up a triage area in front of the ED.
- ED command and control center should be set up.

Types of urban disasters

Terrorism is more likely in urban areas
- Mass-casualty terrorist bomb: Some define this as > 30 casualties (Note that, in Israel, a mass-casualty incident [MCI] is defined as greater than 4 critical patients or greater than 10 total patients)
- In mass-casualty terrorist bombings most deaths were immediate with few early or late.
- Highest number of immediate deaths in terrorist suicide bombings were on buses or associated with structural collapse.
- Low early mortality in general means that, if a victim gets to the ED, resources should be maximized for that victim.

Blast injury
- **Primary:** Blast wave injuring hollow organs including intestinal perforation, blast lung, and tympanic-membrane perforation.
  - Highest rate is with confined-space bombings, especially terrorist-suicide bombings.
- **Secondary:** from shrapnel and debris either primary from the bomb or from secondary shrapnel.
  - Highest rates with open air injuries.
- **Tertiary:** from victim being thrown; associated with all bombing subgroups. Includes traumatic amputations, fractures, solid-organ injuries.
- **Quaternary:** from structural collapse or fires.

ED Issues
- Highest injury severity scores (ISS) in confined-space bombings on buses.
- Burn victims more frequent in confined-space events.
- Inverse relationship between ED utilization and immediate mortality.
- Factors affecting maximum number utilizing ED:
  - Number of immediate survivors.
  - Hospital proximity to the bombing site.
  - Distribution by EMS to the various hospitals.
  - Number of available EDs.
- Admission rates highest for confined space and terrorist-suicide bombings.

Earthquakes
- Crush injury and crush syndrome: lower extremities 74 percent, upper extremities 10 percent, and trunk 9 percent
- Incidence of crush syndrome 2–15 percent
- Half who develop crush syndrome develop acute renal failure (ARF).
- Half of those with ARF need dialysis.
- A certain percentage of victims with crush syndrome victims will need fasciotomy.

Hurricanes and floods
- Theoretically have a certain amount of time to plan.
- Have to deal with the issue of damage to the medical infrastructure itself.
- Casualty collection points and mass-casualty triage.
- Most injuries are wounds and lacerations, strains, sprains.
- Consider carbon monoxide poisoning due to placement of generators indoors.
- Infectious disease can be caused by contaminated flood water–V. vulnificus and leptospirosis.

Infectious disease
- Due to increased density in urban areas, there is an increased risk of epidemics.
- Centers for Disease Control and Prevention (CDC) is part of the Department of Health and Human Services.
- Includes the Coordinating Center for Infectious Disease (CCID)
- And the Coordinating Office for Terrorism Preparedness and Emergency Response (COPTER).
- Strategic National Stockpile (SNS) includes antibiotics antidotes and antitoxins as well as life support medical supplies.
- Once federal and local officials agree, then free life-saving medications and supplies can be delivered to local communities.

Radiation emergencies
- Could be from an accident at a nuclear site, dirty bomb, or act of war.
- CDC partners with numerous other agencies including FEMA, FBI, and the Agency for Toxic Substances and Disease Registry (ATSDR)—part of the HHS.
- Involved in protecting people from radioactive fallout and supplying equipment and monitoring devices.
- Establish an exposure registry.

Suggested readings

Arnold J et al. (2003). Mass-casualty, terrorist bombings: Epidemiological outcomes, resource utilization, and time course of emergency needs (Part 1). *Prehospital and Disaster Medicine* 18(3): 220–234.

Briggs S. (2006). Earthquakes. *Surgical Clinics of North America* 86(3): 537–544.

Ciottone Gary et al. (2006). *Disaster Medicine*. Philadelphia, PA: Mosby Elsevier.

Halpern P et al. (2003). Mass-casualty, terrorist bombings: Implications for emergency department and hospital emergency response (Part II). *Prehospital and Disaster Medicine* 18(3): 235–241.

http://www.bt.cdc.gov

http://www.fema.gov/emergency/usr/index.shtml

Sever MS, Vanholder R, Lameire N (2006, March). Management of crush-related injuries after disasters. *The New England Journal of Medicine* 354(10): 1533–4406.

Shatz David et al. (2006). Response to hurricane disasters. *Surgical Clinics of North America* 86(3): 545–555.

Terrorism

Frederick M. Burkle, Jr.

Terrorism

Terrorism is recognized as a subset of complex humanitarian emergencies (Chapter 20). Acts of terror occur on a daily basis in many countries of the world (Figure 46.1). Of 2010's most failed nations, 6 out of 10 (Somalia, Sudan, Democratic Republic of the Congo, Iraq, Afghanistan, Pakistan) suffer daily acts of terrorism.

Definition

The international community has been slow to formulate a universally agreed, legally binding definition. A 2004 United Nations Secretary General report described terrorism as any act "intended to cause death or serious bodily harm to civilians or noncombatants with the purpose of intimidating a population or compelling a government or an international organization to do or abstain from doing any act." Yet, no single definition satisfies all acts of terrorism.

Origins of terrorism

Much of the world's population has experienced a decline in public health infrastructures, systems, and economic, social, political, and developmental protections. Acts of terrorism have roots in social movements that seek change in government-led societies or in preventing change they oppose. Initially this process seeks resolution and change through peaceful grievances and demands. Splintering groups may break away from peaceful pursuits for change, first as simple protestors and then as nonstate foot soldiers who provoke a police- action response. Violence may continue to escalate. State repression (violence used by the state to put down challenges) and a reactionary self-defense for the cause can lead to more sophisticated forms of violence and mobilization of new followers. As the political struggle rages, mass appeal increases the population base and rages against those who do not join the cause. Terrorism occurs when the violence indiscriminately targets the innocent.

Historically, pre-September 11 acts of terrorism were limited to national causes within national borders. In most instances, the terrorists represented splinter groups that stemmed from social movements formed to draw attention to unaddressed economic, development, and social needs of a specific country.

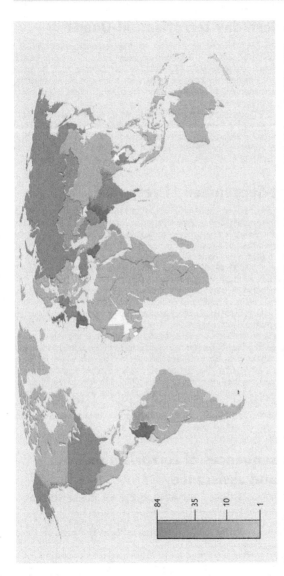

Figure 46.1 Number of terrorist incidents: 2000–2008. This map was modified from the original that was published February 8, 2009 by Wikimedia Commons, released into worldwide public domain by its author Emilfaro. Map created by Arthur Gunn (GunnMap_Icon.svg). Available free at http://gunn.co.nz/map.

84
35
10
1

Modern day terrorism: Al-Qaeda

Al-Qaeda (AQ) historically differs from other terrorist groups in that it is not country focused. It represents a global radical Islamic force that recruits and acts worldwide. AQ's 2010 master tactician is an American citizen. AQ has equally targeted centers for moderate Islamic teachings and governance. AQ's motivation is to control a population, not to obtain territory or resources.

In Iraq, AQ quickly grew brutal, overpowered other Iraqi insurgent groups, declared an Islamic state, and enforced a severe form of Islamic law. There is no specific government or nation associated with AQ, yet it has a deep presence in Afghanistan, Pakistan, Somalia, Yemen, Iraq, Mali, Sudan, and the Sahara, and cells of influence in many countries of the Western world.

Post-September 11 response

Coalition forces went into Afghanistan in 2001 to attack AQ, destroy its safe haven and prevent further terrorist attacks. This remains the stated objective of the Afghan campaign even though AQ is no longer in Afghanistan and moved their safe haven to Northwestern Pakistan. Coalition military efforts in Afghanistan have switched to AQ's Taliban sponsors—estimated to number 30,000–40,000 fighters, 2,200 regional commanders, and 170 key leaders, although much is left to conjecture.

International security forces "stability and reconstruction operations" include elements of traditional combat, counterterrorism, peace making/peace keeping, counterinsurgency, nation building, monetary development assistance, and disaster relief.

Targets of terrorism are picked for a reason and commonly focus on local civilian points of resistance and structures of the state. In situations, such as Afghanistan, acts expanded to target the innocent whom terrorists feel are equally guilty. Aid agencies can easily become targets along with the populations they are trying to help. In 2009, 4 female aid workers from the NGO International Rescue Committee were assassinated because they were considered "part of the occupation," and in 2010, 10 medical team members of an NGO with a 40-year presence in the country were assassinated for being "spies."

Consequences of terrorism on aid and assistance

Capacity to gather, assess, and analyze data on the effectiveness of AQ is impeded as the security situation and allegiances on the ground shift among the many stakeholders. This is negatively influenced by refusal of the Afghan government, the UN, and the International Security Assistance Forces (ISAF) to release detailed data on attacks or their consequences. Requests for access are routinely denied. In mid 2010, insurgents are active in 33 of 34 provinces; up to 70 percent of 368 districts are deemed too dangerous to visit for data gathering. The humanitarian space has shrunk considerably. As such, all data and analysis should be interpreted with caution.

Status summary of functional areas of aid and assistance

The primary functional areas greatly impacted by terrorism are human security, health, food security, education, and women's rights.

Human security

In 2010:

- Half of all suicide attacks occur in the southern provinces of Afghan. Most victims are civilians with 67–70 percent killed by insurgents.
- Suicide bombings tripled; assassinations increased by 49 percent over 2009, and IEDs or roadside bombs increased by 94 percent.
- From March–June 2010, 332 children were killed or maimed, 60 percent by insurgents.
- A marked increase in attacks on schools, teachers, and pupils occurred in Afghanistan; abduction of students as suicide bombers in Pakistan also increased.
- The Afghan NGO Safety Office confirmed insurgent attacks on aid workers increased 49 percent over 2009; expatriate humanitarian organizations primarily field Afghan workers and have either restricted their movements or closed projects altogether.

Health

In both Iraq and Afghanistan, the prolonged and highly organized terrorism led to a state of pervasive insecurity and a catastrophic deterioration of public health and social protections (Figure 46.2). Obtaining accurate data is especially difficult in prolonged terrorist environments.

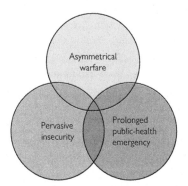

Figure 46.2 Current unconventional wars and conflicts, including terrorism, have three major interdependent and inseparable components that need equal monitoring, attention, and measurement. Reprinted from *The Lancet*. Burkle FM Jr. Measuring humanitarian assistance in conflicts. *Lancet* 2008; 371(9608): 189–90, with permission from Elsevier.

- The Ministry of Public Health in Afghanistan is notable in requiring that all NGO and other health programs conform to an integrated Basic Package of Health Services (BPHS) that focus on essential-health and public-health services most likely to mitigate direct and indirect mortality and morbidity; in 2010, 85 percent of the population currently have BPHS access.
- According to the 2008 *State of the World's Children* report, the modeled projections for 2008 of under-age-5 mortality rate (U5MR) stood at 257 per 1,000 live births, and the infant mortality rate (IMR) at 165 per 1,000 live births. They essentially had not changed since 2000.
- A 2010 Johns Hopkins study further analyzed the 2006 multistage cluster Afghanistan Health Survey of the rural population in 29 of 34 provinces (did not cover urban areas or highly unsafe regions) suggesting an adjusted (underreported for females) U5MR of 209 and IMR of 191.
- Schools remain the one place where most children receive basic health care and health education.

Food insecurity

In a 2009 report, food security had deteriorated in 25 of 34 Afghan Provinces.

- About 36 percent of the population lives below the poverty line and cannot afford basic necessities.
- Afghanistan ranks last among supplies in basic food staples in 163 countries and the only non-African nation among the 10 most food-insecure countries of the world.
- Up to 60 percent of children under age 5 are chronically malnourished.

Education

Advances in education are particularly threatening to Islamic and other terrorist groups worldwide:

- Schools and teachers are increasingly attacked as symbolic targets in religious or ideological conflicts: In Colombia, 360 teachers have been assassinated by Revolutionary Armed Forces of Colombia (FARC) and National Liberation Army (ELN) terrorists in the past decade. In Thailand, Muslim separatists demanding a Sharia-law sultanate routinely target teachers and schools.
- Education of girls and female teachers is highly threatening to AQ and other Islamic separatists. The intimidation of academics works to silence political opponents and restricting human-rights campaigns.
- A 2010 UN OCHA report states that half of schools in Afghanistan do not fit minimum standards for health and safety. School attendance is as low as 50 percent or more.

Women's rights

- During the rule of the Taliban (1996–2001), women were treated worse than at any time in the history of Islam. With the fall of the Taliban in 2001, the political and cultural position of Afghan women substantially improved, allowing them to return to work and serve in important position in the government. These successes remain fragile.

- According to the 2007 United Nations Development Program (UNDP), 90 percent of adult Afghan women are illiterate, and 75 percent of the girls attending primary school drop out before the fifth grade.
- A 2006 survey reported that violence against women is prevalent, extreme, systematic, and unreported. Sexual violence against girls, institutionalized through "traditions" such as child marriage, remains widespread.
- Suicide among young women is increasing, a number choosing self-immolation to escape the harsh realities of their lives.

Suggested readings

The Asia Foundation. Afghanistan in 2009: A survey of the Afghan people. Available at http://asiafoundation.org/resources/pdfs/Afghanistanin2009.pdf.

Burkle FM Jr. (2005, January). Integrating international responses to complex emergencies, unconventional war, and terrorism. *Crit Care Med 33*(1): S7–12.

Burkle FM Jr. (2008, January). Measuring humanitarian assistance in conflicts. *Lancet 371*(9608): 189–190.

Marks TA, Gorka SL, Sharp R. (2010) Getting the next war right: beyond population-centric warfare. *Prism; 1*(3): 79–96.

Viswanathan K, Becker S, Hansen PM, et al. (2010). Infant and under-five mortality in Afghanistan: Current estimates and limitations. *Bull World Health Organ 88*: 576–583.

Chapter 47

Public media relations

Tyeese Gaines Reid

Introduction

When crises occur that affect the public, there is both an urgency and necessity to disseminate information as quickly as possible

Media outlets strive to provide the public with frequent, up-to-date information. Health and governmental agencies strive to keep the public abreast of advisories, evacuation routes, and recovery efforts. Appropriate collaboration with media outlets can significantly aid public-health efforts during a crisis.

An organization's Public Information Officer (PIO) is the liaison between the organization and the general public, typically utilizing media outlets. A PIO's main goal is to gather accurate information and promptly disseminate that information in an organized, strategic, and informative manner. This dissemination can occur in anticipation of a crisis, such as a hurricane watch, or to notify victims after the crisis occurs.

Predetermined PIOs typically work full-time in communications or public relations, and have had extensive training on how to effectively work with media outlets. Sometimes, particularly in health organizations, a PIO may be designated at the last minute, with little to no media experience. This chapter serves as a quick guide for any PIO or public relations professional planning to head a disaster media initiative.

Preparation

Designate roles and responsibilities

Based on available manpower, designate the following roles and responsibilities. If manpower is limited, the PIO should include these duties in their job description.

Public Information Officer

- Coordinates communication efforts and acts as spokesperson for governmental or health organizations.
- Carefully protects the image they project on behalf of the organization.

Spokesperson

- Acts as the face of the organization, fielding questions from media contacts and making appearances.
  - Look for a representative who has public speaking experience.
  - Consider selecting the person with the best public-speaking skills over the highest-ranking officer in the organization.
  - A bilingual spokesperson may become helpful for non-English media outlets or for a bilingual audience when an interpreter is not available.

Event coordinator

- Schedules and publicizes press conferences.
- Coordinates multiple media interviews.
- Creates a shift schedule for multiple spokespersons, including an organized plan for handing off responsibilities between teams
- Schedules tours of damaged areas for the media.

- • If space is limited, allow one representative from each genre of media with the expectation that the representative will share with colleagues.
- Provides necessary material and equipment, including podium and audiovisual equipment.
- Decides on an appropriate space, considering size, background, echoes, and lighting.
- Makes press materials available to the media.

News desk
- Takes calls from media outlets.
- Disseminates basic information to the press.
- Manages real-time Internet updates.
- Keeps media outlets abreast of preparedness and awareness campaigns.

Public inquiries
- Answers main phone lines or hotlines.
- Fields questions.
- Collects information from general public.
- Disseminates updates.

News monitors
- Monitors various news outlets, particularly stories highlighting the organization.
  - • Important to prevent misinformation.
  - • Provides a chance to correct inaccuracies in the next interview.

Research your audience

Who is your audience?
- Education level:
  - • The average American has a sixth-grade reading level. Choose your words accordingly.
- What language do they speak?
- Age range?
- Gender?
- Demographics: Families, single professionals, college students, or a combination?
- Economic status?

What does your audience care about?
- Recent issues?
- News coverage?
- Polls, surveys?
- Letters to the editor?

Where is your audience?
- Members of the local, affected community?
- Loved ones in other parts of the world?

What does your audience need to know?
- General information:

- Course of events.
- Casualties, death toll.
- Overall plan.
- Forecast.
- Recovery efforts.
- Notices:
  - Escape routes.
  - Shelter locations.
  - Curfews.
  - Hotlines.
  - Available resources.
  - Preferred methods to check the status of victims.
- Advisories
  - Contaminated food.
  - Harmful substances.
  - Appropriate use of medical services.

What media outlets reach your audience?

- Mainstream media.
- Community outlets.
- Niche markets.
- Non-English media outlets.

Special populations

- Special needs (Braille, large print, American Sign Language).
- Disabilities.
- Non-English speakers.
- Pet owners.
- Children.

Gathering information

Sources

- Governmental agencies (health department, FEMA, mayor's office, etc.).
- On-scene responders (EMS, firefighters, police).
- Relevant experts.
- National Weather Service.
- Medical journals.
- Community organizations.
- Media reports.

PIO training

- Basic community public information and statistics.
- Incident Command System (ICS) courses.
- Press release writing.
- Interview basics.
- Disaster drills.

Materials

Keep a prepacked disaster media bag with necessary items. The Federal Emergency Management Agency (FEMA) GoKits is one good example:

- Laptop with external storage devices.
- Maps.

- Personal digital assistant (PDA), cell phone.
- Fax machine.
- Letterhead.
- Office supplies.
- Camera.
- Contact lists.
- Radio with extra batteries.
- Prescripted announcements.
- Prescripted press releases.
- Organization policies.
- Organization disaster plan.

Dissemination

Different types of information are appropriate for each phase of a crisis or disaster.

Preparedness
- Press releases.
- Weather advisories.
- Preparedness fairs.
- Brochures.

During or following the incident

Internal communication
Typically, internal communication is first priority, but it can be performed simultaneously with external communication.
- Employees
  - Details, impact of events.
  - Reassurance.
  - Ongoing efforts.
  - Actions that employees should take (staying home, versus reporting to work to assist).

External communication
- General public.
- Victims.
- Community leaders.
- Nongovernmental organizations (NGOs).
- Volunteers.

Methods
The highest-yield method of external communication is via media outlets, however, a multifaceted approach will ensure greater success. Consider limitations in accessibility (power outages, phone tower disruption, lack of internet access), and plan alternatives.
- Press releases.
- Television.
- Radio.
- Newspapers.
- Web sites.
- E-mails, faxes.
- Texts.
- Government and police memorandums.
- Emergency Alert System.
- Reverse 911.
- Loud speakers.
- Door-to-door.
- Meetings.
- Press conferences.
- Newsletters.
- Word of mouth (community groups, churches).

Press releases

Public relations personnel and public information officers (PIOs) use press releases to communicate to the media, and occasionally, the public. Media outlets use press releases to remain abreast of newsworthy topics and events they may choose to cover.

Press releases are written in layman's terms and include quotes from important officials and experts. See Box 47.1. Expect that news outlets will copy directly from your press release word for word. For that reason, releases should be written in "newsy" format, providing the journalist with enough information to write at least one basic story.

Every journalist will spin the same topic differently. So, even if you write a complete and thorough press release, journalists may still call for updates occurring since the release or additional quotes.

General format:
- Standard press releases are 300 to 800 words.
- Left-justified, single-spaced.
- Do not type in ALL CAPS.
- Keep paragraphs as short as possible.
- Place one line of space in between each 1- to 2-sentence paragraph.
- Only use plain text, so the release can be easily e-mailed (no images or fancy graphics).

Content:
- Headline
  - Headlines are typically 80 characters or less.
  - The headline should immediately grab your target audience's attention.
  - Look at newspaper headlines for examples.
- Date and time of planned release.
- Contact
  - Organization name
  - Name, e-mail address, and phone number of the organization's public-relations contact.

Box 47.1 How to format a press release

HEADLINE
FOR IMMEDIATE RELEASE
Month, Day, Year

Organization
Contact: Full name
(xxx) xxx-xxxx

Synopsis (optional)
Location (city, state) — Lead paragraph.
2–3 paragraphs of body text, including quotes.

Boiler plate, including organization mission, and current contact information including e-mail.

- Synopsis (optional)
  - A 1- to 4-sentence synopsis of the topic.
  - Similar to headlines, synopses are longer and written in sentence format.
- Lead
  - Lead sentences are typically 25 words or less.
  - Opening line should be interesting and engaging.
  - Lead with the best information, even if it requires further explanation later.
  - Unlike a thesis or term paper with a slow introduction, followed by facts that build up to a strong conclusion, put the best information upfront in the first two sentences.
  - Ask yourself, why does this matter today?
- Body
  - Used to explain the lead in greater detail.
  - Remember the 5 W's and How (Who, What, Where, When, Why and How?). See Creating the Story, under Talking to the Media, later in this chapter.
- Quotes
  - Quotes from officials or spokespersons are mandatory.
  - Use the body text to explain facts. Use quotes to personalize, display authority, or show authority.
  - It may be odd to write your own quotes. Ask someone to interview you if you run into trouble.
  - Use quotes from multiple sources, if possible. Make sure each quote adds something different. Not just repeating information found elsewhere in your release.
  - Quotes should be full sentences. See Delivering a Sound Byte, under Talking to the Media later in this chapter.
- Boiler plate
  - An italicized blurb that includes the official summary of your organization's efforts. It is the very last paragraph in the release.
  - Include the most accurate and easily accessible contact information.
- General Tips
  - Use present tense.
  - Use active verbs.
  - Use layman's terms.
  - Be concise. Avoid unnecessary adjectives or redundant expressions (use stand instead of stand *up*).
  - Write with a conversational tone.
  - Check spelling.
  - Pick your angle and focus the release on that one angle. Other releases can cover the other angles. Do not try to cram too much information into a single release.
  - Drier, factual, or chronological information goes toward the end.

Design strategic dissemination efforts

Consider which avenues provide the highest yield. Have prescripted press releases.
- E-mail is a rapid and efficient way to distribute press releases and newsletters.
- Web sites make large amounts of information accessible to a large amount of the public.
- Utilize community figures to help spread information.

Talking to the media

The most effective utilization of media outlets for public-health crises includes a team of PIOs, officials, and media personnel collaborating harmoniously. The primary goal of a PIO when working with media outlets is to accurately distribute information about a crisis while providing the journalist with an interesting story.

Media's impact

As PIOs provide information to the public via media reports, it is important to understand both the positive and negative impacts on the community as a whole.

Psychological effects

- Media reports can help by providing accurate information to anxious viewers.
- Posttraumatic stress disorder (PTSD) is not uncommon, especially among pediatric viewers watching repetitive, disturbing images related to catastrophic events.
- Mass Psychogenic Illness (MPI)
  - Symptoms (with no organic cause) brought on or exacerbated by media reports.
  - Cases associated with supposedly toxic Coca-Cola in Belgium (1999), a chemical odor smelled at a Tennessee school (1998), adverse reactions to vaccinations in Jordan (1998), and the hospitalization of 600 children in Japan after watching a popular cartoon animation on television (1997).
  - After Chernobyl (1986), media reports were found to have done more harm, providing incorrect information and causing mass hysteria.

Box 47.2 PIO preparation

30-Minute PIO preparation
- 5W's (Who, What, Where, When, Why) and How
- Basic community data
- Hot topics in the community
- Local media contacts
- Names of top community officials (memorize or make a cheat sheet)
- Upcoming plans
- Advisories

During the interview:
- Provide proven facts, cite sources when appropriate.
- Never say "No comment."
- Speak with emotion and compassion.
- Nothing is ever "off the record."
- Speak in full sentences.
- Do not read from your cheat sheet. Only glance down sparingly.
- Watch nervous habits such as, "um," "like," or talking with fast-moving hands.
- Wear solid colors that complement skin color.
- Consider light makeup to cover blemishes and outline eyes (♂ as well as ♀).

Negative outcomes and responsibility
- Both journalists and PIOs are concerned with negative outcomes from media attention.
  - Studies have shown that reports alone are unlikely to cause panic.
  - No need to withhold facts, but be careful to present accurate information.
  - Aim to present information strategically.

Public opinion and policy
- Media has been shown to shape public opinion and policy.
- Most notably, coverage of Hurricane Katrina recovery efforts helped shape subsequent federal emergency management responses.
- There was also a significant effect on the public's opinion of FEMA.

Trust
- Accurate and timely information invokes public trust for that particular agency or organization throughout the disaster.
- Public trust becomes increasingly important in the face of conflicting information from various sources.
- The public may also not heed a warning if it is preceded by too many false alarms.

Suggested readings

Barnes MD, Hanson CL, Novilla LMB, et al. (2008). Analysis of media agenda setting during and after Hurricane Katrina: Implications for emergency preparedness, disaster response, and disaster policy. *Am J Public Health* 98: 604–610.

Dilling S, Gluckman W, Rosenthal MS, et al. (2006). Media relations. In Ciottone G, ed., *Disaster Medicine*, pp.124–129. Philadelphia: Elsevier-Mosby.

FEMA. (2007). Basic guidance for public information officers (PIOs), the national incident management system (NIMS). FEMA 517.

Lowrey W, Evans W, Gower KK, et al. (2007). Effective media communication of disasters: Pressing problems and recommendations. *BMC Public Health* 7:97.

Vasterman P, Yzermans CJ, Dirkzwager AJE. (2005). The role of the media and media hypes in the aftermath of disasters. *Epidemiol Rev 27*: 107–114.

Ultrasound in disaster medicine

Krithika M. Muruganandan
Sachita Shah

Introduction

Over the years, the use of ultrasound has extended beyond the traditional hospital setting to disaster relief, military medicine, austere/resource-poor settings and prehospital care. In a mass casualty event or disaster, the surge in volume of critically ill and injured patients remains a challenge. It is necessary to quickly and efficiently identify these patients among the masses in order to direct them to prompt resuscitation and care. Point-of-care ultrasound has gained momentum due to its versatility and durability. Its technology has developed rapidly, enabling lightweight, portable and sturdy machines. In published literature, there are reports of the utility of ultrasound in several natural disasters including the earthquakes in Turkey (1999), China (2007), and Haiti (2010), the mudslides in Guatemala (2005), and the cyclone in Australia (2007). Ultrasound has proven to be useful in these harsh environments both locally and internationally and can aid in the clinical care of trauma and medical patients.

Extended focused assessment with sonography for trauma

E-FAST (Extended Focused Assessment with Sonography for Trauma) has been used routinely in the management of trauma patients in the emergency department and is often an extension of the physical exam. In a disaster setting, this test is arguably the most important ultrasound exam a clinician can know and perform. E-FAST is a rapid noninvasive way to evaluate patients with thoracoabdominal trauma answering the following clinical questions:

- Is there free fluid in the peritoneum?
- Is there a pericardial effusion/tamponade?
- Is there a hemothorax?
- Is there a pneumothorax?

In the peritoneal cavity, ultrasound identifies blood pooling in dependent areas: Morrison's pouch (between the liver and kidney), the splenorenal/perisplenic space, and the inferior portion of the pelvis (pouch of Douglas). E-FAST also includes cardiac and lung views to identify thoracic injuries.

The E-FAST scan can be performed rapidly, in less than three minutes. It has also been shown to decrease time to operative intervention and decrease hospital length of stay. The sensitivity of E-FAST scans in detecting intraperitoneal hemorrhage ranges from 65 to 95 percent and its specificity is approximately 98 percent. The volume of intraperitoneal blood necessary for detection is approximately 200–300 cc. In addition, ultrasound is more sensitive than a supine chest radiograph in diagnosing pneumothorax and can detect a small hemothorax of as little as 30 cc. Clinically, the E-FAST scan is particularly beneficial in evaluating the hypotensive trauma patient.

E-FAST is ideal in a disaster setting for multiple reasons. When rapidly evaluating multiple severely injured patients, E-FAST can serve as a triage tool to identify severe life-threatening injuries. In a facility with operative capacity, these patients can then be directed to lifesaving surgical interventions including exploratory laparotomy, chest-tube thoracostomy, or pericardiocentesis. E-FAST is also valuable in a resource-poor setting where there is limited access to computed tomography and plain-film radiography.

E-FAST has some limitations, including its inability to identify retroperitoneal hemorrhage, bowel injury, diaphragmatic injury, and encapsulated solid organ injury. Its ability to visualize deep structures is limited by obesity and subcutaneous emphysema. Blood, urine, and ascites are indistinguishable by ultrasound, therefore, clinical correlation is necessary if intraperitoneal fluid is detected. In some cases, peritoneal aspiration may be indicated to make a definitive diagnosis. And finally, a negative E-FAST does not reliably exclude a serious thoracoabdominal injury since the scan may have been performed when there was insufficient intraperitoneal blood for ultrasound detection. Therefore, in a patient with a negative E-FAST, consider serial ultrasound exams if their condition deteriorates.

Indications for E-FAST
- Blunt thoracoabdominal trauma.
- Penetrating thoracic trauma.
- Unexplained hypotension.

Equipment
- Ultrasound machine, gel.
- Curved or phased array probe, frequency 2–5 Hz.
- Linear probe, 7–12 Hz (pneumothorax exam)

E-FAST – procedure, 5 Views
Patient position: supine
  Note: Blood appears black (anechoic) on ultrasound.

1. Right upper quadrant, Morrison's pouch.
- Place the probe at the right midaxillary line between the 9th and 12th rib with the probe marker toward the patient's head.
- Check for fluid (black/anechoic stripe) between liver and kidney.
- Slide the probe toward the patient's head to evaluate for blood (hemothorax) above the right diaphragm.
- Placing the patient in Trendelenburg position may increase test sensitivity.
- See Figure 48.1.

2. Left upper quadrant, perisplenic/perirenal
- Place the probe at the left midposterior axillary line between the 8th and 10th rib with marker toward the patient's head.
- Check for blood around the spleen, between the spleen and diaphragm, and between the spleen and kidney.
- Slide the probe toward the patient's head to evaluate above the left diaphragm for hemothorax.
- See Figure 48.2.

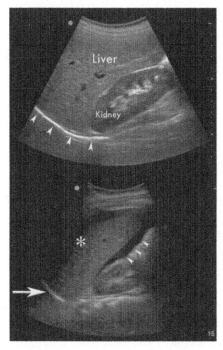

Figure 48.1 FAST right upper quadrant: The top image represents normal right upper quadrant with the kidney and liver labeled. Small arrow heads are pointing to the diaphragm. The lower image is a positive FAST where the large arrow points to the diaphragm, and small arrow heads point to the anechoic stripe between liver and kidney representing intraperitoneal hemorrhage. Reproduced with permission from Partners in Health. Manual of Ultrasound for Resource-Limited Settings, 2011.

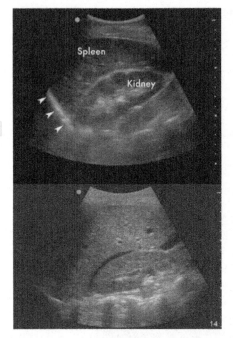

Figure 48.2 FAST left upper quadrant: The top image represents a normal left upper quadrant with the spleen and kidney labeled. Small arrow heads are pointing to the diaphragm. The lower image is a positive FAST with an anechoic stripe between the spleen and kidney representing intraperitoneal hemorrhage. Reproduced with permission from Partners in Health. Manual of Ultrasound for Resource-Limited Settings, 2011.

3. Subxiphoid, pericardium
- Place the probe inferior to the xiphoid process and costal margin with the probe marker toward the right side. Angle the probe upward toward the heart.
- Check for an effusion in pericardial space, between the liver and the right ventricle.
- Alternate View: Parasternal long-axis view (if subxiphoid view is inadequate). Place the probe in the 3rd/4th intercostals space, left of the sternum with the probe marker toward the right shoulder. Look for effusion in the anterior/posterior pericardium.
- See Figure 48.3.

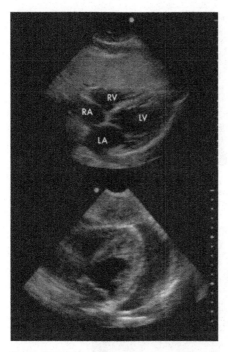

Figure 48.3 FAST subxiphoid pericardial view: The top image is a normal subxiphoid view with right atrium (RA), right ventricle (RV), left atrium (LA), and left ventricle (LV) labeled. The lower image represents a positive FAST with a circumferential anechoic stripe around the heart representing a pericardial effusion. Reproduced with permission from Partners in Health. Manual of Ultrasound for Resource-Limited Settings, 2011.

4. Suprapubic, pelvic cul-de-sac
- Place the probe midline, superior to the symphysis pubis visualizing bladder in sagittal and transverse plane
- Check for blood in the dependant area of the pelvis: recto-uterine pouch in females, and the rectovesical pouch in males (Pouch of Douglas).
- See Figure 48.4.

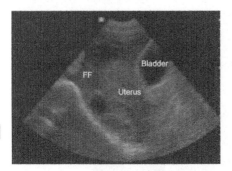

Figure 48.4 FAST Pelvis: The above image represents a positive FAST with the bladder, uterus and free fluid (FF) labeled. Reproduced with permission from Partners in Health. Manual of Ultrasound for Resource-Limited Settings, 2011.

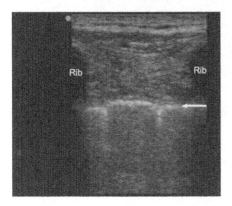

Figure 48.5 FAST Anterior Thorax: The above image represents a normal lung without a pneumothorax. The ribs are labeled and the pleura is marked with an arrow. Notice the comet tails, the white vertical lines descending from the pleural line. Reproduced with permission from Partners in Health. Manual of Ultrasound for Resource-Limited Settings, 2011.

5. Anterior Thorax, Pneumothorax

- Linear probe (6–10 Hz).
- Place the probe in the sagittal plane at the midclavicular line, 2nd intercostal space with the probe marker toward the patient's head.
- Check for lung sliding (movement along the pleural line) and comet tails (bright white lines descending from pleural line) with respiration.
- The absence of these two findings indicates a pneumothorax.
- Repeat at the 3rd, 4th, 5th intercostals space bilaterally.
- See Figure 48.5.

Other uses for ultrasound in resource-poor settings

Deep vein thrombosis

Evaluating for DVT is useful in patients with crush injuries or prolonged immobilization. The linear vascular probe is used to identify the common femoral vein and superficial femoral vein at the level of the inguinal crease and the popliteal vein in the popliteal fossa. Vein compressibility is evaluated by placing direct pressure on the vein. Absence of normal compressibility indicates DVT. Color flow and Doppler can also be used to evaluate for DVT.

Orthopedic injuries

In the absence of plain radiograph, ultrasound can be used to identify displaced fractures. Using the linear probe and sliding along injured area, ultrasound can detect cortical disruptions at the fracture site along with associated hematoma. Ultrasound-guided hematoma blocks can then be performed that may be useful for fracture-reductions and pain control.

Soft tissue

The linear probe can be used to evaluate pathology in the soft tissue. Ultrasound can differentiate cellulitis from abscess by identifying fluid collections in abscesses compared with the classic cobble stone pattern that is seen in cellulitis. Ultrasound can also evaluate cysts and foreign bodies.

Intravenous catheter placement

If the traditional IV approach as failed, the linear probe can assist in IV catheter placement. The target vein (which is compressible and nonpulsatile) is identified by ultrasound and the needle is advanced under direct ultrasound visualization. This technique limits injury to surrounding structures (arteries or nerves) and improves success rate in cannulation of the vessel. This is used for both central and peripheral venous access.

Echocardiography, inferior vena cava

Ultrasound evaluation of the heart and inferior vena cava (IVC) can be useful in determining the volume status of a patient. Multiple views of the heart are used in evaluating left ventricular function and cardiac contractility. IVC collapsibility with inspiration of greater than 50 percent correlates with intravascular volume depletion. Both these parameters can be used to guide resuscitation efforts.

Nerve block

Ultrasound guided nerve blocks can be used to provide regional anesthesia in complex laceration repairs, orthopedic fracture/dislocation reductions, and operative procedures. Forearm and brachial plexus nerve blocks are useful for upper extremity injuries and femoral and popliteal nerve blocks are useful for lower extremity injuries. This provides an alternative to general anesthesia and is useful in a resource-poor setting with minimal anesthesia support. Ultrasound guided nerve blocks also improve success rates and decrease complication rates.

Suggested readings

Ma J (2003). *Emergency Ultrasound.* New York: McGraw-Hill.
Noble VE (2007). Manual of emergency and critical ultrasound. New York: Cambridge University Press.
Shah S. (2011). Manual for ultrasound in resource limited settings. *Partners in Health USA.* Available at http://parthealth.3cdn.net/3ad982b2456f524cf8_kxvm6qpr9.pdf.
www.emsono.com
www.sonoguide.com

Disaster informatics

Kenneth A. Williams

Definition

Informatics is the study of information acquisition, processing, management, organization, and delivery. Computers are used to manage complex systems, but increasingly, in this rapidly evolving discipline, these operations can be carried out using handheld and other smart devices. Disaster informatics is the application of these concepts to disaster prevention, response, recovery, and mitigation.

Introduction

Disasters raise many information-management challenges. In a broad sense, most disasters do not involve injury or illness; they primarily involve finance, damaged or challenged resources, behavior, relationships, or other aspects of human and business efforts. This type of disaster may involve data and information management. For example, release of damaging or confidential information to the media, loss of computer files, or errors in information systems can be devastating to businesses, hospitals, governments, or individuals. This type of disaster however, is beyond the scope of this book, and this chapter will focus on disaster informatics as a resource during medical-disaster management.

Informatics in disaster management

Complete reliance on electronic/computer information management systems should be avoided. Just as with other aspects of disaster management, redundancy, reliability, and flexibility in information management are keys to success. Both electronic and paper systems with independent backup of important information will assure continuity of operations in most circumstances. The following are some aspects of disaster management where information systems are important.

Responder issues
- Recruiting.
  - Forming teams of the needed composition.
- Credentialing.
  - Assuring valid credentials in the necessary fields.
- Training and competency
  - Adult education and competency tracking.
- Preparation.
  - Acquiring and cataloging equipment, briefings.
- Deployment.
  - Travel plans, credentials, disaster site arrival logistics.
- Accountability.
  - Responder location, status, availability.
- Operations.
  - Documenting and communicating rescue and care of victims, access to information resources from command structure, media, and personal sources (family and others not deployed).
- Rehabilitation.
  - Determining fitness, screening for illness/injury.
- Repatriation and debriefing.
  - Travel, counseling, acquisition of knowledge for future responders.

Patients and victims
- Personal communication and information access.
  - Calls for assistance, knowledge about the incident.
- Family/group coordination.
  - Reassurance information, family or group connection.
- Personal data challenges.
  - Loss of personal financial, business, or other data and related devices.

Patient care
- Location and rescue.
  - Search and location of patients.
  - Hazard and other rescue information.
- Tracking.
  - Triggers for event-related patterns (outbreaks, hazardous materials exposures).
  - Location of patients and their flow through the response system.
- Documentation.
  - Medical care records.

- Diagnostics.
  - Access to images, test results, etc.
- Reference access.
  - Medical information, literature, and expert consultation via telemedicine.
- Therapy and education.
  - Use of information technology to educate patients and provide therapy.

Incident management team
- Resources.
  - Amount, location, type of resources.
- Command and control.
  - Communication with responders, media, resources.
- Logistics.
  - Coordinating search, resource supply and deployment, weather effects, etc.
- Finance
  - Donations, tracking of expenses, allocation of revenue, justification of expenditures.
- Operations.
  - Daily incident operations.
- Safety.
  - Hazards, care of equipment, disease risks, weather, responder fatigue, etc.
- Mitigation and prevention.
  - Automated sensors, detectors, monitors.

Wireless Internet and cellular-telephone access ideally should be part of typical disaster management. These resources should be part of an integrated communications and informatics system involving data servers and software to enhance response. Importantly, sole reliance on any one of these systems should be avoided—redundancy is key. Devices exist (see Figure 49.1) that can provide these information services in remote areas via satellite or microwave link. Responders, managers, and others can share information via a variety of devices. These devices are evolving rapidly and continue to offer improved speed, longevity, and flexibility. Various technologies also now exist to *acquire* data; share, *coordinate*, transmit disaster data (including images, geographic location, resource material etc.); and *analyze* this data for responder, management, and other purposes (see Figure 49.2).

In addition to direct use of informatics by the disaster response system, those affected by a disaster as victims, patients, or local residents can benefit both themselves and the response if they have ready access to information services. Traditionally, local residents perform many of the immediate rescue, coordination, and sheltering aspects of disaster response. Engaging these people through distributed information systems by providing accurate and timely information will enhance their ability to assist themselves, their families, and their neighbors. Current technologies allow these local residents to provide feedback to the response system

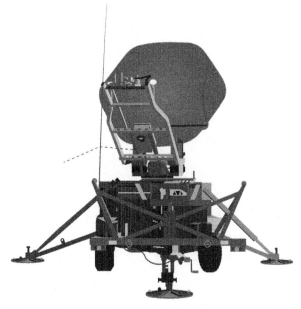

Figure 49.1 Remote interoperable communications.

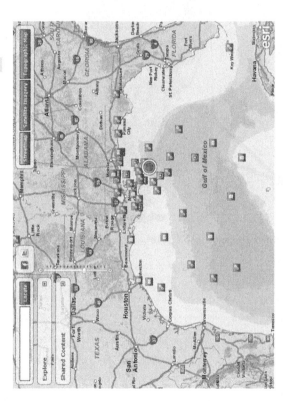

Figure 49.2 Gulf-oil-spill data mapping to assist with disaster response. Reprinted with permission from Esri: www.esri.com/services/disaster-response/gulf-oil-spill-2010/index.html.

(by e-mail, text, or cellular phone, for example), thereby also engaging them as sources of valuable information for rescue, logistics, response, and outbreak monitoring.

Suggested readings

For more information on medical informatics, see www.AMIA.org

For more information on new radio technologies, see:

http://www.swri.org/3pubs/ttoday/Summer07/Software.htm http://www.project25.org/

http://www.its.dot.gov/ng911/

For more information on graphic (map) information systems, see: www.esri.com

For information on informatics for disaster victims, see http://redcrosschat.org/about-the-emergency-social-data-summit/

http://www.its.dot.gov/ng911/

Chapter 50

Palliative care in disaster medicine

Michelle Daniel

David C. MacKenzie

Introduction

- Disasters, both large and small, are likely to yield victims who may have survived the initial insult, but who are not expected to survive long term.
- Although the primary goal of a coordinated disaster response is to maximize the number of lives saved, a secondary, but no less important goal, should be to provide the maximal amount of physical and psychological comfort to those who are suffering and dying.
- Palliative care is an ethical, humane, and appropriate care option for patients not designated to receive life-saving or curative treatment.
- Palliative care is a valuable component of treatment for *all* patients, as even those who are not expected to die deserve to have their suffering addressed.
- To date, little has been written about the role of palliative care in disasters. Further discussion and research is needed to help refine its role in the response rubric.

Defining palliative care

Having a clear understanding of what palliative care is, and what palliative care is not, is critical to the successful incorporation of palliation into a disaster response.

Palliative care is:
- Evidence-based care focused on the aggressive management of symptoms and the relief of suffering.
- Care that honors the humanity of the sick and the dying through medical, social, spiritual, and psychological support.

Palliative care is not:
- Abandonment.
- Elimination of treatment.
- Euthanasia.

These definitions are critical to public and provider acceptance of palliation as a treatment modality during times of crisis.

In our everyday practice, providers are accustomed to patients choosing whether they wish to receive life-sustaining interventions or palliation. During disasters, resource scarcity will force providers to adopt a more utilitarian approach. In attempting to achieve the greatest good for the greatest number of people, victims who are not expected to survive should be triaged to receive palliative care only.

Triage incorporating palliative care concepts

Most traditional triage schemes do not incorporate palliative care concepts. Multiple different triage schemes exist worldwide. The one most widely used during disaster response is the START system (Simple Triage and Rapid Treatment.) The START system segregates victims into four color-coded categories:

- Expectant (black) patients are those who are dead, or who are not expected to survive. They have catastrophic injuries requiring extensive medical treatment that exceeds the medical resources available.
- Immediate (red) patients are those deemed to have life threatening or moderately severe injuries requiring immediate intervention. They are treatable with a minimum of time, personnel, and supplies, and they have a good chance of recovery.
- Delayed (yellow) patients are injured, but not expected to die or worsen significantly if treatment is delayed.
- Ambulatory (green) patients are the walking wounded who require only minor treatment.

In practice, some patients categorized as immediate may need to be managed as expectant if the medical resources needed to treat them are not available in the disaster aftermath. All patients in the expectant and many of the patients in the immediate categories should be assigned to receive palliative care.

In addition to these critically injured short-term survivors, other patients in the population with preexisting illnesses will be severely affected by the shifts in standards of care and scarcity of health-care resources. These patients may include, but are not limited to, previously ventilator-dependent patients, the terminally ill, and the extremely old and frail. These patients may all benefit from a focus on palliative care.

These difficult triage decisions pose substantial challenges to all involved. Emergency providers must recognize that some people who might survive under different circumstances will now die. Resisting designating people as unlikely to survive, and attempting to save everybody, can exacerbate an already overwhelmed medical system. Incorporating palliative care as a viable and humane treatment option may reduce health-care provider and public resistance to such designations.

Triage schemes that incorporate palliative care as a treatment option will work most effectively when:

- They are publicly transparent, straightforward, fair, valid, and consistent across settings.
- They are flexible enough to adapt to changing circumstances (patients who were expected to die may unexpectedly do well, and their category should change accordingly. As new resources become available, a patient's category may also change from expectant to immediate.)

- Communication lines are open regarding resources that *will be* available. This is critical to appropriate patient assignation to triage categories. Unfortunately, this is often very difficult to achieve in real time, and decisions must be made with the best available information.
- Difficult triage decisions are shared by a small group of providers instead of being made by individuals. This distributes the burden of decision making and may reduce the psychological stress felt by health-care professionals after the event.

Once a triage decision has been made to focus on palliative care, time and resources should not be wasted on interventions unlikely to improve a patients' comfort.

Planning and surge capacity

Comprehensive disaster plans should incorporate palliative care surge capacity into their response strategies. On any given day, 1–2 percent of the population is in need of palliative services. In the wake of a disaster, this percentage could increase significantly. Stockpiles of supplies and training of providers in advance of a crisis will improve the response. The following supplies should be stockpiled:

- Personal protective equipment.
- Essential palliative care medications (see later section)—controlled substances such as narcotics and benzodiazepines may require special security measures to be in place.
- Butterfly needles, transparent film dressings, syringes, patient controlled analgesia (PCA) pumps, oral droppers.
- Incontinence supplies.
- Beds or cushioned surfaces.

Identification of providers

Providers of palliative care should be identified and trained before an event. People already working in hospice settings, on interdisciplinary palliative care teams, or in nursing homes may be designated for leadership roles.

Once a mass casualty event has occurred, skilled health-care providers may be deployed to treat the most "medically salvageable." Clergy, social workers, and even laypersons can be recruited to provide comfort care. Many will already have skills that lend themselves to ministering to the dying. Although it may be difficult for physicians and nurses to accept, their time may be best spent in the first hours to days following a disaster training others to provide needed repetitive care, rather than ministering to patients themselves. Laypeople can be trained to safely administer the majority of palliative medications. Focusing on medications that can be administered by topical patches or oral droppers (instead of by intravenous or subcutaneous routes), will reduce the amount of skilled health-care interventions required, and facilitate administration by families or other volunteers.

Sites of care

Palliative care can occur anywhere, but creating sites designated for comfort care makes logistical sense. This could occur at the scene, within a hospital, or at an alternative care site (ACS.)

On-scene segregation of patients triaged to receive palliative care only:

• Provides for clear identification of those designated for expectant management.
• Allows comfort-care resources to be focused in one geographic area.
• Ensures that valuable ambulance services are not used on patients unlikely to benefit from transport.
• May help contain exposure to pathogens or radiation to the scene.

Segregation of patients to a specific ward within a hospital similarly helps identify the goals of care, and allows for the geographic concentration of resources (e.g., social work, clergy) When these patients are intermingled with general ward patients, they are more likely to receive interventions that are not focused on their comfort (e.g., blood-pressure medications, lipid-lowering drugs, blood draws, tests, and procedures) that have no effect on their long-term outcome.

Sending patients designated as palliative-care only to alternative care sites is another possibility. This has the advantage of freeing up hospital beds for medically salvageable patients. Nursing homes, churches, large public buildings, or even patients' homes are possibilities. If ACSs are to be used, palliative-care stockpiles should be accessible from these sites. Flexibility must exist within the system such that patients can be transferred out to higher levels of care should their triage status change. Barriers to this approach include public resistance to the overt rationing of health-care resources. Ensuring the public understands that these patients will receive aggressive treatment of their symptoms and suffering and that they will not be abandoned, is critical to the success of any palliative-care site.

Common symptoms requiring palliation

Common symptoms encountered in patients requiring palliation include:
- Pain (may be mild to severe; bony, visceral, or neuropathic).
- Shortness of breath.
- Pulmonary secretions, including terminal respiratory congestion (death rattle).
- Nausea and vomiting.
- Diarrhea.
- Constipation.
- Incontinence.
- Fever.
- Anxiety.
- Depression.
- Delirium.
- Insomnia.
- Restlessness.
- Fatigue.
- Skin wounds and breakdown.
- Itching.
- Sweating.
- Dry mouth.
- Anorexia.
- Cough.
- Hiccups.

Patient assessment should identify symptoms that can be treated with medication, nursing care, and psychosocial support. Aggressive symptom management is a core element of palliative care. When medications are dosed carefully, and patients reassessed regularly, caregivers can generally titrate medication doses to the desired effect. In some instances, the medication doses required to relieve suffering may inadvertently hasten death. The ethical principle of "double effect" suggests this may be permissible in the context of end-of-life care, if the caregiver's *intent* is symptom palliation and not euthanasia.

Essential medications for palliative care

Table 50.1 Essential medications for palliative care

Drug	Indication	Adult Dose
Acetaminophen / Paracetamol	Pain: mild to moderate Fever	650 mg PO or PR q4 hours PRN
Amitriptyline	Depression Neuropathic pain	25–150 mg PO qd
Bisacodyl	Constipation	10 mg PO or PR PRN
Carbamazepine	Neuropathic pain	200 mg PO bid
Citalopram	Depression	20 mg PO qd
Codeine	Cough Diarrhea	30 mg PO q4 hours PRN
Dexamethasone	Anorexia Nausea/vomiting Cerebral/spinal metastases Bowel obstruction by tumor	4–8 mg PO q12–24 hours
Diazepam	Anxiety	2.5–5 mg PO or IV q6–8 hours
Diclofenac	Pain: mild to moderate	50 mg PO q8 hours
Diphenhydramine	Nausea Itching	25–50 mg PO or IV q6 hours
Fentanyl	Pain: moderate to severe	25–50 mcg/hr patch q72 hours, or 25–75 mcg IV PRN
Gabapentin	Neuropathic pain	300 mg q8 hours
Halperidol	Delirium Terminal restlessness Nausea	2.5–5 mg PO or IM PRN
Hysocine/ Scopolamine	Nausea/vomiting Visceral pain	1 patch q3 days (hydrobromide) 0.6 mg IM, SC, or IV q8 hours (butylbromide) 10–20 mg PO, IM, SC, or IV q4 hours
Ibuprofen	Pain: mild to moderate	200–600 mg PO q6 hours
Loperamide	Diarrhea	2 mg PO PRN
Lorazepam	Anxiety	0.5–2 mg PO or IV PRN
Megestrol	Anorexia	800 mg PO qd
Methadone	Pain: moderate to severe	5–10 mg PO q4–8 hours
Metoclopramide	Nausea/vomiting Hiccups	10 mg PO or IV q8 hours

Table 50.1 (Contd.)

Drug	Indication	Adult Dose
Midazolam	Anxiety	1–2 mg PO or IV PRN
Mineral oil enema	Constipation	118 mL PR
Mirtazapine	Depression	15 mg qHS
Morphine	Pain: moderate to severe	5–10 mg PO, IV, or PR PRN
	Dyspnea	
Octreotide	Vomiting/diarrhea	100 mcg SC q 8 hours
Oral rehydration salts	Diarrhea	As directed by kit
Oxycodone	Pain: moderate to severe	5–10 mg PO q4 hours
Prednisolone	Anorexia	10 mg PO q8 hours
Senna	Constipation	2 tablets PO qd
Tramadol	Pain–mild to moderate	50–100 mg PO q6 hours
Trazodone	Insomnia	25–75 mg PO qHS
Zolpidem	Insomnia	5–10 mg PO qHS

- Many palliative-care medications come in liquid form and may be administered by dropper to patients otherwise unable to take medications by mouth.
- The least resource-intensive route of administration should be chosen whenever that route is adequate for symptom control.
- Families and laypersons may be quickly trained to administer topical, oral, and even rectal medications.
- Some medications and supplies (e.g., PCA pumps) are likely to be in short supply even with the best of plans. Flexibility in the choice of drugs and an emphasis on the augmentation of comfort through nonpharmaceutical means is helpful.

Pediatric considerations

Provision of palliative care for a pediatric population poses unique challenges, even when optimal resources are available. These barriers may be exacerbated after a disaster, or in a resource-limited setting. Disease states that may not typically be considered palliative may be triaged as such following a disaster. Providers may be reluctant to identify or label a child as best served by palliative care, but they should not be swayed from appropriate triage, particularly in the postdisaster context. A child's triage category should be reassessed at regular intervals to determine if their clinical status or resource availability has changed.

Several principles differentiate pediatric palliative care from the care of adults.

- Children may have physiologic reserve that frail adults do not possess. Alternatively, they may be at greater risk if they are malnourished or have preexisting disease.
- Infants and young children may be unable or less likely to express specific complaints, complicating attempts to provide targeted symptom relief.
- Caregivers may over- or underestimate discomfort.
- Pediatric patients have a variable understanding of disease and death in both physical and psychological dimensions. Understanding will vary with developmental stage. The permanence of death is typically not understood until at least 5–7 years of age.
- Children will communicate, and should be engaged and assessed, in light of their developmental level. In settings with sufficient resources, engaging children with opportunities for nonverbal forms of expression and play is standard of care.
- Parents should be directly involved with the care of their children, if culturally appropriate.
- Medication administration may be more difficult, as some children will be unable to swallow pills. Topical, liquid, and chewable formulations are desirable.
- Pediatric medications should be dosed by weight, rather than by standard initial doses. Children can have wider variability in metabolism and elimination of drugs than adults; titration to effect requires careful observation.
- A dying or critically ill child is a unique source of stress and grief for family members and caregivers alike. Whenever possible, psychosocial support should be offered to those caring for palliative pediatric patients.
- Disaster-response team planners should consider specific inclusion of caregivers with pediatric experience.

Suggested readings

Agency for Healthcare Research and Quality (2005). Altered standards of care in mass casualty events. *AHRQ* 05-0043. Available at http://www.ahrq.gov/research/altstand/altstand.pdf. Accessed November 9, 2010.

Bogucki S, Jubanyik K (2009). Triage, rationing, and palliative care in disaster planning. *Biosecur Bioterror* 7(2): 221–224.

De Lima L (2007). International Association for Hospice and Palliative Care list of essential medicines for palliative care. *Ann Oncol 18* (2): 395–399.

Himelstein BP, Hilden JM, Boldt AM, Weissman D (2004). Pediatric palliative care. *N Engl J Med 350:* 1752–1762.

International Association for Hospice and Palliative Care Essential Medicines for Palliative Care List. http://www.hospicecare.com/resources/pdf-docs/iahpc-essential-meds-en.pdf

Matzo M, Wilkinson A, Lynn J, Gatto M, Phillips S (2009). Palliative care considerations in mass casualty events with scarce resources. *Biosecur Bioterror* 7(2): 199–210.

World Health Organization (2006, November). Definition of palliative care. Available at http://www.who.int/cancer/palliative/definition/en/ (Accessed November 9, 2010).

World Health Organization (2004, June). Integrated management of adult and adolescent illness: Palliative care: Symptom management and end of life care. Available at http://www.who.int/3by5/publications/documents/en/genericpalliativecare082004.pdf (Accessed November 15, 2010).

Chapter 51

Seasonal risks and variations of an aerosolized bioterror attack

Ryan Tai

Selim Suner

Overview

Biological agents can be dispersed by various routes, including aerosolization of infectious particles, contamination of water supplies, and dissemination of infected vectors or reservoirs. However, it is difficult to achieve significant mortality and morbidity with contamination of water sources with biological agents. Often, water sources are treated with chlorine and germicidal radiation. Additionally, enough infectious particles must be released into the water source to achieve a concentration that can cause substantial morbidity and mortality. Dissemination of pathogens through release of contaminated vectors or reservoirs often yields unpredictable results. Aerosolized release of pathogens is effective, can affect a large population, and may easily overwhelm local and even regional medical resources.

The impact of an aerosolized biological weapons attack varies according to a variety of factors, including weaponization techniques, the strain of the biological agent, the method of aerosolization, and the meterologic factors at the site of dissemination. Meterologic factors including UV radiation, temperature, and relative humidity are primary determinants of pathogen survival after aerosolization. Other factors including wind, temperature inversion, and precipitation may also affect the impact subsequent to the release of the biological agent.

Meterologic factors also play an important role in the physical decay of aerosolized particles. For example, aerosolized particles must be between 1 to 5 micrometers to ensure that particles are suspended in the air for a long enough period of time to enter and colonize the terminal respiratory tract. However, at levels of relative humidity above 75 percent and temperatures above 40 degrees Celsius, aerosol particles tend to aggregate together.

UV radiation

- Biological agents are generally susceptible to the germicidal effects of UV radiation. Typically, DNA absorbs UV radiation at a wavelength between 260 to 265 nm. As a result, pyrimidines dimerize and cellular replication is hindered. With the exception of *Bacillus anthracis*, almost all potential bioterror agents are susceptible to the germicidal effects of solar UV. Different bacteria have different susceptibilities to UV radiation. Resistant bacteria can repair damaged DNA through photoreactivation or dark repair. Other factors that affect susceptibility to UV inactivation include aerosolization techniques, size of the particles, strain of the pathogen used, temperature, and initial bioburden.

Table 51.1 Susceptibility of CDC Category A agents to UV radiation

Agent	Susceptibility
Anthrax	Relatively resistant
Botulinum	Susceptible to inactivation
Plague	Susceptible to inactivation
Tularemia	Susceptible to inactivation
Smallpox	Susceptible to inactivation
VHF	Susceptible to inactivation

Temperature

- Biological agents are generally susceptible to inactivation at high temperatures. Temperature also plays an important role in the physical decay of aerosolized particles. For example, temperature inversion can facilitate the dissemination of aerosolized pathogen. Temperature inversion occurs when cold air is trapped below a layer of warm air. As a result, aerosolized particles remain concentrated near the breathable atmosphere. Temperature inversion occurs most often during dusk, night, and dawn. Additionally, during the winter months, the lower ambient air temperature can significantly strengthen the effects of temperature inversion.

Table 51.2 Susceptibility of CDC Category A agents to temperature

Agent	Susceptibility
Anthrax	Resistant to extremes in temperatures; however, temperature inversion effect present with cold ambient temperatures facilitates dissemination of anthrax particles.
Botulinum	Optimal survival at lower temperatures
Plague	Optimal survival at lower temperatures
Tularemia	Optimal survival at lower temperatures between −7 and 3 degrees Celsius
Smallpox	Optimal survival at lower temperatures
VHF	Optimal survival at lower temperatures

Relative humidity

Biological agents are usually susceptible to desiccation. However, at high levels of relative humidity, particle size usually increases, which results in higher pathogen decay. Higher levels of relative humidity may also protect pathogens from the germicidal effects of UV radiation.

Table 51.3 Susceptibility of CDC Category A agents to relative humidity

Agent	Susceptibility
Anthrax	Relatively resistant to the effects of relative humidity; however, high levels of relative humidity may promote survival at high temperatures.
Botulinum	Optimal survival at low levels of relative humidity.
Plague	Optimal survival at low levels of relative humidity; however, with high levels of UV radiation, higher levels of relative humidity is protective.
Tularemia	Optimal survival at low levels of relative humidity; however, with high levels of UV radiation, higher levels of relative humidity is protective.
Smallpox	Optimal survival at low levels of relative humidity; however, with high levels of UV radiation, higher levels of relative humidity is protective.
VHF	Optimal survival at low levels of relative humidity.

Wind

At wind speeds below 5 mph, aerosols are not widely disseminated, and at speeds above 25 mph, the physical integrity of the aerosols is compromised.

Precipitation

Precipitation is a less critical meterologic factor in determining survival of aerosolized pathogens. Snow or rain may wash out aerosolized infectious particles from the atmosphere; however, since the atmosphere contains very minimal amounts of precipitation, the overall effect of precipitation on the survival of aerosolized particles is negligible.

Determining seasonal risks

- Levels of relative humidity, temperature, and UV radiation vary according to the season for each geographic area. At locations farther away from the equator, seasonal variations in meterologic factors are more pronounced; therefore, the variations in the seasonal risks of a biological weapons attack is also more significant.
- Typically, levels of relative humidity, UV radiation intensity, and temperatures are lower during the winter months. Additionally, temperature inversion effect is more pronounced during the winter, and wind speeds are often higher during the winter.
- As a result, the impact of a biological weapons attack with CDC category A agents are more significant during the winter.

Table 51.4 Seasonal risks of a biological weapons attack

Agent	Winter	Spring	Summer	Fall
Anthrax	Very High Risk	High Risk	High Risk	High Risk
Botulinum	High Risk	Moderate Risk	Low Risk	Moderate Risk
Plague	High Risk	Moderate Risk	Moderate Risk	Moderate Risk
Tularemia	High Risk	Moderate Risk	Moderate Risk	Moderate Risk
Smallpox	High Risk	Moderate Risk	Moderate Risk	Moderate Risk
VHF	Moderate– Low Risk	Low Risk	Very Low Risk	Low Risk

Suggested readings

Ciattone G, ed. (2006). *Disaster Medicine*. St. Louis, MO: Mosby.

Jae Hee Junga C, Jung Eun Leeb, Sang Soo Kima. (2009, August). Thermal effects on bacterial bio-aerosols in continuous air flow. *Science of The Total Environment* 407(16): 4723–4730.

Sinclair Ryan, Boone Stephanie A., Greenberg David, Keim Paul, Gerba Charles P. (2008, February). Persistence of category A select agents in the environment. *Applied and Environmental Microbiology* 74(3): 555–563.

Chapter 52

Legal aspects of disaster medicine

Gabrielle Jacquet

David Bouslough

Introduction

The impact of federal and state emergency laws on governments' ability to respond to declared emergencies has been the subject of extensive analysis and scholarship. The impact of the same types of laws at the local level has received markedly less attention even though the localities are routinely on the front lines of emergency response efforts. Additionally, international laws are becoming increasingly important as relief organizations respond more and more frequently to natural disasters.

Laws that normally promote health in nonemergencies will often impede the protection of health during emergencies. Underlying a response to a disaster is a dichotomy: the medical community's understanding that medical care delivery will necessarily change (i.e., less efficiency, use of alternate care sites/venue change, rationing of supplies), while the affected public holds heightened expectations for standards of care (i.e., increased efficiency, increased accessibility, and additional help finding missing persons.)

Given the immense variability of legal systems and their approach to dispensing justice at the local, state, federal, and international levels, it is important to address these issues at multiple levels of government. An understanding of basic legal definitions is of utmost importance. See Table 52.1.

Table 52.1 General Health-care Legal Concepts

Legal Concept	Definition/Explanation
Autonomy	The unimpaired patient has a fundamental right to decide what medical care (if any) he or she will receive
Consent	The unimpaired patient agrees to the action, care, or opinion proposed by the healthcare provider.
Implied Consent	The presumption of consent for impaired, intoxicated, or critically ill or injured patients who cannot reply for themselves.
Emergency Exception	This concept provides for the care, rescue, and decontamination of patients without obtaining consent when health-care provider's obligation to the rights of many supersede the rights of the individual.

Principles of liability in disaster

- Negligence: Medical negligence is the act or omission in treatment of a patient by a medical professional, which deviates from the accepted medical standard of care. A physician who fails to provide a surgical patient with sufficient, appropriate aftercare is an example of negligence.
- Duty of care: The duty of care is one component of the law of negligence. In order to establish a defendant's liability in negligence, all four of the following requirements must be met:
  - The defendant must owe the plaintiff a duty of care (responder established a relationship with the patient that created duty).
  - The defendant must fail to meet the standard of care established by law (breach).
  - The plaintiff must have suffered a legally recognized injury or loss.
  - The defendant's conduct must have been the actual and legal cause of the plaintiff's injury.

The American Medical Association has established an ethical duty for physicians to provide assistance to individuals requiring emergency care.
- Standards of Care:
  - Legal Standard of Care: The legal definition of *standard of care* refers to the degree of care or skill that a reasonable practitioner would exercise acting under the same or similar circumstances.
  - As the legal standard of care definition implies, there is no single standard that can be expected at all times. This built-in flexibility, therefore, defies the formation of a subsequent definition of *altered* standards of care, like those expected during an emergency. Despite the obvious challenge of creating a definition, the Institute of Medicine published a consensus definition for *Crisis Standards of Care* in September 2009.
  - Crisis Standards of Care: Crisis standards represent

    a change in usual health care operations and the level of care it is possible to deliver, which is made necessary by a pervasive (e.g., pandemic influenza) or catastrophic (e.g., earthquake, hurricane) disaster.
    This change…is justified by specific circumstances and is formally declared by a state government, in recognition that crisis operations will be in effect for a sustained period. The formal declaration…enables specific legal/regulatory powers and protections for health care providers in the necessary tasks of allocating and using scarce medical resources and implementing alternate care facility operations.

  - International Care Standards: The international standard of care is quite different than the U.S. legal definition.

In 1997 a group of humanitarian NGOs and the Red Cross and Red Crescent movement formed The Humanitarian Charter 3, which is based on the principles and provisions of international humanitarian law, international human rights law, refugee law, and the Code of Conduct for the International Red Cross and Red Crescent Movement and NGOs in Disaster Relief. It describes the core principles that govern humanitarian action and reasserts

the right of populations affected by disaster, whether natural or man-made (including armed conflict), to protection and assistance. See Table 52.2. It also reasserts the right of disaster-affected populations to life with dignity. It affirms the fundamental importance of the following principles:
- The right to life with dignity.
- The distinction between combatants and noncombatants.
- The principle of nonrefoulement.

The Sphere Project also outlines specific minimum standards in disaster response:
- Water, sanitation, and hygiene promotion.
- Food security, nutrition, and food aid.
- Shelter, settlement, and nonfood items.
- Health services.

Table 52.2 Minimal standards common to all sectors—the Sphere Project

Participation	The disaster-affected population actively participates in the assessment, design, implementation, monitoring, and evaluation of the assistance program.
Initial Assessment	Assessments provide an understanding of the disaster situation and a clear analysis of threats to life, dignity, health, and livelihoods to determine, in consultation with the relevant authorities, whether an external response is required and, if so, the nature of the response.
Response	A humanitarian response is required for situations in which the relevant authorities are unable and/or unwilling to respond to the protection and assistance needs of the population on the territory over which they have control, and when assessment and analysis indicate that these needs are unmet.
Targeting	Humanitarian assistance or services are provided equitably and impartially, based on the vulnerability and needs of individuals or groups affected by disaster.
Monitoring	The effectiveness of the program in responding to problems is identified and changes in the broader context are continually monitored, with a view to improving the program, or to phasing it out as required.
Evaluation	There is a systematic and impartial examination of humanitarian action, intended to draw lessons to improve practice and policy and to enhance accountability.
Aid worker competencies and responsibilities	Aid workers possess appropriate qualifications, attitudes, and experience to plan and effectively implement appropriate programs.
Supervision, management, and support of personnel	Aid workers receive supervision and support to ensure effective implementation of the humanitarian assistance program.

General theories of liability protection

- General Immunity: The volunteer has no liability in lawsuits resulting from the authorized emergency response effort provided, excepting willful misconduct, gross negligence, or bad-faith efforts.
- Sovereign Immunity: Lawsuits against government, including local officials and/or employees, are restricted. Sovereign immunity is subject to exceptions and defined further by state law.
- Indemnification: Indemnification refers to the practice of the local or state government paying the damages associated with successful lawsuits against volunteer health professionals (VHPs) in authorized response efforts. See Tables 52.3 and 52.4.

Table 52.3 Legislation and Common Law Acts/doctrines affecting liability protection

Legal Doctrine	Synopsis	Protections
Good Samaritan Laws	Protecting those volunteers who choose to serve and tend to others who are injured or ill.	Volunteer care providers are protected from liability resulting from harm done to the injured or ill
Volunteer Protection Act of 1967	No volunteer of a nonprofit organization or governmental entity will be liable for harm caused by an act or omission of the volunteer on behalf of the organization or entity.	Immunity for volunteers of nonprofits, not the organization
Federal Tort Claims Act	A mechanism for compensating people who have suffered personal injury by the negligent or wrongful action of employees of the U.S. government. Health centers are considered Federal employees and are immune from lawsuits, with the Federal government acting as their primary insurer.	Federal employees are immune from lawsuits involving negligence. Employees of eligible health centers are immune from medical malpractice suits. Eligible health centers are immune from medical malpractice suits.
Stafford Disaster Relief & Emergency Assistance Act	Legislation to provide an orderly and continuing means of assistance by the federal government to state and local governments in carrying out their responsibilities to alleviate the suffering and damage that result from disasters	Immunity from liability for the federal government for emergency management.

Table 52.4 Legislation and Common Law Acts/doctrines affecting liability protection

Legal Doctrine	Synopsis	Protections
Homeland Security Act of 2002	The Act establishes the Department of Homeland Security, and defines protections for the federal government and response actors.	Government and responders are protected from liability in response to the threat of terrorism.
Military Claims Act	Military personnel families (nonactive duty personnel) who are injured at an American military hospital outside the U.S. and its territories may file a claim for compensation from their military branch of service.	Monetary awards for damages due to medical negligence.
State Created Danger Doctrine	State officials and agencies will be liable if they create a dangerous environment resulting in harm of the third party (i.e., reckless car chase injuring a bystander).	Citizens injured due to state actor negligence. A legal exception to the general constitutional rule that the state has no duty to protect someone from injury at the hands of a third person.
Sanders Court Decision	Attempts to further interpret the "special relationship doctrine" that attaches liability to government agents when they impose limitation on an individual's freedom, to protect them from harm (i.e., medical restraints, quarantine).	Rights of injured parties who are restrained by government emergency responders.

Legal challenges at each regulatory level

- Local: The concept of Home Rule allows localities to take legislative or other action on issues of local concern without relying upon a specific grant of authority from the state. The amount or percentage of home rule enjoyed by local governments varies widely state to state. Local governments are often endowed with special emergency powers triggered by official emergency declarations. These declarations are the cornerstone of emergency responses that require reshaping the legal environment to prioritize important response objectives. The ability of localities to invoke emergency powers, deploy VHPs, and provide liability protections stems from their local home-rule power.
- State: Localities with weak home rule are susceptible to considerably greater control by the state; this situation can negate the need for local ordinances to address policies that are already addressed at the state level. Conversely, more burden of responsibility for legislative emergency preparedness rests with state agencies and actors.
- Federal: The Federal Emergency Management Agency (FEMA) is the federal agency responsible for coordinating emergency planning, preparedness, risk reduction, response, and recovery.
- International: In 2007, the 30th International Conference of the Red Cross and Red Crescent unanimously adopted the Guidelines for the domestic facilitation and regulation of international disaster relief and initial recovery assistance: IDRL Guidelines. The IDRL Guidelines help governments be better prepared for the common legal problems in international response operations. Using the Guidelines, governments can avoid needless delays in the dissemination of humanitarian relief while ensuring better coordination and quality of the assistance provided.

Planning recommendations for legal aspects of emergency response

- Volunteer Health Professionals (VHP): Volunteerism by qualified health-care providers is dependant on several assurances that legal planners should take into consideration. Table 52.5 presents these recommendations.

- Emergency Service Organizations (ESO)

Any organization providing emergency services should actively plan for the legal ramifications of providing such services. Table 52.6 outlines a risk-management approach to identifying and addressing these issues.

Table 52.5 Legal recommendations for states utilizing VHPs in health emergencies

1.	Incorporate advanced registration systems and protocols into the legal system.
2.	State and federal laws should ensure robust privacy protection regarding the use and maintenance of registry information.
3.	Define a "floor" of legal protection for volunteers, and encourage its uniform adoption across state lines.
4.	Expand the scope and breadth of types of volunteers registered to ensure a broad workforce capable of a comprehensive and coordinated effort.
5.	Laws must ensure a balance between civil liability protections for VHPs and their host entities, and alternate mechanisms to compensate injured patients.
6.	Enact laws to provide defence services for VHPs involved in lawsuits specific to care rendered in an emergency.
7.	Enact laws and regulations providing for license portability during emergencies.
8.	Ensure workers compensation protection for VHPs.
9.	Ensure re-employment rights for VHPs if they are employed outside the federal government.

Adapted from: Hodge J, et al. The legal framework for meeting surge capacity through the use of volunteer health professionals during public health emergencies and other disasters. Wayne State Univ. Law School, Legal Studies Research Paper Archive, No. 08-06, Dec 2005.

Table 52.6 Applying a risk management approach to legal issues

1. Characterize the hazards—this means knowing and understanding the relevant law. Seek legal advice if necessary.

2. Define your expectations—this may involve asking what your people, your stakeholders, your community, and your regulators expect from you. What standard are you required to comply with?

3. Determine your vulnerability—know what legal issues or standards you are unable to comply with.

4. Analyze your risks.

5. Evaluate and rank your risks.

6. Identify and evaluate your legal mitigation plan

7. Be aware that any documents created during a risk management audit may become publicly available through a "Freedom of Information" request. Discuss this risk with your lawyers.

Reprinted with permission from Dunlop C. Legal Issues in Emergency Management: Lessons from the last decade. *Australian Journal of Emergency Management* 19(1) 2004: 26–33.

- Scarce resource allocation
ESOs are aware that, in an emergency, staffing and supply concerns rank highly on the priority list. Legal principles of scarce-resource allocation decision making are outlined in Box 52.1.

- State Immunity Provisions
Significant variability in legal protection exists at local and state levels.
  • Immunity from liability is generally given to health-care providers performing duties required by state or local law including:
  • Disease surveillance and reporting.
  • Quarantine.
  • Immunity from liability generally not given in cases of:
  • Criminal act.
  • Gross negligence.
  • Willful misconduct.

- Proactive Legal Planning in Emergency Preparedness
It is advisable that each Emergency Preparedness Committee (EPC) incorporate legal planning into all Emergency Action Plan (EAP) development efforts. It is the EPC and its members living in a given municipality and state that are most aware of local and state legislation. During planning proceedings, committees are encouraged to develop a compilation of questions, comments, and concerns related to the regulatory requirements currently in place that would either need to be waived or amended in order for the planned emergency response to be effective. Legal consultation can aid

Box 52.1 Legal and ethical principles guiding the decisions for allocation of scarce resources in public-health emergencies

Obligations to community
1. Maintain transparency (e.g., openness and public accessibility) in the decision-making process at the state and local levels.
2. Conduct public-health outreach to promote community participation in deliberations about allocation decisions.

Balancing personal autonomy and community benefit
3. Balance individual and communal needs to maximize the public health benefits to the populations being served while respecting individual rights (to the extent possible), including providing mitigation for such infringements (e.g., provide fair compensation for volunteers who are injured while rendering emergency care or services for the benefit of the community).
4. Consider the public-health needs of individuals or groups without regard for their human condition (e.g., race/ethnicity, nationality, religious beliefs, sexual orientation, residency status, or ability to pay).

Good preparedness practice
5. Adhere to and communicate applicable standard-of-care guidelines (e.g., triage procedures), absent an express directive by a governmental authority that suggests adherence to differing standards.
6. Identify public -health priorities based on modern, scientifically sound evidence that supports the provision of resources to identified people.
7. Implement initiatives in a prioritized, coordinated fashion that are well targeted to accomplishing essential public-health services and core public-health functions.
8. Assess the public-health outcomes following a specific allocation decision, acknowledging that the process is iterative.
9. Ensure accountability (e.g., documentation) pertaining to the specific duties and liabilities of people in the execution of the allocation decision.
10. Share personally identifiable health information—with the patients' consent where possible—solely to promote the health or safety of patients or other people.

Reprinted with permission from Barnett D, et al. Resource Allocation on the Frontlines of Public Health Preparedness and Response: Report of a Summit on Legal and Ethical Issues. *Public Health Reports 124*(2009): 295–303.

in the review of these issues, and refined lists of legal questions should be forwarded to official governmental preparedness representatives or committees at the state level. The following example is one compiled by a community hospital during the planning stages for a regional pandemic influenza emergency response. See Box 52.2.

Box 52.2 Regional Pandemic Influenza Legal Concerns, by Topic

- Liaison
  - Review EMS transportation regulations within and between municipalities.
  - Non-EMS drivers utilized for EMS transport.
  - Non-EMS vehicles utilized for EMS transport.
  - Transportation regulations to and from alternate care sites.
  - Vehicle and driver standards, regulations, and licensure.
  - Private ambulances company memo of understanding (MOU), use, and standards of transport care.
  - Pronouncing death: regulations about who may, and where the body must be.
  - Transportation of deceased.
  - Security and storage of the deceased, municipal police surge limitations.
  - Central 911 operator use for transport directions: hospital versus ACS.
- Information
  - Pandemic application of HIPAA regulations.
  - Interoperable and transmunicipality radio frequencies for police, fire.
  - Ethics of withholding/editing information for public release.
- Safety
  - Transmunicipal cooperation and support: police.
  - Deputizing community members for law enforcement.
  - Regulations for prolonged detention of prisoners versus community release.
- Operations
  - Utilizing nonlicensed and noncredentialed personnel to provide patient care in hospitals and nursing homes
  - The determination of standards of care: who, when, consensus issues.
  - Documentation requirements for patients receiving care at an ACS.
  - Utilizing nonpharmacy personnel to dispense medications at a hospital or ACS.
  - MDS completion for noncritical patients cared for at a nursing home.
  - RN supervision regulations for nursing homes: same or relaxed.
  - Nursing home square footage for determining reasonable patient housing.
  - Relaxing supply and food-storage requirements.
  - Storage space surge capacity, regulation changes for use of nonapproved spaces if needed.
  - Pandemic clinical protocol development, adjustment and regulation: who, when, how.
  - Immunization requirements for clinicians, volunteers, patients of all acuity, and per location (hospital, ACS, NH).
  - Quality care data collection: continued, amended, or aborted.
  - Nursing-home feeding, license renewal, and care-plan requirements.

Source: The Miriam Hospital, Regional Pandemic Influenza Plan, August 2010, Lifespan Health System.

Conclusion

No matter the degree of preparation, one can never be entirely ready for a disaster. Due to the significant variability in legal protections at the local, state, federal, and international levels, one must know the legal and ethical ramifications involved before a disaster occurs. Being armed with this knowledge will ensure that the best relief and aid can be given with minimal legal obstacles or complications.

Suggested readings

Anderson ED, Hodge JG (2009). Emergency legal preparedness among select US local governments. *Disaster Medicine and Public Health Preparedness 3*: S176–S184.

Barnett D, et al. (2009, March–April). Resource allocation on the frontlines of public health preparedness and response: Report of a summit on legal and ethical issues. *Public Health Reports 124*: 295–303.

Dunlop C. (2004). Legal issues in emergency management: Lessons from the last decade. *AJEM 19*(1): 26–33.

Hodge J, et al. (2005, December). The legal framework for meeting surge capacity through the use of volunteer health professionals during public health emergencies and other disasters. Wayne State Univ. Law School, Legal Studies Research Paper Archive, No. 08-06.

Hoffman S, et al. (2009, June). Law, liability, and public health emergencies. *Disaster Medicine and Public Health Preparedness. 3*(2): 117–125.

http://www.iom.edu/Reports/2009/DisasterCareStandards.aspx

The Humanitarian Charter. Available at http://www.sphereproject.org/component/option,com_docman/task,doc_view/gid,5/Itemid,203/lang,english/.

Sphere Project Handbook, Chapter 1, pp. 21–50.

Sphere Project Handbook, Chapters 2–5, pp. 51–249.

Walker AF. (2002). The legal duty of physician and hospitals to provide emergency care. *CMAJ 166*(4): 465–469.

Mechanical and Structural Disasters

Land

Air and Sea

Natural Disasters

Human Caused Disasters

Man-made threats: an overview

Alex Garza

Overview

Man-made disasters are events which, either intentionally or by accident cause severe threats to public health and well-being. Because their occurrence is unpredictable, man-made disasters pose an especially challenging threat that must be dealt with through vigilance, and proper preparedness and response. They can generally be thought of in two broad categories with frequent comingling of both categories

Sociological hazards
- Crime.
- Arson.
- Civil disorder.
- Terrorism.
- War.

Technological hazards
- Chemical, Biological, Radiation, Nuclear and Explosive (CBRNE).
- Industrial Hazards:
  - Fuel or chemical spills.
  - Electrical outages.
- Structural Hazards:
  - Building or bridge collapse.
  - Aircraft or other transportation failings.

Human error does not fit neatly into these two categories but is recognized as a major contributor to man-made disasters.

Although much of this text is devoted to intentional acts of destruction, it is important to remember that the majority of disaster scenarios will not involve acts of terrorism. Man-made disasters are usually technical or human failures with catastrophic results.

Because of this likelihood, it is important to prepare and train for all hazards.

Succeeding in "routine" disasters, such as multivehicle motor crashes, will better prepare the response for intentional events.

Terrorism

The unlawful use of force or violence against persons or property to intimidate or coerce a government or civilian population in the furtherance of political or social objectives.

FBI

The purpose of terrorism is to terrorize.

Attributed to Mao TseTung

Classic terrorism
- Limited objectives
  - Usually political
- Limited range of weapons
  - Guns and bombs

Modern terrorism
- Variety of actors.
- Multinetworked organizations.
- Religious nexus.
- Rogue or near-failed states.
- Asymmetric warfare is common.
- Blurring of crime and terrorism.
- Evolution of cyber threats.
- Evolving technical expertise on CBRNE from rogue states.

Challenges
- Recognizing an attack (or outbreak).
- Lack of Weapons of Mass Destruction (WMD) knowledge/experience.
- Lack of personal protective equipment (PPE) and doctrine for its use.
- Security/crowd control issues.
- Issues of quarantine.
- Staffing/resources.
- Speed of decision cycle.

Situational recognition
- An intentional attack may present no discernable signature.
- Recognition of terrorist nexus may be delayed.
- Fog, friction, noise.
- Significant consequences.
- Multiple levels of government/disciplines.

Bioterrorism

History

- **1346–1347** Mongols catapult corpses contaminated with plague over the walls into Kaffa (in Crimea), forcing besieged Genoans to flee.
- **1710** Russian troops allegedly use plague-infected corpses against Swedes.
- **1767** During the French and Indian Wars, the British give blankets used to wrap British smallpox victims to hostile Indian tribes.
- **1863** The U.S. War Department issues General Order 100, proclaiming "The use of poison in any manner, be it to poison wells, or foods, or arms, is wholly excluded from modern warfare."
- **1916–1918** German agents use anthrax and the equine disease, glanders, to infect livestock and feed for export to Allied forces. Incidents include the infection of Romanian sheep with anthrax and glanders for export to Russia, Argentinian mules with anthrax for export to Allied troops, and American horses and feed with glanders for export to France.
- **June 17, 1925** "Geneva Protocol for the Prohibition of the Use in War of Asphyxiating, Poisonous, or Other Gases, and of Bacteriological Methods of Warfare" is signed; not ratified by U.S. and not signed by Japan.
- **1937** Japan begins its offensive biological weapons program. Unit 731, the bioweapon (BW) research and development unit, is located in Harbin, Manchuria. Over the course of the program, at least 10,000 prisoners are killed in Japanese experiments.
- **1942** U.S. begins its offensive biological weapons program and chooses Camp Detrick, Frederick, Maryland as its research and development site.
- **May, 1945** Only known tactical use of a BW by Germany. A large reservoir in Bohemia is poisoned with sewage.
- **June, 1966** The United States conducts a test of vulnerability to covert BW attack by releasing a harmless biological simulant into the New York City subway system.
- **November 25, 1969** President Nixon announces unilateral dismantlement of the U.S. offensive BW program.
- **1975** U.S. ratifies Geneva Protocol (1925) and biological weapons convention (BWC).
- **1978** In a case of Soviet state-sponsored assassination, Bulgarian exile Georgi Markov, living in London, is stabbed with an umbrella that injects him with a tiny pellet containing ricin.
- **April 2, 1979** Outbreak of pulmonary anthrax in Sverdlovsk, Soviet Union. In 1992, Russian president Boris Yeltsin acknowledges that the outbreak was caused by an accidental release of anthrax spores from a Soviet military microbiological facility.
- **1984** The Dalles, Oregon. Intentional salmonella release in salad bars.
- **1995** Aum Shinrikyo releases sarin in Tokyo, has arsenal of biological weapons.

- **1996** Dallas, Texas, Shigella found in microlab donuts, 12 ill (4 hospitalized).
- **2001** Anthrax attacks infect 22 people, killing at least five.

Classification of bioterrorism

- Small-Scale Bioterrorism:
  - Common pathogens.
  - Unlikely to be identified as bioterrorism.
- Larger-Scale Bioterrorism:
  - Identified package/parcel (low risk).
  - Identified mechanical device (higher risk).
  - Unidentified release (human cases); need sentinel cases to identify that release occurred.

Biologics as weapons: desired properties;

- Infectious via aerosol.
- Organisms fairly stable in environment.
- Susceptible civilian populations.
- High morbidity and mortality.
- Person-to-person transmission (smallpox, plague, VHF).
- Difficult to diagnose and/or treat.
- Potential for widespread dissemination.
- Psychological effect.
- Perpetrators escape easily.
- No treatment or vaccine.

Methods of dissemination

- Aerosol
  - The ideal aerosol contains a homogeneous population of 2 or 3 micron particulates that contain one or more viable organisms.
  - Maximum potential for human respiratory infection is via a particle that falls within the 1 to 5 micron size.
- Ingestion.
- Cutaneous.

Detection of outbreak

- Epidemiologic or syndromic based.

Epidemiologic:

- Large epidemic with high illness and death rate.
- Multiple, simultaneous outbreaks.
- Multidrug-resistant pathogens.
- Infection nonendemic for region.
- Sick or dead animals.
- Epidemiological Information.
  - Travel history.
  - Infectious contacts.
  - Employment history.
  - Activities over the preceding 3 to 5 days.

Epidemiologic clues to a bioterrorism event (BT)event E clues
- Point source Exposure
  - Low attack rates in "protected" areas.
  - High attack rate among Exposed.
- Compressed Epidemic curve.
- Young and healthy die.
- Exotic—Unusual illness, season, location
  - Tularemia in 2000.
- Epizootic (Animals also acquiring disease).

Syndromic
- Respiratory symptoms predominate.
- Infection nonendemic for region.
- Delivery vehicle or intelligence information.

Syndromes that may be associated with bioterrorism
- Pulmonary:
  - Fever.
  - Cough.
  - Myalgias.
  - Hypoxia.
- Rash and fever:
  - Vesicular.
  - Petechial.
- GI:
  - Fever.
  - Nausea/vomiting.
  - Diarrhea ?bloody.
- Neurologic:
  - Headache (HA) fever, bulbar palsy, encephalopathy.
- Septic Shock:
  - Disseminated intravascular coagulation (DIC).
  - Organ failure.

Typical incubation periods
- <1 day:
  - Staphylococcal enterotoxin B.
- <1 week:
  - Anthrax.
  - Plague.
  - Tularemia.
  - Venezuelan equine encephalitis (VEE).
  - Botulism.
- >1 week:
  - Brucellosis.
  - Q fever.
  - Smallpox.
  - Eastern equine encephalitis/Western equine encephalitis (EEE/WEE).
  - Viral hemorrhagic fever (VHF).
  - Anthrax.

Differences between chemical and biological attacks
- CHEMICAL:
  - Rapid onset (obvious).
  - Field first response.
  - Police and Fire.
  - EMS.
  - Decontamination is critical.
  - Antidotes.
- BIOLOGICAL:
  - Slow onset (insidious).
  - Medical response.
  - Hospital.
  - Office.
  - Decontamination is less useful.
  - Antibiotics and vaccines.

Suggested readings

Brennan RJ, Waeckerle JF, Sharp TW, Lillibridge SR (1999) Chemical warfare agents: emergency medical and emergency public health issues. *Ann Emerg Med 34: 191–204.*

Inglesby Thomas V, Henderson Donald A, Bartlett John G, Ascher Michael S, Eitzen Edward, Friedlander Arthur M, Hauer Jerome, McDade Joseph, Osterholm Michael T, O'Toole Tara, Parker Gerald, Perl Trish M, Russell Philip K, Tonat Kevin (1999). Anthrax as a biological weapon: Medical and public health management. *JAMA Working Group on Civilian Biodefense 281:* 1735–1745, 2127–2137.

Ryan Jeffrey, Glarum Jan. (2008). *Biosecurity and bioterrorism: Containing and preventing biological threat.* Waltham, MA: Elsevier Press.

Wilkening DA (2006). Sverdlovsk revisited: Modeling human inhalation anthrax. *Proc Natl Acad Sci. USA 103*(20): 7589–7594.

Zubay, Geoffrey (2005). *Agents of bioterrorism: Pathogens and their weaponization.* New York: Columbia University Press.

Biological
Disasters

Anthrax

Jason Bellows

Bacillus anthracis

The only obligate Bacillus pathogen in vertebrates. It is primarily a disease in herbivores such as cows, goats, and sheep. Animals contract the disease by ingesting spores on forage plants. At body temperature in the nutrient rich environment of the host, dormant spores are converted by a process termed *germination*.

Sporulation ultimately occurs in the animal carcass when conditions are unfavorable or nutrients are exhausted. After decay, the spores return to the soil and complete the anthrax life cycle.

Epidemiology

Historical importance

Anthrax has been an agent of disease throughout human history. The classic black eschar of cutaneous anthrax is derived from the Greek *anthracos* meaning "coal."

- 5th & 6th plagues described in Exodus.
- Medieval times—The "Black Bane."
- Wool-sorter's disease.
- Rag-picker's disease.
- Agent from which Sir Robert Koch developed germ theory of disease.
- Louis Pasteur developed the first known vaccines in 1881.

At-risk human populations

- Those in contact with grazing animals.
- Prior to 2001, only 18 cases were recorded in the United States.
- 82 reported cases of inhalational anthrax from 1900–2005 globally

Anthrax in modern day

The Soviet Union in the 1970s had a large anthrax weaponization program. An epidemic occurred in Sverdlovsk, Russia in 1979. Citizens living in the city became sick after the accidental release of "weaponized" anthrax spores from a Russian military compound.

- 60 to 100 deaths.
- Deaths occurred up to 5 km from the release site.
- Animal deaths were reported 40 km away.

Agent of biological warfare

- Designated a "Category A" biologic-threat agent.
  - Highest level threat potential.
- Has been used as a terror agent on a small scale.
- No examples of use as a weapon of mass destruction.
- Difficult to "weaponize" spores; purified in a dry powder.
- Report by the WHO in 1970 estimated that if technical difficulties in preparation and execution were overcome, the release of 50 kg of anthrax spores would cause death or incapacity in more than 40 percent of the population within a 2 km radius.
- Congressional Office of Technology Assessment analysis in 1993, with the same proviso, concluded that between 130,000 and 3 million fatalities would result from the release of 100 kg of anthrax spores upwind of Washington, DC.

2001 U.S. anthrax attacks

During a 7-week period in 2001, letters laced with anthrax were mailed to New York City, Washington DC, and Lantana, Florida. The perpetrator of attacks had access to a virulent strain which was present at both the U.S.-vaccine-production facility at BioPort and 19 other laboratories.

- Particles passed through pores of envelopes.
- Particles aerosolized when pressed by postal facility sorting machines.
- Contaminated offices of targeted individuals.

- 22 people diagnosed with anthrax infection.
- 11 confirmed as inhalational anthrax with 5 deaths.
- 11 cutaneous cases; 7 confirmed, and 4 suspected.

Pathogenesis

Endotoxins

Clinical features are produced by two endotoxins. Endotoxins are binary and full virulence of anthrax requires both.

- Virulence genes are located on two plasmids
- Genes code for two toxin complexes (see Box 54.1).
- Poly-D-glutamic acid capsule, which protects spores from host phagocytosis.
- Once in the alveoli, most of the spores are rapidly phagocytosed by alveolar macrophages, the primary site of spore germination.
- Spore laden macrophages are transported through pulmonary lymphatics to hilar and mediastinal lymph nodes, leading to severe mediastinal hemorrhage and necrosis.
- The lung parenchyma usually shows little or no pneumonia. Massive bacteremia and toxemia ensue.
- Anthrax spores may remain latent for weeks or months after inhalation.
- Humans are moderately resistant to anthrax.
- Particle size must be less than 5 microns to reach the alveoli.
- LD50 approximately 2,500 to 55,000 spores.
- Person to person transmission has not been documented.

Box 54.1 Anthrax endotoxins

Edema Toxin = Edema Factor + Protective Antigen

Lethal Toxin = Lethal Factor + Protective Antigen

Clinical features

Cutaneous anthrax

Cutaneous anthrax is the most common form of infection, accounting for 90–95 percent of all anthrax infections within the United States. Spores are usually introduced through breaks in the skin, but biting flies may transmit the disease.

- After 2–5 days: painless, pruritic papule with a ring of vesicles.
- 6–7 days: papule ulcerates, dries, blackens, and forms an eschar.
- 80–90 percent of the cases are self-limited.
- Select cases can progress to fatal septicemia.

Treatment consists of local wound care. Fever and lymphangitis usually point to secondary infection. Surgical debridement is contraindicated unless treated with antibiotics. Circumferential lesions on the extremities could lead to compartment syndrome requiring fasciotomy.

Intestinal anthrax

Intestinal anthrax is analogous to cutaneous, but on intestinal mucosa. Generalized disease develops with spread from mucosa to lymphatic system.

- 2.5–5 percent of naturally occurring cases.
- Infected by the consumption of contaminated food.
- Clinical manifestations occur 2–5 days after ingestion.
- Death rate ranging from 25–60 percent.
- Infection may result in oropharyngeal edema and respiratory compromise requiring surgical airway.
- Involvement of lower gastrointestinal tract may require surgical exploration and resection of affected segments.
- GI ulceration and necrosis, hematemesis, coffee-ground emesis and bloody diarrhea often develop, and intestinal perforation may occur.

Pulmonary anthrax

Inhalation anthrax accounts for 2.5–5 percent of the cases occurring sporadically. Spores are optimal in size to reach the alveolar space. Alveolar macrophages transport spores to mediastinal lymph nodes, where they may germinate. Clinical course is biphasic in nature with an incubation period followed by fulminant disease.

- Incubation period of 4–6 days.
- Initially an influenza-like illness lasting 4 days.
- May improve briefly before fulminant course.
- Fulminant period features sudden onset of hyper acute illness.
- Dyspnea, cyanosis, high fever, and disorientation.
- Rapidly enlarging pleural effusions and marked mediastinal expansion.
- Progresses to septic shock, coma, and death, most within 24 hours.
- At time of death, live bacilli account for 30 percent of a person's blood weight.

An inhaled spore may be cleared by being expelled through the bronchus, or destroyed by macrophages. Disease will occur if at least one spore germinates before it is cleared, provided antibiotics are not circulating at the time of germination. Experimental studies with rhesus monkeys suggest that the clearance rate is in the order of 7 percent per day. Other studies suggest that only 15 percent of all inhaled spores are delivered to the lungs.

Meningoencephalitis
- Reported to occur in up to 50 percent of cases of fulminant anthrax.
- Mode of entry can be via the cutaneous or inhalation route.
- Is associated with statistically higher hazard ratio for death.

Diagnosis

Workup of a febrile patient presents a unique challenge. Most lethal form of inhalation anthrax present in the prodromal stage with nonspecific symptoms. During the 2001 outbreak, 4 of 11 patients diagnosed with inhalation anthrax were initially sent home with a diagnosis of "viral syndrome," bronchitis, or gastroenteritis. See Box 54.2.

- An important diagnostic clue appears to be heart rate, which was elevated in all patients during the 2001 attacks.
- Dyspnea, abnormal chest auscultation, and nausea with vomiting are signs and symptoms more likely evident in inhalational anthrax.
- Rhinorrhea, coryza, and sore throat are far more common in influenza.
- It is more difficult to discern inhalational anthrax from community acquired pneumonia (CAP) than from influenza on the basis of clinical presentation. See Box 54.3.

Prodromal phase

- Initial labs are mostly nonspecific.
- Median WBC of 9,800 with elevated neutrophil and band forms.
- Mildly elevated liver-function tests.
- PaO_2 less than 70 mmHg in some patients.
- Most rapid diagnosis by Gram stain.
- Nasal-swab tests can reveal the presence of anthrax spores, but a positive test only confirms exposure, not infection.
- The FDA has approved a rapid blood test to help confirm the diagnosis of anthrax.
- The assay detects antibodies to a component of the anthrax toxin and can be completed in less than an hour.

Box 54.2 Common presenting symptoms and signs

- Abnormal temperature (81%)
- Abnormal lung findings (80%)
- Fever or chills (67%)
- Tachycardia (66%)
- Fatigue or malaise (64%)
- Cough (62%)
- Dyspnea (52%)

Box 54.3 Initial laboratory workup

- Complete blood counts
- Liver function tests
- Arterial blood gas
- Blood cultures with Gram stain
- Influenza and respiratory syncytial virus (RSV) testing may be helpful

Fulminant phase
- Median WBC of 26,400.
- Low CSF glucose level with marked infiltration of leukocytes.
- Presence of elevated red-blood-cell count in CSF or gross blood.

Radiographic evaluation
- Chest radiograph findings were abnormal in all 10 patients during the 2001 attacks.
- During the prodromal stage, the chest radiograph may provide the first clues, albeit subtle ones.
- The most common findings are a widened mediastinum or bilateral hilar enlargement.
- Pleural effusions and mediastinal contours may rapidly enlarge over hours or days.
- Differential diagnosis of mediastinal widening includes tuberculosis, sarcoidosis, histoplasmosis, lymphoma, tumors, and aneurysm.
- Noncontrast computed tomography may provide the most convincing evidence of disease.
- Mediastinal and hilar lymphadenopathy, pleural effusions, perihilar infiltrates, and mediastinal edema may be seen.
- Increased attenuation of the mediastinal fat is compatible with extension of toxin-induced nodal edema.
- CT manifestations are nearly pathognomonic of inhalational anthrax.

Box 54.4 Common chest radiograph findings

- Prominent peribronchovascular markings
- Pleural effusions
- Peribronchovascular airspace opacities may be evident
- Extensive consolidations are not characteristic

Treatment

Antibiotics
- Medical management is the mainstay of therapy.
- Anthrax shows sensitivity to a wide array of antibiotics.
- Anthrax is resistant to 3rd and 4th generation cephalosporins as well as trimethoprim-sulfamethoxazole.
- The 2001 strain produced an inducible beta-lactamase, thus penicillin was not recommended for treatment.

2001 Bioterrorism strain sensitivities:
- Chloramphenicol.
- Ciprofloxacin.
- Clindamycin.
- Doxycycline.
- Erythromycin.
- Gentamicin.
- Imipenem.
- Penicillins.
- Rifampin
- Tetracyclines.
- Vancomycin.

▶ **CDC Recommendations**
- Combination antibiotic therapy of ciprofloxacin (or doxycycline) plus rifampin and clindamycin on the basis of anecdotal evidence from the 2001 U.S. experience.
- If central nervous system involvement is suspected, doxycycline should not be used due to poor penetration.
- Other popular fluoroquinolones have shown promise in animal studies, but have not been approved by the FDA.
- Febrile patients should not be treated with oral antibiotics for "presumed" anthrax.

It should be noted that the "weaponization" of anthrax may also include the genetic manipulation of its genome. Therefore, it may be unwise to assume that future strains may have similar sensitivities. There has been a report of a genetically engineered strain with resistance to tetracyclines and penicillins.

Box 54.5 CDC recommended antibiotic therapy
- Treatment for 60 days
- Ciprofloxacin or Doxycycline + Rifampin + Clindamycin
- If suspected CNS involvement:
  - Add Vancomycin, Chloramphenicol or Imipenem

Length of therapy
- Antibiotic therapy is recommended for 60 days.
- Support for prolonged therapy derives from animal models and observation from the outbreak in Sverdlovsk, Russia, both showing long retention time.
- Studies have shown that 17 percent of monkeys treated for 30 days after inhalational challenge relapsed after antibiotic therapy was discontinued.

Prophylaxis
- Antibiotics are ineffective against spores that may lay dormant.
- Prophylaxis depends upon the incubation period, which accounts for the risks of spore germination and spore clearance.
- In animal models, antibiotic prophylaxis is effective, vaccination is not.
- No cases of anthrax in persons receiving prophylaxis during US attacks.
- 60 days of antibiotic prophylaxis is considered adequate.

Surgical management
- Pleural fluid drainage is associated with decreased mortality.
- In a review of all 82 case reports (1900–2005) increasing time to pleural fluid drainage was associated with statistically higher hazard ratio for death.
- Two patients survived after progressing to the fulminant phase, both received multidrug antibiotic regimens and pleural fluid drainage.

Outcomes

- Overall mortality rate of 85 percent.
- Mean time from symptom onset to death is 4.8 days.
- Fulminant phase is almost uniformly fatal.
- Factors associated with increased hazard ratios for death.
  - Treatment with antiserum alone or single antibiotic therapy.
  - Increasing time to initiation of antibiotics.
  - Advancing age.
  - Development of meningoencephalitis.
- Mortality from anthrax during the 2001 U.S. attack (45%) was substantially lower than that reported historically (89–96%).
  - This is attributed to the rapid provision of antibiotics and supportive care in modern intensive-care units.
- U.S. 2001 patient's median time from symptom onset to antibiotics was 4.7 days.
  - The U.S. 2001 patients who received antibiotics in 4.7 days or sooner had a 40 percent mortality rate.
  - If antibiotic therapies were initiated after 4.7 days, then the mortality rate was 75 percent.

Control

Anthrax vaccine for humans has been in use since 1959. Biothrax is currently the sole licensed anthrax vaccine in the United States and has been available since 1970. Efficacy may be affected by genetic engineering.

> Box 54.6 Anthrax vaccine
>
> • Cell-free filtrate
> • Attenuated, nonencapsulated strain
> • 6 doses over 18-month period
> • Booster doses at 1-year intervals
> • In monkeys, is protective against amounts 900 times the LD50

Suggested readings

Abramova FA, Grinberg LM et al. (1993). Pathology of inhalational anthrax in 42 cases from the Sverdlovsk outbreak of 1979. *Proceedings of the National Academy of Sciences 90*, 2291–2294.

Barakat LA, Quentzel HL, et al. (2002). Fatal inhalational anthrax in a 94-year-old Connecticut woman. *JAMA 287*: 863–868.

Binkley CE, Cinti S, et al. (2002). Bacillus anthracis as an agent of bioterrorism: A review emphasizing surgical treatment. *Annals of Surgery 236*: 9–16.

Borio L, Frank D, et al. (2001). Death due to bioterrorism-related inhalational anthrax: Report of two patients. *JAMA 286*: 2554–2559.

Brookmeyer R, Johnson E, Bollinger R. (2003). Modeling the optimum duration of antibiotic prophylaxis in an anthrax outbreak. *Proceedings of the National Academy of Sciences 100*: 10129–10132.

Bush LM, Abrams BH, et al. (2001). Index case of fatal inhalational anthrax due to bioterrorism in the United States. *NEJM 345*: 1607–1610.

Centers for Disease Control and Prevention. (2001). Considerations for distinguishing influenza-like illness from inhalational anthrax. *JAMA 286*: 2537–2539.

Cinti SK, Saravolatz L, et al. (2004). Differentiating inhalational anthrax from other influenza-like illnesses in the setting of a national or regional anthrax outbreak. *Archives of Internal Medicine 164*: 674–676.

Culley NC, Pinson DM, et al. (2005). Pathophysiological manifestations in mice exposed to anthrax lethal toxin. *Infection & Immunity 73*: 7006–7010.

Deziel MR, Heine H, et al. (2005). Effective antimicrobial regimens for use in humans for therapy of Bacillus anthracis infections and postexposure prophylaxis. *Antimicrobial Agents & Chemotherapy 49*: 5099–5106.

Frazier AA, Franks TJ, Galvin JR (2006). Inhalational anthrax. *Journal of Thoracic Imaging 21*: 252–258.

Friedlander AM. (2002). Diagnosis and treatment of cutaneous anthrax. *JAMA 288*: 43–44.

Holty JE, Bravata DM, et al. (2006). Systematic review: A century of anthrax cases from 1900 to 2005. *Annals of Internal Medicine 144*: 270–280.

Mayer TA, Bersoff-Matcha S, et al. (2001). Clinical presentation of inhalational anthrax following bioterrorism exposure: Report of two surviving patients. *JAMA 286*: 2549–2553.

Meyer MA. (2003). Neurologic complications of anthrax: A review of the literature. *Archives of Neurology 60*: 483–488.

Meyerhoff A, Murphy D. (2002). Guidelines for treatment of anthrax. *JAMA 288*: 1848–1849.

Mina B, Dym JP, et al. (2002). Fatal inhalational anthrax with unknown source of exposure in a 61-year-old woman in New York City. *JAMA 287*: 858–862.

Quintiliani R Jr, Quintiliani R. (2003). Inhalational anthrax and bioterrorism. *Current Opinion in Pulmonary Medicine 9*: 221–226.

Stephenson J. (2004). Rapid anthrax test approved. *JAMA 292*: 30.

Steward J, Lever MS, et al. (2004). Post-exposure prophylaxis of anthrax in mice and treatment with fluoroquinolones. *Journal of Antimicrobial Chemotherapy 54*: 95–99.

Wilkening DA. (2006). Sverdlovsk revisited: Modeling human inhalation anthrax. *Proceedings of the National Academy of Sciences 103*: 7589–7594.

Botulism

Daniel Fagbuyi

Introduction

- Botulism is a clinical syndrome caused by botulinum toxin, a potent neurotoxin produced by anaerobic, spore-forming bacterium *Clostridium botulinum (C. botulinum)*.
- Botulism was first described in the late 1700s during the Napoleonic War as a result of poverty and substandard sanitary measures.
- During that period, smoked blood sausages were the primary source of botulism and culminated in many deaths in Europe.

Botulism is derived from the Latin word for sausage, *botulus*

- Today, botulinum toxin has many medical uses that involve alleviating or weakening spasticity of specific muscle groups, in addition to the popular use of Botox for cosmesis.
- Although there are fewer than 200 cases of all forms of botulism reported annually in the United States, there is a growing concern for the use of botulinum toxin as a potential bioterrorism agent.
- It is of paramount importance that medical personnel be cognizant of the clinical manifestations of botulism in order to promptly identify cases, institute life-saving measures, and notify authorities.
- Botulinum toxin, with its ease of dissemination, aerosol transmissibility, toxicity at low doses, potential for social disruption, public panic, public health impact, and capability for causing high morbidity and mortality, has been labeled a Category-A biological agent in the United States.
- *C. botulinum* is ubiquitously found in soil and aquatic sediments.
- Botulinum toxin is one of the most potent lethal neurotoxins known
- (1 gram of evenly dispersed and inhaled crystalline botulinum toxin could kill more than 1 million people).
- Seven antigenic neurotoxin types exist (A–G). Neurotoxin types A, B, and E account for nearly all human cases.

Pathophysiology

- Absorbed toxin binds to nerve-cell-ending receptors, is internalized within the neuron, and culminates in irreversible presynaptic blockade of acetylcholine neurotransmitter release at all neuromuscular junctions, ganglionic synapses, and postganglionic parasympathetic synapses.
- Toxin impairs the ability of neural cell intracellular calcium ions to trigger exocytosis of acetylcholine neurotransmitter release.

Clinical features

- Signs and symptoms mainly include cranial dysfunction with subsequent descending motor paralysis sparing the sensory system.
- Incubation period ranges from 6 hours to 10 days, although clinical manifestations are typically noted within 24 to 72 hours of neurotoxin exposure and include:
  - Ptosis.
  - Dysphagia.
  - Dry mouth.
  - Diplopia.
  - Dysarthria.
  - Fatigue.
  - Generalized weakness.
  - Constipation.
  - Dyspnea.
  - Nausea and vomiting.
  - Abdominal cramps.
  - Diarrhea.
  - Urinary retention or incontinence.
  - Sore throat.
  - Paresthesias.

Clinical syndromes

Although all have similar clinical features, there are seven clinical botulism syndromes described.
- Food-borne botulism (classic)
  - Preformed neurotoxin is ingested.
  - Food is undercooked and contains clostridial spores that vegetate and produce neurotoxin.
  - *C. botulinum* spores are hardy and can survive temperatures below 120°C.
  - Example—home-canned foods.
  - Worldwide most common form of botulism observed.
- Infant botulism
  - *C. botulinum* colonizes the intestine of infants less than 1 year old and produces neurotoxin in vivo (a combination of bacterial infection/neurotoxin intoxication).
  - Spores germinate and produce neurotoxin in the infant's gastrointestinal (GI) tract as a result of lack of protective bacterial flora and reduced levels of clostridial-inhibiting bile acids, especially when compared to adults.
  - Example—Honey consumption in children under one year of age is a significant risk factor (neurotoxin type B) in about 25 percent of cases. Home/industrial construction is also a risk factor.
  - Honey consumption is not recommended in United States for infants less than 1 year old.
  - *Manifestations include*
  - Poor suck/gag/swallow.

- Hypotonia.
- Weak cry.
- Ptosis.
- Loss of neck control.
- Lethargy.
- Somnolence.
- Constipation.
- Irritability.
- Ocular abnormalities.
- Hypotension.
- Tachycardia.
- Neurogenic bladder.
- Progressive descending paralysis.
- Seizures.
- Respiratory failure.
- Most common form of botulism in the United States since 1980.
- Adult intestinal toxemia botulism (hidden or intestinal colonization botulism)
  - Similar to infant botulism.
  - Colonization of adult intestines that have anatomical or functional abnormalities with production of neurotoxin.
  - Examples—Antibiotic or other antimicrobial exposure, achlorhydria, inflammatory bowel disease or prior surgery, may result in altered GI flora permitting colonization with Clostridia → neurotoxin production.
- Wound botulism
  - Usually described among intravenous drug users; injection sites become infected with multiple organisms including *C. botulinum*.
  - Tissue necrosis and anaerobic conditions that exist with abscess formation enable spore germination and production of neurotoxin within the wound.
  - Example—Exposed wound becomes contaminated with *C. botulinum* →produces neurotoxin with systemic manifestation of botulism syndrome.
- Inhalational botulism
  - Not a natural mode of transmission; few cases have occurred.
  - Clinical picture similar to food-borne botulism as evidenced by accidental exposure in veterinary workers and experimentally, in primates and mice
  - Neurotoxin A in mice has produced severe lung injury including alveolar hemorrhage and interstitial edema, in addition to botulism syndrome.
  - A bioterror attack would likely involve aerosolization or food contamination with botulinum toxin.
- Iatrogenic (inadvertent) botulism
  - Accidental occupational exposure in laboratory workers or exposure during administration of botulinum toxin for medical indications.

- Rarely does iatrogenic exposure result in full-blown botulism, although there are few case reports.
- Neurotoxin likely entered the blood stream resulting in systemic symptoms

Differential Diagnosis for suspected botulism

Table 55.1 Clinical features of infant botulism.

Weak cry
Weakness/hypotonia
Lethargy/somnolence
Irritability
Hyporeflexia
Poor oral feeding/weak sucking
Reduced gagging and/or sucking reflex
Swallowing difficulties
Poor head control
Facial weakness
Ocular abnormalities (mydriasis, ptosis)
Dry mouth
Pharyngeal erythema
Constipation
Ventilatory (respiratory) difficulty
Cardiovascular abnormalities (hypotension, tachycardia)
Neurogenic bladder
Seizures (rare)

Reprinted from Caya JG, Agni R, and Miller JE. Clostridium botulinum and the Clinical Laboratorian: A Detailed Review of Botulism, Including Biological Warfare Ramifications of Botulinum Toxin. *Arch Pathol Lab Med.* 128(6) 2004:653–662, with permission from Archives of Pathology & Laboratory Medicine. Copyright 2004, College of American Pathologists.

Diagnosis/investigations

- High index of suspicion required.
- Clinical diagnosis (thorough history and physical exam).
- Stool cultures, wound culture, electromyography 20–50Hz (rapid repetitive electromyography) are confirmatory.
- Possibly excluded/included by performing Imaging studies (MRI, CT), Lumbar puncture with CSF studies, Porphyria evaluation, Toxicology screen, Edrophonium (Tensilon) challenge test.

Management

- Airway, breathing, and circulation are first priority.
- Protection and control of airway by intubation and mechanical ventilation.
- Supportive care; mainly ventilatory support in severe botulism.
- Cardiovascular support as necessary.
- Frequent neurological assessments.
- Antibiotic use should be limited to treatment of infections and wound botulism.
  - Metronidazole is the drug of choice for wound infection; other antibiotic such as polymyxin B, aminoglycosides, and clindamycin should be avoided as they have intrinsic neuromuscular blocking properties and may exacerbate neurotoxin release.
- Baby BIG (human botulinum immune globulin) should be administered immediately to infants 1 year old or less with botulism.
- Human-derived antitoxin preparation.
  - Prevents progression of paralysis and affords less severe course averting the need for intubation and mechanical ventilation.
- Equine-derived trivalent antitoxin (A, B, E) should be administered immediately to children over 1 year old and adults.
  - 15–25 percent experience side effects like serum sickness and anaphylaxis.
  - Prevents progression of paralysis and affords less severe course averting the need for intubation and mechanical ventilation.
  - Most effective when given within the first 24 hours of neurotoxin exposure as it neutralizes only toxins not bound to neural tissue.
  - Not recommended in infant botulism because of safety concerns.
- Psychological evaluation and counseling should be initiated to treat psychological depression.
- Vaccine prophylaxis in the acute setting is futile.
- Protective immune response to the vaccine may take up to 6 months.
- Decontamination
  - Standard precautions should be observed.
  - No isolation required for hospitalized patients.
  - Secondary spread from patient to health-care provider is unlikely.
  - The toxin is sensitive to heat, sunlight, chlorine, soap, and water.

Suggested readings

Arnon SS, Schechter R, Inglesby TV, et.al. (2001, February). Botulinum toxin as a biological weapon: Medical and public health management. *JAMA* 285(8): 1059–1070.

Caya JG, Agni R, Miller JE (2004, June). Clostridium botulinum and the clinical laboratorian: A detailed review of botulism, including biological warfare ramifications of botulinum toxin. *Arch Pathol Lab Med* 128(6): 653–662.

Chapter 56

Plague

Korin Hudson

Introduction

Plague is a severe bacterial infection caused by the gram-negative bacillus Yersinia pestis. Y. pestis causes three distinct forms of disease in humans: bubonic plague, pneumonic plague, and septicemic plague. Other forms of the disease including ocular plague and plague meningitis have also been observed but are far less common.

The bacteria Y. pestis most commonly exists in rodents such as prairie dogs, squirrels, and rats. However, Y. pestis may also be found in other small mammals such as cats. The bacteria are most commonly transmitted from the host animal to humans by fleas. Direct contact, animal bites, or exposures to sick animals or infected carcasses may also lead to spread of the disease in humans.

Endemic plague is seen in the southwestern United States (Colorado, New Mexico, Arizona, and California), Southeast Asia, India, parts of the former Soviet Union, and parts of Africa. Hikers, campers, veterinarians, and owners of infected animals, especially those living in, or visiting, endemic areas are at risk for contracting plague especially during warm, wet summer months.

Plague is also considered a potential bioterrorism agent because of its pathogenicity, transmissibility, and virulence.

A sudden influx of previously healthy patients presenting with severe pneumonia and/or gram negative septicemia, should raise the suspicion of a possible plague.

Bubonic plague

Bubonic plague can be acquired naturally, or as a result of a bioterrorist attack. The natural form of the disease generally develops secondary to a bite from an infected flea. See Box 56.1.
- Most common form of naturally occurring plague.
- The incubation period is 4–7 days with abrupt onset of symptoms.
- Signs and symptoms include:
  - Malaise.
  - Myalgias.
  - High fever.
  - Headache.
  - Tachycardia.
  - Buboes—large tender regional lymph nodes (usually inguinal or axillary nodes), that develop near the site of the bite/inoculation. These buboes are the hallmark of this form of the disease.
- The mortality rate of bubonic plague is low (1–15%) when treated early, but rises to 40–60 percent when untreated.
- Untreated, bubonic plague can progress to septicemic and occasionally to pneumonic plague within 2–6 days. In such cases, death rates increase precipitously.

Pneumonic plague

Pneumonic plague is a severe, fulminant respiratory illness that results from direct contact with an infected individual and generally develops via droplet transmission from person to person. See Box 56.1.

- Signs and symptoms include:
  - High fever.
  - Myalgias.
  - Malaise.
  - Chest pain.
  - Productive cough.
  - Hemoptysis.
  - GI symptoms (nausea, vomiting, abdominal pain, diarrhea)
- If not treated within 24 hours of onset, pneumonic plague rapidly progresses to septicemia, leading to acral cyanosis, respiratory failure, circulatory collapse, and death.
- Even with prompt treatment, the mortality rate for pneumonic plague is approximately 15 percent. Untreated, the mortality rate may be as high as 50–90 percent.
- Pneumonic symptoms may also develop in patients with the septicemic form of the disease.

Septicemic plague

Septicemic plague occurs when the Y. pestis bacteria multiply in the blood stream causing bacteremia and severe sepsis. See Box 56.1.

- Incubation period of 1–6 days.
- Sudden onset and rapid progression of symptoms.
- Initial signs and symptoms include:
  - Fever/chills.
  - Malaise.
  - Abdominal pain.
  - Shock.
  - Coagulopathies—Bleeding underneath the skin, from mucous membranes, or from other organs may occur and may result in disseminated intravascular coagulation (DIC), necrosis of small vessels, and purpura.
  - Acral cyanosis/necrosis—distal extremities such as the fingers, toes, and nose may become gangrenous. This development of dark, necrotic tissue led to the term "black death," the name given to the disease during a pandemic in the Middle Ages.

Primary septicemic plague
- Results from direct inoculation of the bacteria into the bloodstream, typically via the bite of an infected animal or flea or from direct contact with infected tissues.

Secondary septicemic plague
- Occurs when there is progression of disease and dissemination of bacteria following an initial bubonic or pneumonic presentation of disease.

Septicemic plague is rarely transmissible human to human, but may become extremely contagious if pulmonary symptoms develop. In both primary and secondary septicemic plague, the mortality rate is approximately 40 percent when treated promptly. In untreated cases, the mortality rate approaches 100 percent.

Box 56.1 **Associated signs and symptoms that may assist in differentiating various forms of plague.**

Bubonic
- Myalgias
- Headache
- Tachycardia
- Painful regional lymph nodes (buboes) in the groin, axilla, or neck
- Petechial or purpuric eruptions
- Papule, pustule, vesicle, bulla, or ulcer may be present at the site of the flea bite (up to 25% of cases)

Pneumonic
- Extreme weakness
- Chest pain
- Cough
- Shortness of breath
- Rapidly developing pneumonia
- Sputum may be bloody or watery
- History of airborne exposure
- Recent history of tender, matted, regional lymph nodes

Septicemic
- Shock
- Purpura
- Skin necrosis
- Acral cyanosis or gangrene
- Mucous membrane bleeding
- Hematuria
- Epistaxis
- Oral mucosal bleeding
- Vaginal bleeding
- Rectal bleeding
- Evidence of flea bites, which may appear as small ulcerations, pustules, papules, vesicles, or bullae
- Buboes—do not develop in primary septicemic plague, but may precede the symptoms of severe sepsis in secondary sep-ticemic plague.
- Coagulopathies/Disseminated Intravascular Coagulation (DIC)
- Ecthyma-like lesions

Diagnosis

Differential diagnosis
- Acute meningococcemia.
- Acute respiratory distress syndrome.
- Cat-scratch disease.
- Cellulitis.
- Chancroid.
- Cryoglobulinemia.
- Disseminated Intravascular Coagulation (DIC).
- Ecthyma gangrenosum.
- Inhalational anthrax.
- Gas gangrene.
- Legionnaires' disease.
- Lymphogranuloma venereum.
- Mycobacteria marinum.
- Necrotizing fasciitis.
- Pneumonia.
- Q Fever.
- Ricin Inhalation.
- Septic shock.
- Tick-borne diseases.
- Tularemia.

Lab tests

In cases of severe disease, there may be laboratory evidence of multi-organ failure.

Routine laboratory testing should include:
- Complete blood count.
- Coagulation profile.
- Chemistry panel.
- Liver function panel.
- Urinalysis.
- Cultures of blood and urine as well as cultures of sputum, CSF, and aspirate from buboes when present.
- Gram stain of infected body fluids (blood, sputum, CSF, bubo aspirate) may show Gram-negative bacilli.
- Specialized staining with Wright's, Giemsa, or Wayson stains reveal a classic "closed safety pin" appearing bipolar shaped bacteria.

It is important that the laboratory be notified that plague is suspected as special handling of samples is recommended during certain tests, special tests may be useful, and cultures grow optimally at 28°C.

Special diagnostic testing is available at some laboratories including state health departments and the United States Centers for Disease Control and Prevention (CDC). Such tests include a direct fluorescent antibody stain, which may provide rapid diagnosis when performed on blood, sputum, or bubo aspirate samples. When suspicion for plague is high, the local health department and/or the CDC should be notified immediately.

Imaging

In cases of pulmonary disease, chest radiographs may reveal patchy bilateral alveolar infiltrates with or without hilar adenopathy. Pleural effusions may be seen in up to 50 percent of patients.

Vaccine

In the past, killed-whole-cell and live-attenuated vaccines have been used with varying degrees of efficacy and safety. Several prospective vaccines are in development, most using protective plasmid-specific protein antigens. However, currently a plague vaccine is not commercially available in the U.S.

Treatment

Care for patients with plague is primarily supportive. Patients with pneumonic and/or septicemic plague will likely require management in an ICU setting. Patients may require respiratory support and mechanical ventilation as well as fluid resuscitation and pharmacologic blood-pressure support.

Antibiotic treatment should begin immediately within 24 hours of initial symptoms whenever possible. Persons who have had close contact with infected patients should be rapidly identified and evaluated and should begin prophylactic antibiotic therapy immediately.

See Box 56.2 and Box 56.3.

Adult Treatment Recommendations

Box 56.2 Antibiotic recommendations for adults in cases of known or suspected plague

First line antibiotic therapy for all types of plague
- Streptomycin 1 g IM twice daily for 10 days.
  - Not recommended for pregnant women.

OR
- Gentamicin 5 mg/kg IM or IV once daily or 2 mg/kg loading dose followed by 1.7 mg/kg IM/IV three times per day for 10 days.

OR
- Doxycycline 100 mg IV twice daily or 200 mg IV once daily for 10 days.
  - If gentamicin not available or oral antibiotics must be used.

OR
- Ciprofloxacin 400 mg IV twice a day for 10 days.
  - Other fluoroquinolones may be used at appropriate dosing.

AND
- In cases of suspected plague meningitis, add Chloramphenicol: 25 mg/kg IV 4 times daily for 10 days.
  - Concentrations should be maintained between 5 and 20 ug/ml, concentrations greater than 25 ug/ml can cause irreversible bone marrow suppression.

Post exposure prophylaxis for adults:
- Doxycycline 100 mg PO twice daily for 7 days.

OR
- Ciprofloxacin 500 mg PO twice daily for 7 days.

Adapted from: Inglesby, TV, Dennis, DT, Henderson, DA, et al. (2000), "Plague as a Biological Weapon: Medical and Public Health Management. Working Group on Civilian Biodefense, *JAMA, 283*: 2281. (Note: IM indicates intramuscularly, IV-intravenously, and PO- orally.)

Pediatric treatment recommendations

Box 56.3 Antibiotic recommendations for children in cases of known or suspected plague

First line antibiotic therapy for all types of plague:
- Streptomycin 15 mg/kg IM twice daily for 10 days.
  - Maximum dose 2 g per day.

OR

Gentamicin 2.5 mg/kg IM or IV three times per day for 10 days (adjust for renal function).

OR

- Doxycycline:
  >45 kg, give adult dosage.
  <45 kg, 2.2 mg/kg IV twice daily for 10 days.
  - Maximum 200 mg/day.

OR

- Ciprofloxacin 15 mg/kg IV twice daily for 10 days.
  - Maximum daily dose 1 g.

AND

- In cases of suspected plague meningitis, add Chloramphenicol, 25 mg/kg IV 4 times daily for 10 days.
  - Concentrations should be maintained between 5 and 20 ug/ml, concentrations greater than 25 ug/ml can cause irreversible bone marrow suppression.
  - Consult Infectious Disease specialist for dosing recommendations.

Post Exposure Prophylaxis for pediatrics:
- Doxycycline:
  > 45 kg use adult dose.
  <45 kg use 2.2 mg/kg PO twice daily for 7 days.

  OR
  Ciprofloxacin 20 mg/kg PO twice.

Adapted from: Inglesby, TV, Dennis, DT, Henderson, DA, et al. (2000), "Plague as a Biological Weapon: Medical and Public Health Management. Working Group on Civilian Biodefense, *JAMA, 283*: 2281. [Note: IM indicates intramuscularly, IV-intravenously, and PO-orally.]

Isolation/precautions

Health-care providers should use standard contact and droplet isolation precautions. This includes isolating the patient from other patients. All health-care providers should wear gowns, gloves, and a mask when in contact with any infected patient or any patient with a suspected diagnosis of plague. Patient transport should be limited as much as possible in cases of confirmed or suspected plague.

According to the CDC, there is a U.S. Public Health Service requirement that all cases of suspected plague must be reported to local/state health departments. The diagnosis must be confirmed by the CDC and in accordance with International Health Regulations; the CDC reports all U.S. cases of plague to the World Health Organization (WHO).

In the United States, per Title 42 US Code Section 264, plague is a federally quarantineable disease, empowering the CDC to detain, medically examine, or conditionally release individuals reasonably believed to be carrying a communicable disease.

Plague in a terrorist attack

Plague is classified as a Category A bioterrorism agent because of its ease of dissemination, contagiousness, and high mortality rate. There are several ways that plague might be used in a terrorist attack including aerosol release of bacteria, release of infected fleas, or intentional human spread.

In the event of intentional dissemination, plague bacteria would most likely be released in an aerosol form, resulting primarily in the highly lethal and contagious pneumonic form of the disease. In an aerosol attack, bubonic plague would not likely immediately result, but may occur later in the outbreak due to secondary transmission by fleas.

A release of infected fleas may also lead to an outbreak of disease in humans, likely the bubonic form initially, but perhaps progressing to an outbreak of the pneumonic or septicemic forms of the disease.

Conclusion

Plague is an ancient disease with very modern implications in endemic areas and with its potential use as a bioterrorist weapon. Rapid identification of signs and symptoms, as well as prompt diagnosis and treatment of disease can minimize mortality.

Suggested readings

Center for Infection Disease Research and Policy. Accessed 8/22/2010: Available at www.cidrap.umn.edu/content/bt/plague/biofacts/plaguefactsheet

Centers for Disease Control. Accessed 8/22/2010. Available at www.cdc.gov/ncidod/dvbid/plague

Gage K (2007). Plague and other Yersinia infections. In Goldman L, Ausiello D, eds., *Goldman: Cecil Medicine*, 23rd ed. Philadelphia, PA: Saunders/Elsevier.

Inglesby TV, Dennis DT, Henderson DA, et al. (2000). Plague as a biological weapon: Medical and public health management. *JAMA Working Group on Civilian Biodefense 283*: 2281.

Prentice MB, Rahalison L. (2007). Plague. L:ancet 369: 1196.

Chapter 57

Smallpox

David R. Lane

Overview

- Smallpox is one of six diseases classified as Category-A bioterrorism agents, and is caused by variola, a DNA virus in the genus orthopox.
- Although eradicated from human populations in 1980 after a concerted global effort directed by the WHO, the variola virus is maintained in two separate secured stockpiles in the United States and in the Russian Federation. It is a human disease with no known animal reservoir.
- After September 11, 2001 and the subsequent anthrax releases in the United States, there has been concern that the variola virus may become available to terrorist groups with the capacity to create aerosolized forms of the virus.
- Released onto a now largely unvaccinated public, the variola virus has the potential to create a smallpox outbreak with significant social, political, and economic impact.

Transmission

- Transmission of smallpox person to person requires direct, prolonged face-to-face contact, or contact with contaminated bodily fluids or objects such as bedding or clothing.
- Rarely is transmission airborne, and the large majority of aerosolized virus would be inactive within 24 hours.
- An infected person is most contagious from the onset of rash until the final smallpox scab falls off. There is no evidence of transmission during the incubation period or prodromal period.
- Transmission rates are high in household contacts, with documented attack rates of approximately 50 percent.

Signs and symptoms

- The incubation period is approximately 2 weeks (range 7–17 days), during which the victim is asymptomatic and not contagious.
- This is followed by a prodrome lasting 2–4 days of high fevers, malaise, myalgias, and headaches. The patient may have vomiting and abdominal pain. The patient is not contagious during the prodrome.
- A macular rash develops, primarily on the face and oropharynx, and then progresses over 24 hours to the palms and soles, arms, and then trunk and legs.
- Over 4–5 days, the lesions progress from papular, to vesicular, then finally to deep, round, hard, pustular lesions that scab over and ultimately leave permanent pitted scars.
- Smallpox lesions are differentiated from varicella lesions in that they are all:
  - Of the same age.
  - Characteristically deep.
  - Predominantly on the face and extremities.
- Varicella lesions are of:
  - Varying ages.
  - Superficial.
  - More prominent on the trunk.
  - Associated with a milder prodromal illness.
- The illness has a 30 percent mortality rate in unvaccinated individuals, and a <1 percent mortality rate in vaccinated individuals.
- Atypical presentations including hemorrhagic smallpox (mucosal bleeding) and malignant smallpox (lesions do not progress past macular) have much higher fatality rates—nearly 100 percent.

Diagnostic testing

- Differential diagnosis for the rash includes varicella zoster virus (VZV), disseminated herpes virus (HSV), measles, enterovirus, parvovirus B, rubella virus, and molluscum contagiosum.
- CDC algorithm is available to evaluate an acute rash illness suspicious for smallpox. Available at: http://www.bt.cdc.gov/agent/smallpox/diagnosis/riskalgorithm/. Accessed December 6, 2010.
- Laboratory confirmation of smallpox involves PCR of variola DNA in a clinical specimen, or isolation of the variola virus from a clinical specimen with variable PCR confirmation. If there is an outbreak, after laboratory confirmation of one case, cases fitting the clinical description are considered smallpox until proven otherwise.
- The laboratory technology is not typically available in hospital laboratories, but rather samples should be forwarded by local public health officials to the appropriate state and national testing facilities, with biosafety level 4 capacity.
- Complete blood count with differential is likely to reveal a lymphocytosis.

Management

- Smallpox has no specific treatment. Supportive care including intravenous fluids, analgesics, and antipyretics can be offered to victims.
- Patients should be quarantined: in hospital settings and patients should be fitted with an N-95 mask and placed in a negative pressure room for respiratory isolation. In a large outbreak, patients may be quarantined in their homes or in specific facilities.
- Antibiotics may be needed for secondary skin infections. The infected patient should be kept in isolation for 17 days or until the scabs dry up and fall off.
- Research is being conducted with new antiviral agents, but currently they are still experimental.

Epidemic prevention

Isolation and vaccination

- The theory of "ring vaccination," in which smallpox victims are identified and isolated, and then all significant contacts of that victim are immediately vaccinated and monitored, was successful in eradicating smallpox in human populations. It is the model on which public-health preparedness is based in the event of a terrorist smallpox attack. However, there are limitations to ring vaccination in a large outbreak, and population-wide vaccinations would be considered.
- Vaccine immunization with live vaccinia virus vaccine is thought to provide three to five years of high-level immunity. Vaccinia is significantly preventive if given within three days of exposure, and somewhat preventive if given within four to seven days after exposure.
- Complications of the vaccine included generalized or progressive vaccinia, eczema vaccinatum, and postvaccination encephalitis. Vaccinia immunoglobulin has some utility in serious vaccine reactions.
- The vaccine is contraindicated in nonemergent situations in patients who are:
  - Immunosuppressed.
  - Pregnant or breastfeeding.
  - Under the age of 1 year.
  - Affected by atopic dermatitis or eczema.
  - Allergic to vaccine components.

Suggested readings

Henderson et al. (1999). Smallpox as a biological weapon. *JAMA 281*: 2127–2137.
Sidell FR, Takafuji ET, Franz DR, eds. (1989). *Medical Aspects of Chemical and Biological Warfare*. Chapter 27: Smallpox. Washington, DC: McGraw Hill Professional.
United Kingdom Department of Health. Guidelines for Smallpox Response and Management in the Post-Eradication Era, vol. 2.
http://www.cdc.gov (Accessed December 4, 2010).
http://www.smallpox.gov (Accessed December 4, 2010).
http://www.who.int (Accessed December 4, 2010).
http://www.bepast.org (Accessed December 4, 2010).

Chapter 58

Tularemia

Michael Sean Antonis

History of tularemia

Tularemia was first isolated by McCoy and Chapin in 1912 as the causative agent of a disease in ground squirrels located in Tulane County, California. The origins of tularemia have been proposed as far back as the biblical plague of the Philistines around the second millennium BC. This facultative, gram negative, intracellular coccobacillus causes a zoonotic disease in humans as accidental hosts. Several formulations of disease names have been proposed such as Francis' disease, Deer-fly disease, rabbit fever, trappers' ailment, and O'hara's disease.

Epidemiology

Subspecies of tularemia
- Two most common
- Tularensis (Type A)
  - Most virulent type; causes 90 percent of all North American tularemia infections.
  - Dry environmental conditions.
- Holarctica (Type B)
  - Geographically in Europe and former Soviet Union.
  - Damp environmental conditions.

Clinical manifestations

- The clinical spectrum ranges from an asymptomatic illness to septic shock and death.
- Before antibiotics the mortality from tularemia approached 33 percent.
- With symptom recognition and treatment mortality is now ~ 3 percent.
- *F. tularensis* is a highly virulent organism, requiring only 10–50 organisms to produce clinical illness.

Common signs and symptoms

Most to least common
- Lymphadenopathy.
- Fever.
- Pharyngitis.
- Ulcer/Eschar/Papule.
- Nausea and Vomiting.
- Hepatosplenomegaly.

Symptom onset
- Patients infected with Francisella species present with abrupt onset of fever, chills, headache, and malaise, after an incubation period of 2–10 days up to 2–3 weeks.
- Other symptoms and signs are related to portal of entry and the principal organ system involved.

Clinical syndromes

Ulceroglandular (60–80%)
- Occurrence: animal bite, intimate handling of animals, tick exposure
- Fever, single erythematous papulo-ulcerative lesion with single eschar.
- Tender regional lymphadenopathy.
- Progression: portal of entry develops into papule that progresses to a slowly healing ulcer.

Glandular (3–15%)
- Single or multiple lymph nodes without skin lesions.
- Differential diagnosis: cat-scratch disease, malignancy, mycobacterium infection, lymphogranuloma venerum, streptococcal or staphylococcal lymphadenitis, fungal infection, plague, lymphoma.

Typhoidal (1%)
- High-grade fever with sepsis.
- CSF shows mononuclear pleocytosis.
- Relative bradycardia, GI symptoms, pulmonary infiltrates.

Pneumonic (5–10%)
- Caused by airborne (lab workers) or hematogenous spread (more common).
- Presents similar to typhoidal form with predisposition for elderly and increased mortality.
- Radiographs:
  - Patchy unilateral or bilateral infiltrates.
  - Lobar or segmental opacities.
  - Hilar adenopathy.
  - Pleural effusion.
  - Cavitary lesions and miliary patterns.
- Nodular infiltrate + pleural effusion = tularemia or plaque pneumonia.
- Clinical presentation + Chest x-ray cannot distinguish from community acquired pneumonia.

Oropharyngeal (1–4%)
- Caused by ingestion of poorly cooked wild animal meat or water.
- Fever and exudative pharyngitis unresponsive to penicillin

Oculoglandular (1–2%).
- Special form of ulceroglandular caused by direct inoculation of the eye by fingers after preparing contaminated meat.
- Conjunctival erythema with chemosis and vascular engorgement.

Diagnosis

Laboratory testing
- WBC counts may be ↑, but normal differential.
- Moderately ↑ESR.
- Abnormal liver functions in 50 percent of cases.
- Histology of lymph nodes similar appearance to TB or cat-scratch fever.
- Cultures negative due to fastidious nature of organism and culture media must contain cysteine.
- Must notify laboratory workers when culture is ordered for Tularemia as biosafety level-3 precautions must be observed.

Note: despite difficulties in isolating tularemia in the lab, Francisella is a hardy organism in nature persisting in mud, water, or animal carcasses for weeks.

Serologic testing
- Most published experience with serum agglutination testing.
  - A single titer of 1:160 with supporting clinical evidence.
  - Fourfold increase in acute vs. convalescent serum is the gold standard confirmatory testing.
  - Disadvantage: requires a two- to four-week interval test that will delay diagnosis and treatment.
  - Antibody titers will remain elevated for years after exposure.
  - Single high antibody titer is nonspecific.
  - Agglutination testing is NOT a screening tool.
- Strategy based on screening with ELISA and confirmation by western blot has been a recent update for suggestion of diagnosis.

Reportable disease

- The Centers for Disease Control removed Tularemia from reportable disease list in 1995, restored it in 2000. Now classified as a Category-A bioterror agent.

Pathogenesis

- Low infective dose enters macrophage as an intracellular parasite causing apoptosis, then escapes from cell with minimal inflammatory response.
- Cell-mediated response: crucial for elimination and provides life-long immunity in 2 weeks after onset of clinical disease.
- Humoral response: limited value to eliminate bacteria, but agglutinating antibodies can be detected for diagnosis in one week.

Routes of transmission

- Direct Contact: hunters of infected rodents and lagomorphs usually through abraded skin, but may infect through intact skin.
- Vectors: arthropods (insects and ticks) and flies (horse and deer flies).
- Inhalation (smallest infective dose): laboratory workers (most commonly) and farmers. Recently, multiple cases of exposure in landscapers mowing grass in Martha's Vineyard, Massachusetts, United States.
- Ingestion: infection through contaminated water occurred in Turkey and Southern Europe in WWII.
- No human-to human-transmission.

Treatment

The cornerstone of treatment is early diagnosis and implementation of appropriate antimicrobial therapy. No controlled prospective trials have defined the efficacy or various drug regiments or the optimal duration of therapy.

Antimicrobial therapy

- Streptomycin: (97% cure rate with no relapses).
  - 10 mg/kg IM every 12 hours for 7–10 days in adults.
  - 30 mg/kg IM in two divided doses for 7 days in children.
  - Used in most critically ill patients.
- Gentamicin: (86% cure rate with 6% relapse rate).
  - 3–5 mg/kg IM or IV every 8 hours for 7–10 days in adults.
  - 6 mg/kg/day with peak serum levels one hour after IV administration of greater than 7 mg/mL in children.
  - Used in critically ill patients.
- Tetracycline: (88% cure rate with 12% relapse rate)
  - 500 mg orally 4 times a day for 14 days.
  - Not for use in children.
  - May substitute doxycycline 100 mg 2 times a day.
  - Common for relapses due to bacteriostatic nature.
- Chloramphenicol: (77% cure rate with 21% relapse rate)
  - 25–60 mg/kg per day IV in 4 divided doses for 14 days.
  - Common for relapse due to bacteriostatic nature.
- Ciprofloxacin: mixed results with high rate of relapse.

Special populations

- Pregnancy: Streptomycin or Chloramphenicol drugs of choice.
- Meningitis: Chloramphenicol at 50–100 mg/kg and Streptomycin.

Bioterrorism and tularemia

The ease of production, low infective dose, aerosolization of small particles, and difficulty with immediate diagnosis make tularemia an attractive option for terrorists.

- Human volunteers subjected to the minimal infective dose of aerolsized 0.7 micrometer particles showed 16 of 20 exposed volunteers developed systemic infection after an incubation period of 4–7 days.
- In 1970, a WHO published report estimated that an aerosolized dispersal of 50 kilograms of virulent *F. tularemia* over a metropolitan area of 5 million inhabitants would result in 250,000 incapacitating causalities with over 19,000 deaths.
- The former USSR, as part of the BIOPREPARAT program, incorporated extensive research into developing Tularemia into weapons for war that included antibiotic resistant and increased survivability strains.
- A high-resolution multiple-locus-variable-number tandem repeat analysis (MVLA) typing method for *F. tularensis* has been developed.
  - Powerful tool in understanding the natural population of Tularemia endemic to a particular area.
  - Crucial in forensic determination of suspected perpetrators of a bioterrorism attack.

Vaccines

- The live vaccine for *F. tularensis* was used to a large extent in the former Soviet Union with good clinical results. The Soviet-borne vaccine was used for at-risk personnel in the United States and western Europe, but was unlicensed because:
  - Genetic background for the attenuation and protection unknown.
  - Live vaccine strain retains high virulence upon testing in mice.
  - Vaccine also exhibits phase variation allowing a spectrum between immunogenic protection, a disease state, or no response.

Live Vaccine Strain (LVS)

- *Francisella tularensis* live vaccine has been developed that is well tolerated and highly immunogenic when administered to rabbits.
- The comprehensive toxicological and immunological study of *F. tularensis* LVS in the rabbit model has proved adequate to assess the safety and immunogenicity in human candidates at this time.

Suggested readings

Eliasson H, Broman Tina, Forsman Mats, et al. (2006, June). Tularemia: Current epidemiology and disease management. *Infect. Disease Clinics of N.A.* 20(2): 289–311.

Enderlin G, Morales L, Jacobs RF, et al. (1994). Streptomycin and alternative agents for the treatment of tularemia: Review of literature. *Clin Infect Dis* 19: 42–47.

Pasetti M, Cuberos L, Horn, TL, Shearer JD, et al. (2008). An improved Francisella tularensis live vaccine strain is well tolerated and highly immunogenic when administered to rabbits in escalating doses using various immunization routes. *Vaccine* 26: 1773–1785.

Chapter 59

Viral hemorrhagic fevers

Amy M. Stubbs

Background

- Hemorrhagic fever viruses (HFVs) are a diverse group of RNA viruses that have the potential to cause severe illness and could be a major public-health threat if used as a weapon.
- Most are highly virulent, have potential to be disseminated by aerosol, cause high morbidity and/or mortality, and require special measures to control spread.
- For theses reasons, many of the HFVs are classified as Category-A agents by the CDC, meaning that they are considered to have high potential for bioterrorism and could pose a major public-health threat.
- HFVs cause a clinical illness known as viral hemorrhagic fever (VHF) that can be difficult to recognize and diagnose in certain settings.
- Early recognition and reporting of possible infection is key to the containment and management of a possible attack or outbreak; a high index of suspicion is required.
- Treatment is largely supportive; ribavirin may be useful with certain viruses.
- *Strict isolation and protective measures* for infected patients and their health-care providers must be implemented as soon as suspicion exists for infection.

History

- To date, there have been no uses of HFVs in terrorist attacks.
- Several countries, including the United States and Russia, have weaponized certain viruses.
- Most countries have destroyed or stopped production of this type of weapon as a result of the Biological Weapons Convention.
- The Japanese terrorist group Aum Shinrikyo unsuccessfully attempted to obtain and weaponize Ebola, and most experts agree that further efforts by other groups will likely occur.
- Outbreaks in endemic areas have been sporadic and impact has been variable.

Epidemiology

- Geographic distribution known for most HFVs; cases outside known region, if patient has not traveled to endemic area, should raise suspicion for deliberate infection.
- Zoonotic life cycles with seasonal variation; most are initially spread through bites of infected insects or contact with animal waste.
- No person-person transmission during the incubation period of the illness has been reported.
- The multiple viruses known as HFVs are members of one of four families (see Table 59.1):
  - Filoviridae.
  - Arenaviridae.
  - Bunyaviridae.
  - Flaviviridae.

Table 59.1 Current HFV threats and their associated clinical illness

Family	Virus	Clinical Illness
Filoviridae	Ebola	Ebola hemorrhagic fever
	Marburg	Marburg hemorrhagic fever
Arenaviridae	Lassa	Lassa fever
	New World Arenaviridae includes:	
	Machupo	Bolivian hemorrhagic fever
	Junin	Argentine hemorrhagic fever
	Guanarito	Venezuelan hemorrhagic fever
	Sabia	Brazilian hemorrhagic fever
Bunyaviridae	Rift Valley fever	Rift Valley fever
	Crimean-Congo hemorrhagic fever	Crimean-Congo hemorrhagic fever (CCHF)
	Agents of hemorrhagic fever with renal syndrome (hantaviruses)	Hemorrhagic fever with renal syndrome (HFRS)
Flaviviridae	Yellow fever	Yellow fever
	Dengue	Dengue fever, Dengue hemorrhagic fever (DHF), Dengue shock syndrome (DSS)
	Kyasanur Forest disease	Kyasanur Forest disease (KFD)
	Omsk hemorrhagic fever	Omsk hemorrhagic fever (OHF)

Filoviridae
- Sub-Saharan Africa (Ebola, Marburg).
- Reservoir and vector unknown; likely zoonotic
- Transmitted through close personal contact, body fluid, or mucosal exposure; airborne transmission rare but thought possible.

Arenaviridae
- West Africa (Lassa), South America (Junin New World).
- Rodents are chronically infected.
- Spread primarily through contact (inhalation, ingestion, or cutaneous) with infected rodent waste; has been transmitted person-person through infected body fluids; airborne transmission is suspected in a few cases.

Bunyaviridae
- Africa (Crimean-Congo Hemorrhagic Fever [CCHF], Rift Valley Fever), Asia (CCHF, Hemorrhagic Fever with Renal Syndrome [HFRS]), Middle East (CHHF, Rift Valley), Europe (CCHF, HFRS).
- Domestic animals (cattle, sheep, etc.) often infected and serve as amplifying hosts.
- Mosquito bites (Rift Valley), tick bites (CCHF), rodent waste (HFRS); direct contact with infected animals or aerosolization of virus from infected animals also a mode of transmission; person-to-person rare but thought possible.

Flaviviridae
- Africa (Dengue, yellow fever), Asia (Omsk Hemorrhagic Fever [OHF], Dengue), India (KFD), Americas- South and Central (Dengue, yellow fever).
- Rodents are hosts to OHF and KFD.
- Mosquito bites (Dengue, yellow fever), tick bites (OHF, [KFD]); transmission via aerosol reported in laboratory workers.

There have been a few isolated outbreaks of Dengue in North America. The *Aedes Aegypti* mosquito, a known vector, is found in south/southeastern U.S. states.

Pathophysiology

- All of the HFVs are small RNA viruses that have the ability to affect multiple organ systems and most produce a profound viremia.
- All are capable of causing increased vascular permeability, microvascular damage, and bleeding diatheses, though their mechanisms and propensity for specific organ systems may vary.
- Exact mechanisms for all are not known due to the difficulty of studying these dangerous pathogens during outbreaks.
- Most known data is from the results of observation, experience, and animal studies.

Filoviridae

- Directly cytotoxic,
- Causes release of cytokines and inflammatory mediators
  - Leads to tissue damage.
  - Systemic inflammatory response.
  - Coagulopathy.
  - Impaired immunity.

Arenaviridae

- Induce inflammatory mediators from macrophages leading to:
  - Platelet dysfunction.
  - Widespread tissue infection.
  - Minimal histologic damage.

Bunyaviridae

- Poorly understood.
- Evidence for direct cellular damage leading to:
  - Coagulopathy.
  - Hepatic damage in Rift Valley fever and CCHF.
  - Renal damage in HFRS.

Flaviviridae

- Yellow fever causes direct cellular damage.
- Dengue causes intense immune response.
- OHF and KFD are poorly understood.
  - Leads to organ failure.
  - Hemorrhage.
  - Shock.
  - Yellow fever virus is hepatotropic.

Clinical presentation

- Will vary with each virus, but all typically cause multi-system illness, fever, and bleeding diathesis to some degree.
- Mode of transmission and severity of illness varies with each infection.
- Most have zoonotic life-cycles and have limited treatment options, making early recognition and prevention key in the management of an outbreak.
- CCHF and HFRS not currently considered a significant threat for bioterrorism due to difficulties with replication in culture, which is considered necessary for weaponization.
- Dengue cannot be transmitted by aerosol, therefore, it is not currently considered a biologic weapon threat, however, it remains a major public-health problem with ongoing epidemics around the world.

Diagnosis

- VHF must be suspected in any patient presenting with severe illness, fever ≥101°F (38.3°C) of <3-weeks duration, with no predisposing factors to hemorrhagic manifestations who has any 2 of the following:
  - Hemorrhagic or purpuric rash.
  - Epistaxis.
  - Hematemesis.
  - Hemoptysis.
  - Melena/hematochezia.
  - Other hemorrhage without an alternative diagnosis.
- Recent travel to endemic regions, close personal contact with known VHF patients, or exposure in a laboratory setting should obviously raise suspicion level.
- In the case of deliberate infection, historical factors will be less helpful.
- A high index of suspicion must remain, but more common or probable disease processes should be sought and treated as well.
- The history, physical exam, and laboratory findings may provide clues to the diagnosis.
- Radiological tests may be helpful to rule out other conditions or to assess severity of illness.
- Only tests for the specific viruses will provide a definitive diagnosis.

Clinical features

- Early presentation can resemble other viral syndromes with nonspecific symptoms such as fever, malaise, and myalgias.
- As illness progresses, multiple organ systems may be involved and patient's condition may progress to fulminant shock and organ failure.
- Presentation and severity varies with each illness.
- Fever, headache, and myalgias are virtually universal in VHFs; characteristic features of each illness are listed in Table 59.2.

Table 59.2 Clinical features

Pathogen	Incubation period	Onset	Signs & Symptoms	Mortality
Filoviridae				
Ebola	2–21 d	Acute	• Conjunctivitis • Abdominal pain • Nausea and vomiting • Pharyngitis • Diffuse maculopapular rash on day 3–5 • Diffuse bleeding/ DIC (GI, gingival, conjunctival) • Shock, organ failure	50–90%, depending on subtype
Marburg	3–14 d	Acute	• Similar to Ebola, rash more prominent on trunk	21–90%
Arenaviridae				
Lassa	5–16 d	gradual	• Exudative pharyngitis • Conjunctivitis • Retro-orbital pain • Facial and neck swelling • Encephalitis, • Pleural and pericardial effusions • ARDS • Hemorrhagic manifestations occur, but less common	1% overall, ~80% of those infected have mild disease, but of those hospitalized with severe form, ~20% die
New World	7–14 d	Gradual	• Similar to Lassa • Also facial flushing often seen • CNS dysfunction (tremors, myoclonus, seizures) • Hemorrhage more common than in Lassa	10–30%

Table 59.2 (Contd.)

Pathogen	Incubation period	Onset	Signs & Symptoms	Mortality
Bunyaviridae				
CCHF	1–3 d	Acute	• Neck and back pain, • Flushing • Mucosal and skin petechiae • Altered mentation • Mood changes • Melena • Epistaxis • Hematuria • Gingival bleeding • Hepatitis • Multiorgan failure	9–50%
Rift Valley	2–6 d	biphasic	• Usually mild • Biphasic fever • hepatitis/jaundice • Encephalitis • Retinitis • Hemorrhage in severe form	1%
HFRS	7–14 d	acute	• Truncal pain • Visual changes • Nausea and vomiting • Flushing • Conjunctivitis • Hypotension • Shock • ARF in severe form	1–15% depending on virus type
Flaviridae				
Dengue	3–14 d	acute	• Eye pain • Nausea and vomiting • Maculopapular rash • Severe abdominal pain • AMS • Shock and bleeding diathesis in Dengue Hemorrhagic Fever (DHF) → Dengue Shock Syndrome (DSS)	<1% with good supportive care; up to 10% if progression to DSS

Table 59.2 (*Contd.*)

Pathogen	Incubation period	Onset	Signs & Symptoms	Mortality
Yellow Fever	3–6 d	biphasic	• Initially fever, back pain, malaise, n/v • Remission or jaundice, hemorrhage, • Bradycardia/dysrhythmias • Hematemesis • AMS/seizures • Coma	15–50%
OHF	2–9 d	acute	• Flushing • Splenomegaly • Lymphadenopathy • Papulovesicular lesions on soft palate • Pulmonary and CNS involvement	0.5–10%
KFD	2–9 d	acute	• Similar to OHF, but biphasic • Recovery or second phase 1–3 weeks later • Meningoencephalitis	3–10%

Diagnostic testing

General laboratory tests
- Hematology.
  - Cell count and differential.
  - Thrombocytopenia, leukopenia typical for most.
  - Anemia variable; dependent on degree of hemorrhage.
  - Can see leukocytosis in Lassa fever.
- Metabolic.
  - Azotemia common.
  - Liver-function tests.
  - Elevated transaminases typical for most.
  - Elevated bilirubin with Rift Valley fever and yellow fever.
- Coagulation and/or DIC panel.
  - Prolonged bleeding time, PT/INR/APTT.
  - Elevated fibrinogen degradation products, low fibrinogen.
- Urine.
  - Proteinuria, hematuria common.
- Pan-culture.
  - Blood, urine, sputum.
- Lumbar puncture.
  - Consider if meningitis is in differential.
  - Not advised if patient is coagulopathic.
- If VHF suspected, weigh risk/benefit ratio to patient and health-care staff carefully.

Radiologic tests
- To rule out other causes for illness.
- CXR to evaluate for:
  - Pneumonia.
  - Pulmonary manifestations also seen in some VHFs.
- CT head to evaluate for intracranial hemorrhage.
- Disease-specific testing.

Health alerting

- Contact local public health authorities as soon as suspicion for diagnosis of VHF exists.
- Contact CDC for specific instructions on specimen preparation and shipping (**CDC Special Pathogens Branch 404-639-1115**).
- Specimens must be sent to CDC or U.S. Army Medical Research Institute of Infectious Diseases (USAMRIID); the only biosafety level-4 (BSL-4) labs in United States.
- Antigen detection by ELISA or RT-PCR most useful tests in acute setting.
- CDC is able to have preliminary diagnosis in approximately one working day if advance notice is given regarding arrival of specimens.

Management

In the acute management of an outbreak, whether deliberate or naturally occurring, early recognition, good supportive care, and strict infection-control precautions are key interventions.

Treatment
- If the diagnosis of VHF is in question initially, which is likely in the index case of an event, a patient with fever and shock will likely need broad spectrum antibiotics to cover bacterial sepsis.
- Aggressive supportive care.
- Maintain adequate circulatory volume with isotonic fluids, vasopressors may be necessary.
- Correct electrolyte abnormalities.
- Transfusion/blood products as needed—*No anticoagulants.*
- Mechanical ventilation as necessary.
- Hemodialysis for renal failure.
- Acetaminophen only for fever; *NSAIDs/ASA contraindicated.*
- Carefully weigh risk/benefit ratio to patient when considering invasive procedures.
- Patient with VHF of unknown etiology:
  - Ribavirin should be initiated until definitive results are available.
  - Shown to be effective in bunyaviruses and arenaviruses only (discontinue if patient found to have other infection).
  - 30 mg/kg IV loading dose (2 g max) →16 mg/kg IV 4 times daily x 4 days (1 g/dose max)→ 8 mg/kg IV 3 times daily x 6 days (500 mg/dose max).
  - Mass-casualty setting: 2000 mg po x 1→ 1200 mg/day po in two divided doses (≥75 kg) or 1000 mg/day in two divided doses (≤75 kg) x 10 days.
  - Possible teratogen, but should be considered in pregnant patients due to severity of illness.

Safety precautions
- Controlling spread is vital.
- Notify hospital infection control and local public-health authorities immediately.
- Notify lab personnel or others who may come in contact with patient's body fluids; additional lab precautions are needed.
- Minimize contact with staff/visitors—only essential personnel.
- Strict hand hygiene, before and after patient contact; wash before and after removing goggles/face shields to minimize mucous membrane exposure.
- Place patient in negative pressure/respiratory isolation; in mass casualty situation, group patients together in separate wings with separate air-handling systems.
- Establish designated area for applying and removing protective gear.

- Keep patient care equipment in room (stethoscopes, etc.).
- Protective equipment:
  - Double glove.
  - Face shield, goggles/eye protection.
  - Impermeable gown; leg and shoe covers.
  - N-95 (HEPA) or powered air-purifying respirator (PAPRS); both shown to be effective.

Prophylaxis

- No vaccines currently available in United States.
  - Yellow fever live attenuated 17D vaccination available in some endemic areas.
- High-risk exposures: anyone exposed in biological attack or anyone with mucous membrane contact or body fluid exposure with infected person.
  - Medical evaluation and follow-up.
  - Should be monitored for symptoms; including temperature check twice daily.
  - Skin should be washed immediately with soap and water, mucous membranes should be irrigated copiously.
  - Prophylactic Ribavirin controversial; not currently recommended.

Future issues

- Multiple vaccines currently in development; several proven effective in animal studies.
- Treatments currently being investigated include Interferon-β and Activated protein C.

Suggested readings

CDC Special Pathogens Branch. Available at http://www.cdc.gov/ncidod/dvrd/spb/index.htm.
CDC and WHO. Infection control for viral hemorrhagic fevers in the African healthcare setting. Available at http://www.cdc.gov/ncidod/dvrd/spb/mnpages/vhfmanual.htm.
USARMIID *Blue Book* 6th ed.: *Medical Management of Biological Casualties Handbook.* Available at http://www.usamriid.army.mil/education/instruct.htm.

Chapter 60

Other biological agents

Lawrence Proano

Robert Partridge

Introduction

A large number of biologic agents of various types could be used for a terrorist attack. The CDC has classified biologic agents according to lethality,
ease of dissemination, and potential for weaponization. The agents most
likely to be weaponized, with the highest mortality rates requiring a major
public-health response, and causing the greatest fear in a population are
Category-A biologic agents. These have been covered in preceding chapters. This chapter will focus on Category-B and C biologic agents. These
agents have been given a lower priority for public-health preparations but
are no less important. A natural, unintentional, or bioterrorist-related outbreak could result in a medium- to large-scale disaster and significant civil
disruption.

- Category-B agents are described as being moderately easy to
  disseminate, and would result in moderate morbidity and low
  mortality. Diagnosis and disease surveillance of these agents is likely to
  be slower and more difficult.
- Category-C agents are pathogens that are not known to have
  previously been weaponized but have potential to be used as biological
  agents because of availability, ease of production and delivery, and high
  morbidity and mortality.

This chapter will discuss the characteristics of selected Category-B and C
agents, potential for weaponization and dissemination, clinical presentations, treatment, surveillance, and public-health response.

Category-B biologic agents

- Coxiella Burnettii (Q fever): presents with fever, chills, headache, pneumonia. Difficult to recognize as BT agent due to long incubation period 10–40 days. Serologic identification. Illness duration 10–14 days, very low mortality. Treatment and prophylaxis with doxycycline. No vaccine available in United States.

- Brucella species (brucellosis): presents with fever, chills, anorexia, and malaise. Incubation period 5–60 days. Illness persists weeks to months untreated. Mortality low. Identification by blood culture or serology. Treatment and prophylaxis with rifampin plus either doxycycline or fluoroquinolone.

- Burkholderia mallei (glanders): presents with tender skin nodules, septicemia, pneumonia. Incubation period 10–14 days. Illness duration days to weeks; mortality high >50 percent, usually within 7–10 days. Identification by blood culture or serology. Treatment with doxycycline, trimethaprim/sulfamethoxazole (TMP/SMX), chloramphenicol. Prophylaxis with doxycycline or TMP/SMX.

- Alphaviruses (Venezuelan encephalitis, Eastern Equine Encephalitis (EEE), Western Equine Encephalitis (WEE): presents with fever, headache, myalgias, encephalitis. Incubation period short, 2–6 days. Illness duration days to weeks. Mortality low. Serologic identification. Treatment supportive. Live vaccine available but many side effects.

- Rickettsia Prowazekii (Epidemic Typhus): presents with sudden onset of headache, chills, fever, myalgias, and extreme fatigue. In half of cases, a rash develops after 4–6 days, with pink macules on the upper trunk and extremities, spreading to the entire body, but sparing the face, palms, and soles. Incubation period 1–2 weeks. Illness duration days to weeks. Mortality high. Serologic identification. Treatment with doxycycline. No commercial vaccine, but experimental vaccines used by military.

- Chlamydia Burnetti (psittacosis): presents with acute or subacute onset of a mild flulike illness with fever, chills, headache anorexia, pharyngitis, and photophobia. Alternatively, may present with a virulent atypical pneumonia symptoms. Incubation period 1–4 weeks. Illness duration is 2–3 weeks. Mortality high in severe untreated infections. Treatment is with doxycycline. No vaccine available.

- Bunyaviruses (California encephalitis): presents with fever, chills, headache, nausea, vomiting, and abdominal pain, progressing to a picture of encephalitis. Incubation period 3–7 days. Illness duration is 10–14 days. Mortality is low, but morbidity high. Treatment supportive.

- Flaviviruses (West Nile Virus, Japanese encephalitis, St. Louis encephalitis): presents with flulike symptoms, including fever, anorexia, nausea, vomiting, myalgias, headache, back pain, and retro-orbital headache. Severe cases involve profound weakness, paralysis, stupor, and coma. A maculopapular or morbilliform erytematous rash may be present on the trunk and extremities. Incubation period 5–15 days. Illness may be subclinical. Duration ranges from days to weeks. Mortality low, except in severe cases. Vaccine available for Japanese encephalitis. Treatment supportive.

Food- or water-borne agents

- Salmonella species Presents with fever, nausea, often diarrhea. Human-to-human transmission. Incubation and disease duration short, 1–3 days. Very low mortality. Stable in food and water. Treatment mostly supportive. Quinolones, azithromycin used in treatment and prophylaxis. Oral and parenteral vaccines available.
- Shigella dysenteriae Presents with fever, nausea, cramps, and diarrhea. Human-to-human transmission. Incubation 1–3 days. Disease duration 1–3 weeks. Low mortality. Stable in food and water. Stool-culture identification. Treatment mostly supportive. Quinolones, TMP/SMX, azithromycin used in treatment and prophylaxis. Vaccines experimental.
- Escherichia coli O157:H7 Presents with bloody diarrhea, fever, hemolytic-uremic syndrome (HUS) in 6 percent, especially children. Human-to-human transmission. Incubation and disease duration 1–3 days. Mortality low. Stable in food and water. Identification by stool culture. Treatment supportive, avoid antibiotics, antimotility agents. Prophylaxis with quinolones.
- Vibrio cholerae: presents with copious watery diarrhea. Incubation 4 hours–5 days. Disease duration 1 week or more. Low mortality with treatment, high without. Treat with fluids, ciprofloxacin, or doxycycline. Prophylaxis with ciprofloxacin, doxycycline. Vaccine available, low effectiveness.
- Cryptosporidium parvum. Presents with diarrhea, cramps. Human-to-human transmission. Incubation 1–3 weeks. Duration of illness 1–3 weeks. Very low mortality. Diagnosis by stool acid-fast stain. Supportive treatment; azithromycin or paromomycin may be used in treatment and prophylaxis.
- Giardia lamblia: Presents usually with insidious onset of watery, foul smelling diarrhea, and abdominal cramps. Incubation period is 1–2 weeks. Duration of illness is 3–10 weeks. Mortality very low. Diagnosis by stool exam, stool antigen detection, stool culture, or serum serology. Treatment is with metronidazole.
- Entamoeba histolytica: Presents most commonly with the gradual onset of bloody diarrhea, abdominal pain. If amebic liver abscess formation, presents with fever and right upper quadrant pain. Incubation period 2–4 weeks, but wide spectrum from days to years. Duration of illness is weeks. Mortality rate variable, high with necrotizing colitis or amebic liver abscess.
- Ricin toxin (castor beans) Presents with fever, dyspnea, vomiting, diarrhea, shock. Incubation period 4 hours to 1 day. Duration of illness days, death in 10–12 days. High mortality. Serologic diagnosis, specialized lab. Treatment supportive.
- Epsilon toxin (Clostridium perfringens) Presents with diarrhea, cramps, nausea. Incubation period hours. Duration of illness one day. Very low mortality. Diagnosis ELISA testing of stool. Treatment supportive.
- Staphylococcus enterotoxin B presents with fever, headache, vomiting, diarrhea, myalgias, cough. Incubation period 3–12 hours after inhalation or ingestion. Duration of illness 1–3 days. Mortality very low. Urine antigen diagnosis. Supportive treatment .

Category-C biologic agents

- Nipah virus: Presents with encephalitis. Aerosol or contact transmission. Incubation period: 1–2 weeks. Illness duration: 2–4 weeks. Mortality common. Serologic identification in blood or CSF (level-4 lab). Treatment supportive, ribavirin may help.
- Hantavirus presents with fever, myalgias, dyspnea. Incubation <1 week. Illness duration days to weeks. Mortality high. Identification by serology or PCR. Supportive care.
- Tick-borne hemorrhagic fever (Crimean-Congo Hemorrhagic Fever[CCHF]): Presents with headache, fever, back pain, arthralgias, nausea, and vomiting. Conjunctivitis, pharyngitis, and palatal petichiae are common. Jaundice, neurologic changes, and bleeding diatheses sometimes follow. The incubation period is 1–3 days. Illness duration is 1–3 weeks. Supportive treatment. Mortality is high. There is no vaccine available.
- Tick-borne encephalitis: Presents with fever and headache, infrequently progresses to encephalitis. Incubation: 1–4 weeks. Duration of illness: weeks. Overall mortality low. 20 percent with encephalitis die. Serologic identification. Supportive treatment. No vaccine available in the United States.
- Yellow fever (Flavivirus). Presents with fever, headache, myalgias, jaundice. Incubation 3–6 days. Illness duration weeks. Mortality is common. Serologic identification, rarely isolated from blood. Supportive treatment. Effective attenuated vaccine available.
- Chikungunya fever (Flavivirus). Presents with chills, fever, nausea, vomiting, headache, severe joint pain, and sometimes rash. Incubation period 2–5 days. Fever lasts days but severe joint pain may last months. Mortality low. Serologic or RT-PCR identification. Treatment is supportive. No vaccine available.
- Multidrug resistant TB Presents with fever, cough. Respiratory transmission. Incubation and disease duration weeks to years. Both treated and untreated mortality common. Sputum acid-fast bacillus (AFB) identification. Treatment and prophylaxis with combination drug therapy. Bacillus of Calmette and Guérin (BCG) vaccine available, low effectiveness.

Suggested readings

Moran GJ (2002, May). Threats in bioterrorism. II: CDC category B and C agents. *Emerg Med Clin North Am* 20(2): 311–330.

Pappas G, Panagopoulou P, Christou L, Akritidis N (2006, June). Category B potential bioterrorism agents: Bacteria, viruses, toxins, and foodborne and waterborne pathogens. *Infect Dis Clin North Am* 20(2): 395–421.

Tucker, Jonathan B. (2000). *Toxic Terror: Assessing Terrorist Use of Chemical and Biological Weapons. BCSIA Studies in International Security.* Cambridge, MA: Belfer Center for Science and International Affairs. John F. Kennedy School of Government, Harvard University. Available at http://www.bt.cdc.gov/agent/agentlist-category.asp. Last accessed January, 2011.

Chemical
Disasters

Asphyxiants

Zaffer Qasim

Introduction

Asphyxiants are a group of agents characterized collectively by their ability to impair oxygen carriage and utilization at the cellular level with resultant tissue hypoxia. Common agents include carbon monoxide and hydrogen cyanide. Other potential agents the provider should be aware of include hydrogen sulfide and sodium azide.

Exposure scenarios

Cyanide is commonly utilized in numerous industrial processes. Along with carbon monoxide, exposure is likely as an inhalational agent during industrial accidents or at fire scenes. Situations in which patients experience nonspecific symptoms followed by rapid deterioration (knockdown) are highly suggestive of an exposure to asphyxiants. Rarely, asphyxiants may contaminate food and be ingested.

In the setting of terrorism, the likely asphyxiant due to its lethality and availability is cyanide. Annually, about 1.84 billion pounds of hydrogen cyanide are produced worldwide for use in a variety of industries. Cyanide, therefore, has a high potential for theft for criminal use. The 2002 robbery of 10 tons of cyanide in Mexico (ultimately recovered) raised concerns about a possible terrorist attack in the United States.

To date, no successful terrorist attack has been reported using cyanide, though use during warfare is well described.

Pathophysiology of exposure

Common properties

Asphyxiants alter hemoglobin's (Hb) ability to either carry (carbon monoxide) or utilize (cyanide) oxygen. The result is a dependence on anaerobic metabolism, which produces a profound lactic acidosis. Organ systems most dependent on aerobic metabolism (CNS, cardiovascular system) will manifest symptoms first.

Specific agents

Carbon monoxide (CO)
- Binds reversibly to Hb to form carboxyhemoglobin (COHb)
- 250x higher affinity for Hb than O_2
- Results in leftward shift of oxyhemoglobin dissociation curve.
- Also binds with high affinity to cardiac myoglobin → depressed cardiac function.

Cyanide (CN)
- Principally binds to the ferric component of cytochrome oxidase → inactivation of oxidative phosphorylation at the mitochondrial level.
- Binding is reversible.
- All tissues affected.

Hydrogen sulfide (H_2S)
- Similar to CN.
- Main mechanism is cytochrome oxidase binding and dysfunction.
- Highly lipid soluble.
- Locally irritating to exposed mucous membranes.

Sodium azide
- Irreversibly binds to cytochrome oxidase.
- Highly water soluble.

Cyanide

Exposure potential

CN is common in industry (e.g., electroplating, jewelry manufacturing). Hence, exposure is mainly from industrial fires. Gaseous exposure produces the most rapid onset of symptoms. In 2006, a Rhode Island firefighter died and several colleagues tested positive for CN poisoning after working at several civilian fire scenes in close succession.

Due to its wide availability, its potential for use in a terrorist incident is increased. In 1995, the terrorists involved in the Tokyo subway Sarin gas attack had also planned to utilize CN-releasing devices in a separate incident. In 2002 in Rome, terrorists were arrested for planning to poison the U.S. Embassy's water supply with CN.

Naturally occurring sources of CN include apricots and almonds.

Clinical presentation

The nervous and cardiorespiratory systems are primarily affected.

The classic bitter-almond smell may be reported by up to 50 percent of patients.

The clinical presentation is dependent on rate, type, dose, and route of exposure.

CNS signs and symptoms include:
- Headache.
- Dizziness.
- Confusion.
- Seizures.
- Coma.

Cardiorespiratory signs and symptoms include:
- Shortness of breath.
- ↑ respiratory rate.
- ↑ or ↓ heart rate.
- Persistent hypotension.
- Pulmonary edema.
- Apnea and cardiac arrest.

Diagnostic tests
- Pulse oximetry readings may be falsely elevated.
- Arterial blood gases show a metabolic acidosis with a reduced arterial-venous oxygen saturation difference (usually <10%).
- Serum lactate levels are markedly ↑.
- CN levels are not widely available and take time to obtain; do not wait for this when clinical suspicion is high.
- Also check the carboxyhemoglobin (concurrent CO poisoning) and methemoglobin levels.

Mortality
- Significant inhalational exposure (median lethal concentration and time [LCt50] is about 2500 mg min/m^3) causes death within minutes.
- Significant oral exposure (LD50 is about 50 mg/kg) causes death from 30 minutes to several hours.

Mass-casualty considerations

- Cardiovascular collapse at the scene carries a very poor prognosis and the expectant category should be considered.
- Not all received patients will require antidote because many fatalities will occur at the scene.
- Receiving hospitals must be able to provide mechanical ventilation and advanced circulatory support.

Treatment

- Decontamination procedure and requirement of personal protective equipment (PPE) will vary and depend on route of exposure.
- Remove the patient from the hazardous environment as soon as possible.
- Administer high-flow oxygen early with or without advanced airway maneuvers as indicated.
- Provide continuous hemodynamic monitoring during transport and in hospital.
- Provide supportive care, which may involve use of mechanical ventilation and vasopressors.
- Administer antidote early in appropriate cases.

Antidote

Cyanide Antidote Kit (CAK)—contains sodium thiosulfate, sodium nitrite, and amyl nitrite.

- The nitrites induce methemoglobinemia, which combines with CN to release cytochrome oxidase.
- Thiosulfate converts CN to thiocyanate which is renally cleared.
- Crush amyl nitrate pearls and use as an inhalant as a temporizing measure until IV access is established.
- Use sodium nitrite (3% solution, 10 mL over 5 minutes) in conjunction with thiosulfate (25% solution, 50 mL over 10 minutes) through separate lines.
- Precautions: avoid inducing methemoglobinemia in patients with ↑ HbCO (i.e., do not administer nitrites, though thiosulfate can be given).
- May cause profound hypotension.

Hydroxocobalamin (Cyanokit)

- Forms cyanocobalamin, which is renally excreted.
- Give 5g IV over 5 minutes.
- May be combined with sodium thiosulfate (through a separate line) for synergy of action.
- May cause transient hypertension (potentially beneficial) and discoloration of urine and skin.

Outcomes

- Untreated severe exposure is fatal.
- Rapid identification and treatment carries a good prognosis.
- Neurologic sequelae (including Parkinsonian syndromes) can occur 7–10 days after exposure.

Carbon monoxide

Exposure potential

A tasteless, colorless gas produced from incomplete combustion of organic substances. Exposure is mainly unintentional, more common in winter, and should be suspected in people living in enclosed spaces with inadequate ventilation. Sources can include:
- Fires.
- Faulty gas heaters.
- Car exhausts.
- Paint stripper.

CO is the most common fatal occupational inhalation in the United States, and may coexist with cyanide poisoning.

Clinical presentation

Early symptoms can be nonspecific:
- Headache (most common).
- Dizziness.
- Nausea.

Continued exposure leads to:
- Confusion and memory loss.
- Lethargy.
- Gait disturbance.
- Visual impairment and nystagmus.
- Incontinence.

Signs of severe toxicity include:
- Altered mental status and unconsciousness.
- Noncardiogenic pulmonary edema.
- Myocardial infarction.
- Skin pallor (rarely cherry-red skin).
- Hypotension.
- Brisk reflexes.
- Increased muscle tone.

Standard pulse oximetry is misleading and should not be relied upon. As standard oximeters only measure bound Hb (regardless of what it is bound with), readings are falsely ↑ despite the presence of significant hypoxemia.

Diagnostic tests

- Measure COHb level: may not correlate well with clinical symptoms and be misleading if patient has already received high-flow oxygen. Levels >15 percent suggest significant exposure. Levels up to 10 percent may be normal in smokers
- Specific CO-pulse oximeters are available and can rapidly identify significant exposure
- Arterial blood gas (ABG) may show a lactic acidosis. PaO_2 levels should be normal.

Treatment
- Promptly remove the patient and yourself from the source.
- Maintain a patent airway and apply high-flow O_2. Unconscious patients will require intubation.
- Continue O_2 therapy until the patient is asymptomatic and COHb levels are <10 percent (<2% if there is significant cardiorespiratory comorbidity).
  - The elimination half-life at room air is ~4 hrs; with 100 percent O_2 is ~1 hr; with O_2 at 3 atmospheres ~20 minutes.
- Provide supportive therapy to correct the metabolic acidosis.
- Monitor neurologic function closely as cerebral edema may develop.
  - Mannitol may be required.

Hyperbaric oxygen therapy
- Controversial as no determined survival advantage.
- No standard selection criteria exist; discuss individual cases with your local hyperbaric center especially in the setting of coma, pregnancy, and cardiac or neurologic complications.
- Balance the benefits of hyperbaric treatment with the time delay required in identifying a center, initiating treatment, and the complications of therapy (decompression sickness, gas embolism, barotrauma).

Outcomes
- Dependent on exposure levels and clinical presentation.
- High COHb levels are associated with a poor outcome.
- Abnormal brain imaging may predict persistence of neurologic problems.

Hydrogen sulfide

Exposure potential
- Colorless, flammable gas smelling of rotten eggs (which may not be detected by the olfactory nerve in high-concentration exposures).
- Forms through the fermentation of organic matter.
- Used in many industrial processes (especially the petroleum industry) so has a potential for terrorist use due to availability.
- Mainly an inhaled poison, though dermal exposure may occur.

Clinical presentation

Early identification is important, as high-concentration exposure can be rapidly fatal.
　　Initial symptoms may be vague and nonspecific:
- Headache.
- Cough.
- Lethargy.

Significant exposure presents with:
- Tachypnea and dyspnea.
- Hemoptysis/acute lung injury.
- Confusion and dizziness.
- Altered mental status including coma.
- Seizures.
- Cardiopulmonary arrest.

Diagnostic tests
- ABG will show a metabolic acidosis with ↑ lactate levels. As with cyanide poisoning, there may be ↓ arterial-venous oxygen saturation difference.

Mortality
- LC50 is 800 ppm after 5 minutes exposure.

Treatment
- Appropriate PPE should be used and the patient removed from the toxic environment as soon as possible.
- Maintain a patent airway.
- Provide high-flow oxygen through a tight fitting mask with reservoir or via mechanical ventilation if indicated.
- Consider hyperbaric oxygen therapy, though this has only anecdotal supportive evidence.
- Induce methemoglobinemia by giving 10 mL of 3 percent sodium nitrite solution over 5 min.
- Provide supportive therapy to correct the metabolic acidosis.
- Administer bronchodilators if necessary to counteract the respiratory irritant effect. Monitor for acute lung injury.
- Monitor for ophthalmic injury ("gas eye").
- Identify and treat any concurrent injuries the patient may have sustained.

Outcomes
- With adequate, early treatment, prognosis is good, even in high-level exposure.

Sodium azide

Exposure potential
- Colorless azide salt produces hydrazole gas, which is highly toxic.
- Found in industry primarily as a propellant in car airbags and airplane escape chutes. Other uses include explosive production and as a preservative in the biochemical industry.
- Exposure is primarily unintentional. Incidents of intentional contamination of drinks in Japan (1998) and the United States (2009), although affecting small numbers of civilians, demonstrate the potential for terrorist use on a larger scale.

Clinical presentation
Rapid onset of:
- Cough and rhinorrhea.
- Conjunctivitis.
- Tachypnea.
- Tachycardia and hypotension.
- Confusion, agitation and vertigo.

This can progress quickly to:
- Coma.
- Cardiac arrest.

Diagnostic tests
- ABG will show a metabolic acidosis with ↑ lactate levels. There may be ↓ arterial-venous oxygen saturation difference.

Treatment
- Ensure personal safety when evacuating the patient from the exposed environment.
- Be wary that exhaled breaths from the patient may contain hydrazole gas and can contaminate medical personnel.
- Maintain a patent airway.
- As with other asphyxiants, provide supportive treatment for the metabolic acidosis.
- Hypotension may be resistant to fluids and even vasopressors.
- Little evidence supports the effectiveness of the traditional antidotes used in cyanide toxicity in sodium azide poisoning, likely due to its irreversible binding to cytochrome oxidase.

Outcome
- Delayed hypotension (>1 hour after exposure) is a poor prognostic sign
- Prognostication is difficult even for low-dose exposure.

Suggested readings
Varon J, Marik PE, Fromm RE, et al. (1999). Carbon monoxide poisoning: a review for clinicians. J Emerg Med 17: 87–93.
Buckley NA, Isbister GK, Stokes B, et al. (2005). Hyperbaric oxygen for carbon monoxide poisoning: A systematic review and critical analysis of the evidence. Toxicol Rev 24:75–92
Cummings TF (2004). The treatment of cyanide poisoning. Occup Med 54: 82–85.

Chapter 62

Blistering agents

Jacob Kesterson

Background

Blistering agents, or vesicants, are chemical-warfare agents that produce significant burns and blisters upon exposure but have low overall mortality. The most well-known vesicants are sulfur mustard, lewisite, and phosgene oxime. Sulfur mustard is the prototypical agent. It was first used during World War I and is well-described in the literature. Less information is available for other vesicants. Lewisite has had very little battlefield use and phosgene oxime has had none.

Potential exposure

Although terrorist use of blistering agents is a concern, exposure is more likely to be related to accidental or occupational contact with storage containers. Exposure can occur with direct contact with the liquid or solid forms, but is more likely due to vapor.

Properties

Sulfur mustard (H)

- Oily liquid with low volatility at cool temperatures, but vaporizes readily in hotter climates.
- Lethal dose of mustard is ~7 grams (enough to cover 25 percent of total body surface area).
- All symptoms of mustard exposure present in a delayed fashion.

Lewisite (L)

- Oily, colorless liquid.
- Characteristic odor of geraniums.
- More volatile and persistent at cooler temperatures than sulfur mustard.
- Lethal dose is 2 grams.
- Unlike mustard, symptoms occur within minutes of exposure.

Phosgene oxime (CX)

- Yellowish-brown liquid.
- Not a true vesicant because it does not produce vesicles. Better described as an urticant or nettle agent.
- Able to penetrate garments and rubber.
- Produces symptoms immediately.

Signs and symptoms

- Ocular and cutaneous symptoms are the most common followed closely by respiratory symptoms.
- Other systems may occasionally be affected, especially at high doses.
  - Cutaneous symptoms occur following vapor exposure.

Cutaneous symptoms

Sulfur Mustard

- Erythema begins 4–8 hours after exposure, followed by vesicles in 12–18 hours.
- Warm, moist areas such as the perineum and axilla are more vulnerable.
- Vesicles coalesce into blisters over days.
- Lesions are superficial, translucent, and 0.5 to 5 cm.

Lewisite exposures

- Cause immediate pain and central blistering.

Phosgene exposure

- Causes immediate pain followed by erythema and urticaria that later progress to a dark eschar.

Ocular exposure

- Leads to tearing, conjunctivitis, eyelid edema, and blepharospasm.
- Corneal edema and sloughing can occur hours later with large exposures.
- Injuries from lewisite are less severe because of severe blepharospasm which prevents further exposure.

Inhalation symptoms

- Leads to respiratory symptoms such as sore throat, hoarseness, cough, bronchospasm, dyspnea, and hemorrhagic bronchitis.
- Pulmonary edema may occur after lewisite or phosgene oxime.

Ingestion symptoms

- May cause vomiting but is not usually a prominent symptom.

Systemic effects

- Leukopenia and pancytopenia may occur days after sulfur mustard exposure.
- Lewisite can cause capillary leak with shock.

Differential diagnosis

- Thermal burns.
- Other chemical burns.
- Pemphigus or pemphigoid.
- Stevens-Johnson syndrome and toxic epidermal necrolysis (TEN).
- Staphylococcal scalded skin syndrome.
- Mycotoxin exposure.

Diagnosis

- Characteristic skin findings associated with ocular and respiratory symptoms are the most reliable method of diagnosis.
- Large numbers of casualties from a common exposure could suggest vesicant exposure.
- Differentiating between sulfur mustard and lewisite injuries is based on the time from the exposure until symptoms occur.
- There is no practical laboratory test to establish the diagnosis of vesicant exposure. Leucopenia may be seen days after sulfur mustard exposure.
- Mustard and lewisite can be detected in tissues or urine, but only at specific CDC laboratories.
- Urinary arsenic excretion may be helpful in identifying lewisite exposure.

Treatment

- Decontamination reduces continued exposure and protects health-care workers. It should be done within 1–2 minutes.
- Decontamination may not be helpful if delayed because of rapid absorption or evaporation. It can be done with dry powder, soap and water, or resin decontaminants.
- No specific antidotes exist for sulfur mustard or phosgene oxime exposure.
- Povidone iodine ointment may help protect the skin if applied within 20 minutes of sulfur mustard exposure.
- British Anti-Lewisite (BAL, dimercaprol) binds arsenic and may decrease symptoms of lewisite exposure.
  - Administered intramuscularly and should be given within 15 minutes of exposure.
- Supportive care is the mainstay of treatment.
  - Burns should be managed with analgesia, infection control, and fluid replacement.
  - Eyes should be irrigated thoroughly, followed by antibiotics and steroids.
  - Bronchodilators and humidified air may help bronchospasm and wheezing.
  - Patients with ocular or airway symptoms and those with moderate to severe skin exposure should be hospitalized.

Outcomes

- Mortality is low (~2%) and usually delayed (>4 days).
- Most deaths are due to respiratory insufficiency or infection/sepsis.
- Most burns resolve completely by 2–10 weeks.
- Mustard burns heal more slowly than similar thermal burns. Prolonged hospitalization may be required.
- Ocular symptoms usually resolve in 1–2 weeks.
- Visual defects and cutaneous scarring may rarely be persistent and significant.
- There is a slight increase in certain cancers after sulfur mustard exposure.
- There are no human data on long-term effects of lewisite or phosgene oxime exposures.

Suggested readings

Sidell FR, Urbanetti JS, Smith WJ, et al. (1997). Vesicants. In: Zajtchuk R, Bellamy RF, eds. *Textbook of Military Medicine. Part I: Medical Aspects of Chemical and Biological Warfare*, pp. 197–228., Falls Church, VA: Office of the Surgeon General, Dept of the Army.

McManus J, Huebner K (2005). Vesicants. *Crit Care Clin* 21, 707–718.

Organophosphates/ nerve gases

Payal Sud

David C. Lee

Introduction

Organophosphates (OPs) are phosphoric acid esters used as pesticides. These compounds have four oxygen atoms surrounding a central phosphorus atom. Since they directly affect the CNS, they are often described as "nerve gases."

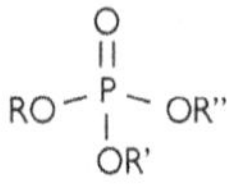

$$RO-\overset{\overset{\displaystyle O}{\|}}{\underset{\underset{\displaystyle OR'}{|}}{P}}-OR''$$

Figure 63.1 Organophosphate molecule.

History

Organophosphates (Ops) were initially developed as insecticides but were found to be too harmful to humans. They have been weaponized and multiple nations stockpile these chemicals for military use. In the 1990s, a particular organophosphate, Sarin, was used in terrorist attacks on civilian populations in Japan.

Mechanism of action

- Acetylcholine (ACh) binds to nicotinic and muscarinic receptors at sympathetic neurons, parasympathetic neurons and at the neuromuscular junction.
- Acetylcholinesterase (AChE) hydrolyzes ACh into inert acetic acid and choline.
- OPs bind to and inhibit the action of AChE and this causes inhibition of breakdown of acetylcholine at muscarinic and nicotinic receptors by AChE. Thus, OP poisoning leads to cholinergic excess.
- Certain OPs bind to AChE irreversibly in a process called aging. If this occurs, de novo synthesis of AChE is required to replenish stores and restore function.

Signs and symptoms

- Cholinergic excess often presents in a typical syndrome. However, the specific type of OP, lipid solubility, route of exposure, and dose of the compound all determine the signs and symptoms encountered. A mnemonic for cholinergic excess is DUMMBBBELSS:
- D—Diarrhea
- U—Urination
- M—Miosis
- M—Muscle cramps
- B—Bradycardia
- B—Bronchorrhea
- B—Bronchoconstriction
- E—Emesis
- L—Lacrimation
- S—Salivation
- S—Sweating
- Of all the effects of cholinergic excess, the most important are the "killer B's"—Bradycardia, Bronchorrhea and Bronchoconstriction.
- Sudden death can occur with CNS toxicity presenting with agitation, coma, and seizures.

Management

Decontamination

- Personal protective equipment (PPE): Nitrile, neoprene or butyl rubber gloves are recommended because several OPs can penetrate latex and vinyl gloves. Leather agents should be discarded well because they absorb OPs. Hair may need to be cut because shampooing may not remove all OPs.
- Activated charcoal (AC) can adsorb some OPs and, therefore, a single dose of 1 g/kg of AC is recommended for ingested exposures.
- Antidotes:

Atropine

- Atropine is a competitive inhibitor of ACh at muscarinic receptors. The goal of atropinization is a reduction of pulmonary secretions and improvement of respiratory status.
- Atropine should not be discontinued solely due to tachycardia. Tachycardia may be a result of hypoxia due to bronchorrhea and may be improve with continued atropine dosing.
- The starting dose of atropine is 0.5–1 mg in adults and 0.02 mg/kg in children (minimum dose of 0.1 mg) and each subsequent dose must be doubled every 2–3 minutes. The minimum dose (0.5 mg in adults and 0.1 mg in children) is necessary to avoid paradoxical bradycardia. Massive doses of atropine are typically required to achieve drying of secretions.

Pralidoxime (2-PAM, Protopam)

- Pralidoxime binds to OP-bound AChE and causes dissociation of the OP-pralidoxime portion of the complex, regenerating active AChE.
- Pralidoxime also binds to OPs that have not yet bound to AChE and prevents the OP from binding AChE.
- Pralidoxime may be ineffective if OP-AChE complexes have aged. Various OPs age at different rates. Pralidoxime therapy may be started even if the patient presents late.
- Pralidoxime and atropine have different mechanisms of action and act synergistically.
- The adult loading dose of pralidoxime is 1–2 grams in 100 mL of normal saline over 15–30 minutes. Subsequently, either this dose can be repeated every 6–12 hours or a drip started at 500 mg/hour. The pediatric loading dose is 25 mg/kg (maximum dose of 1 g/dose) and then repeated every 6–12 hours. Another option is a loading dose of 20–40 mg/kg over 30–60 minutes and then a drip at 20 mg/kg/hour.

Benzodiazepines

- Benzodiazepines can be used in severe cases to attenuate CNS stimulation and to control seizures.

Delayed toxicity

Intermediate syndrome (IMS)

- This occurs 24–96 hours after exposure and presents with muscle weakness without fasiculations and the typical cholinergic toxidrome. Other symptoms of IMS include cranial nerve palsies, areflexia, respiratory depression, and preserved sensation and sensorium. This syndrome starts after the initial cholinergic signs and symptoms have resolved with atropine and pralidoxime therapy.
- Diagnosis of IMS is primarily clinical, although EMGs can be used to show attenuation in response after repeated stimulation.
- Treatment is supportive and requires close attention to managing the airway. Pralidoxime can be used.

Suggested readings

Flomenbaum N, Goldfrank L, et al.(eds.). (2006). Pesticides in *Goldfrank's Toxicologic Emergencies*, 8th edition. New York: McGraw-Hill.

Okumura T, Suzuki K, Fukuda A, et al. (1998). The Tokyo subway sarin attack: Disaster management, part 1: Community emergency response. *Acad Emerg Med* 5:613–617.

Okumura T, Suzuki K, Fukuda A, et al. (1998). The Tokyo subway sarin attack: Disaster management, part 2: Hospital response. *Acad Emerg Med* 5:618–624.

Chapter 64

Cyanide and other chemical agents

Kavita Babu

Jason Hack

Background

Cyanide

The use of cyanide as an agent of chemical warfare dates to the Franco-Prussian war. Cyanide gas was used in trench warfare during World War I, and employed in the mass murder of concentration camp victims during World War II under the name Zyklon B. Potassium cyanide was used in the mass suicide at Jonestown in 1978, while cyanide-tainted acetaminophen led to a massive investigation and widespread panic in 1982. Cyanide gas was also reportedly deployed against the Kurds during the Iran-Iraq war in the early 1980s. However, the vast majority of today's cyanide exposures result from inadvertent occupational exposures, or smoke inhalation during house fires.

Opioid agents

High-potency opioid gases are considered potential incapacitating agents in modern chemical warfare. In 2002, more than 800 Russian theatergoers were taken hostage by Chechen rebels. During the attempted rescue of hostages, a chemical agent was employed that subsequently resulted in the death of more than 100 people. In the days following this tragedy, the Russian Ministry described the use of a fentanyl derivative during the rescue attempt.

Sedative and incapacitating agents

There are many different types of gases that may be classified as sedating or incapacitating agents, including 3-quinuclidyl benzilate (QNB), Agent 15, LSD, benzodiazepine gases, and inhalational anesthetics. Whereas most of these gases would be required in prohibitively high concentrations for a large-scale attack, the use of the QNB is suspected to have been used in both Mozambique and Bosnia.

Hemolytic agents

Arsine and stibine represent two important chemical threats. These gaseous forms of arsenic and antimony, respectively, are highly toxic. Although these gases cause similar effects (massive hemolysis with resulting anemia and organ dysfunction), arsine toxicity occurs more often. Mass poisoning with these agents could result in a crippling shortage of blood products.

Properties

Cyanide
- Includes hydrogen cyanide (AC) and cyanogen chloride (CK).
- Exposures may occur via inhalation or dermal absorption of liquid.
- Poisons electron transport chain and uncouples oxidative phosphorylation.
- In high concentrations, may cause death within minutes.
- 50 percent of population can detect scent of "bitter almonds."

Opioid gases
- Include agents like carfentanil, sufentanil, alfentanil, and remifentanil.
- Carfentanil 10,000 times more potent than morphine.
- Acts at opioid receptor.s
- Onset of symptoms within minutes of exposure.

Sedative (incapacitating) gases
- QNB competitively inhibits muscarinic receptors, resulting in typical anticholinergic symptoms.
- QNB onset within hours, but symptoms may persist for days.
- LSD produces hallucinations by acting a 5-HT$_{2A}$ receptors.
- Benzodiazepines produce sedation via agonism at GABA receptors.

Hemolytic gases
- Arsine and stibine toxic in low concentrations.
- Arsine associated with characteristic garlic-like odor.
- Produce oxidant stress and red-cell lysis.
- Onset of symptoms may be delayed by hours.

Signs and symptoms

Cyanide
- In low concentrations, may cause vertigo, dyspnea, and headaches.
- Progression to seizures, coma, dysrhythmias, hypotension, and severe acidosis.
- Cyanogen chloride also produces mucous membrane irritant effects.

Opioid gases
- Classic triad of central nervous system depression, miosis, and respiratory depression.
- Pupils may be midsized to dilated if other exposures or severe hypoxia.
- Hypoxia may precipitate dysrhythmias.

Sedative (incapacitating) gases
- QNB may cause dramatic and persistent hallucinations.
- Associated findings include picking at clothing, muttering delirium, mydriasis, tachycardia, and hypertension.
- Characteristics of LSD exposure include vivid hallucinations, synesthesias (confusion of the senses), tachycardia, and hypertension.
- Benzodiazepine exposure results in sedation and possible respiratory compromise.

Hemolytic gases
- Severity of symptoms dependent on time and intensity of exposure
- Early symptoms (within hours of exposure) include headache, nausea, fatigue, and weakness.
- Massive intravascular hemolysis produces dark urine.
- Late symptoms (within days of exposure) include oliguria and renal failure.

Differential diagnosis

Cyanide
- Sodium azide.
- Carbon monoxide.
- Carbon dioxide.
- Aluminum and zinc phosphide.
- Phosphine.
- Simple asphyxiants.
- Rotenone.
- Malonate.

Opioid agents
- Clonidine.
- Phenothiazines.
- Anoxic brain injury from simple asphyxiants.
- Nerve agents (produce coma, miosis, and bradycardia).

Sedative and incapacitating agents
- Opioid gases.
- Heat stroke.
- Carbon monoxide.
- Carbon dioxide.
- Simple asphyxiants.

Hemolytic agents
- Nitrites and nitrates.
- Cyanide.
- Pyrogallic acid.
- Phenol.
- Phosphine.

Diagnosis

Cyanide
- Clinical finding most suggestive of cyanide intoxication includes unconsciousness or severe air hunger despite normal O_2 saturation.
- Laboratory findings suggestive of cyanide toxicity include anion gap metabolic acidosis and increased serum lactate.
- Elevated venous oxygen secondary to decreased oxygen extraction ("arterialization").
- Whole blood or serum cyanide levels aid detection, but not routinely available; both may be elevated in smokers.
- Semiquantitative cyanide detection kits commercially available to assess presence of cyanide.

Opioid agents
- Can be suspected if large number of patients with typical findings of miosis, coma, and respiratory depression.
- Traditional urine drug screening for opioids will NOT detect fentanyl and derivatives.

Sedative and incapacitating agents
- No routine tests available to detect QNB, Agent 15, LSD, benzodiazepine gases, or halothane.

Hemolytic agents
- Findings suggestive of hemolysis include anemia, elevated lactate dehydrogenase (LDH, marker of red cell turnover), elevated total and indirect bilirubin, elevated blood urea nitrogen (BUN) and creatinine.
- Spot urine and blood arsenic levels commercially available.

Treatment

- The most important priority in approaching patients exposed to these gases is protection of rescuers. All prehospital providers must be vigilant about personal protective equipment to prevent becoming symptomatic themselves.

Cyanide

- Treatment is indicated for any patient with coma, acidosis, hypotension, air hunger, or serum lactic acid > 8 mmol/L.
- Two treatment options available: cyanide antidote kit and hydroxocobalamin (see Table 64.1 for dosing and adverse effects associated with treatment).
- In suspected cyanide toxicity, patients must be treated before confirmatory testing is received; delay in treatment can result in death.

Opioid agents

- Naloxone or airway management and ventilation
- are indicated for hypoxia, bradypnea, or apnea.
- Naloxone may also be considered for reversal of central nervous system depression.
- Naloxone can be delivered intramuscularly, intravenously, or via nebulizer (if patient breathing).
- Initial dose of 2 mg, followed by repeated 2 mg doses until response. High potency opioids may require large doses.
- Naloxone's onset of action is rapid (seconds to minutes); duration of action is 30 to 60 minutes, depending upon administration route.

Table 64.1 Cyanide Antidotes, Dosing and Adverse Effects

		Adult Dose	Pediatric Dose	Adverse Effects
Cyanide Antidote Kit				
	Amyl Nitrite	One perle held near patient's mouth for 30 seconds	Same	Hypotension
	Sodium Nitrite	300 mg iv over 3–5 mins	10 mg/kg iv over 3–5mins	Hypotension
	Sodium Thiosulfate	12.5 grams	400 mg/kg	Hypotension
Hydroxo-cobalamin		5 grams iv over 15 minutes; a second dose may be required	Not defined; 70 mg/kg used previously	Rash, reddish discoloration of skin, interference with laboratory assays

Sedative and incapacitating agents

- Supportive care indicated for incapacitating gases.
- May require emergency airway management and ventilation.
- Can use benzodiazepines for sedation of agitated or hallucinating patients.
- Avoid antipsychotics, such as haloperidol, in cases of suspected QNB-induced hallucinosis and agitation, because they may worsen symptoms.

Hemolytic agents

- Transfusion may be required to support patients with anemia.
- If available, exchange transfusion with plasma exchange associated with best outcomes.
- Urinary alkalinization, mannitol, and diuretics of unproven benefit in improving oliguric renal failure.
- Hemodialysis may be required for patients with acute renal failure.

Outcomes

Cyanide

- Asymptomatic patients may be discharged after six hours of observation
- All symptomatic patients should be treated in an intensive care unit setting.

Opioid agents

- Observe all patients who receive naloxone for a minimum of six hours for recurrence of symptoms.

Sedative and incapacitating agents

- Observe until resolution of symptoms.
- QNB-induced symptoms may persist for days.

Hemolytic agents

- Observe all patients with history of arsine or stibine exposure for 24 hours for delayed onset of hemolysis.
- Observe all patients with hemolysis for 72 hours for development of renal failure.

Suggested readings

Wax PM, Becker CE, Curry SC. (2003). Unexpected "gas" casualties in Moscow: A medical toxicology perspective. *Ann Emerg Med.* May *41*(5):700–705.

Mather LE, Woodhouse A, Ward ME, et al. (1998, Jul). Pulmonary administration of aerosolised fentanyl: pharmacokinetic analysis of systemic delivery. *Br J Clin Pharmacol.* 46(1):37–43.

Wilkinson SP, McHugh P, Horsley S, Tubbs H, Lewis M, Thould A, et al.(1975, Sep 6). Arsine toxicity aboard the Asiafreighter. *Br Med J.* 3(5983):559–563.

Hay A. (1998, Apr–Jun). Surviving the impossible: The long march from Srebrenica. An investigation of the possible use of chemical warfare agents. *Med Confl Surviv.* 14(2):120–155.

Holstege CP, Bechtel LK, Reilly TH, Wispelwey BP, Dobmeier SG.(2007, May). Unusual but potential agents of terrorists. *Emerg Med Clin North Am.* 25(2):549–566; abstract xi.

Chapter 65

Pulmonary agents

Bryan Fisk

Background

Pulmonary agents (also known as choking agents, lung-damaging agents, and toxic inhalants) refer to those chemicals that result in injury primarily via their effects on the lungs.

- Pulmonary agents were first used on the battlefield in large scale during WWI.
- On April 22, 1917, the Germans released chlorine gas from thousands of nonexplosive cylinders at Ypres, Belgium. The gas cloud blew over British soldiers and created numerous casualties.
- Shortly afterwards, the Allies deployed primitive emergency protective masks and launched their own chlorine attack against the Germans at Loos.
- Phosgene, the other historically important pulmonary agent in offensive use, was first used by Germany at Verdun in 1917, also with later use by both sides.
- Although there have been instances of use of other types of chemical warfare agents by militaries since WWI, there is little documentation of the further use of pulmonary agents.
- Episodes of chemical warfare since WWI typically involved the use of vesicants or nerve agents.
- There is increasing acceptance by terrorist groups throughout the world for utilizing chemical agents.
- In 2007, Al Qaeda terrorists began using chlorine gas attacks in Iraq.
  - Attacks were carried out by combining chlorine gas cylinders with vehicle-borne improvised explosive devices, or truck bombs.
  - The choice of chlorine by the terrorists was most likely due to its availability as an industrial chemical.
  - Thought the lethality of the attacks were not high, they met goals of producing a psychological impact of terror and increasing the strain on the medical infrastructure to respond to the much higher numbers of injured and panic-stricken.
- A terrorist group will often use chemical agents as a means of instilling widespread fear, garnering publicity for their cause, creating a negative economic impact by halting activity in a city, and paralyzing medical systems.
- Despite the real concern for the nefarious use of pulmonary agents on the populace, the average health-care provider is much more likely to encounter casualties of these agents after an accidental exposure.
- Chlorine and phosgene, their chemical derivatives, and numerous other pulmonary toxicants (i.e., hydrochloric acid, sulfur dioxide, diphosgene, etc.), are widely used for industrial purposes and exposure can occur after an industrial accident.
- Exposure to these other chemicals can present similar to chlorine and phosgene exposures.
- Accidental exposure may also occur in and around the home.
- Common sources in this setting are household bleach and chlorine tablets used to clean swimming pools.

- Since pulmonary agents as a group have similar clinical presentations and similar requirements for supportive care, this discussion will focus on chlorine and phosgene as representative agents. See Box 65.1. Phosgene is also discussed as a vesicant in Chapter 62.

Overview

- Pulmonary agents tend to be volatile substances and are encountered as either vapors or gases.
- Volatility refers to a substance's tendency to evaporate or vaporize at a relatively low temperature and is a major factor in the degree of persistence of a chemical agent.
- Vapor is the gaseous form of a substance that occurs at a temperature below its boiling point.
- Because vapors and gases are easily dispersed, they are also more difficult to deploy offensively in an effective fashion due to their lack of persistence.
- This factor is a major reason they have not been a choice for military operations since WWI.
- Doses of exposure to pulmonary agents are expressed as the concentration-time product (Ct).
- Ct is calculated by the concentration of an agent (mg/m^3) multiplied by the duration of exposure (minutes).
- *Haber's rule* refers to the understanding that similar biological effects can be expected to result from exposures to the same agent with varying concentrations and times as long as the Ct is similar.
  - This rule does not hold true for all agents and is valid only over a finite range of concentrations and times for a given agent.
  - Haber's rule does not take into account minute ventilation (respiratory rate x tidal volume) of an exposed individual.
  - The inhalational exposure for an individual who is exerting himself and breathing heavily will be much greater at the same Ct then someone who is not.

Box 65.1 Specific characteristics of chlorine vs phosgene

CHLORINE
- Yellow-green gas at standard temperatures and air pressures.
- Denser than air, accumulates in low lying areas.
- Pungent odor detectable below toxic threshold (Parrish).
- Water soluble, cause injury from upper to lower respiratory tract.
- Damage mediated by hydrochloric acid, hypochlorous acid, oxygen free radicals.

PHOSGENE
- Colorless gas at standard temperatures and air pressures.
- Denser than air, accumulates in low lying areas.
- Odor of sweet, newly mown hay, not reliable for detection below toxic threshold.
- Less water soluble, tends to spare upper respiratory mucosa.
- Damage due to both acylation of proteins and lipoids and formation of hydrochloric acid.

Clinical effects

The various classes of chemical warfare agents are categorized by their predominant physiologic effects. As such, pulmonary agents (classically known as choking agents) have their greatest clinical effect on lung function.

- Inhalation of pulmonary agents can result in injury anywhere along the respiratory tract.

Biochemical effects

- Pulmonary agents take place at exposure but the clinical symptoms may be delayed for hours and progress over time.
- Damage with chlorine inhalation is related to hydrolysis and the formation of hydrochloric and hypochlorous acids.
- Phosgene also reacts with water to form hydrochloric acid.
  - Phosgene is less water soluble.
  - Reaction more often occurs at the terminal bronchioles and alveoli where the movement of molecules is slower and allows for greater contact time.
  - Another mechanism of injury is acylation and subsequent denaturation of cellular proteins and lipoids.
- Both agents cause a chemically induced injury to bronchioles and alveoli leading to the loss of tight junctions at the cellular level.
  - There is increased permeability at the alveolar-capillary membrane.
  - Permeability is exacerbated by release of inflammatory cytokines from immune cells responding to the initial injury.
  - There is formation of edema and cellular exudates that flood the alveoli.
  - This permeability-type pulmonary edema is known as *acute lung injury* or *acute respiratory distress syndrome* depending on the severity hypoxemia.
- Because of the water solubility of chlorine, these reactions can readily occur on moist mucosal membranes from the nostrils to the alveoli with subsequent epithelial damage.

Symptoms

- Because of chlorine's water solubility, it will cause immediate irritation of the proximal airway mucosa including.
  - Lacrimation,
  - Nasal and ocular irritation.
  - Burning sensation of mucus membranes.
- Phosgene will often spare the proximal airway mucosa at lower concentrations due to its lower solubility.
- Higher levels of exposure of either can result in early hoarseness and inspiratory stridor that may signal impending loss of an airway.
- Progressive symptoms of the lower airways with either agent include:
  - Chest tightness.
  - Progressive dyspnea.
  - Cough.
  - Hemoptysis.

Physical findings
- Findings on physical exam may include:
  - Tachypnea.
  - Hypoxia evident by cyanosis and/or pulse oximetry.
  - Wheezing and crackles.
- Lower-respiratory symptoms and findings are usually delayed and may develop anywhere from 30 minutes to 48 hours afterwards, depending on severity of exposure.
- Even after a potentially lethal exposure to a pulmonary agent, clinical evidence of physiologic damage may be delayed for 4–6 hours.
- Observation and reassessment for at least 4–6 hours before discharge of an asymptomatic patient is required.
- Normal arterial-blood-gas values at 4–6 hours and a clear chest x-ray at 8 hours are strong indicators that the patient is highly unlikely to have had a lethal exposure.
- The latency period to onset of overt clinical signs and symptoms is correlated with prognosis, with worse prognosis in early onset.

Chest radiograph findings
- Early after exposure, the chest radiograph may appear normal.
- Pulmonary edema is progressive and radiographic evidence may lag behind respiratory symptoms.
- As clinical symptoms progress, the radiographic appearance may change to include:
  - Diffuse nodular opacities.
  - Patchy consolidation.
  - Diffuse bilateral fluffy infiltrates.
- There may also be signs of air trapping in the presence of persistent airway hyperreactivity and obstruction.
- In the absence of concomitant cardiac pathology or volume overload, there should not be evidence of vascular congestion.
- Radiographic changes will usually improve over 3 to 5 days unless pneumonia develops.

Treatment

Initial response

- The fact that an emergent incident involved the intentional or accidental release of toxic chemicals may not be immediately known.
- It is important to be aware of possible indicators of chemical weapons usage so that responders can take appropriate precautions.
- Indicators of a potential chemical weapons incident are listed in Box 65.2.
- Before entering a potentially hazardous site, responders must put on appropriate personal protective equipment (PPE) (see Table 65.1). PPE is also discussed in Chapter 35.
- The first step in patient care is to remove the casualties from the toxic environment.
- Most, if not all, ambulatory casualties would have likely self-evacuated the scene by this time, and remaining casualties will be either nonambulatory or trapped in some fashion.
- For those who are freed from trapping and subsequently ambulatory, it is medically preferred to have the casualty of a pulmonary agent exposure carried from the scene if feasible.
  - This is due to findings from WWI, when it was noted that physical exertion lead to exacerbation and increased severity of respiratory symptoms after a gas exposure.
  - The feasibility of this approach will depend on the number of casualties, the number of rescuers, and other physical factors that would lead to significantly greater time in the hot zone.
  - An air-purifying respirator (gas mask) or supplemental oxygen via a tight-fitting face mask should be applied to the casualty during evacuation, if available.

Triage and decontamination

- After evacuation from the hot zone, a quick triage of casualties should be performed.
- At this time, any immediately life-threatening issues with airway, breathing, or circulation should be dealt with.

Box 65.2 Indicators of a Potential Chemical Weapons Incident (U.S. Army SBCCOM).

- Explosion with little or no structural damage
- Reports of a device that dispersed a mist or vapor
- Multiple casualties exhibiting similar symptoms
- Mass casualties with no apparent reason or trauma
- Reports of unusual odors, liquids, spray devices, or cylinders
- Dead animals
- Discarded personal protective equipment (PPE)

Table 65.1 Environmental Protection Agency (EPA) Levels of Chemical PPE.

Level	Protection Afforded	Situation For Use	Components
Level A	Vapor, gas, solids, and liquid protection	Required for entry into areas of high contamination with significant risk of inhalation, skin, mucous membrane, and/or eye exposure	Fully encapsulated suit with pressure-demand, full-face SCBA, inner chemical-resistant gloves, and chemical-resistant safety boots
Level B	Liquid splash protection, with same respiratory protection as Level A but suit without vapor protection	When the threat has been identified and is associated with liquid and not vapor contact	Suit, pressure demand, full facepiece SCBA, inner chemical-resistant gloves, chemical-resistant safety boots, and hard hat
Level C	Same level of skin protection as Level B, but a lower level of respiratory protection	Appropriate for use when the hazard is identified and known to be in effective range of filters	Full facepiece, air purifying, canister-equipped respirator, chemical-resistant gloves and safety boots
Level D	No respiratory protection, and minimal skin protection	When the atmosphere contains no known hazards	Coveralls, safety boots/shoes, safety glasses or chemical splash goggles

- If none are present or once they have been addressed, decontamination of the casualty should proceed immediately to minimize further injury.
- The initial step in decontamination is the removal of clothing, which will eliminate any trapped gas or vapor.
- Contact lenses should be removed.
- For a pure-gas or vapor exposure, this may be sufficient for decontamination.
- In general, it is safest to perform skin decontamination if possible.
- This is performed with copious soap and water, with particular attention to areas of skin folds.
- Triage should be repeated after decontamination and patients evacuated to an appropriate medical treatment facility based on priority.

Definitive treatment
- There are no specific antidotes available for the medical treatment of casualties after an exposure to a pulmonary agent.
- Medical treatment is focused on limiting the degree of damage to the respiratory system and on supportive care.
- Continuation of bed rest must be enforced for patients with moderate or greater exposure due to the risk of exacerbation of respiratory failure with exertion.

Primary survey
- Airway:
  - The patency of an airway could be endangered by the presence of copious secretions that the patient is unable to clear.
  - Be aware of impending laryngospasm heralded by hoarseness or stridor.
  - Agents that affect the proximal airway, like chlorine, can result in upper airway edema that threatens airway patency.
  - The development of respiratory failure from acute lung injury is progressive with time.
  - Sudden death soon after intense exposures can result from laryngospasm or upper airway obstruction.
  - The patient should be intubated immediately if there is any doubt regarding maintenance of airway patency.
- Breathing
  - Assessment of breathing includes noting the presence of bronchospasm, hypoxia, or an elevated work of breathing.
  - Patients with wheezing on exam or an elevated pCO_2 on arterial blood gas evaluation should be treated with bronchodilators.
  - Consider the addition of intravenous corticosteroid therapy if the bronchospasm is severe (i.e., methylprednisolone in doses similar to an asthma exacerbation).
  - Supplemental oxygen should be supplied to all patients, with the severity of hypoxemia dictating the mode of delivery.
  - O_2 via nasal cannula may be sufficient for mild decreases in oxygen saturation that are readily reversed.
  - Significant O_2 desaturations indicate severe exposure that will worsen over time requiring early intubation.
  - Patients presenting with increased work of breathing not readily responsive to bronchodilator therapy, or those who demonstrate evidence of fatigue require early intubation.
  - Given the nature of the lung injury, a low-tidal-volume strategy should be selected in accordance with the findings of the ARDSNET trial.
  - The preferred mode of mechanical ventilation is volume-assist-control a targeted tidal volume of 6 ml/kg (predicted body weight).
  - The setting of the positive end expiratory pressure (PEEP) is set in relation to the FiO_2 (a higher FiO_2 requirement results in setting a higher PEEP).
  - Maintain plateau pressures below 30 cm of water to limit the risk of barotrauma.

- Potential salvage modes of ventilation include high frequency oscillatory ventilation (HFOV) and airway pressure release ventilation (APRV).
- Close attention must be paid to detect evidence of barotrauma as soon as possible given the need for high airway pressures in severe exposures.
- Additional salvage therapies for refractory hypoxemia include the addition of inhaled nitric oxide and prone positioning.
- Circulation
  - Exposure to a pulmonary agent will not generally cause vascular collapse evident at presentation.
  - If exposure was explosive in nature, sources of hypotension should be elucidated according to trauma protocols.
  - The presence of respiratory failure may lead to a hypoperfusing dysrhythmia or cardiac arrest.
  - The patient with moderate to severe exposure is at risk for the development of hypotension over the ensuing hours.
  - As the lung injury progresses and vascular permeability increases, fluid will shift from the intravascular space to the pulmonary interstitium and alveoli.
  - The intravascular depletion may result in a hypoperfused state.
  - Fluid replacement goal is to provide adequate replacement without excessive fluid, which will worsen pulmonary edema.
  - In a patient with normal renal function, this is best achieved by following urine output with the goal of achieving a rate of 0.5 ml/kg/hr.
  - Following the central venous pressure (CVP) can provide additional data to assist in resuscitation.
  - Mechanically ventilated patients CVP goal will be 3 to 4 mm Hg higher than in a patient who is not mechanically ventilated.
  - In the patient with acute or chronic kidney disease, the CVP or pulmonary artery occlusion pressure may be needed to guide fluid replacement.

Other therapies

Diuretics
- The use of diuretics may decrease the degree of pulmonary edema and improve lung function in patients with acute lung injury.
- Their use in the early period mandates close monitoring of intravascular pressures via central venous pressure or pulmonary artery occlusion pressure measurements to avoid excessive diuresis.
- The use of scheduled albumin dosing along with titrated furosemide has shown promise in the treatment of acute lung injury in patients who are also hypoproteinemic.

Steroids
- Steroid therapy limits the inflammatory cascade that can worsen the severity of pulmonary edema.
- There are several reports of animal studies that support the beneficial effects of corticosteroid therapy with chlorine exposure, most frequently with inhaled delivery and administration immediately or shortly after exposure.
- Based on the experimental data, it is reasonable to consider the initiation of corticosteroid therapy at the time of presentation for patients with moderate to severe chlorine exposure.
- If used, they should not be instituted late and there is little data for long-term use for this indication.

Nebulized sodium bicarbonate
- Nebulized sodium bicarbonate is theoretically beneficial in chlorine exposure.
- Chlorine is converted to hydrochloric acid, the intent is to deliver sodium bicarbonate to the distal airways to neutralize the acid and prevent further injury.
- There are several case reports and series that describe experience with the treatment. Although the use of the treatment appears to be safe, there is not good evidence that it appears to be beneficial.
- There is insufficient data to recommend for or against the routine use of nebulized sodium bicarbonate after chlorine exposure.
- If the decision is made to utilize this therapy, the greatest theoretical benefit would be expected to be seen with administration at presentation.

N-acetylcysteine and ibuprofen
- One of the mechanisms of phosgene-mediated lung injury is the reduction of glutathione and subsequent peroxidation of lipids.
- Several studies in animal models have investigated the hypothesis that intratracheal supplementation and repletion of glutathione can counteract these effects and demonstrated promising results.
- Ibuprofen has also been investigated as a peroxidation inhibitor in a rat model and was found to decrease pulmonary edema after phosgene exposure.
- Comparable human doses (25–50 mg/kg) to those used in experiments are much higher than approved dosing levels.

Patient outcomes

- Pulmonary effects of chlorine and phosgene typically resolve over 3–5 days after exposure
- Casualties who survive 48 hours have a very good prognosis.
- Patients who have not improved significantly by the fourth day, particularly in the presence of fever, leukocytosis, and purulent sputum, should be evaluated for the presence of bacterial superinfection and treated with appropriate antibiotics if indicated.
- The underlying lung injury and mechanical ventilation are both risk factors for the development of pneumonia.
- A minority of casualties may go on to develop persistent changes noted by spirometry that are consistent with obstructive airway dysfunction, restrictive airway dysfunction, or both.
- Symptoms of reactive airway dysfunction syndrome may become chronic.
- The majority of patients who survive will have complete resolution of their symptoms.

Suggested readings

Acute Respiratory Distress Clinical Trials Network. (2000). Ventilation with lower tidal volumes as compared with traditional tidal volumes for acute lung injury and the acute respiratory distress syndrome. *New Eng J Med* 342:1301–1308.

Acute Respiratory Distress Clinical Trials Network. (2006). Comparison of two fluid-management strategies in acute lung injury. *N Engl J Med* 354:2564–2575.

Army Soldier and Biological Chemical Command (2000, Nov). *Domestic Preparedness Program. Chemical Weapons Improved Response Program (CWIRP) Guidelines for Responding to a Chemical Weapons Incident.* Aberdeen Proving Ground, MD.

Borak J, Diller WF (2001) Phosgene exposure: Mechanisms of injury and treatment strategies. *J Occ Env Med* 43:110–119.

Department of Justice, National Institute of Justice Law Enforcement and Corrections Standards and Testing Program. (2002 Nov). Guide for the selection of personal protective equipment for emergency first responders. *NIJ Guide 102–00*, I:1–15.

Evison D, Hinsley D, Rice P. (2002). Chemical weapons. *BMJ* 324:332–335.

Kanne JP, Thoongsuwan N, Stern EJ. (2006). Airway injury after acute chlorine exposure. *Amer J Roent* 186:232–233.

Parrish JS, Bradshaw DA. (2004).Toxic inhalational injury: gas, vapor and vesicant exposure. *Resp Care Clin* 10:43–58.

Urbanetti JS. (1997). Toxic inhalational injury. In: *Textbook of Military Medicine* series. Part I, *Medical Aspects of Chemical and Biological Warfare*, pp. 1247–1270. Washington, DC: Office of the Surgeon General.

Wang J, Zhang L, Walther SM. (2004, Apr). Administration of aerosolized terbutaline and budesonide reduces chlorine gas-induced acute lung injury. *J Trauma* 56:850–862.

Riot control agents

Steve Go

Overview

The use of chemical means to subdue civil disturbances by law enforcement agencies in the United States has been on the increase since the 1920s, with a parallel rise worldwide since the 1950s. In contrast to other classes of chemical warfare agents, riot control agents (RCAs) and their delivery methods are specifically designed to incapacitate targets with minimal injury and no permanent harm. To this end, RCAs typically have a rapid dissemination and onset of action, short duration of effect, and low toxicity.

Major classes of RCAs
- Peripheral Chemosensory Irritant Chemicals (PCICs)
- Dye markers
- Malodorous substances
- Central neuropharmacological agents
- Obscuring cloud smokes

The most common RCAs used domestically in the United States are the PCICs; therefore, this chapter will focus primarily on these.

Chemicals used as RCAs
- Chlorobenzylidenemalononitrile (CS).
- Chloroacetophenone (CN) ("mace").
- Dibenzoxasepine (CR).
- Oleoresin capsicum (OC) (commonly found in "pepper spray").
- Pelargonic acid vanillylamide (PAVA) ("synthetic capsaicin").
- Chloropicrin (PS).
- Diphenylaminearsine (DM) (currently banned in most countries).

Signs and symptoms

- The time of symptom onset is within seconds.
- Duration is typically 10 minutes to one hour.
- PCICs primarily affect the skin and mucus membranes, eyes, and lungs, but systemic effects can occur as well.

Cutaneous

- Pain and stinging or burning sensation.
- Local skin erythema.
- Skin vesiculation (associated with OC).
- Pruritis.
- Buccal irritation.
- Rhinorrhea.
- Drooling and excess salivation.

Ocular

- Excess tearing (hence the term "tear gas").
- Pain.
- Blepharospasm.
- Photophobia.
- Periorbital edema.
- Conjunctival edema (chemosis).
- Conjunctival erythema.
- Increased intraocular pressure (associated with CR).
- Corneal abrasions (associated with OC).

Respiratory

- Dyspnea.
- Stinging.
- Chest tightness or pain.
- Breath holding.
- Laryngospasm.
- Wheezing.
- Sneezing.
- Coughing.
- Increased secretions.

Systemic (seen especially with DM)

- Transient hypertension.
- Transient bradycardia or tachycardia.
- Headache.
- Malaise.
- Nausea and vomiting.
- Abdominal cramping.
- Diarrhea.

The clinical effect of PCICs on the intended targets is influenced by a number of factors including:

- Environment (effect increases with temperature and humidity).
- Concentration of PCICs (effect increases with concentration).

- Preexisting medical conditions in the targets (respiratory effects may increase with preexisting lung disease).
- Crowd motivation and distracters (effect decreases with increased crowd motivation and distracters).
- PCIC exposure can also result in severe allergic reactions.
- Additional injuries can occur depending on the delivery method (e.g., projectile-related injuries, carrier solvent-related toxicity, etc.).
- The flammability of some agents (particularly CS) can also contribute to target injuries.
- Some PCIC agents, notably OC and CN, have also been implicated in patient deaths.
- Teratogenicity and carcinogenicity of various PCICs have been investigated but definitive evidence of potential causation is currently lacking.

Triage

- Patients should be triaged appropriate in mass casualty incidents per generally accepted principles.
- Other potential injuries should be considered in PCIC exposed patients.

Decontamination

- Except in cases of the most trivial exposures, patients should be undressed and briefly given cold-water decontamination in the field, if possible, or at the hospital *before* entry into the ED because agents can affect ED personnel and patients during an internal secondary decontamination
- Hot water and soap can cause secondary contamination as particulate PCICs dissolve in the irrigant.
- In the majority of cases, water decontamination will suffice, but some experts have recommended an alkaline solution.
- Those performing the primary decontamination should wear appropriate protective equipment (including respirators and eye protection).
- Patients requiring showers should be warned that PCICs from their hair may cause transient increased symptoms as it is washed away.
- Any contaminated clothing or possessions should be bagged and stored safely.
- If the patient has isolated ocular exposure to OC or PAVA, then whole body decontamination is probably not indicated, but copious ocular Morgan lens irrigation with normal saline should be performed.
- Although some controversy exists, in general, contact lenses should be removed and discarded prior to decontamination, as lenses can retain residual PCICs, resulting in continued exposure.

History

- After the patient is decontaminated, a thorough history should be taken, paying particular attention to:
  - Type and duration of exposure.
  - Potential for secondary injuries (projectile, falls, trauma).
  - Current symptoms with emphasis on skin, ocular, and respiratory symptoms.
  - Past history of respiratory, cardiac, and ocular diseases (including glaucoma).
  - Tetanus status should be assessed.
- Although accidental (and potentially occult) exposures and ingestions of PCICs have been reported, most often the mode and nature of the exposure is self-evident from the patient's history.
- For cases in which exposure occurs due to a law enforcement or military action, representatives of the responsible agencies should be urgently requested to provide information regarding the exact agent(s) used. This is important because there exists a possibility that novel, unfamiliar RCAs may be introduced during these actions.

Physical examination

- A thorough physical examination should be performed, paying particular attention to:
  - Vital signs.
  - Respiratory status.
  - Ocular exam, including a slit-lamp examination with fluorescein stain (performed after irrigation).
  - Skin exam.
  - General exam for occult trauma.

Treatment

Treatment is largely symptomatic and supportive, but general principles include:

Triage
- Patients should be triaged appropriate in mass casualty incidents per generally accepted principles.
- Other potential injuries should be considered in PCIC-exposed patients.

Cutaneous
- Decontamination is the key. Rubbing affected areas should be avoided to prevent further contamination.
- Diphoterine® has been reported to be efficacious in chelating PCICs in cutaneous and ocular exposures.
- Hypersensitivity reactions.
- Tetanus vaccination should be updated.
- Skin lesions secondary to perforation with embedded PCICs (especially CN) should be sought, because they may result in chronic lesions. These lesions may require referral to a dermatologist.

Ocular
- Decontamination (see earlier) is suggested for significant exposures.
- Diphoterine® (see earlier) may be useful as well.
- Slit-lamp microscopy should be performed in all patients to detect injuries (especially corneal abrasions) and foreign bodies on the lid margins or under the eyelids.
- Increased ocular pressure in patients with preexisting glaucoma should be managed in consultation with an ophthalmologist.

Respiratory
- Preexisting pulmonary conditions may be exacerbated by PCICs and require standard treatments (e.g., bronchodilators, steroids).
- Laryngotracheal bronchitis can result from severe exposures and may require bronchodilators, steroids, and prophylactic antibiotics.
- High concentration exposure to PCICs may precipitate reactive airways dysfunction syndrome (RADS), an asthma-like syndrome that can occur ≤24 hours after exposure to toxic gases.
- Acute treatment is similar to that of asthma, but this syndrome may persist for years from a single acute exposure.

Systemic
- Systemic allergic reactions should be treated aggressively, and treatment may include epinephrine, histamine blockers, and corticosteroids.
- Patients with preexisting cardiovascular disease should be evaluated and treated for acute coronary or cerebrovascular events, as these may be precipitated by the stress of the inciting events.

Disposition

- Patients with persistent allergic symptoms, respiratory symptoms, or significant injuries or sequelae associated with the inciting event should be hospitalized
- A low threshold for consultation of toxicologists, ophthalmologists, and pulmonary/critical care specialists should be maintained in these cases.

Suggested readings

Alberts WM, Brooks SM (1996). Reactive airways dysfunction syndrome. *Curr Opin Pulm Med* 2: 104–110.

Ballantyne B (2006). Medical management of the traumatic consequences of civil unrest incidents: Causation, clinical approaches, needs and advanced planning criteria. *Toxicol Rev* 25: 155–197.

Blaho K, Stark MM (2000). Is CS spray dangerous? CS is a particulate spray, not a gas. *BMJ* 321: 46.

Brown L, Takeuchi D, Challoner K (2000). Corneal abrasions associated with pepper spray exposure. *Am J Emerg Med* 18: 271–272.

Chapman AJ, White C (1978). Death resulting from lacrimatory agents. *J Forensic Sci* 23: 527–530.

Hall AH, Blomet J, Mathieu L (2002). Diphoterine for emergent eye/skin chemical splash decontamination: A review. *Vet Hum Toxicol* 44: 228–231.

Hill AR, Silverberg NB, Mayorga D, Baldwin HE (2000). Medical hazards of the tear gas CS. A case of persistent, multisystem, hypersensitivity reaction and review of the literature. *Medicine* 79: 234–240.

Lazarus AA, Devereaux A (2002). Potential agents of chemical warfare. Worst-case scenario protection and decontamination methods. *Postgrad Med* 112: 133–140.

Nehles J, Hall AH, Blomet J, Mathieu L (2006). Diphoterine for emergent decontamination of skin/eye chemical splashes: 24 cases. *Cutan Ocul Toxicol* 25: 249–258.

Olajos EJ, Salem H (2001). Riot control agents: Pharmacology, toxicology, biochemistry and chemistry. *J Appl Toxicol* 21: 355–391.

Sanford JP (1976). Medical aspects of riot control (harassing) agents. *Annu Rev Med* 27: 421–429.

Stahl CJ, Young BC, Brown RJ, Ainsworth CA, (1968).Forensic aspects of tear-gas pen guns. *J Forensic Sci* 13: 442–469.

Steffee CH, Lantz PE, Flannagan LM, Thompson RL, Jason DR (1995). Oleoresin capsicum (pepper) spray and "in-custody deaths." *Am J Forensic Med Pathol* 16: 185–192.

Stein AA, Kirwan WE (1964). Chloracetophenone (tear gas) poisoning: A clinicopathologic report. *J Forensic Sci* 9: 374–382.

Solomon I, Kochba I, Eizenkraft E, Maharshak N (2003). Report of accidental CS ingestion among seven patients in central Israel and review of the current literature. *Arch Toxicol* 77: 601–604.

Warden CR (2005). Respiratory agents: Irritant gases, riot control agents, incapacitants, and caustics. *Crit Care Clin* 21: 719–737, vi.

Watson WA, Stremel KR, Westdorp EJ (1996). Oleoresin capsicum (Cap-Stun) toxicity from aerosol exposure. *Ann Pharmacother* 30: 733–735.

Weigand DA (1969). Cutaneous reaction to the riot control agents CS. *Mil Med* 134: 437–440.

Explosives

Matthew Gratton

Overview

There has been much written about the risks of attack with weapons of mass destruction (WMD) specifically referring to the use of biologic, chemical, or nuclear weapons. However, as witnessed by the 1995 Oklahoma City bombing, the 2002 Bali Nightclub bombing, the 2004 Madrid train bombing, and the 2005 London tube bombing, as well as multiple other bombings throughout the world, the most likely type of WMD attack is with a conventional explosive device. In the United States alone, from 1983 through 2002, there were 36,110 bombing incidents with 5,931 injuries and 699 deaths.

The treatment of casualties due to explosions can no longer be considered the exclusive realm of military physicians. All physicians must be familiar with the effects of these weapons. Most of the injuries seen after high-explosive detonations comprise conventional blunt, penetrating, and thermal trauma well known to out-of-hospital personnel, emergency physicians and trauma surgeons. This chapter will concentrate on issues not as well known, particularly primary blast injury.

Essential concepts

Brief bomb physics

High-order (HE) explosives

- High-order (HE) explosives undergo a near instantaneous transformation to highly pressurized gases that expand outward and produce a supersonic pressure wave.
- This "blast wave" travels outward and causes an almost instantaneous increase in air pressure ("overpressure") followed by a decrease to a subatmospheric pressure.
- The magnitude of the blast wave decreases exponentially from the focus of the blast in the open air, but in an enclosed space or near walls or corners there can be reverberations that can dramatically increase the amplitude, and thus the destructive potential, of the wave.

Low-order (LE) explosives

- Low-order (LE) explosives do not produce over pressurization waves but both HE and LE explosions do produce a "blast wind."
- This blast wind is characterized by movement of air that can propel an individual causing impact with the ground or a stationary object.

Types of blast injury

Primary
- Caused by direct effects of the over- and underpressurization (blast) wave.
- The effects are concentrated at the junctions of tissues with different densities, particularly at air-fluid interfaces.

Ear
- The tympanic membrane (TM) will rupture with an overpressure of as little as 5 pounds per square inch (psi) above atmospheric pressure.
- Is the most common primary blast injury (PBI).
- Results in impaired hearing.
- Decreased hearing as well as tinnitus and vertigo can result from sensorineural injury, which is usually reversible.
- Ossicular chain, oval and/or round window disruption can also occur.
- Decreased hearing can be a problem for patient care (difficult to obtain a history and/or instruct a patient) and for scene management (difficult for those involved to hear instructions).
- Ruptured TM does not correlate well with primary blast injury to other organs and should not be used to predict injury.
- An intact TM makes other primary blast injury less likely, but does not rule them out (2, 3, 5).

Lung
- Overpressure causes tearing of alveoli and capillaries resulting in hemorrhage, pulmonary contusion, and edema; pneumothorax, pneumomediastinum, and potentially systemic air embolism.
- Symptoms and signs may include dyspnea, cough, and chest discomfort as well as tachypnea, decreased breath sounds, and rales or wheezing.
- If injury progresses, then hemoptysis and cyanosis as well as signs and symptoms of simple or tension pneumothorax and hemothorax may occur.
- Pulmonary injury is the most common life-threatening manifestation of PBI.
- Body armor does not protect from pulmonary blast injury.
- Air embolism from pulmonary damage may manifest with symptoms consistent with MI, stroke, or spinal cord injury due to obstruction of myocardial, cerebral, or spinal vessels by air.
- Apnea, bradycardia, and hypotension have been described due to exposure of the thorax to PBI. This is thought to be mediated by vagal nerve stimulation and can complicate management decisions.

Abdomen
- Overpressure may cause perforation, hemorrhage, or contusion and mesenteric tears, likely due to shearing forces.
- If immediate perforation occurs, the colon is most likely to rupture, followed by the small bowel.
- Delayed perforation can occur due to ischemia leading to infarction.
- Solid organs can also be injured.

- Symptoms range from simple abdominal pain and tenderness to signs of an acute abdomen and/or hemorrhagic shock.
- Most abdominal injuries post blasts are due to typical penetrating or blunt trauma.

Brain

- Concussions are common. Transient loss of consciousness, headache, dizziness, lethargy, and depression may occur.
- In the past, these injuries were typically attributed to associated blunt or penetrating trauma.
- Evidence from blast victims wearing body armor lends credence to there being a direct effect from the blast.

Eye

- Pure PBI to the eye is likely rare, but blunt and penetrating eye injury is extremely common.

Bone

- Overpressure can cause fractures in long bones with traumatic amputation completed by the blast wind.
- Traumatic amputations due to PBI have a very poor prognosis due to the high likelihood of multiple other injuries.

Secondary

- Caused by missiles distributed by the explosion.
- These objects include parts of the casing of the explosive device as well as items that may have been embedded in the device (nails, screws, ball bearings, etc) and environmental debris that may be scattered by the explosion.
- These objects cause injury by directly penetrating and tearing tissue (wound tract) as well as by creating temporary cavities that can shatter inelastic tissue (solid organs, bone).
- Signs and symptoms are determined by the location of the penetration and size and energy of the missile.
- Penetrating injuries from missiles are the most common injuries seen after intentional explosions.
- Blast-wave effects and blast-wind effects diminish in intensity in a shorter distance than missiles hurled by the explosion.
- Those closer to the blast are more likely to be killed instantly due to combined effects.

Tertiary

- Caused by the displacement of individuals by the blast wind.
- This results in typical blunt trauma (or penetrating trauma if the patient is impaled on an object.)
- Signs and symptoms are determined by the body part/s impacted.
- Structural collapse is often included here and can result in crush injury, crush syndrome, and compartment syndrome.

Crush injury

- A part of the body is entrapped between solid objects, which compress the part leading to cell injury and/or death.

Crush syndrome

- Condition that may result when the entrapped part is released and blood flow is reestablished.
- Edema develops in the part that may cause hypovolemia from fluid shifting out of the intravascular space.
- In addition, intracellular products are released into the systemic circulation, which includes myoglobin (rhabdomyolysis), potassium, lactic acid, and other products potentially resulting in acute renal failure, acidosis, and cardiac-rhythm disturbances.

Compartment syndrome

- Damaged muscle becomes edematous and pressure rises as it is compressed within its fibrous sheath.
- Increased pressure causes decreased perfusion leading to muscle death.
- Clinical manifestations include pain out of proportion to physical findings, tense compartment.
- Paresthesias, and pulselessness are late findings.

Quaternary

- All other effects including burns, toxic inhalation, radiation exposure from a dirty bomb, etc. are in this category.

Burns

- Many bombs do not cause fires because available oxygen is depleted due to the explosion.
- Flash burns may occur.
- If a secondary fires occurs, such as with incendiary bombs, (Molotov cocktails, white phosphorous) burns and smoke inhalation may occur.

Exacerbation of medical illness

- Asthma, COPD, angina, or essentially any other chronic illness can be exacerbated.

Mental-health problems

- Most stress reactions are expected and normal and can be handled with supportive care.
- Mental-health follow-up should be made available to patients and staff.

Initial evaluation and treatment

Because the majority of injuries will be typical blunt or penetrating trauma, initial evaluation and management of individual casualties should follow the tenants of Advanced Trauma Life Support (ATLS) which includes airway management (with cervical spine control if indicated), breathing, circulation with hemorrhage control, and neurologic evaluation with appropriate treatment rendered as problems are found, followed by a secondary survey. Evaluation and treatment issues specific to primary-blast injury follow.

If the injuries involve a combat or tactical environment, then the tenets of Trauma Combat Casualty Care should initially be followed (these will be described later).

Ear
- Most TM ruptures heal with expectant treatment (keep the auditory canal clean and dry.)
- Some recommend antibiotic ear drops if there is blood or debris in the canal.
- All should be referred to an otolaryngologist for follow-up.
- Middle- or inner-ear injuries should also be referred.

Lung
- Oxygen saturation and chest x-ray evaluation should be used liberally.
- Blast lung is a complex injury that warrants treatment in an intensive care setting and is generally treated similarly to pulmonary contusion.
- High flow oxygen by appropriate means and avoidance of fluid overload are important. (However, fluid resuscitation may be indicated due to concomitant injury.)
- If intubation and positive pressure ventilation are necessary, high inspiratory pressures should be avoided if possible.
- Attention to the possibility of simple or tension pneumothorax as well as arterial air embolism is critical.
- Immediate chest decompression for pneumothorax as indicated.
- If air embolism is suspected, 100 percent oxygen administration and placement in the left lateral decubitus or prone position followed by hyperbaric chamber utilization are indicated, whenever possible.

Abdomen
- Evaluation should proceed as for typical blunt or penetrating trauma including serial exams and close observation.

Brain
- Evaluation should proceed as for typical blunt or penetrating trauma.
- CT scan for significant loss of consciousness or signs of a space occupying lesion.
- In disasters with multiple patients needing imaging, delaying CT for less acute concussion injuries is reasonable.

Eye
- Although primary blast trauma to the eye is probably infrequent, secondary trauma from missiles is extremely common.
- If there is any suspicion of a penetrating globe injury, the eye should be protected from any compression, including vigorous examination, with an eye shield or other noncompressing device (i.e., Styrofoam cup taped over the eye).

Multicasualty incident concepts

- All hazards planning should emphasize the fact that terrorism by explosion is much more likely than by nuclear, biologic, or chemical means.
- Information from the scene must include the location of the event.
  - Enclosed-space bombings (i.e., bus) increase the likelihood of primary blast injury and the likelihood of needing endotracheal intubation and chest-tube placement.
  - Building collapse increases the likelihood of crush and compartment syndrome.
  - Open-air bombing makes penetrating injury most likely.
- Accurate triage is extremely important when treating mass casualties, with scarce resources.
  - An experienced clinician (RN or MD) should be used in this position.

Suggested readings

Arnold JL, Halpern P, Tsai MC (2004). Mass casualty terrorist bombings: A comparison of outcomes by bombing type. *Ann Emerg Med* 43(2): 263–273.

Born CT, Briggs SM, Ciraulo DL, et al (2007). Disasters and mass casualties: II. Explosive, biologic, chemical, and nuclear agents. *J Am Acad Orthop Surg* 15: 461–473.

Centers for Disease Control and Prevention, Atlanta. Explosions and blast injuries: A primer for clinicians. http://www.bt.cdc.gov/masscasualties/explosions.asp. {Excellent summary with links to other disaster and WMD related material} (Accessed July 29, 2008).

Centers for Disease Control and Prevention, American College of Emergency Physicians. Bombings: Injury patterns and care. http://www.bt.cdc.gov/masscasualties/bombings_injurycare. asp. {One or three hour PowerPoint presentations of blast related medical material} (Accessed July 30, 2008).

DePalma RG, Burris DG, Champion HR, et al (2005). Blast injuries. *N Engl J Med* 352(13): 1335–1341.

Garner J, Brett SJ (2007). Mechanisms of injury by explosive devices. *Anesthesiology Clin* 25: 147–160.

Kapur BG, Hutson R, Davis MA, et al (2005). The United States twenty-year experience with bombing incidents: Implications for terrorism preparedness and medical response. *J of Trauma* 59(6): 1436–1444.

Leibovici D, Ofer NG (1999). Eardrum perforation in explosion survivors: Is it a marker of pulmonary blast injury? *Ann Emerg Med* 34(2): 168–172.

Wightman JM, Gladish SL. Explosions and blast injuries. *Ann Emerg Med* 37(6): 664–678.

Mass shootings

Joseph A. Salomone, III

History

Mass shootings date back as far as the early 1900s, and probably date back to the invention of firearms. The most resent reports and discussion of mass shootings often indicate the mid-1960s as the point when these events increased in frequency. The numbers of killed and injured as a result of mass shootings has increased with the advent of "repeating" or automatic weapons.

Definition

Mass shootings have been defined as incidents with more than five casualties perpetrated by one or more assailants acting in unison over a period of less than 24 hours.

Patterns of injury and mortality

- Approximately 94 percent of deaths occurred on scene, whereas only about 6 percent died after reaching medical facilities.
- Overall dead to wounded ratio is 1.2 to 1, much higher than documented military experience.
- Handguns were used as primary weapon 36 percent of the time (78% semi-automatic), rifles 53 percent of the time (81% semi-automatic), and shotguns 11 percent of the time.
- Shotguns had highest fatality rate, followed by handguns, then rifles, primarily because shotguns and handguns were used as close range weapons.
- Mortality rates by anatomic region were head (95%), chest (75%), neck (58%), abdomen (25%).

Timing

- Most incidents occur in very short time spans.
- Range from a few minutes to less than an hour.
- Most victims are wounded during the first few minutes.
  - This short time frame is relevant for incident response and planning.
  - Even in well-organized urban settings, response of tactical and medical teams will take longer than the duration of most mass shooting incidents.

Incident preparation

Planning and training
- Preplanning is key with coordination of on-scene personnel and/or security, local law enforcement, tactical response, EMS agencies, and receiving facilities.
- Schools and campuses should have emergency response and notification procedures.
- Integrated training exercises are essential for success.
- Concept of operation (COA) and scene management with defined perimeters, "zones of care" and command structures.
  - Hot zone—immediate and direct threat.
  - Warm zone—threat may exist but is not immediate or direct.
  - Cold zone—the operational safe zone outside outer perimeter.
- Operational Security (OPSEC) concerns for local-response planning and implementation must be taken into account to prevent perpetrators from circumventing planned responses.
- Awareness of lessons from previous responses.

Response

General
- First-arriving-units response and situational evaluation is critical.
- Concept of "windshield survey."
- Anticipate the unexpected.
- Immediate interagency cooperation is essential.
- Adhere to Incident Command System (ICS) structure once able.
- Rapid implementation of community-disaster procedures as needed.
- Public-safety responders may become victims, information should be disseminated to all those involved in the incident.
- Integration of tactical medical-response personnel with law enforcement is important.
- Preparation for crisis management post incident.

Out of hospital
- Scene security determination is key, begins with remote observation.
- Assure that the scene is secured by law enforcement before entering.
  - In active shooter scenario, law enforcement may stage medical personnel away from the scene.
- First-arriving medical personnel should concentrate on triage and correcting any immediate life threatening injuries if they have safe access to victims.
- A quick estimation of patients including severity should be accomplished for subsequent dispersal of patients to hospitals.
  - Immediate and continued communication and coordination with base-station physician/emergency department is essential for deploying needed personnel and equipment.
  - Minimize the number of personnel communicating from the scene to avoid confusion.

- Upon arrival of other EMS personnel, a specific command structure should be developed in accordance with principles of ICS.
- EMS Command should set up triage, treatment, and transport officers.
- Ingress and egress routes for EMS transport units should be identified and executed.
  - If the shooter is still active, the need to minimize risk of personnel is paramount and may require law-enforcement personnel bringing patients to EMS units from a distance.
  - Aeroevacuation should be delayed in an active shooter scenario unless a secure landing zone can be established safely away from the scene.

Tactical medical response

- Importance of tactical medical personnel to support responding teams and provide immediate care even in "hot zone."
- Making a tactical medical assessment using Counter Narcotics and Terrorism Operational Medical Support (CONTOMS) RAM (Risk Assessment Methodology) or similar is important.
- Maximize opportunity to extract and treat medically salvageable victims while minimizing risk to providers and responding personnel.
- Observation of breathing and respiratory rate.
- Observation of exsanguinating hemorrhage.
- Note obvious wounds and other injuries particularly those incompatible with life.
- Acoustic observation for detectible speech or other sounds.
- Risk-benefit assessment with command prior to extraction.
- Limited care focused on management of immediate life threats.
- Appropriate but limited airway management.
- Standard adjuncts.
- Rescue airways.
- Alternative endotracheal intubation methods.
- Hemorrhage control with use of tourniquets or pressure/hemostatic dressings.
- Chest decompression with needles or other devices.
- Coordination with Special Response Teams (SRT or SWAT).

Regional coordination

- Early activation and use of regional-emergency-response plans.
- On-scene command and emergency operations center communication and coordination.
- Regional resources and receiving centers early activation.

Suggested readings

"A time Line of Recent Worldwide School Shootings." Infoplease. (2000–2007). Pearson Education, publishing as Infoplease http://www.infoplease.com/A0777958.html (Accessed Nov 11, 2008).

Chapman S, et al. (2006). Australia's 1996 gun law reforms: Faster falls in firearm deaths, firearm suicides and a decade without mass shootings. *Inj Prev 12*: 365–372.

Coupland RM, Meddings DR (1999) Mortality associated with use of weapons in armed conflicts, wartime atrocities and civilian mass shootings: literature review. *BMJ* 319(7207):407–410.

Stein TM (2007). *Mass Shootings in Disaster Medicine*, 2nd ed. Hogan DE and Burstein JL, eds. Philadelphia, PA: Lippincott Williams & Wilkins.

Nuclear terrorism and disasters

Justin S. Gatewood

Introduction

Detonation of a nuclear device uses fission and fusion of radioactive materials to release vast quantities of thermal and radiation energy in the form of a massive explosion. The amount of energy released by such an explosion is referred to as the *yield* and is most commonly expressed in equivalent of tons of TNT.

A nuclear device may take the form of a thermonuclear weapon or an improvised nuclear device (IND), the former having yields ranging between tens of kilotons and several megatons, and the latter usually having less. Whereas nuclear weapons are made by any of the nuclear states, an IND is a nuclear weapon illicitly obtained from such a state, or an explosive weapon fabricated from illicitly obtained fissile material.

Although less likely during the current era of nuclear disarmament, detonation of a nuclear device, either in an act of aggression by a nuclear state or terrorist group, would constitute a major catastrophe yielding several thousands if not millions of dead and injured.

Table 69.1 Capability of states possessing nuclear weapons

Country	Number of active warheads	Est. destructive power (Mt**)
NPT* States		
China	176	294
France	300	55
Russian Federation	4,600	1273
United Kingdom	160	n/a
United States	2,468	n/a
Non-NPT States		
India	40–50	0.8–1
North Korea	Unknown	Unknown
Pakistan	24–48	0.6–1
Undeclared*		
Israel	200–400	940

*International Nuclear Non-Proliferation Treaty
** Millions of tons of TNT equivalent
***Although known to possess nuclear weapons, maintains a policy of nuclear opacity.
Source: The Nuclear Threat Initiatve.

Blast injury

Approximately 50 percent of energy dispersed by a nuclear detonation takes the form of blast waves.

Direct blast wave

- Extremely high temperatures and pressures cause a hydrodynamic front that radiates outward from the center of the explosion at very high velocities.
- The immediate rise in pressure over that of atmospheric pressure caused by compression of air immediately ahead of the front results in an *overpressure*.
- Peak overpressures in the vicinity of the blast are proportional to the distance from, altitude and yield of the detonation.
- Tympanic membrane (TM) rupture: 0.3–1.4 atm peak overpressure; lung injury: 1.4–2.7 atm. Therefore, evidence of TM rupture should prompt suspicion of lung injury.
- Lung injury is a significant cause of morbidity/mortality and may manifest as pulmonary contusion, pulmonary edema/hemorrhage, hemo/pneumothorax, or air emboli.
- Median lethal dose (LD_{50}) (due to overpressure alone) = approx. 3 atm peak overpressure, roughly the peak overpressure felt 0.4 miles from ground zero caused by detonation of 1 MT bomb at 1.4 mile altitude.

Indirect blast wave

- Drag forces cause high velocity winds varying with distance from blast, altitude of blast, and weapon yield.
- Penetrating trauma secondary to generation of missiles by flying debris.
- Blunt trauma caused by crush injury from flying objects and actual displacement of the human body over considerable distances (translational injury).
- Estimated wind velocity at 1.1 miles from 1 megaton (MT) detonation is 400 mph.

Prompt radiation

- Ionizing radiation mostly in the form of neutron and gamma radiation created by fission or fusion reactions (usually expressed in Gray units, Gy).
- Accounts for approx. 5 percent of energy released during detonation.
- Amount of radiation decreases with increasing distance from ground zero.
- Injury is proportional to received dose of whole-body radiation, causing acute radiation syndromes:
  - Nausea, vomiting, and diarrhea, usually within hours.
  - Hematopoietic depression with fever, impaired wound healing, bleeding complications, and anemia (days to weeks).
  - CNS signs/symptoms (ataxia, confusion) and cardiovascular collapse within hours of very high exposure.
  - $LD_{50(60\ days)} \approx 2.5$–5 Gy.

Thermal radiation

Approximately 35 percent of energy from a nuclear detonation is released in the form of thermal energy. This energy is composed of the electromagnetic radiation emitted from the fireball and decreases with increasing distance from ground zero. Injury occurs predominantly via two mechanisms:

Flash burns
- Burns caused by absorption of thermal energy through exposed skin, proportional to duration of exposure (seconds), and thermal energy per exposed area.
- Clothing can provide partial shielding, the extent of which depends upon the material and color of the clothing.

Flame burns
- Burns from flames caused by thermal ignition of environmental objects, including clothes.

Flash blindness
- This occurs when large amounts of electromagnetic radiation in the visible light spectrum saturate the retina, bleaching visual pigments.
- Effects last seconds to minutes and vary with ambient light preceding the detonation.
- Although uncommon, retinal scarring may also occur, causing permanent visual impairment.

Fallout

- Fallout refers to the radiation hazard caused by atmospheric dispersal of residual nuclear particles after detonation.
- These particles, many of which are long-lived radioisotopes, find their way, by local or meteorological dispersal, into soil and water sources.
- They may then cause external radiation exposure or internal hazard if they are inhaled or ingested.
- Depending on the level of exposure, in the short term, those exposed may experience varying degrees of radiation sickness.
- Long-term effects, which are often radioisotope specific, include oncogenesis, teratogenesis/infertility, radiodermatitis, and cataract formation.

Radiologic dispersal device

- Also known as a "dirty bomb" this is the most likely form of nuclear terrorism.
- Basically a conventional explosive device used to disperse radioactive material over many city blocks.
- Americanum-241, cesium-137, cobalt-60 and strontium-90 are potential isotopes for use in such a device because they have relatively long half-lives, have common industrial uses, and could be obtained in small, relatively unsecured amounts.
- Extent of contamination depends on size/sophistication of the bomb, isotope used and weather conditions/topography.
- The **majority** of acute morbidity/mortality is secondary to **traumatic injury**, especially penetrating trauma, shrapnel, and thermal burns.
- **Acute radiation syndrome is unlikely**.
- Lasting effects would be psychological and economic because the contaminated area may need to be abandoned for months/years until decontamination is complete.

Simple radiologic device

- A device containing radioactive material that might be left in a highly populated or strategic location.
- Americanum-241, cesium-137, cobalt-60, and strontium-90 are potential isotopes.
- Because the material is not physically dispersed, radiologic contamination is minimal.
- Although physical injury would not be anticipated, such an event may cause significant immediate and long-term psychological effects within a community.

Nuclear reactor core damage

- A nuclear reactor is any device in which a nuclear fission chain reaction occurs under controlled conditions so that the heat yield can be harnessed or the neutron beams utilized.
- There are 104 commercial reactors in the United States.
- Reactors are composed of multiple units of radioactive (usually uranium) fuel cells and neutron-absorbing control rods housed behind several feet of concrete and steel.
- Although their sound construction, high security, and sophisticated safety systems make them relatively secure, terrorists may attempt to breach the coolant system using large amounts of explosives or an airplane as a missile.
- If significant damage did occur, the most likely result would be local fallout generated by a radioactive plume.

Response to nuclear incident

- Because any act of nuclear terrorism would be considered an incident of national significance, the initial response would consist of the coordinated efforts of multiple federal agencies as outlined by the National Response Framework (NRF).
- Federal agencies would then simultaneously coordinate with state, local, and nongovernmental agencies according to the National Incident Management System (NIMS).
- A list of the coordinating agencies, although not exhaustive, includes the following:

Federal agencies
- Department of Homeland Security (DHS): coordinates the Federal response to any deliberate nuclear/radiologic incident.
- Department of Health and Human Services (DHHS): utilizes the National Disaster Medical System (NDMS) to augment State and local medical response capability.
- Federal Bureau of Investigation (FBI): deploys a Disaster Squad to identify injured persons and Hazard Materials Response Unit to collect evidence.
- Department of Defense (DOD): provides military assistance to civilian authorities.
- Department of Energy (DOE): involved in mitigating hazards caused by incidents involving DOE-controlled facilities or materials.
- Environmental Protection Agency (EPA): provides environmental response to inland (non-coastal) incidents.
- Nuclear Regulatory Commission (NRC): provides support to DHS for incidents involving commercial nuclear reactors.

State and local agencies
- Emergency Medical Service first responders.
- Local fire department.
- Law-enforcement agency.
- Search-and-rescue teams.
- Health department.
- HAZMAT teams.

Nongovernmental agencies
- American Red Cross.
- Volunteer disaster medical assistance teams (DMATs) under the jurisdiction of DHHS.
- Urban Search and Rescue (USAR) (Deployed by FEMA).

Patient transport and triage

After control of the scene and safe perimeters are established, efforts should be focused on the prompt transport of patients to definitive medical care.

- Patient transport
- Before arriving at the scene, first responders should put on personal protective equipment (PPE) as well as personal dosimeters.
- The overwhelming majority of radiation hazard during a nuclear incident comes from the radiation source itself. Although the surface of the patient may be contaminated with radioactive material, patients themselves should not be considered radioactive.
- Stabilization and transport of *unstable patients* (those with respiratory distress, signs/symptoms of shock, altered mental status or who have sustained life/limb threatening injuries) to the Emergency Department *should not be delayed by a radiologic survey or decontamination procedures.*
  - Limited preliminary decontamination and radiation containment may be performed en route if it does not delay patient care or transport.
- *Stable patients* should be moved to central location upwind of the radiation source and *undergo a preliminary radiologic survey, decontamination* (discussed separately in Chapter 70: Radiologic Terrorism.) and *final radiologic survey* before being transported to the Emergency Department.
  - Survey and decontamination may also be performed at a designated staging at the hospital outside the Emergency Department.
- Cover burns and open wounds with a clean, dry dressing.
- Personal belongings should be placed in containers marked "Radioactive" and be tagged with the patient's name.
- Care should be taken not to cross-contaminate patients.

Triage

Prehospital

- Initial prehospital triage should follow standard conventional trauma/ burn triage algorithms.
- Deficits in the primary survey should be presumed to be secondary to trauma and not radiation.
- Although combined conventional/radiation triage algorithms do exist, they are not useful immediately after an incident because reliable methods of determining acute whole-body radiation doses are not available until the patient reaches the hospital.

In hospital

- Once the estimated radiation dose has been determined by biodosimetry (time to onset of vomiting, lymphocyte depletion kinetics or presence of chromosome dicentrics, discussed separately in Chapter 70: Radiologic Terrorism), Table 69.2 may be used to further triage patients.

Table 69.2 Revised triage of patients with conventional injury after estimated whole-body radiation dose.

Conventional triage category before estimated radiation dose	Revised triage category after estimated whole-body radiation dose		
	<1.5 Gy	1.5–4.5 Gy	>4.5–10 Gy
Immediate	Immediate	Immediate	Expectant
Delayed	Delayed	Variable	Expectant
Minimal	Minimal	Follow treatment guidelines for ARS* when dose >3 Gy	
Expectant	Expectant	Expectant	Expectant
Absent	Ambulatory monitoring	Routine care and hospitalization as needed	

*Acute radiation sickness

Source: Waselenko JK, Mac Vittie TJ, Blakeley WF, et al. (2004). Strategic National Stockpile Radiation Working Group. Medical management of the acute radiation syndrome: recommendations of the Strategic National Stockpile Radiation Working Group. *Annals of Internal Medicine* 140: 1037-1051.

Suggested readings

Cerveny, TJ, Walker RI, and Zajtchuk R, eds. (1989). *Medical Consequences of Nuclear Warfare* (Textbook of Military Medicine Series). Washington, DC: Borden Institute.

Strategic Stockpile Radiation Working Group (2004). Medical management of the acute radiation syndrome: Recommendations of the Strategic National Stockpile Radiation Working Group. *Annals of Internal Medicine; 140*: 1037-1051.

US Army Field Manual 4-02. (2001, Dec 20). Treatment of Nuclear and Radiological Casualties. FM 4-02.283 / NTRP 4-02.21 / AFMAN 44-161(I) / MCRP 4-11.1B

Radiological terrorism

D. Adam Algren

Radiation background/epidemiology

The threat of potential terrorist attacks has increased awareness regarding the possible use of radiation as a weapon. This has led to increased federal, state, and local government planning and training to address this threat. The extent of injury, casualties, and radiation exposure would vary depending on the device used. Likewise, the general public's lack of knowledge and misperception of the actual threat posed by a radiation event would likely result in a significant number of psychological casualties and hysteria.

Five methods that could be employed for dispersal of radiologic agents include:

- Simple radiological device.
  - Higher probability.
  - Medical radiotherapy sources (Cesium-137).
  - Industrial radiography sources (Cobalt-60, Iridium-192).
  - External and/or internal contamination.
- Radiological dispersion device.
  - Higher probability.
  - Multiple simple radiological devices packaged with conventional explosives.
  - Blast/thermal injuries in addition to radiation exposure/contamination.
- Nuclear reactor sabotage.
  - Low probability.
  - Direct breech of containment vessels presents greatest threat.
  - Significant long-term environmental contamination.
- Improvised nuclear device.
  - Low probability.
  - Crude nuclear device.
  - "Suitcase bombs."
- Conventional nuclear weapon detonation.
  - Low probability.
  - High magnitude event with significant number of casualties and extensive environmental contamination.

The Radiation Emergency Assistance Center/Training Site (REACTS) of the U.S. Department of Energy reports that between 1944 and 2005 there were 428 major radiation events worldwide. There were 3,050 significant human exposures resulting in 134 fatalities. A majority of events involved industrial radiography or medical radiotherapy sources. Although reported, use of radiation as a terrorist weapon has not been confirmed.

Radiation physics and pathophysiology

There are five types of ionizing radiation (Table 70.1). Exposure can occur via irradiation or contamination. Irradiation is an exposure that does not result in transfer of radioactive material. Contamination with radioactive material results in ongoing exposure (external or internal) and risks potential radiation exposure to other individuals.

Radiation injury and damage to biological tissues can be classified as deterministic or stochastic. Deterministic effects are those that are dependent on the radiation dose (e.g., acute radiation sickness, local radiation injury). A threshold dose is required to develop clinical effects and the severity of the effect increases with an increasing dose. Stochastic effects are those that occur independent of dose (e.g., cancer). These effects occur randomly; however, the probability of occurrence increases as the radiation dose increases.

Radiation exposure results in cellular dysfunction. The energy imparted results in free-radical formation. This leads to DNA damage and injury to cell structures. Lower exposures are often amenable to cellular-repair mechanisms, however, once a cell has been exposed to a critical dose, cell death occurs as free-radical injuries overwhelm cellular-repair mechanisms. The cells most susceptible to radiation are those with high mitotic activity, including white blood cells, intestinal lining, endothelium, connective tissue, muscles, and nerves.

Table 70.1 Types of ionizing radiation

	Particle Type/ Energy	Penetration	Tissue Damage	Shielding
Alpha	2 protons and 2 neutrons High energy	Short—a few cm in air, several microns in tissue	High, if internalized	Easily shielded
Beta	High-energy electron Energy varies	Moderate— several meters in air, several millimeters in tissue	Varies	Easily shielded
Gamma and X-rays	Electromagnetic energy High energy	Significant— many meters in air	High	Difficult to shield
Neutrons	Neutral particle emitted from nucleus High energy	Significant	High—can induce radioactivity	Difficult to shield

Radiation units

RAD (Radiation Absorbed Dose)
- United States unit of measurement.
- Amount of energy actually absorbed into material.
- Does not describe biological effects.

REM (Roentgen Equivalent Man)
- U.S. unit of measurement.
- Quantifies biological effect/damage to tissues.
- REM = RAD x Q (Q= quality factor that is unique to the specific radiation).

Gray (Gy)
- International unit.
- Amount of energy absorbed into material.
- 1 Gray = 100 Rads.

Sievert (Sv)
- International unit.
- Quantifies biological effect/damage to tissue.
- 1 Sievert = 100 Rem.

Radiation detection instruments

Geiger Mueller detectors are handheld instruments that are widely available and useful for surveying for radioactive contamination. Prior to use determine the following:

- Check the instrument battery and calibration
- Determine the background radiation level
- If alpha particles are suspected leave the probe uncovered
- If beta or gamma particles are suspected the probe may be covered to prevent contamination.
- Adjust the multiplier value on the instrument as needed to appropriately and consistently identify contamination present
- Patients should be surveyed in a slow and thorough fashion (See below).
- Particular attention should be given to open wounds as these could harbor radioactive material/contamination.

Acute radiation syndrome

Acute Radiation Syndrome (ARS) is an acute or subacute, systemic illness that occurs following radiation exposure. ARS results in a characteristic clinical syndrome that evolves over hours to days. There are several phases in the evolution of ARS (Table 70.2):

- **Prodromal:** Occurs within the first 48 hours.
  - Nausea, vomiting, diarrhea.
  - Lymphopenia—the Andrews curve (Figure 70.1) is a useful tool that uses the absolute lymphocyte count to predict the severity of radiation injury.

Latent: Lasts hours up to 21 days. No significant signs or symptoms are present. Prodromal symptoms diminish.

- **Manifest Illness:** Multi-organ system involvement.
  - Bone marrow suppression (leucopenia, anemia, thrombocytopenia).
  - Infections.
  - Bleeding (gastrointestinal).
  - Vomiting, diarrhea.
  - CNS—confusion, seizures, altered level of consciousness.
- **Recovery**: Increased risk of malignancies.

Table 70.2 Acute Radiation Syndrome

	Severity and Radiation Dose Exposure (Gy)				
	Mild (1–2)	Moderate (2–4)	Severe (4–6)	Very Severe (6–8)	Lethal (>8)
Mortality	0%	0–50%	20–70%	60–80%	100%
Vomiting					
Onset	> 2 hours after exposure	1–2 hours after exposure	<1 hour after exposure	<30 minutes after exposure	<10 minutes after exposure
Incidence	10–50%	70–90%	100%	100%	100%
Diarrhea			Mild	Severe	Severe
Onset	None	None	3–8 hours	1–3 hours	<1 hour
Incidence			<10%	>10%	100%
Headache	Minimal	Mild	Moderate	Severe	Severe
Onset			4–24 hours	3–4 hours	1–2 hours
Incidence			50%	80%	80–90%
Level of Consciousness	Normal	Normal	Normal	May be altered	Unconsciousness within minutes
Body Temperature	Normal	Elevated	Fever	High fever	High Fever
Onset		1–3 hours	1–2 hours	<1 hour	<1 hour
Incidence		10–80%	80–100%	100%	100%
Medical Response	Outpatient observation	In-patient observation at general hospital	Treatment in specialized hospital	Treatment in specialized hospital	Palliative care

Source: International Atomic Energy Agency. Diagnosis and Treatment of Radiation Injuries. Safety Reports Series No. 2. Vienna: IAEA; 1998.

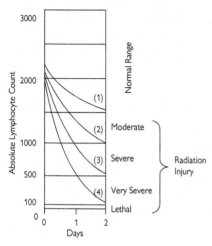

Figure 70.1 Andrews curve

Local radiation injury

Local Radiation Injury (LRI) is the effect/injury ("radiation burn") that occurs to the skin, soft tissues, muscle, and/or bone following a localized exposure to radiation. LRI can occur with or without ARS. See Table 70.3.

Table 70.3 Local radiation injury

Dose (Gy)	Injury	Timing
3	Epilation	Approximately 17 days
6	Erythema	Hours to weeks
10	Dry desquamation without blister formation	2–3 weeks
>20	Moist desquamation with blister formation	2–8 weeks
>50	Necrosis	Weeks to months

Emergency medical management

Radiation protection

As with any hazardous materials incident, it is imperative to protect emergency medical personnel. These measures will protect/limit radiation exposure:

- Decrease quantity of radioactive material present.
  - Decontaminate victims (remove clothing and wash with soap/water) and remove material from area. All contaminated water runoff should be collected if possible.
  - Only patients who have been contaminated (not irradiated) with radioactive material require decontamination.
  - The goal is to decontaminate to the background radiation rate. However, this can be difficult even following multiple attempts. In these cases, a level that is twice the background rate is acceptable.
- Decrease time of exposure.
  - The dose is proportional to the time exposed.
  - Rotate workers in shifts and use dosimeters to limit exposure.
- Increase distance of radioactive material.
  - Most effective. The dose is inversely proportional to the square of the distance. Doubling of distance from material decreases dose fourfold.
- Use shielding
  - Typical universal precautions are effective shielding for alpha and beta particles.
  - Universal precautions provide adequate shielding for those personnel taking care of exposed victims.
  - Lead can shield some x-rays. Neutrons and gamma rays are not easily shielded.

Medical management of radiation victims and ARS

- Perform a radiation survey (front and back) and decontaminate the patient carefully (Figure 70.2). All contaminated clothing should be double bagged and removed from the area.
- Re-survey patients following decontamination
- Treat conventional injuries first (prior to decontamination if life threatening).
- Obtain a history regarding the incident and identity/amount of source material involved.
- Identify (including time of onset) early symptoms or signs of radiation injury.
- Perform a through physical exam.
- Obtain baseline laboratory studies.
- Obtain CBC with differential every 6 hours for at least 48 hours to follow the absolute lymphocyte count.
- Begin 24-hour collection of urine and feces for radioassays.
- Consider cytogenetic dosimetry/chromosomal aberration analysis.
- Any surgery or procedures should be performed early (within the first 48 hours). Beyond 48 hours victims are at high risk for infection and impaired wound healing.

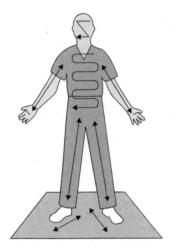

Figure 70.2 Survey for external contamination

- Consider prophylactic treatment with antibiotics, antivirals, and antifungal agents.
- Transfuse with blood and platelets as needed.
- If exposure > 2 Gy consider early treatment with granulocyte colony stimulating factor (G-CSF).
- For exposures >6 Gy consider bone marrow transplant.

Medical management of internal contamination

Internal contamination (inhalation or ingestion) with radionuclides necessitates chelation to hasten excretion and decrease radiation exposure. The agents that can serve as antidotes include:
- Zinc or calcium DTPA (IV) for Americium, Californium, Curium, Plutonium.
- BAL (intramuscular) for Polonium.
- Potassium Iodide (oral) for Iodide-125 or Iodide-131.
- Prussian Blue (oral) for Cesium-137.
- Aluminum antacids (oral) for Strontium.
- Sodium bicarbonate (IV) for Uranium.
- IV fluids/water diuresis for Tritium.

Medical management of local radiation injury (LRI)
- Protect the involved area.
- Provide meticulous wound care.
- Encourage smoking cessation.
- Ensure adequate nutrition.

- Treat infections early.
- Treat pain aggressively.
- Avoid surgical procedures if possible.
  - It can be difficult to know where to debride because LRI can evolve slowly over weeks to months.
  - Surgery may worsen outcome as wounds heal poorly and are at increased risk of infection.

Response to a radiation incident

- Malicious use of radiation as a weapon would constitute an act of terrorism and would necessitate immediate notification of local, state, and federal law enforcement as well as public-health agencies.
- For incidents that are not related to terrorism the institution's radiation safety officer (RSO) should be notified. The RSO can help coordinate and determine the necessary response.
- REACTS can also serve as a valuable resource in the management of radiation events. REACTS is available 24 hours a day to provide a wide variety of consultative services. They have a multidisciplinary team that can assist with dose assessments, triage, and treatment of radiation victims.
- REACTS emergency phone number: 1-865-576-1005.

Suggested readings

Berger ME, Christensen DM, Lowry PC, et al (2006). Medical management of radiation injuries: Current approaches. *Occup Med* 56: 162–172.

Bushberg JT, Kroger LA, Hartman MB, et al (2007). Nuclear/radiological terrorism: Emergency department management of radiation casualties. *J Emerg Med* 32: 71–85.

Koenig KL, Goans RE, Hatchett RJ (2005). Medical treatment of radiological casualties: Current concepts. *Ann Emerg Med* 45: 643–652.

Waselenko JK, MacVittie TJ, Blakely WF (2004). Medical management of the acute radiation syndrome: Recommendations of the Strategic National Stockpile Radiation Working Group. *Ann Intern Med* 140: 1037–1051.

Mechanical
and Structural
Disasters

Land

Automobile disasters

Andrew Milsten

Introduction

Motor vehicle crashes (MVCs) are the leading cause of death among people under 40 years of age. In the United States in 2009, approximately 37,000 people died in MVCs, and approximately 3 million were injured. The annual U.S. MVC fatality rate has been slowly declining since peaking in 1990 at 44,000 deaths. The disability and financial consequences of these crashes are substantial. Despite improved safety features and driver awareness, major highway disasters resulting in fatalities and severe injuries continue to occur worldwide (Figure 71.1). The geographic variability in fatal MVCs has been partially attributed to the differences in available emergency medical services (EMS) and trauma care.

The prehospital care and ultimate management of MVC victims in mass casualties presents a unique challenge. Studies of emergency medical system response to multiple casualties at the scene of MVCs have shown that the triage process is complex, and must incorporate evidence-based physiologic cues and situational variables to determine casualty priority.

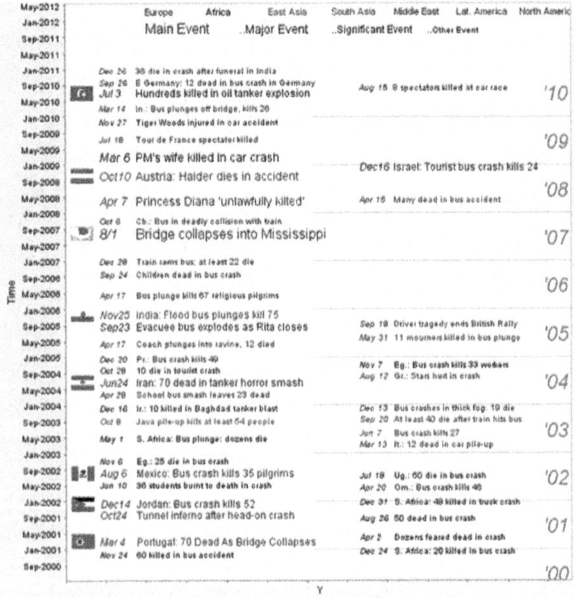

Figure 71.1 Major highway disasters 2000–2010. Reprinted with permission from MapReport.com at www.mapreport.com/subtopics/d/c.html.

Proper scene triage includes a consideration of the following:
- Specific interventions.
- Transport methods.
- Treatment locations.

Several studies identify an association between motor-vehicle-related mortality and available prehospital resources. Therefore, particularly in major highway disasters, it is essential to assess local emergency response as well as motor vehicle fatality data and existing trauma systems in order to optimize treatment and minimize preventable deaths.

The fundamental components of a trauma system include:
- Injury prevention.
- Prehospital care.
- Acute-care facilities.
- Posthospital care.

The demographics of a region also must be taken into account when estimating the prevalence and severity of motor-vehicle-related trauma. This includes:
- Age of drivers.
- Use of alcohol or other intoxicant.
- Average speed.
- Collision severity.

Motor-vehicle-injury patterns

In frontal collisions, unrestrained occupants continue to move forward as the vehicle comes to a stop. The initial impact against the interior of the vehicle is often the lower extremities, resulting in fractures or dislocations of the ankles, knees, femurs, or hips. As the body continues to move, the head, cervical spine, and torso strike the windshield and steering column. In the upper body, there may be rib fractures, sternal fractures, myocardial or pulmonary injury. As the head strikes the windshield, cervical spine injuries, facial fractures, and traumatic brain injury may result. With a lateral impact or rollover collision, the occupant may sustain a wide range of injuries as multiple parts of the body strike the interior of the vehicle. The occupant is also at greater risk of ejection from the vehicle.

The use of a seat belt has been estimated to offer a 75% reduction in fatalities and a 30 percent reduction in any injury following an MVC. Frontal air bags can protect against facial, head, and chest injuries, but only after a head-on collision or impact within 30 degrees of a head-on collision.

In a study of automobile passengers injured in an MVC from 1996–2002, the distribution of specific injuries were analyzed both in restrained and unrestrained drivers. Injuries were classified according to the Abbreviated Injury Scale and the Injury Severity Score. Of the 10,338 restrained and unrestrained casualties studied, 1,599 were children and 8,739 were adults. See Table 71.1.

This study revealed that children under 15 years of age were more likely to suffer a head or abdominal injury. Over half the injuries to young children are head injuries. This may be explained by the relatively high center of gravity of children, the resultant tendency of children to fall head first during a fall, and the lack of strength and coordination of the upper extremities to protect the head. The most likely reason for increased abdominal injuries is the inappropriate use of seatbelts or failure to use child safety seats when needed for smaller children.

Table 71.1 Distribution of injuries of automobile passengers in MVCs

| | Restrained Passengers | | Unrestrained Passengers | |
	Children (n = 1033)	Adults (n = 6535)	Children (n = 566)	Adults (n = 2204)
Head	263 (25.46%)	1069 (16.36%)	176 (31.1%)	672 (30.05%)
Chest	150 (14.52%)	1916 (29.32%)	36 (6.36%)	359 (16.29%)
Abdomen	93 (9.0%)	390 (5.97%)	27 (4.77%)	118 (5.35%)
Spine	155 (15.0%)	2260 (34.58%)	57 (10.07%)	554 (25.14%)

Motor vehicle trauma in rural areas

Although only one-third of the U.S. population lives in rural areas, over one half of motor vehicle related deaths occur in these areas. Most trauma research has been conducted on urban trauma systems, particularly Level I trauma centers. Despite efforts to apply trauma system development to areas outside urban areas, rural trauma continues to be a major public-health problem.

The mortality rate of rural vehicle trauma is approximately twice that of urban vehicle trauma (29.5/100,000 MVCs vs.16.3/100,000 MVCs). The most frequently cited reasons for this difference in casualties include a shortage of trauma surgeons, neurosurgeons, nurses, prehospital personnel, and trauma centers in addition to longer response and transport times. In addition to an expansion of existing trauma systems, more specific prospective studies need to be performed to identify additional prehospital factors contributing to higher mortality. To date, it is unclear whether increased resource deployment would have a significant effect on rural MVC-related mortality.

Emergency action for highway disasters

A highway disaster involving multiple victims and multiple motor vehicles may require significant emergency medical resources. In addition to alerting the emergency medical services dispatcher, a survey of the wreckage by helicopter may be helpful for a complete assessment of the disaster. If the disaster occurs along a highway between two different communities, it may be necessary to coordinate with a second emergency response system so that the responders can approach from both directions. This is particularly helpful with disasters occurring over divided highways and responders are needed on both sides of the disaster scene.

Strategies for reducing motor vehicle fatalities

Many studies have been performed which detail the extent to which increased speed leads to increased injuries and fatalities. For example:

- States with speed limits of greater than 65 mph had approximately 13 percent more traffic fatalities than states with a maximum speed of 65 mph.
- It is estimated that a nationwide speed limit of 65 mph would save almost 3,000 lives per year.
- Increased traffic enforcement by local police departments reduces driving speeds and fatalities, but this reduction appears to be transient, lasting a maximum of 8 weeks after initiation.
- The costs of enforcement must be weighed against the estimated mortality benefit.
- The time of injury may provide a teaching moment, particularly for alcohol related MVCs. Engaging emergency patients in brief interventions prior to discharge has shown to decrease the risk of recurrent injury.
- In the future, it may be possible to improve EMS response time using automatic crash notification systems capable of making predictions about MVCs with a high probability of serious injury.
- It has been estimated that with a notification time of 1 minute and a response time of 15 minutes, between 2,000 and 3,000 lives could be saved annually using automatic crash notification technology.

Several safety improvements have been suggested to prevent the highway disasters. These include:

- Prohibiting hand-held cell phone usage by drivers (DC, California, Connecticut, New Jersey, New York, Oregon, and Washington require hands-free devices). It has been estimated that cell phone use is responsible for approximately 1.6 million crashes per year.
- Prohibiting all cell-phone usage and texting by junior operators.
- Improve child occupant protection by requiring booster seats for children up to age 8.
- Enacting legislation that reduces alcohol-related accidents such as zero blood alcohol requirements for repeat offenders, license revocation for refusing or failing sobriety tests, increased sobriety checkpoints.
- Enacting seat belt laws that allow do not restrict officers from observing another offense first (primary enforcement).
- Improve motorcycle safety by requiring helmets, which comply with Department of Transportation Motor Vehicle Safety Standards.

Suggested readings

Kramer, W (2009). *Disaster Planning and Control*. Tulsa, OK: PennWell.
National Transportation Safety Board. Available at: http://www.ntsb.gov/.
US Dept of Transportation. Available at: www.dot.gov.

Bus disasters

Kerry K. McCabe

Megan L. Salinas

Considerations regarding bus disasters

- Collisions or bombings
- Mass casualty incidents (MCIs)
- Differing populations and circumstances: bus, coach, school bus, or charter bus
- Collisions—more likely blunt trauma
- Bombings—confined space blast injuries

Collisions

- Statistics.
  - Yearly average of nine fatalities on school buses and four on motor coaches in the United States. Statistically, buses are much safer than automobiles.
- Bus collisions are more likely to occur with automobiles and are more likely to happen in dry weather.
- No restraints on buses.
  - Thus passengers are more likely to be ejected in a collision.
  - In the EU, restraints are required in all new buses built.
- Compartmentalization.
  - Seats are strong, closely spaced together, high-backed, well padded, and designed to absorb energy.
  - Doesn't protect in lateral impact or rollovers.
  - Patients are injured when they fall out of the compartment.
- Egress.
  - May be difficult for passengers to escape if bus is lying on its side, is upside down, or submersed in water.
  - Emergency exit windows may be heavy to lift.
- Extrication.
  - Requires extra training by rescue personnel as roofs are reinforced, seats are closer together making it more difficult to enter and extract.

Bus and coach collisions

- Compared with automobiles, buses have a larger mass and lower center of gravity.
- Fatalities often are the result of ejection.
- Occupants seated within the direct line of impact are most severely injured.
- Rollovers are most dangerous.
- Mechanisms of injury.
  - Projection: interactions/collisions between passengers inside the coach.
  - Ejection or partial ejection.
  - Intrusion/structural deformation.
- Bus versus coach. See Table 72.1.

Table 72.1 Comparison of Bus and Coach Collisions

Bus	Coach
• City bus	• Touring or traveling long distances
• Urban	• Greater speeds
• Lower speed	• Seated passengers
• More likely to have an incident	• More serious incidents
• More internal movement of passengers	• May be in rural or remote locations
• More passengers standing	• Charter buses may be full of elderly passengers
• Standing passengers: worse injuries. Head is heavier—it tilts the body forward, impact is with the cranium.	

School bus collisions
- Black stripes on school buses are impact rails to absorb energy.
- Occupants seated within direct line of impact are also the most severely injured.
- Rollovers cause the most injuries.
- Head, neck, shoulder injuries most predominant in rollovers.
- May be challenging for prehospital personnel or medical centers not accustomed to seeing and treating children.
- May also have a very detrimental effect psychologically.

Terrorist bombings involving buses

Characteristics
- Setting.
  - Usually city bus, urban environment, busy, populated time, and environment.
- Mechanism.
  - Suicide bombers versus remote detonation—Suicide bombers tend to be more precise in their targets and timing.
  - Usually employ improvised explosive devices (IEDs).
  - Often are packed with fragments of metal, such as nails, screws, bolts, ball bearings.
  - May also be contaminated with hazardous material.
- Scene Safety
  - Secondary devices may be planted to be detonated later, intending to injure responders.
  - Perpetrators, assailants, sharpshooters.
  - Structural or building collapse.
  - Contaminated patients, environment, or air.

Principles of response
- Personal Protective Equipment (PPE).
- Incident Command System (ICS).
- Contain the scene.
  - Crime scene—limit access in or out.
  - May be difficult as typically urban environment.
- Decontamination.
  - If necessary.
- Preserve evidence.
- Triage.
- Identify and account for victims.
- Patient self-referral.
  - Up to 75 percent of patients will self-refer to hospital.
  - ½ of casualties will present in first hour after event
  - Severely injured present later.

Injury patterns
- Injury type will depend on:
  - Magnitude of blast.
  - Nature of device.
  - Method of delivery.
  - Presence of shrapnel.
    - High-mass objects can cause great damage.
  - Confined versus open space.
    - Pressure waves are reflected off walls.
  - Distance.
  - Effect of blast waves inversely related to third power of distance from explosion.
  - Protective barrier.

Types of blast injuries

- Primary injury: Blast waves → overpressure causes blunt injuries and barotraumas.
  - Only seen in certain types of explosives classified as high order.
  - Injuries may have delayed presentation.
  - Examples:
    — Blast lung (pulmonary edema).
    — Pulmonary contusion.
    — Pneumothorax.
    — Brain injury.
    — Tympanic membrane rupture.
    — Middle-ear damage (fracture or dislocation of ossicles).
    — Hollow-abdominal-organ perforation.
    — Abdominal hemorrhage.
    — Blast injury to eye: ruptured globe, serous retinitis, hyphema.
- Secondary injury: Wounds from flying debris.
  - Most likely to cause death.
  - Objects follow an unpredictable path through the body.
  - Objects do not pass through but are retained in body.
  - External signs may be minimal.
  - Clothing may offer some protection: head, neck, hands at increased risk.
  - Wounds are contaminated and may contain pieces of flesh if mechanism is suicide bomber.
    — There is no case report of transmission of a blood-borne disease in this manner.
  - Examples:
    — Penetrating injuries
    — Fractures
    — Soft tissue injury
    — Amputations—associated with significant concurrent trauma, exsanguination, and worse prognosis.
- Tertiary injury: Blast wind throws patient causing forceful impact.
  - Examples:
    — Traumatic brain injury.
    — Skull fracture.
    — Fractures.
    — Pneumothorax.
- Quaternary injury: Other injuries.
  - Examples:
    — Heat.
    — Radiation.
    — Burns.
      - Burns from the explosive itself tend to be flash burns over exposed skin.
      - More severe in confined space & if vehicle catches on fire.
    — Crush injury.
    — Crush syndrome.
      - Less likely, more often seen in building collapse.

- — Inhalation injury.
  - – Not very common.
- — Exacerbations of prior medical conditions such as asthma/ COPD, angina.
- Confined-space blast injuries
  - Carry higher mortality. Overall injuries are more severe.
  - Primary—Blast lung, hollow viscus rupture, tympanic membrane (TM) rupture.
    - — More likely to have primary blast injury than victims of open-air blasts.
    - — More likely to have pulmonary injuries than TM rupture.
  - Secondary—Penetrating injuries to head, eye, chest, abdomen.
  - Tertiary—Amputation, fractures of face, ribs, pelvis, spine.
  - Quaternary—Crush injuries, burns.
    - — Confined-space patients suffer larger burn body surface area (BSA).
- Treatment of blast injuries.
  - Transfer to a trauma center, occasionally burn center.
  - Advanced Trauma Life Support (ATLS) protocols.
  - Full exposure and examination.
  - Repeatedly reexamine patients for injuries because presentation may be delayed.
  - Pregnant women 2nd or 3rd trimester: Check for abruption & admit to Labor and Delivery (L&D) for fetal monitoring.
- Psychological Issues
  - Mass-casualty incidents are very detrimental psychologically.
  - Victims, witnesses, and responders will be affected.
  - There are immediate as well as delayed effects.
  - Psychological complaints can include normal grieving, acute stress disorder, posttraumatic stress disorder (PTSD), or depression.
  - Psychosomatic complaints may also be seen in survivors after the event.

Suggested readings

Albertsson P, Falkmer T (2005). Is there a pattern in European bus and coach incidents? A litera-ture analysis with special focus on injury causation and injury mechanisms. *Accident Analysis & Prevention* 37: 225–233.

Centers for Disease Control and Prevention (2009). Blast injuries: Fact sheets for professionals. Available at http://www.bt.cdc.gov/mass casualties/blastinjuryfacts.asp.

DePalma RG, et al. (2005). Blast injuries. *NEJM 352*: 1335–1342.

Lapner PC, Nguyen D, Letts M (2003). Analysis of a school bus collision: Mechanism of injury in the unrestrained child. *Cam J Surg 46*: 269–272.

Leibovici D, et al. (1996). Blast injuries: Bus versus open-air bombings—A comparative study of injuries in survivors of open-air versus confined-space explosions. *J of Trauma: Injury, Infection, and Critical Care 41*: 1030–1035.

National Transportation Safety Board (1999). Bus crash worthiness issues: Highway special investi-gation report—NTSB/SIR-99/06. Available at http://www.ntsb.gov/publictn/1999/SIR9904.pdf.

Fires

Ian Greenwald

Matthew Bitner

Fireground operations and evolution

To combat the inherently dangerous and often chaotic nature of structural firefighting, a systematic and stepwise approach is taken by fire/rescue crews operating on the scene of fire-related emergencies.

Fireground operations begin with a careful 360-degree scene assessment performed by the first-arriving unit(s). This assessment is succinctly broadcast to other responding units and provides:

• The type and size of structure involved (residential versus commercial).
• Fire condition present (smoke versus fire).
• Entrapment.
• Relevant hazards.

Initial unit on the scene establishes incident command until relieved by a higher-ranking officer or more appropriate unit. It is initially the responsibility of the incident commander to ensure arriving units are directed to appropriate positions on the fireground to maximize function of different types of firefighting apparatuses.

Following the initial scene assessment, fireground operations transition into a rescue mode if life or property is at immediate risk.

Most fire engines/pumpers are equipped with preconnected lightweight hoses (1½" to 1¾") that can be used to quickly mount an interior or offensive attack.

If conditions are unfavorable for an interior attack (i.e., risk of structural collapse) exterior or defensive operations are undertaken with the goal of containing and extinguishing the fire and protecting surrounding structures.

Once the primary seat of fire is extinguished and the structure is searched for fire extension, firefighters progress into a salvage and overhaul mode where the focus becomes property conservation. Overhaul is complete when all units operating on the scene are reequipped and back in service.

Common injury patterns

The occupation of firefighting has a fatality rate approximately three times that of all occupations, which places it in the top-15 occupations at risk of a fatal occupational injury. Illness and injury patterns demonstrate risk begins when fire personnel receive an initial alarm. Sudden awakening from a deep sleep to almost instantaneous maximal physical exertion and stress predisposes firefighters to sudden cardiac events on firegrounds.

Mortality statistics show that fully half of firefighter deaths on firegrounds are from nontraumatic cardiac arrest. Vehicle collisions while responding to fire emergencies represent another 20–25 percent of firefighting deaths. Offensive (interior) firefighting is the most dangerous activity on the fireground and accounts for roughly 20 percent of firefighter deaths. These deaths are attributable to:

- Firefighters becoming caught or trapped in burning structures.
- Running out of air in self-contained breathing apparatuses (SCBAs).
- Thermal injuries.
- Toxic exposures.
- Falls.
- Electrocutions.
- Drowning.

Non-life-threatening injuries include burns and smoke inhalation and a preponderance of myofascial sprains and strains, abrasions, and soft-tissue injuries. Salvage and overhaul phases of fireground operations are associated with frequent injuries, as exhaustion and complacency become major safety factors.

Exhaustion and rehabilitation

Fighting structural fires often requires prolonged on-scene operations lasting several hours and can be associated with extreme physical stress placed on firefighters. A key component of the fireground operations is the establishment of a rehabilitation sector where firefighters can rest, rehydrate, and receive basic nutritional support as well as undergo a basic medical screening exam to ensure they are safe to resume firefighting activities.

Prehospital medical providers' on-scene in a sheltered environment should follow local medical direction protocols and assess each firefighter's vital signs and query them for any complaints. Firefighters with vital signs out of predefined ranges are held back from resuming duties. Those with complaints are transported to the hospital for evaluation. It is mandatory that rehabilitation personnel have the authority and direct line of communication with incident commanders to determine who is fit to return to duty.

Inhalational injuries

Inhalational injuries are common in fire ground operations, ranging from mild to severe. There are generally two categories of injuries commonly seen: thermal injuries and toxin related injuries.

- Thermal injuries occur when the individual inhales heated or superheated air. Superheated air can occur at fire scenes because the air is filled with steam and atmospheric pressures is increased. Although thermal injuries are usually confined to the upper or conducting airways of the respiratory tract, the introduction of steam and superheated air can often result in injury to the lower tract causing an even more severe injury.
- Toxin-related injuries classically referred to smoke inhalation, the presence of carbon monoxide and oxygen depletion in the fire environment. However, smoke is a complex mixture of organic and inorganic compounds that can be an irritant, causing burning or tearing, or it may contain cellular toxins causing significant morbidity and mortality. The composition of smoke has evolved to include new dangers that have been the result of changes and advances in building technologies.

Since the 1800s there have been significant changes in structural design and building materials. With these advances have come new challenges for fire suppression. Materials are burning at higher temperatures and may smolder for longer periods of time releasing toxic substances into the environment. For example, some of the newer plastics used in construction when exposed to high temperatures can release a variety of toxic substances including:

- Highly corrosive hydrogen chloride gas.
- Lethal hydrogen cyanide gas.
- Inorganic acids.

Some of these components have been reported to contribute a significant mortality associated with smoke inhalation deaths.

Burns

Although entire careers are dedicated to the study of burns and the care of burn victims, a basic knowledge of these injuries should be reviewed. It is important to note that in the fire ground setting, one must remember to follow standards of care for evaluation of the traumatic injuries (such as the American College of Surgeons Advanced Trauma Life Support). Following a careful evaluation for other traumatic injuries, one should remember to assess the:

- Extent.
- Severity.
- Associated risk factors of the thermal injury.

The extent of burns classically refers to the calculated body surface area or BSA. This can be calculated by a variety of methods including the "rule of nines" in which the body is portioned off into areas that are fractions or multiples of 9 percent (see Figure 73.1). However, without a rapid reference, the rule of nines can be complex, especially when assessing a pediatric patient.

Some authors, therefore, advocate for the "rule of palms" (see Figure 73.2). In this rule, the palm of the patient represents approximately 1 percent of the patients BSA. However, it is important to remember that the initial evaluation of burns will underestimate the extent of the burn as the burn may not have fully declared itself and may progress with time.

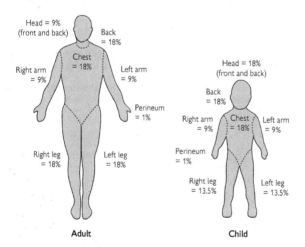

Figure 73.1 Rule of 9's to estimate percent of body surface area burned. Courtesy of Dr. Linda Markell.

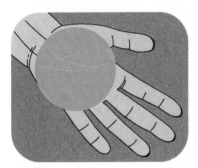

Figure 73.2 Rule of palms.

The severity of the burns again classically refers to the depth of the burn described as:

- 1st degree.
- 2nd degree.
- 3rd degree.

First degree burns are superficial burns that are red and painful and are not blistering. Second degree burns are slightly deeper, penetrating, and blister. They typically have a red base and weep freely. Third degree burns are full thickness burns and typically described as leathery, white, and anesthetic.

Remember to note that burn severity does not typically occur in isolation and various degrees of burns are found concomitantly on the same patient. For example, a 3rd degree burn may be surrounded by an area of 2nd and/or 1st degree burns.

Associated risk factors for burns include both characteristics of the burn as well as characteristics of the patient. Characteristics of the burn that are high-risk factors include location. For example, burns that involve major joints, the face, hands, or genitals are typically considered high risk. Characteristics of the patient that are high risk might include significant co-morbidities such as diabetes.

In the end, a cohesive plan must be in place in advance, to allow for triaging of burn patients to the proper facility with the resources necessary for their care.

Hazardous materials

The presence of a fire scene means that there are hazardous materials present until proven otherwise. The National Fire Protection Association (NFPA), in concert with other agencies, makes recommendations regarding the preparation for, response to, and mitigation of hazardous materials incidents.

Corrosives, hydrocarbons, choking agents, irritants, incapacitating agents, and biological agents/body substances are all potential contaminants at a fire scene.

Toxic exposures at varying doses can produce:
- Immediate or delayed effects.
- Local or systemic reactions.

Perhaps the most significant point is that one must recognize that the potential for exposure to hazardous materials exists. There are many resources that responders can utilize to identify potential threats including local poison centers, hospitals, material safety data sheets, and local hazardous materials response agencies. Additionally, work uniforms and structural firefighting protective clothing may not offer protection to all the substance that can be encountered on a fireground. Firefighters must recognize the limitations of protective equipment and take appropriate precautions.

Suggested readings

Alaire Y (2002). Toxicity of fire smoke. *Crit Rev Tox 32*: 259–289.

American Burn Association. Available at www.ameriburn.org, accessed October 2008.

Federal Emergency Management Agency (2003, April). *Guidelines for HazMat/WMD Response, Planning and Prevention Training*. Available at *www.fema.gov*

U.S. Department of Labor, Bureau of Labor Statistics. Survey of occupational injuries and illnesses. Available at http://www.bls.gov/oes (Accessed October 2008).

U.S. Fire Administration (2004, August). *Firefighter Fatalities in the United States in 1998–2004*. Washington DC.

Chapter 74

Rail disasters

Megan L. Salinas
Kerry K. McCabe

General considerations on rail disasters

Rail disasters pose many challenges for rescuers, prehospital personnel, and hospital-based health-care providers. Unique to rail disasters is the variety of situations that may occur. Some scenarios to consider include the following:

- Rail disasters can include derailment, collision, terrorism.
- Mass Casualty Incidents (MCIs).
- Commuter trains versus freight trains.
- High-speed commuter rails.
- Hazardous materials trains.
- Urban versus rural versus austere.
- Climate may play a role in the accident or the recovery/treatment.
- Challenging for rescuers, for patient care, and for the uninjured.
- Possibility of submersion.
- Passenger trains contain a mixed population—a commuter train may be carrying professionals on their way to work, the elderly, pregnant women, and children, many of whom need special consideration in their management.

Derailment or collision

- In 2007 there were 13,235 total rail crashes/incidents. Total deaths for all railroads was 846 that year, compared to 1,063 in 1997.

Derailments or collisions of passenger trains
High numbers, high speeds
- 173,000 miles of track in the United States.
- Amtrak's Acela Express travels at 135–150 mph.
- Statistics:
  - In 2007, Amtrak had 84 train crashes/incidents with 84 fatalities, or 2.12 accidents per million train miles.
- Sample Incidents:
  - September 1958: Newark Bay, New Jersey. A commuter train derailed into the bay, drowning 48 passengers.
  - September 2008: Los Angeles, California. High-speed commuter train collided with a freight train killing 25 and injuring 135 people. Fifty-one ambulances and five helicopters responded to the scene.
- Access by Responders:
  - If the train crash is on bridge or in a tunnel, responders may have to circumvent the collision, which may delay care.
  - Passengers may have exited both sides of train. Depending on the location of the accident, it may be difficult for personnel to get themselves or emergency vehicles to both sides.
- Scene Safety:
  - Always the prehospital personnel's first concern.
  - Notify Rail Controller early to stop oncoming traffic.
  - Beware of secondary fires.
    - Diesel fuel may ignite. Also, pipelines that may run alongside tracks can be involved. Contact fuel companies to shut off the running fuel.
    - Fire department will need to be involved in fire containment.
  - Electric third rail in some situations may cause additional harm.
  - Collapse of bridges that may have been structurally damaged by a collision.
    - For example, in 1998 in rural Eschede, Germany, a high- speed commuter train collided with a highway overpass causing collapse of the overpass onto the train.
  - Possible hazardous materials situation.
  - PPEs universally required.
- Incident Command System (ICS).
  - The Incident Command System needs a command center established in a secure location.
  - Involved agencies:
    - Police.
    - Fire.
      - City/County.
      - Search and Rescue.
    - EMS.
    - ± Hazardous materials teams.
    - Medical examiner.

- Communication:
  - Surrounding hospitals—communicate the occurrence of the disaster, as well as determine each hospital's capacity.
- Assistance:
  - Request assistance if local agencies are overwhelmed. State and/ or federal agencies may need to be applied to for assistance. Have prior mutual-aid agreements with other local agencies if in rural areas that may only have volunteer agencies.
  - Other agencies—for example, railroad companies may be able to provide helpful information or aid.
- Evidence:
  - Train derailments or collision need to be considered a crime scene. Do not destroy evidence, if possible, while evacuating passengers.
- Extrication:
  - Extrication of passengers may pose a significant challenge. Trains are tall, requiring ladders, particularly if the train has a second story. Stairwells may be crushed, limiting access to the second story. The walls are difficult to cut through. The safety glass of the windows is designed not to break or shatter. Underwater extrication is its own distinct challenge, requiring special teams of rescuers. All conditions require special training for fire and rescue crews. Railroad companies offer such special training.
- Triage:
  - Triage of patients should occur as in any mass-casualty incident. See Triage chapter.
- Injury patterns:
  - Blunt trauma more common.
  - Passengers on trains are more likely to be standing. These patients present with more craniofacial injuries, because their momentum continues after the train stops and the heavier cranium tilts the upper body downward toward impact.
  - Seated passengers will present with thoraco-abdominal injuries. There is a case report of a patient who was seated at table: the impact of the table with the abdomen caused an abdominal vascular injury.
  - Forward -facing patients will present with facial injuries and deceleration injuries (i.e., aortic or mesenteric avulsions).
  - Prolonged extrication time can lead to:
    — Crush syndrome—rhabdomyolysis, hyperkalemia.
    — Exposure—Hypothermia or Hyperthermia.
  - Burns.
  - Potential exposure to hazardous materials.
- Account for and identify victims.
- Noninjured patients
  - Shelter from environment, climate.
  - Food, water.
  - Communication with and between families.
- Transportation of the injured and noninjured.
  - Air, ground EMS, bus, or other train, police, military, bystanders.

- Hospital care.
  - As with any MCI.
  - ICS.
  - Triage.
  - Waiting area for minor patients, separate but near ED.
  - MCI trauma care: damage-control surgery, limited use of limited resources such as laboratory.
- Delayed goals.
  - Restore infrastructure.

Hazardous materials trains

- Background
- Railroads are required by law to transport hazardous materials.
- Statistics
  - 1.7–1.8 million carloads of hazardous materials are transported per year.
  - In 2006, 99.996 percent reached their destination without crash/ incident.
- Sample incidents:
  - January 2005: Graniteville, South Carolina. Collision of two freight trains caused the release of 11,500 gallons of chlorine gas killing 9 people, with 529 seeking treatment.
  - January 2007: Brooks, Kentucky. Twelve hazardous materials cars derailed. These cars contained 1,3-butadiene, cyclohexane, acetone, methyl ethyl ketone, and maleic anhydride, which burned all night. Fifty-three persons were treated for symptoms and 350 were evacuated, and 300 in the surrounding community were ordered to remain indoors.

Disaster management

- Obtain list of hazardous materials from the railroad company.
- Personal Protective Equipment (PPEs).
- Containment:
  - Railroads were designed to travel through the city center, thus increasing risk to residents.
  - Establish a secure zone or perimeter.
  - Air monitoring stations may be useful.
- Decontamination
  - The critical nature of victims' injuries may not allow a formal decontamination.
  - Occasionally, a hose-down between two fire engines may be the best option.
  - See chapter on decontamination techniques.
- Triage
  - Similar to other mass casualty incidents.
- Symptoms from hazardous materials exposure:
  - Eye irritation.
  - Respiratory distress or irritation.
  - Cutaneous manifestations, burns.

- Community Evacuation
  - For gases, volatiles, and fires. Rate of dispersion of chemicals is determined by vapor density and climate: temperature, humidity, wind, terrain.
  - Prompt response in urban environment is mandatory.
  - A community is less likely to be affected by gases during the wintertime if windows are closed or persons are outside for less time.
- Assistance:
  - City, county, or state fire or EMS HazMat teams.
  - American Chemistry Council supports CHEMTREC (Chemical Transportation Emergency Center) with 24-hr information and assistance.
  - Railroads have employees responsible for emergency HazMat response.
  - Environmental Protection Agency (EPA).
- Delayed goals:
  - Clean-up of contaminated soil, water, etc.

Terrorist bombings

- Madrid, Spain:
  - March 11, 2004. Ten improvised explosive devices were detonated on four commuter trains within the span of 15 minutes. The blasts caused 191 casualties and 1,824 wounded.
- Mumbai, India:

July 11, 2006. Seven explosives on seven trains detonated in 11 minutes killed 209 people. King Edward VII Memorial (KEM) hospital received the majority of the casualties, 76 patients. The first victim arrived 30 minutes after event. In the first hour, the hospital received 69 patients. KEM hospital utilized radiography extensively, but the only labs drawn were type and screens.

- Scene safety:
  - Secondary explosives may be planted to be detonated later, intending to injure rescuers and EMS personnel.
  - Bomb squad and police may need to search areas for remaining explosives to be detonated.
- Locations:
  - Train bombings are much more likely to be in urban, heavily populated areas.
  - More victims intentionally injured.
- Access:
  - Because trains are more likely to be targeted while in a city, they are more likely to be in a tunnel during the explosion.
  - Prehospital personnel may arrive on scene earlier if the explosion occurs in town.
- Injury Patterns
  - Blast injuries on trains are very similar to blast injuries on buses.
  - Similar confined space.
  - Explosives on trains may affect more victims.
  - Please see chapter on bus disasters.
- Other Notes
  - Railroads have their own Terrorism Risk Analysis and Security Management Plans that may provide some assistance.

Psychological issues

- In MCIs, the numbers of people affected by the event is increased.
- Those affected include victims, responders, train staff, and witnesses.
- There are immediate as well as delayed effects.
- Psychological complaints can include normal grieving, acute stress disorder or PTSD, or depression.
- Psychosomatic complaints may also be seen in survivors after the event.
- See Chapter 92 on survivor mental health.

Suggested readings

Cryer HG, Eckstein M, Chidester C, Raby S, Ernst TG, et al. (2010). Improved trauma system multi-casualty incident response: Comparison of two train crash disasters. *J Trauma* 68(4): 783–789.

Federal Railroad Administration Office of Safety. Available at www.safetydata.fra.dot.gov (Accessed January 27, 2011).

Chapter 75

Subway disasters

Mazen El Sayed

Andrew Milsten

Subway importance and challenges

- Subways are becoming an essential component in modern urban communities. They provide affordable, rapid, and safe transportation in major cities worldwide. Of the world's largest subway systems, each of the top eleven systems carry more than one billion passengers per year. A recent example is China's restriction of car use and the opening of a $2.3 billion subway line during the Olympics.
- The increasing number of subway riders poses various challenges, most important of which is the ability of cities to expand this transportation network rapidly while trying to fulfill the basic standards of safety.
- Another challenge is that a minor incident in a subway has the potential of becoming a disaster and overwhelming the local EMS resources by easily affecting a large number of passengers: The carrying capacity of a subway car can reach up to 250 passengers (Bombardier T1 subway car in Toronto).

Subway vulnerability and hazards

The complex infrastructure involved in the subway system and the need for reliable energy supplies make subways vulnerable to an array of hazards:

- High speed crashes, and other transportation related injuries. Subways may reach a speed of 60 mph on long stretches between stops and incidents do occur involving derailments and crashes.
- Hazards particular to a subway environment can arise partially due to limited number of underground exits as well as a dependence on ventilation systems.
  - Natural hazards, such as flooding, earthquakes, fires, and gas leaks pose peculiar dangers in underground spaces and subways where passengers and transit workers are at risk of entrapment, submersion, or suffocation. Storm-surge flooding is estimated to threaten up 30 percent of Manhattan's south side including its subway and other transportation systems in the event of a category 3 hurricane hitting New York City.
  - Physical hazards such as noise, vibration, electric shocks, and temperature extremes are present within the subway environment, and their effects on passengers and transit worker are not fully studied.
  - Man-made hazards: including biological hazards (with transmission of airborne diseases such as tuberculosis, and person- or rodent-spread diseases). There are also chemical hazards such as toxic gases, heavy metals, and gas emissions. These particles have been found to be elevated in underground spaces from metal grinding and brakes. Finally crimes ranging from vandalism to homicide as well as suicides are a threat.
  - Terrorist attacks: Radiological, chemical, or bioterrorist attacks have occurred. Subways are especially vulnerable due to lack of security measures that are applied in other mass-transit areas such as airport screening.
- Examples of subway related disasters.
  - New York subway crash in 1995 (1 death and 54 injured) and Tokyo subway train collision in 2000 (4 deaths and 30 injured).
  - King's Cross fire in London underground in 1987 (31 deaths and 60 injured): The fire caused from a discarded match started in a machine room of a wooden escalator and resulted in entrapment of passengers underground.
  - Sarin gas attack in Tokyo in 1995 (12 deaths and 5,000 injured): this event exemplifies the spread of a bioterrorist attack along a subway line from one station to the next with the subway cars serving as carriers of a highly toxic and volatile nerve agent..
  - Train bombing Madrid in 2004 (191 deaths and 2000 injured).This was Spain's worst terrorist attack when 10 bombs exploded on four packed early-morning commuter trains in Madrid.

Disaster preparedness and prevention

The vulnerability and potential hazards found in a subway system highlight the importance of disaster preparedness and prevention. Mitigation efforts should involve the different levels and components of a subway system.

- Steps involving subway network:
  - Planning of infrastructure: Disaster preparedness starts in the early stages of planning the infrastructure of the subway network. Measures include increasing the number of exits, evaluating their locations, and carefully designing all uncovered entrances to underground spaces to minimize the risks of flooding and tunneling of water into the underground network. Routes' design requires extensive study of the surrounding terrain and should take into account the possibility of natural disasters, such as landslides or earthquakes, occurring in the area where the network is being set up. Alternative routes and the ability to seal compartments in an underground system that relies on connectivity are other aspects to be considered.
  - Implementing safety measures: Noise reduction strategies, such as regular wheel maintenance and installing noise absorption systems, are present in newer subway networks. Maintaining clean and compartmentalized ventilation systems is helpful in limiting spread of airborne diseases. Installing surveillance cameras, chemical sniffers, and computer sensors linked to the command center would help with the activation of automatic predesigned protocols for evacuation measures.
  - Establishing an effective communication system that links the subway system with the command center and other EMS resources is a major component of an adequate disaster-response plan.
  - Improving existing systems is essential to cope with the technologic complexity at which new subway systems run. An example is the technology updates of the Washington DC Metro system. Installation of a sensor network and software with live feedback and streaming videos from the subway system to the transit agency and local fire departments allow early detection of an emergency and improve EMS response times.
- Steps involving EMS personnel and transit workers:
  Education and effective training of the transit worker and local EMS personnel in cities with subway systems should incorporate professional training, continuous education, and credentialing with certification programs that focus on disaster preparedness, and include:
  - Creating standardized protocols compatible with the different levels of disasters, and continuously updating and modifying these protocols. This should be done by designated committees with the input from various agencies involved in disaster response. These would include command center, subway engineers, police department, fire department, local EMS agencies and hospitals, etc.
  - Familiarizing transit workers with protocols should help minimize chaos early in the event of a disaster while the planned response is being activated.

- Conducting drills and practicing different disaster scenarios identifies problems with the implementation of predesigned protocols and weaknesses in the planned disaster response.
- Preparing evacuation plans forms an essential component in subway disaster preparedness where the confined nature of underground spaces accentuates the magnitude of minor incidents.
- Steps involving EMS and disaster preparedness agencies:
The EMS agencies response in large cities with complex subway systems should be tailored to be compatible with the underground transport development. This stems from the reasoning that "mega-cities" are more vulnerable to disasters than others with smaller demographic densities and less-complicated transport systems.
  - Education and training of EMS personnel should be addressed with a focus on disaster preparedness and disaster scenario practice.
  - EMS agencies should improve on their ability to mount a quick and effective response in the event of a disaster in addition to maintaining their regular daily activities. This requires both the compatible allocation of EMS resources relative to growth rate of underground transport and the regionalization of response teams (EMS units and hospitals) according to the disaster location within the city.
  - The incorporation of self-dispatched units from neighboring communities or states (e.g., Disaster Medical Assistance Teams [DMAT]) should be considered in the event of a major disaster to prevent overwhelming the local authorities' ability to process these teams.
  - Local hospitals should improve on their surge capacities to accommodate large numbers of victims in the event of a major crisis.
- Prevention of human-caused threats (intentional and unintentional):
The human factor is of utmost importance when it comes to discussing subway-related disasters. Vulnerabilities of subways to natural disasters can be minimized by careful planning and improving the coping capabilities. However, the implementation of measures to reduce human error from transit workers and to prevent terrorists' attacks may have a greater impact on disaster preparedness.
  - At the level of the command center, promoting transit-worker recognition and report of early mechanical or human errors as well as promoting transit-workers' well-being (fatigue awareness) can reduce the possibility of disasters from unintentional mistakes. Monitoring and continuously updating all the preceding safety measures is also the responsibility of the command center.
  - Subway passengers' involvement is essential because previous disaster events have shown that the early stages of disaster response are usually disorganized and led by the victims themselves. Public awareness regarding possible threats (bulletin boards, threat advisory) may improve early detection and reporting of suspicious activities and possible health threats. Public awareness regarding self-triage and self-transport may help limit the chaos that results from a disaster and prevent overwhelming local hospitals with minor injury victims.

- Government involvement in prevention of man-made threats has been growing since the September 11 attack and the increasing worldwide targeting of trains and subways in terrorist attacks. Through developing and implementing risk assessment and surveillance systems, providing funding and equipment to EMS agencies and mass-transit agencies, and finally involving subways and trains agencies in antiterrorism measures (such as random screening of luggage, passenger screening, or setting check points), the government can improve the immunity of subways against terrorist attacks, as is the case with air transport.

Summary

Subways form an integral part of mass transit in developed urban communities. The degree of complexity of operating a subway system and the high number of riders involved make it more vulnerable than other methods of transportation. Disaster preparedness and prevention at the different stages of subway-system development is an essential component for making subways more reliable, safe, and effective.

Suggested readings

American Public Transportation Association. Checklists for emergency response planning and system security. Available at http://www.apta.com/services/safety/checklist.cfm

Bachoual R (2007). Biological effects of particles from the Paris subway system. *Chem Res Toxicol* 20: 1426–1433.

Beijing Subway. Available at http://en.beijingology.com/index.php?title=Beijing_Subway

Colle BA, Buonaiuto F, Bowman MJ, Wilson RE, Flood R, Hunter R, Mintz A, Hill D (2008). New York City's vulnerability to coastal flooding: Storm surge modeling of past cyclones. *B Am Meteorol Soc* 89(6): 829. DOI: 10.1175/2007BAMS2401.1.

Disaster Reduction and the human cost of disaster. IRIN Web Special. Available at http://www.irinnews.org/pdf/in-depth/Disaster-Reduction-IRIN-In-Depth.pdf

Electric Railroaders' Association New York Division Bulletin. AP, *New York Times*, *New York Daily News*, *Newsday*, NY1, WCBS-AM. Available at http://www.nycsubway.org/faq/accidents.html

Federal Transit Administration. Safety and security. Available at http://transit-safety.volpe.dot.gov

Fogarty P, George P (1991). Long term effects of smoke inhalation in survivors of the King's Cross underground station fire. *Thorax* 46: 914–918.

Gershon RR, Qureshi KA, Barrera MA, Erwin MJ, Goldsmith F. (2005). Health and safety hazards associated with subways: A review. *J Urban Health* 82(1): 10–20.

Guth A, O'Neill A (2006). Public health lessons learned from analysis of New York City subway injuries. *Am J Public Health* 96: 631–633.

Jane's Urban Transport Systems (2002–2003). World's largest subway systems. Available at http://www.infoplease.com/ipa/a0762446.html

Los Angeles County Metropolitan Transportation Authority. Available at http://www.metro.net/about_us/library/library.htm

LRTA. A world of trams and urban transit. Available at http://www.lrta.org/world/worldind.html

The MTA Network. Metropolitan Transit Authority. Available at http:// www.mta.nyc.ny.us/mta/network.htm

Okumura T, Takasu N, Ishimatsu S, et al (1996). Report on 640 victims of the Tokyo subway sarin attack. *Ann Emerg Med* 28: 129–135.

Samsone, Gene (1997). *Evolution of New York City Subways: An Illustrated History of New York City's Transit Cars, 1867–1997.* New York: New York Transit Museum Press.

Timeline: Madrid Investigation. Available at http://news.bbc.co.uk/2/hi/europe/3597885.stm

Tokyo Rapid Transit Authority. Available at http://archives.cnn.com/2000/ASIANOW/east/03/07/tokyo.train.05/index.html

Toronto Transit Commission (1998). Subway car: Aluminum class T-1 cars (AC Propulsion). [Pamphlet].

Air and Sea

Aviation disasters

Peter John Cuenca

Jimmy Cooper

Paul T. Mayer

John McManus

Introduction

Aviation travel has significantly progressed in the 100 years of flight history to become the safest form of transportation. In 2007, Americans traveled on over 11 million flights on which there were 91 aviation crashes/incidents. Although aviation accidents are rare, the consequences can be devastating. The tremendous forces involved and with aircraft capacities exceeding 500 passengers create the potential for an instant mass-casualty event. The deadliest disaster in aviation history occurred on March 27, 1977. Known as the Tenerife disaster, 583 people died when a KLM Boeing 747 attempted take-off and collided with a taxiing Pan Am 747 at Los Rodeos Airport.

Epidemiology

Communities near airports must remain vigilant in preparation for response to air-crash emergencies. Approximately 80 percent of all aviation crashes/incidents occur during takeoff or landing, and are often described as resulting from human error. Midflight disasters are rare.

Analysis of National Transportation Safety Board (NTSB) aviation-incident data between 1995 and 2004 revealed that the incident rate for large commercial airlines remained relatively constant at 0.3 to 0.5 incidents per 100,000 departures. The number of incidents has ranged from 30 to 56 per year, with the majority of these being nonfatal injury-only or damage-only incidents. Major and serious aviation crashes/incidents were uncommon (5–16%) with a combined average of 2–6 per year over the 10-year period. The survivability of serious incidents remained relatively high over the decade. There was only 1 fatal incident (5%) out of 19 serious aviation incidents with substantial aircraft damage. However, major crashes with destruction of the aircraft have extremely low survival rates. Review of 18 fatal accidents from 1994 to 2004 showed that there were no survivors in 11 crashes. The 7 incidents with survivors revealed a wide range of fatality rates from 0.3 percent to 98 percent.

Incident actions

Response to aviation accidents follow disaster operation procedures for mass casualty events. Initial actions are dedicated to emergency response by the fire department, law enforcement, and emergency medical services. The Unified Command Post should be established to manage on-scene activities of the incident. An aircraft crash may be scattered over a large geographical area, which may require multiple command posts for scene control. Multiple-casualty incidents in aviation can occur in the remote setting of an airport, which is a restricted space. Access for responders needs to be considered in the disaster planning for the local area. If the aviation accident involves an international flight, emergency personnel must consider news media interest, information flow, and language barriers. As much information as possible, as early as possible, should be given to the ground authorities via the Air Traffic Control or directly to Emergency Services with radio or satellite phone links. Emergency Medical Dispatch should consider direct helicopter transfer to trauma centers after triage. Ground ambulance transfers should be used for the walking wounded after triage.

- After scene stabilization, the National Transportation Safety Board (NTSB) will begin investigative procedures, which may last days to months. They are the lead agency responsible for coordinating the investigation. The Federal Aviation Administration (FAA), law-enforcement agencies and involved airlines are all critical players and aid the investigative process. In today's security situation, all aviation emergencies need to consider terrorist activities as a cause of the incident. If it is determined that a criminal act has occurred, then the Federal Bureau of Investigation assumes the lead role and coordinates efforts in response to potential terrorism.

Clinical aspects

Aviation crashes result in multisystem traumatic injuries from a combination of burns and blunt and penetrating forces. Emergency medical response should focus on the fundamentals of trauma and burn resuscitation to those that survive. A review of 446 large commercial aircraft incidents from 1995 to 2004 revealed that 203 (46%) resulted in nonfatal but serious injuries. Serious injuries were defined as any injury that required hospitalization for more than 48 hours; fracture of any bone (except simple fractures of fingers, toes, or nose); severe hemorrhages; nerve, muscle, or tendon damage; internal organ injury; second- or third-degree burns, or any burns affecting more than 5 percent of the body surface.

Blunt and penetrating forces are the primary mechanisms of injury. Review of 452 fatalities in 289 aircraft crashes/incidents found that polytrauma with vital-organ injury was the most commonly encountered gross pathology finding on postmortem examination. Traumatic pneumonosis (74.8%) and hemorrhage in vital organs (43%) were the common histopathological findings. There is limited data on the distribution of specific injuries in survivors. Injury data coded from discharge summaries for 83 plane crash survivors admitted to 14 different hospitals revealed that

33% sustained intracranial, 39% thoracic, and 27% abdominal/pelvic injuries. Thirty-five percent had spinal fractures, 40% upper-limb fractures, and 70% lower-limb fractures.

Fire and smoke cause significant morbidity and mortality for passengers especially within the confined space of an aircraft. They are a major cause of death from what may have been a survivable crash. Serious inhalation injuries may result from the fire and explosion on impact or exposure to toxic fumes. Initially innocuous appearing throat irritations need to be triaged rapidly and urgently evaluated for early aggressive airway management. Additionally, carbon monoxide poisoning is a major risk for those passengers exposed to smoke and unable to rapidly egress. Patients with respiratory or neurologic symptoms need emergency stabilization and evaluation of carboxyhemoglobin levels.

Barotrauma and hypoxia can occur with rapid decompression of aircraft due to loss of hull integrity and rapid descent. Passengers may experience acute pain as gases trapped within their bodies expand and contract. The most common problems occur with air trapped in the middle ear or paranasal sinuses, which may result in tympanic membrane or sinus rupture. Pain may also be experienced in the gastrointestinal tract with potential for hollow-viscus rupture. The most serious injury is lung barotrauma from the rapidly increasing ambient pressure. This may cause rupture of lung tissue leading to pneumothorax and air-gas embolism.

Key points

- The majority of large commercial aircraft crashes/incidents are nonfatal injury-only or damage-only. Major and serious aviation incidents are uncommon (5–16% of total incidents).
- Survivability of serious crashes/incidents with significant aircraft damage is high, with up to 95% of the serious incidents having no fatalities. However, major crashes with aircraft destruction have extremely low survivability.
- Blunt and penetrating forces are the primary mechanisms of injury. Thermal injuries are also a major cause of morbidity and mortality. Inhalational injury and carbon monoxide poisoning should be considered during the trauma evaluation. Additionally, barotrauma may occur with rapid decompression.
- Terrorist activities may be associated with aircraft crashes. Survivors may need to be questioned and evaluated by law enforcement officials.

Suggested readings

Kramer CF, Thode HC, Kahn J, et al (1995). Adequacy of hospital discharge data for determining trauma morbidity patterns. *Journal of Trauma-Injury Infection & Critical Care* 39(5): 935–940.

Madan R, Subramanya H, Jalpota YP (2006). Retrospective analysis of fatal aircraft accident investigations during the period 1975–2004 : A reality check. *Ind J Aerospace Med* 50(1): 2.

National Transportation Safety Board. Accidents, fatalities, and rates, 2007 preliminary statistics, U.S. aviation. Available at http://www.ntsb.gov/aviation/Table1.htm

NTSB (2007). Annual review of aircraft accident data: U.S. air carrier operations calendar year 2004. Report no. ARC-08-01. Available at http://www.ntsb.gov/publictn/2008/ARC0801.pdf

NTSB. Accidents involving passenger fatalities U. S. airlines (Part 121) 1982–present. Available at http://www.ntsb.gov/aviation/Paxfatal.htm

Helicopter disasters

Peter John Cuenca
Jimmy Cooper
Paul T. Mayer
John McManus

Introduction

Helicopters offer the ability to takeoff and land vertically, hover for extended periods of time, and provide outstanding handling properties under low-airspeed conditions. Vertical flight is an exclusive engineering feat that only helicopters can offer. Today, helicopter uses include transportation, construction, firefighting, search and rescue, and military uses. Because they operate at relatively lower altitudes than airplanes, they are exposed to many hazards beyond those of other flight vehicles. This exposure has led to a higher accident rate for helicopters. In comparison to airplanes, average helicopter crash/incident rate is 7.5 per 100,000 hours of flying, whereas airplane accident rate is approximately 0.175 per 100,000 flying hours.

Based on 2004 United States rates with an estimated 2,225,000 total flight hours, the civilian helicopter crash/incident rate per 100,000 flight hours is 8.09 with a fatal incident rate of 1.48. U.S. civil turbine helicopter crash/incident rate was 5.11 per 100,000 flight hours with a fatal incident rate of 1.21. In comparison, the U.S. Air Carrier incident rate in 2004 was only 0.159 with a fatal incident rate of 0.011. Another relevant comparison is the U.S. general aviation crash statistics to civil helicopter statistics. In 2004 the general aviation rate was 6.22 as opposed to 8.09 for helicopters. In other words, the helicopter crash rate was 30 percent higher. Because helicopters are more prone to crash/incidents, it is important for healthcare providers to have an understanding of the injury patterns that occur with these events.

EPIDEMIOLOGY **643**

Epidemiology

Understanding the epidemiology of helicopter injuries is important. The U.S. Army found that, although 95 percent of the major helicopter crashes/ incidents are survivable, 22 percent of the deaths in all helicopter incidents occur in survivable conditions. Injury patterns in rotary-wing aircraft wire-strike incidents were reviewed by the U.S. Army Safety Center to determine mechanisms of injury. This data revealed that between January 1974 and August 1981 there were 167 wire strikes involving Army helicopters resulting in 60 injuries and 34 fatalities. Updated data on all military rotary-wing aircraft incidents investigated between 1978 and 1982 were analyzed by the Division of Aerospace Pathology to determine the mechanisms of injury to flight-deck personnel. From December 13, 1978 to June 23, 1982, three types of rotary-wing aircraft were in eight fatal crashes. These mishaps accounted for 28 casualties: 14 fatalities, and 14 injuries. Injury pattern analysis revealed:

- Pilots comprised 64.4 percent of the fatalities.
- 100 percent had major head and neck injuries.
- 66 percent having basilar skull fractures.
- Two-thirds had associated mandibular fractures or evidence of impact forces transmitted through the mandible to the skull.
- The same number had wedge-shaped chin lacerations from impact with the cyclic control stick.

Detailed information on the pattern and nature of injuries retrieved from the Federal Aviation Administration's autopsy database for 84 pilots involved in fatal helicopter incidents from 1993 to 1999 identified blunt trauma as the primary cause of death in 88% percent of cases. The most common bone injuries were fractures of the ribs (73.8%), skull (51.2%), facial bones (47.6%), tibia (34.5%), thorax (32.1%), and pelvis (31.0%). Most common organ/visceral injuries included injury to the brain (61.9%), lung (60.7%), liver (47.6%), heart (41.7%), aorta (38.1%), and spleen (32.1%). Injury patterns did not appear to be related to the age of the pilot or the phase of flight of the aircraft. Medical records of 52 aircrew involved in nonfatal helicopter accidents during the period of 2000–2006 were analyzed by the Indian Air Force. Fourteen percent of these personnel did not suffer any injury. Of the 45 aircrew who suffered some form of injury, 8 had multiple injuries resulting in a total of 53 injuries. Of these, 43.4 percent were spinal injuries (n=23) followed by head and face (22.6%, n=12). Sixteen aircrew members sustained 28 vertebral fractures, majority of them located in the thoraco-lumbar region. Although the pilots sustained more spinal injuries, head and face injuries were the leading injuries sustained by the nonpilot aircrew.

Clinical approach

The clinical approach to helicopter disaster patients should follow the standard Advanced Trauma Life Support (ATLS) guidelines as set forth by the American College of Surgeons. The first part of assessing these patients involves a good primary survey assessing patients' airway, breathing and ventilation, circulation with hemorrhage control, disability (neurologic status), and exposure/environmental control. Identification of life-threatening injuries should be performed and simultaneous resuscitation begun.

• *Airway maintenance with cervical spine protection:* The first stage of the primary survey is to assess the airway. If the patient is able to talk, the airway is likely to be clear. If the patient is unconscious, he/she may not be able to maintain his/her own airway. The airway can be opened using a chin lift or jaw thrust. Airway management to include intubation may be required. The high incidence of injury to the mandible in this type of accident should prompt the provider to mange any airway problems quickly and decisively. Difficult airway management techniques such as alternative laryngoscope blades, awake intubation, blind intubation (oral or nasal), fiberoptic intubation, utilizing an intubating stylet, laryngeal mask airway as an intubating conduit, light wand, retrograde intubation, combitube, rigid ventilating bronchoscope, transtracheal jet ventilation, and surgical airway (cricothyroidotomy). While managing the airway, the cervical spine must be maintained in the neutral position to prevent secondary injuries to the spinal cord. As mentioned earlier, data from helicopter accidents in the past demonstrates that those involved with these events are very likely to sustain injuries to the skull, face, jaw, and cervical spine. The neck should be immobilized using a semirigid cervical collar, blocks, and tape.

• *Breathing and ventilation:* The chest must be examined by inspection, palpation, percussion, and auscultation. Subcutaneous emphysema and tracheal deviation must be identified if present. Life-threatening chest injuries, including tension pneumothorax, open pneumothorax, flail chest and massive hemothorax must be identified and rapidly treated. Flail chest, penetrating injuries, and bruising can be recognized by inspection. Injuries to the lung and thoracic cage, including rib fractures should be sought in helicopter-crash victims.

• *Circulation with hemorrhage control:* Hypotension following injury in a helicopter must be assumed to be due to blood loss until proven otherwise. Two large-bore intravenous lines should be established or, if unable to, central venous access should be obtained and crystalloid solution given. If the patient does not respond to this, type-specific blood or O-negative, if type-specific is not available, should be transfused. External bleeding is controlled by direct pressure. Occult blood loss may be into the chest, abdomen, pelvis, or from the long bones especially with high incidence of visceral injury in helicopter-crash victims. Focused Abdominal Sonography for Trauma (FAST) allows rapid and noninvasive determination of the presence of free intra-abdominal fluid. All helicopter-crash patients whose vital signs are stable, should have an assessment for visceral injury to the chest and abdomen with a computed axial tomography scan (CAT or CT scan).

- *Disability (neurologic evaluation)*: A rapid neurological evaluation is performed at the end of the primary survey. Establish the patient's level of consciousness, pupillary size and reaction, lateralizing signs, and spinal cord injury level. The Glasgow Coma Scale is a quick method to determine the level of consciousness, and is predictive of patient outcome. If not done in the primary survey, it should be performed as part of the more detailed neurologic examination in the secondary survey. An altered level of consciousness indicates the need for immediate reevaluation of the patient's airway, oxygenation, ventilation, and perfusion status, as well as assessment with a CT scan of the head. Hypoglycemia, and drugs including alcohol, may also influence the level of consciousness. If these are excluded, changes in the level of consciousness must be considered due to traumatic brain injury until proven otherwise.
- *Exposure/environmental control*: The patient should be completely undressed, usually by cutting off the garments. It is imperative to cover the patient with warm blankets to prevent hypothermia in the emergency department. Intravenous fluids should be warmed and a warm environment maintained.

Upon completion of the primary survey, after resuscitative efforts are well established, and the vital signs are normalizing, the secondary survey can begin. The secondary survey is a head-to-toe evaluation of the trauma patient, including a complete history and physical examination, including the reassessment of all vital signs. Each region of the body must be fully examined. X-rays indicated by examination are obtained. Particular attention to the thoraco-lumbar spine should be made and films of this area performed given the high incidence of injury to this area in helicopter-crash patients. If at any time during the secondary survey the patient deteriorates, another primary survey is performed as a potential life threat may be present.

Key points

- Helicopter disasters produce patients with significant injuries.
- Health-care providers faced with such patients should maintain a high clinical suspicion for injury to the head, brain, cervical and thoracolumbar spine, and visceral injury.
- Immediate airway management with cervical spine immobilization, prompt identification of head injuries, and prompt identification and resuscitation of chest and abdominal injuries and associated hemorrhage should of high priority for providers.

Suggested readings

Farr WD, Ruehle CJ, Posey DM, Wagner GN (1985). Injury pattern analysis of helicopter wire strike accidents. *Aviation, Space, and Environmental Medicine* 56(12): 1216–1219.

Helicopter Association International. Annual U.S. helicopter safety statistics. Available at http://www.rotor.com/Default.aspx?tabid=597

International Helicopter Safety Symposium September 26–29, 2005, Montreal, Quebec, Canada. Executive Summary. Available at http://www.vtol.org/pdf/IHSSSummary.pdf.

Jeevarathinam S, Taneja N, Dahiya YS (2007). A retrospective analysis of injuries among aircrew involved in helicopter accidents. *Indian Journal of Aerospace Medicine* 51(2): 48–53.

Mattox KL (1967). *Injury Experience in Army Helicopter Accidents.* Fort Rucker, AL: Army Board for Aviation Accident Research.

Taneja N, Wiegmann DA (2003). Analysis of injuries among pilots killed in fatal helicopter accidents. *Aviation, Space, and Environmental Medicine* 74(4): 337–341.

Ship disasters

Bradley Younggren

Definition

A ship disaster is any event occurring to a water-borne vessel, which puts the integrity of the vessel, the safety of the cargo, or the safety of the personnel on board at risk.

Background

Ship disasters are not relegated to the tales of antiquity or the black and white photos of turn-of-the-century passenger-ship survivors. In modern times, the record for lives lost at sea in peacetime in a single incident is held by the sinking of the passenger ferry *Dona Paz*, in December 1987 with an estimated 3,132 lives lost. Larger loss of life has occurred in war-time, and though exact numbers are difficult to establish, the sinking of the German liner *Wilhelm Gustloff* in January 1945 resulted in a loss of nearly 10,000 lives. In comparison, in the more famous case of the *Titanic*, 1,489 lives were lost. In a 20-year period between 1978 and 1998, ferry travel was found to be 10 times more dangerous than air travel, and in the developing world, ferry disasters account for the largest loss of life at sea.

Common causes of ship disasters

- Storms.
- Mechanical failure.
- Collisions/grounding.
- Capsizing/foundering.
- Fire/explosions.
- Human error: crew inexperience, poor training, navigation errors, underestimating weather hazards or ship capabilities.
- Piracy and terrorism.

Prevention

Reducing death and injuries associated with ship disasters is best accomplished through preparedness. The International Maritime Organization requires all ships to have a safety and disaster plan, and all ships must have an adequate number of lifeboats stocked with food, water, and medical supplies. Because disasters can occur with amazing rapidity, crew and passenger training and disaster drills are imperative to enable immediate use of emergency equipment (personal flotation devices, life rafts, etc) and to understand actions required in the event of emergency. Additionally, preparations for the next stage of shipboard disaster management should proceed as soon as an emergency has been identified. Communication with surrounding vessels, shore facilities and the Coast Guard should occur immediately to summon aid and improve chances of location and survival in the event of a sinking. Additionally, with issues related to unsafe cargo and piracy, ship security is an increasing component in maritime disaster prevention.

Injuries associated with ship disasters

The most common causes of death are drowning/immersion injuries followed by hypothermia due to exposure to the elements. Other potential injuries include blunt and penetrating trauma from shifting cargo, collisions, or even the capsizing of the vessel. Blast injuries can occur while on the ship, or while floating in the water after the initial incident. Injuries also occur from burns, smoke inhalation, or contamination from oil or other hazardous cargo. Specific injuries germane to ship disasters are covered in detail in the following sections.

Immersion

Four stages of risk are associated with immersion and are caused by cooling of different body regions, starting at the skin and proceeding to deeper tissues. All stages can lead to significant physical or mental impairment which predispose the immersion victim to aspiration and eventual drowning.

Initial responses (0–3 minutes)

Sometimes known as cold-shock response, skin exposure to cold causes immediate vasoconstriction with a subsequent sudden rise in heart rate and blood pressure. Cardiac arrhythmias or ischemia may occur from this sudden increase in work and from catecholamine release or competing vagal stimulation from the dive reflex. Respiratory drive increases involuntarily, and hyperventilation can lead to confusion and contribute to panic. Breath-holding time is significantly reduced and may lead to entrapment within a vessel or aspiration in the first several minutes following immersion.

Short-term responses (3–30 minutes)

Decreasing temperature of muscle, nerves, and joints cause significant reductions in muscle mechanics, nerve conduction, and manual dexterity. This can lead quickly to swim failure or the inability to board a life raft, activate emergency signaling equipment, or perform other life-sustaining tasks.

Long-term responses (>30 minutes)

The thermal conductivity of water is 24 times that of air, and victims immersed in water cool five times more quickly than victims in air at the same temperature. At a brain temperature of 34°C, consciousness becomes impaired, and at 30°C, consciousness is lost. At a cardiac temperature around 32°C, cardiac arrest may occur through ventricular fibrillation. These effects can easily lead to incapacitation and drowning.

Postimmersion responses (during and after rescue)

Roughly 20 percent of immersion victims die shortly before, during, or immediately after rescue. This circumrescue collapse is not completely understood, but it is likely related to the following mechanisms:
- Aggravation of hemorrhage from previous traumatic injury during rescue or with increase in blood pressure.
- Rapid rewarming leading to rewarming collapse.

- Arrhythmia and myocardial ischemia from increased work during rescue.
- Blood pressure collapse from:
  - Hypovolemia secondary to cold diuresis.
  - Reintroduction of gravity on removal from the water.
  - Loss of hydrostatic pressure assisting venous return.

Near drowning

Near drowning is *survival* after aspiration of fluid into the lungs and may occur with volumes as little as 250–500 ml. Aspiration of small amounts of water can damage lung surfactant and lead to small localized areas of collapse. Irritation of lung tissue from contact to water will produce an inflammatory reaction leading to pulmonary edema, which is worsened by osmotic pressure from seawater. The net effect is a decrease in lung-surface area available for gas exchange and the eventual fall in oxygen content in the blood. Rescued victims that have aspirated small quantities of water may initially have no respiratory distress, but may deteriorate over minutes to hours from alveolar collapse and pulmonary edema.

Drowning

Drowning is *death* through suffocation by submersion, though total submersion of the head is not necessary to produce drowning. The lethal dose of aspirated seawater in humans is 22 ml/kg (about 1.5 liters for 70 kg person). Wave splash from waves breaking against the front of a life jacket and washing over the mouth and nose is sufficient to cause drowning.

Injuries associated with delayed rescue

Patients who have a delay in rescue but are able to either remain on a lifeboat or debris will have additional medical problems requiring immediate attention. Dehydration and sunburn can be a significant problem in the victim. Hypothermia from prolonged exposure to the cold air or even frostbite can be seen. Additionally, water-saturated footwear can result in "immersion foot." Malnutrition and behavioral disturbances may also be seen in these victims.

Evacuation and initial treatment

Unless support vessels are nearby or the disaster occurs close to land, evacuation time is likely to be prolonged. Weather may hinder aerial evacuation, casualty recovery by other vessels in rough seas, or the ability of rescuers to locate survivors. Incapacitation from the previously listed stages of immersion-related injury will hinder casualty participation in their own rescue. Immediate treatment goals and evacuation considerations include the following:

- Prevention and treatment of near drowning is the immediate goal at the rescue site with emphasis on maintenance of airway and assisted ventilation and/or oxygenation if possible.
- Cardiac arrest will be difficult to detect, and CPR will be difficult to perform until rescuers can get to more stable treatment platform, and, in general, CPR should not be attempted.
- Horizontal positioning during evacuation and careful handling whenever possible should be attempted to reduce the risk of circumrescue collapse.
- Proper positioning on rescue vessels to minimize risk of hypotension.
  - Helicopter: head forward.
  - Small vessel: feet forward.
  - Recovery position whenever possible to decrease risk of aspiration.
- Prevention of further heat loss if possible.
- Rewarming to commence once aboard a more secure vessel. In general, passive or assisted passive rewarming at a rate of $0.5-1°C$ per hour is safest until a definitive care facility is reached.

Receiving casualties

Receiving facilities will likely have time to prepare for receipt of casualties because of the distance and time involved in evacuation. Special consideration should be paid to the vessel type, cargo, number of crew or passengers, current weather conditions, and facility capacity while planning receipt of casualties. Arrangements should be made to disperse casualties to nearby facilities if mass casualties are expected. Preparations to care for near drowning, trauma, and hypothermia victims should be prioritized. Anticipate the need for advanced airway management and ventilator support as well as active rewarming measures.

Indications for hospital admission

- Persistent changes in mental status.
- Evidence of persistent hypothermia.
- Significant burns from fire or sun exposure.
- Obvious blast injuries or concern for blast injury.
- Near drowning or significant immersion injury.

Conclusion

Though technology and safety standards have decreased loss of life from ship disasters in the developed world, significant deaths are occurring in the developing world. Wartime disasters notwithstanding, ferry disasters have become the most common type of maritime disaster seen in the world. Factors such as inclement weather, overcrowding of vessels, improper cargo storage, and use of substandard or damaged vessels all contribute to ship disasters. Future risks to safety on the high seas are difficult to predict, but terrorism and piracy are already on the rise. Preparation for potential disaster remains the best policy to prevent loss of life in the setting of ship disasters.

Suggested readings

Antosia R (2006). Maritime disasters. In Antosia R, Cahill J, eds. *Handbook of Bioterrorism and Disaster Medicine*, pp. 193–194. New York: Springer Science and Business Media.

Gans L (2006). Maritime disasters. In Ciottone G, ed. *Disaster Medicine*, 3rd ed., pp. 179–881. Phildadelphia, PA: Mosby.

Golden F, Tipton M (2002). *Essentials of Sea Survival*. Frank Golden and Michael Tipton, USA.

Keatinge W R (1965). Death after shipwreck. *British Medical Journal* 2: 1537–1540.

Lawson C (2005). Ferry transport: The realm of responsibility for ferry disasters in developing nations. *Journal of Public Transportation* 8(4): 17–28.

McKnight J, Becker W, Pettit A, et al. (2007). Human error in recreational boating. *Accident Analysis and Prevention* 39: 398–405.

Newman A (1995). Submersion incidents. In Auerbach, ed., *Wilderness Medicine*, 3rd ed., pp. 1209–1230. St. Louis, MO: Mosby.

Oslund S, Brooks C (1995). Survival at sea. In Auerbach, ed., *Wilderness Medicine*, 3rd ed., pp. 1251–1294. St. Louis, MO: Mosby.

Schitzer P, Landen D, Russell J (1993). Occupational injury deaths in Alaska's fishing industry, 1980 through 1988. *American Public Health* 8(5): 685–688.

Natural Disasters

Natural disasters: an overview

Susan Miller Briggs

Introduction

Natural disasters are the result of natural hazards that affect the environment, resulting in significant mortality and morbidity as well as devastating environmental and economic damage. Worldwide, a major disaster occurs almost daily and climate-related disasters requiring international assistance for affected populations occur almost weekly. Floods are one of the most frequent types of natural disasters statistically, whereas earthquakes cause the greatest number of deaths and economic losses.

Vulnerability is an important parameter in determining the impact of a natural disaster. A climate-related hazard will never result in a natural disaster in regions without vulnerability, such as a strong earthquake or volcanic eruption in an uninhabited region of the world. It is anticipated that the number of natural disasters will increase dramatically over the next decade due to increasing population densities in disaster-prone regions (floodplains, vulnerable coastal regions, and near dangerous faults in the earth's crust).

Classification of natural disasters

Natural disasters may be classified as sudden-impact (acute) onset disasters or chronic-onset (slow) disasters. Sudden-onset disasters include the following:

- Earthquakes.
- Tsunamis.
- Tornados.
- Floods.
- Tropical cyclones, hurricanes and typhoons.
- Volcanic eruptions.
- Landslides and avalanches.
- Wildfires.

Chronic-onset disasters include:

- Famine.
- Drought.
- Pest infestation.
- Deforestation.

The following list of deadly natural disasters over the last century illustrates the diversity of natural hazards causing significant loss of human life (estimated death tolls). See Figures 79.1 and 79.2.

- 1931 floods (China): 1,000,000–2,500,000.
- 1970 Bhola cyclone (East Pakistan): 500,000.
- 1976 Tangshan earthquake (China): 300,000.
- 1991 Bangladesh cyclone: 138,000.
- 2004 Indian Ocean Tsunami (Indonesia): 230,000+.
- 2008 Cyclone Nargis (Myanmar): 138,000+.
- 2010 Haiti Earthquake: 220,000+.

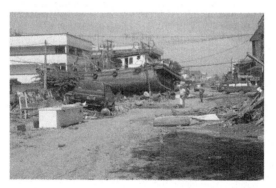

Figure 79.1 Tsunami, Indonesia (2004).

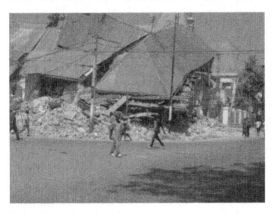

Figure 79.2 Haiti earthquake (2010).

The underlying natural causes of disasters have not changed over the last century. However, the major factors contributing to such disasters, especially in developing countries, are increasing in frequency and severity and include:
- Rapid population growth, especially in low-income populations.
- Environmental degradation resulting from poor land use.
- Human vulnerability resulting from social inequality and poverty.

Sudden-onset natural disasters generally cause significant morbidity and mortality immediately as a direct result of the primary event (e.g., traumatic injuries, crush injuries, drowning) whereas slower-onset disasters cause mortality and morbidity through prolonged secondary effects (e.g., infectious disease outbreaks, dehydration, malnutrition).

Infectious diseases are a prolonged secondary effect of many types of natural disasters (e.g., earthquakes, hurricanes, tsunamis). This situation commonly occurs when there is an interruption of health services, resulting from destruction or lack of predisaster medical and public-health facilities. It is difficult to predict the risk of infectious disease outbreaks after a disaster based only on the magnitude of the disaster. Four factors are important:
- Exposure to new pathogens introduced into a community without preexisting immunity (e.g., floods introducing fungi and mold).
- Altered susceptibilities (e.g., drinking water contamination, increased exposure to vector-borne diseases).
- Increased transmissibility (respiratory and gastrointestinal diseases from populations clustered in close proximity).
- Endemic pathogens (incidence often increases after a natural disaster).

The risk for outbreaks after disasters is low if the medical and public health infrastructure are intact. The risk factors for infectious disease outbreaks are primarily associated with population displacements. Access to safe water and sanitation, the degree of overcrowding, the underlying health status of the population, and the availability of medical and public-health services influence the risk for communicable diseases and death in the affected populations.

Communicable diseases associated with natural disasters include:

- Water-related communicable diseases (diarrheal diseases, cholera, leptospirosis, hepatitis A and E).
- Diseases associated with overcrowding (measles).
- Vector-borne diseases (e.g., malaria, dengue).
- Other diseases (e.g., tetanus, fungal infections).

Psychological trauma and other adverse psychological sequelae are frequently the side effects of natural disasters. These include post-traumatic stress disorder (PTSD), depression, alcohol and substance abuse, domestic violence, suicide, and anxiety. Not all disasters have the same level of psychological impact. Sudden impact disasters have a higher incident of psychological disorders, including PTSD. Disaster characteristics that seem to have the most significant mental- health impact share the following characteristics:

- Little or no warning.
- Serious threat to personal safety.
- Potential unknown health effects.
- Uncertain duration of the event.
- Physical and psychological proximity to the event.
- Exposure to gruesome or grotesque situations.
- Diminished health status.
- Trauma history.
- Degree of community disruption.
- Predisaster family and stability.
- Sensitivity of recovery efforts.

Numerous factors influence mortality and morbidity in natural disasters. Many factors are common to all natural disasters. The following summary highlights the major factors impacting death and injury/disease rates in specific natural disasters.

Earthquakes

Major earthquakes have the potential to be one of the most catastrophic natural disasters. More than a million earthquakes occur worldwide each year, an average of two each minute. Earthquakes of significant size threaten lives and damage property by setting off a chain of events that disrupts all aspects of the environment and significantly impacts the public health and medical infrastructures of the affected region. Earthquakes cause significant blunt and penetrating traumatic injuries. Earthquake-related factors that impact mortality and morbidity include:

• Aftershocks.
• Landslides.
• Hazardous materials.
• Fires.
• Structural factors.

Blunt and penetrating trauma caused by partial or complete collapse of buildings that were not earthquake resistant is the most common cause of injury and death in earthquakes. Demographic factors associated with increased individual risk for death and injury/ disease from earthquakes include individuals over 60 years of age, children, and chronically ill individuals. Lack of mobility, exacerbation of underlying diseases, and inability to withstand major traumatic injury contribute to the increased vulnerability of these groups. Other factors influencing mortality and morbidity are:

• Entrapment of victim (most significant prognostic factor).
• Location of victims within a building at time of disaster.
• Victim's behavior during the disaster.
• Time of rescue.

Volcanic eruptions

Volcanic activity involves the explosive eruption or flow of rock fragments and molten rock in various combinations. Volcanic activity can affect individuals located close to and far away from a volcano. Mortality and morbidity associated with these phenomena depend on the following factors:

• Magnitude of the eruption.
• Local topographic factors.
• Proximity of the population to the volcano.

Toxic gases that form during an eruption are most dangerous near craters or fissures close to the volcano. Because gravity is crucial in determining the flow of volcanic solids and dense gases, people living in low-lying areas and valleys near the volcano are at greatest risk for death and injury. The range of adverse health effects from volcanoes is quite broad. Irritant effects have been reported in the eyes, nose, skin, and upper airways of persons exposed to volcanic dusts and ash particles. Victims can have exacerbation of pre-existing pulmonary diseases or asphyxiate due to inhalation of ash or gases. Victims can sustain injuries from blasts and projectiles of rock fragments, fallen trees or rocks, and collapsed buildings.

Tropical cyclones

Tropical cyclones are among the most destructive weather systems. The terms *hurricane* and *typhoon* are regionally specific names for a strong "tropical cyclone." The impact generally extends over a wide area with deaths, injuries, and property loss resulting from heavy rains and strong winds. See Figure 79.3.

Drowning accounts for over 90 percent of cyclone-related deaths. Regions with overcrowding and inadequate housing are particularly vulnerable to cyclone-related injuries and deaths. Cyclone-related morbidity includes traumatic injuries, gastrointestinal illnesses, and dermal conditions.

Tornados

Winds associated with tornadoes can reach speeds in excess of 250 miles per hour. Agricultural areas tend to be at higher risk for the development of tornados. Individuals are injured or killed by tornadoes when they are struck by flying debris or when their bodies are thrown into stationary objects by high winds. Head injuries, soft tissue injuries and secondary wound infections are common. Stress-related disorders are common.

Risk factors for increased injury and death include:
- Mobile homes.
- Remaining in a vehicle.
- Failing to seek shelter during a tornado warning.
- Unfamiliarity with tornado warning systems.
- Attempting to go kite boarding during a tornado.

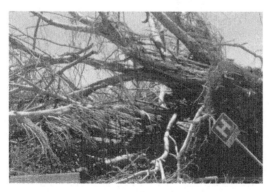

Figure 79.3 Hurricane Katrina (2005).

Floods

Floods are one of the most frequent natural disasters and may accompany other natural disasters such as hurricanes and tsunamis. Flash flooding, such as seen with excessive rainfall or sudden release of water from a dam, is the cause of most flood-related deaths. Many flood victims become trapped in their cars or homes and often drown while attempting to escape. The postdisaster recovery phase can cause significant deaths and injuries/diseases from fires, explosions, gas leaks, downed live wires, and debris. Water-borne diseases are a significant secondary hazard as are vector-borne diseases and skin conditions.

Summary

The morbidity and mortality from natural disasters, especially slow- moving disasters, is frequently underestimated. Undertriage of victims is frequently seen in natural disasters as opposed to overtriage, which is commonly seen in man-made disasters. Infectious and psychological complications are common secondary effects from natural disasters. Disaster preparedness and disaster mitigation are as important as disaster response in the management of natural disasters. Disaster recovery is the most neglected phase of the management of natural disasters. See Figure 79.4.

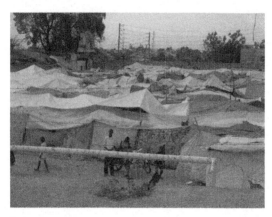

Figure 79.4 Postdisaster camps for displaced persons, Haiti Earthquake (2010).

Suggested readings

Borden KA and Cutter S (2008). Spatial patterns of natural hazards mortality in the United States. *International Journal of Health Geographics* 7:64–78.

Floret JV et al. (2006, Apr). Negligible risk for epidemics after geophysical disasters. *Emerging Infectious Diseases* 12(4):543–548.

Hogan DE and Burstein JL (2002). *Disaster Medicine*. Philadelphia: Lippincott Williams and Wilkins.

Murthy S and Christian MD (2010). Infectious diseases following disasters. *Disaster Medicine and Public Health Preparedness* 4(3): 232–238.

Noji EK, ed. (1997). *The Public Health Consequences of Disasters*. New York: Oxford University Press.

Hays WW (1990). Perspectives on the international decade for natural reduction. *Earthquake Spectra* 6:125–143.

Prager EF. (1999). *Furious Earth, The Science and Nature of Earthquakes, Volcanoes, and Tsunamis*. New York: McGraw-Hill.

Chapter 80

Avalanche

David A. Meguerdichian

Kerry K. McCabe

Background and epidemiology

Critical issues
- Pre-incident preparation
- Post-incident rapid rescue

Decisions must balance the rapid rescue of those injured against the risks to the rescue team.

Avalanche formation
- Snowflakes collect forming a temperature and pressure gradient between the warm ground and cold air.
- Water vapor moves up this gradient until it recrystalizes into a new layer termed a depth hoar—a coarse layer to which snow does not adhere well, thus allowing slippage to occur.
- Typically form above tree line on slopes with a 30–45° angle.
- Higher slopes more likely to create avalanche formation; true up to a 50° angle, at which point snow has difficulty collecting.
- More likely on north and east slopes as southern exposures receive more sunlight in Northern Hemisphere.
- Contributing weather conditions—(1) new snowfall, (2) strong winds, (3) periods of warming and thawing.

Avalanche types: two basic types:
Loose snow avalanche
- Occurs when loose, cohesionless snow cascades down mountain.
- Small amounts of snow.
- Form inverted V shape.

Slab avalanche
- Occurs when poorly anchored layer breaks away down mountain.
- Usually due to weight suddenly being applied to weak layer.
- Size depends on level of the depth hoar and amount of overlying snow.

Epidemiology
- Over 1 million avalanches annually, 100,000 in United States.
- Increased avalanche-related deaths secondary to increased popularity in winter and extreme outdoor sports in North America.
- European casualties decreasing.
- Triggered by skiers, snowboarders, climbers. and snowmobiliers.
- U.S. fatalities: snowmobiling 44 percent, skiers 24 percent, snowboarders 14 percent.
- Most occur between December and April.
- 89 percent of casualties in United States are men.
- Median age of casualties is 31.
- Median annual mortality for 17 countries represented by International Commission for Alpine Rescue (ICAR) = 146.

Event description
- Avalanches can travel at speeds of 90 to 120 km/h.
- Casualties tumble within sea of snow blocks.

- May encounter trees, rocks, or other mountain hazards during descent.
- Casualty can only attempt to grab tree or "swim out" of avalanche.
- Following halt, victim often buried under meters of packed snow.

Avalanche survival strategies

Pre-incident actions:
- Verify local weather conditions prior to back-country travel.
- Train for avalanche analysis and safety-equipment usage.
- Check avalanche hotlines if available.

Self-rescue strategies:
- During event, expand chest to prevent snow compression of thorax.
- Clear air pocket or space in front of mouth to allow for respiration.

Avalanche survival tools

Shovel
- Sturdy and lightweight.

Avalanche rescue beacons
- Developed in 1968.
- Transmit and receive electromagnetic signal at frequency of 450kHz.
- Range of approximately 30 meters.
- Transmit mode activated manually or by avalanche force.
- Ideal for buried victim with no audible or visible signs at the surface.

Long probe poles
- Collapsible devices that extend to three meters.
- Used to detect buried victims.

Artificial air pocket device (AvaLung)
- Breathing tube.
- Separates exhaled air from inhaled air once victim buried.
- Reduces fraction of CO_2 contamination from inspired air.
- Must be inserted into mouth prior to burial from avalanche.

Avalanche airbag
- Rip cord releases compressed nitrogen into 2 airbags on wearer's back.
- Bag keeps individual on top of snow as they are engulfed by avalanche.

Avalanche injuries

Four key forces play into the outcome and survival of the avalanche victim.
- Duration of burial.
- Availability of air.
- Associated trauma.
- Human physiology.

All are the factors important to proper triage and treatment of victims.

Outcome variables

Degree of burial
- Full vs. partial burial.
- Full burial is defined as head and body under snow.
- Partial burial is defined as only part of body under snow after avalanche halts.
- Increased chance of survival with only partial burial.

Air pocket
- Considered to be most important factor linked with survival.
- Defined as cavity in front of mouth or nose of the victim with patent airway.
- Usually only a few centimeters wide; often ice up on inner surface.
- Without air pocket, completely buried victim can only survive 35 min.
- Care must be taken to avoid destruction of air pocket during rescue.
- Dig diagonally toward victim, rather than vertically, to prevent air pocket collapse.

Duration of burial (Fig. 80.1)
- Those rescued within 15 minutes have 90 percent survival probability.
- Precipitous drop in survival probability to 34 percent at 35 minutes due to acute asphyxiation of victims without an air pocket.
- Flattening of survival probability curve between 35 and 90 minutes— latent phase for victims with air pocket.
- Second drop to 7 percent survival at 130 minutes due to slow asphyxia and hypothermia in a closed air pocket.

Associated trauma
- Key factor in outcome for those victims who survive being buried.
- Victim at risk for blunt trauma secondary to encounters with natural obstructions along the mountainside during cascade.
- Closed head injury, pneumothorax, and open fracture are common.

Other pathophysiologic considerations

Circulatory Instability
- Can be triggered at a core temperature of 32°C.
- Results in danger of ventricular fibrillation.
- Reached after 90 minutes of snow burial.

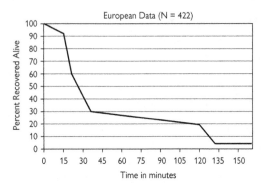

Figure 80.1 Avalanche survival vs. burial time. Reprinted with permission from the Utah Avalanche Center.

Hypothermia
- Body cooling occurs at 3°C/h.
- Initially can act as protective factor in prevention of hypoxic injury.
- Rewarming of asystolic patients is mandatory to pronounce death by hypothermia.
- On-site staging of hypothermia achieved by lay person with criteria created by Swiss Society of Mountain Medicine.
  - Alert, shivering patient—Stage I: 35–32°C.
  - Drowsy, nonshivering patient—Stage II: 32–28°C.
  - Unconscious patient—Stage III: 28–24°C.
  - Nonbreathing patient—Stage IV: <24°C.

Assessment and treatment

Search phase
- Balance rapid rescue versus risk to rescue team.
- 15-minute goal for uninjured companions to rescue buried.
- 90-minute goal for professional team to rescue victims.
- Use search tools and avoid destruction of air pockets.

Assessment of extricated victim
- ABC's—airway, breathing, circulation evaluation.
- Cervical-spine precautions.
- Avoid movement of trunk and large joints as this can promote the flow of cold, peripheral blood to the irritable myocardium, causing arrhythmias.
- Determine responsiveness of patient.
- Remove wet clothing by cutting.
- Measure core temperature—most reliable is esophageal or rectal.
- Stage hypothermia—Swiss Society of Mountain Medicine criteria.
- EKG monitoring during entire rescue, if available.

Airway/breathing
- Immediately establish airway.
- Follow Advanced Cardiovascular Life Support (ACLS) guidelines for victims with airway obstruction or respiratory arrest.
- Intubate unconscious patient with or without vital signs

Circulation
- 85 percent of avalanche victims extricated by rescue teams are in cardiac arrest.
- Cardiac arrest is due to obstructive asphyxia or severe hypothermia in patients with air pocket.
- EM physician should triage asystolic victims.
- Burial time <35 min and/or core temp >32°C—continue ACLS resuscitation.
- Burial time >35 min and/or core temp <32°C:
  - Air pocket present—suspect hypothermia stage IV and continue resuscitation until rewarming by cardiopulmonary bypass.
  - No air pocket and/or airway blocked—terminate resuscitation due to death by asphyxia.
  - Ventricular fibrillation at core temp <28°C—electric defibrillation, continued CPR, and transport to cardiopulmonary bypass hospital.
- Resuscitation medication administration in severe hypothermia patients not recommended—ineffective and can reach toxic levels.

Hypothermia treatment
- Passive rewarming.
  - Removal of wet clothes.
  - Shielding from wind.
  - Application of blankets, aluminum foils, bivouac bags.

- Active external rewarming.
  - Application of heat packs to trunk.
  - Utilization of heat lamps overhead.
  - Provision of warm, sweet drinks to conscious victims.
- Active internal rewarming.
  - Warm humidified oxygen through mask or ET tube.
- Avoid "afterdrop" hypothermia—results from rewarming of extremities with resultant recirculation of cold peripheral blood and subsequent decline in core body temperature.
- Hospital active internal rewarming:
  - Warm IV fluids—avoid lactated Ringer's solution as poorly metabolized in hypothermia.
  - Warm lavage of peritoneum, pleural cavity, and gastric mucosa.
  - Cardiopulmonary bypass.
- Extracorporeal blood warming with cardiac bypass is gold standard of treatment, but not routinely available. Active and passive external rewarming is most practical.
- Rewarming should continue until core temperature of 35°C or spontaneous circulation resumes.

Mountainside triage
- Rapid triage of multiple victims is critical.
- Death determination on-scene limits misuse of resources and limits risk to rescue team during extrication.
- Burial time, presence/absence of air pocket, and core body temperature used to determine death (see Fig. 80.2).

Pitfalls
- Inadequate training or avalanche preparation by back-country enthusiast.
- Improper rescue techniques.
- Destruction of victim's air pocket.
- Improper treatment of hypothermic victims.
- Improper triage of avalanche victims.

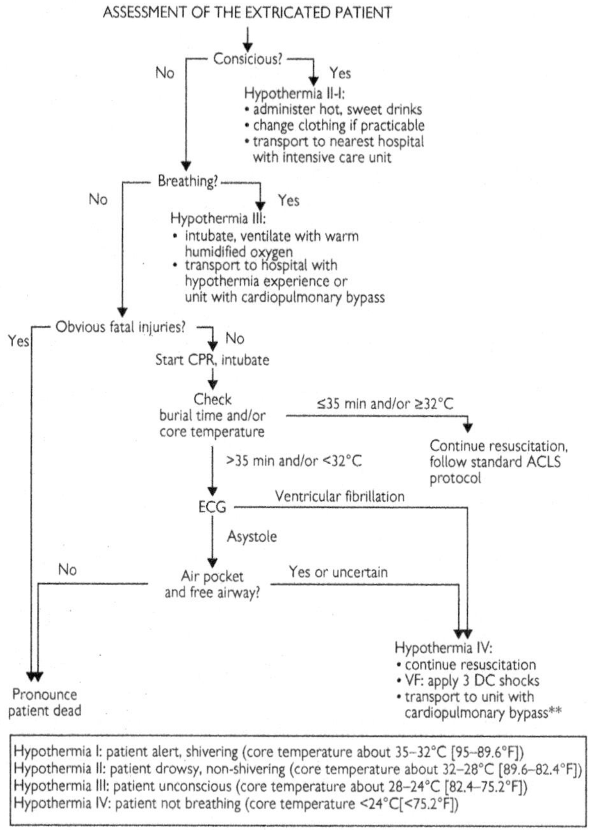

ASSESSMENT OF THE EXTRICATED PATIENT

Conscious?
- No
- Yes

Hypothermia II-I:
- administer hot, sweet drinks
- change clothing if practicable
- transport to nearest hospital with intensive care unit

Breathing?
- No
- Yes

Hypothermia III:
- intubate, ventilate with warm humidified oxygen
- transport to hospital with hypothermia experience or unit with cardiopulmonary bypass

Obvious fatal injuries?
- Yes
- No

Start CPR, intubate

Check burial time and/or core temperature
- ≤35 min and/or ≥32°C
- >35 min and/or <32°C

Continue resuscitation, follow standard ACLS protocol

ECG
- Ventricular fibrillation
- Asystole

Air pocket and free airway?
- No
- Yes or uncertain

Hypothermia IV:
- continue resuscitation
- VF: apply 3 DC shocks
- transport to unit with cardiopulmonary bypass**

Pronounce patient dead

Hypothermia I: patient alert, shivering (core temperature about 35–32°C [95–89.6°F])
Hypothermia II: patient drowsy, non-shivering (core temperature about 32–28°C [89.6–82.4°F])
Hypothermia III: patient unconscious (core temperature about 28–24°C [82.4–75.2°F])
Hypothermia IV: patient not breathing (core temperature <24°C[<75.2°F])

Figure 80.2 Assessment of extricated patient. Reprinted with permission from Brugger H, Durrer B, Adler-Kastner L, Falk M, Tschirky F (2001). Field management of avalanche victims. *Resuscitation* 51: 7–15.

Suggested readings

Boyd J, Haegeli P, Abu-Laban RB, Shuster M, Butt JC (2009). Patterns of death among avalanche fatalities: A 21 year review. *CMAJ 180*(3): 507–512.

Brugger H, Durrer B (2002). Position paper: On-site treatment of avalanche victims ICAR-MEDCOM-recommendation. *High Altitude Medicine & Biology 3*(4): 421–425.

Brugger H, Durrer B, Adler-Kastner L, Falk M, Tschirky F (2001). Field management of avalanche victims. *Resuscitation 51*: 7–15.

Brugger H, Durrer B, Adler-Kastner L (1996). On-site triage of avalanche victims with asystole by the emergency doctor. *Resuscitation 31*: 11–16.

Hohlrieder M, Brugger H, Schubert HM, et al. (2007). Pattern and severity of injury in avalanche victims. *High Altitude Medicine & Biology 8*(1): 56–61.

Lane AQ, Eischen J (2007). Avalanches. In Hogan DE, Burstein JL, eds. *Disaster Medicine*, pp. 248–255. Philadelphia, PA: Lippincott Williams & Wilkins.

McIntosh SE, Grissom CK, Olivares CR, et al. (2007). Cause of death in avalanche fatalities. *Wilderness and Environmental Medicine 18*: 293–297.

Online Information at Utah Avalanche Center. Available at http://utahavalanchecenter.org/

SATSIE Avalanche Studies and Model Validation in Europe. European Commission – Fifth Framework Programme. EU Contract no. EVG1-CT2002-00059.

Tracy JA (2006). Avalanche. In Ciottone G, ed. *Disaster Medicine*, pp. 514–516. Philadelphia, PA: Mosby.

Cold weather

Peter John Cuenca

Jimmy Cooper

Paul T. Mayer

John McManus

Introduction

Since the time of Hippocrates and Aristotle, cold-related injuries have resulted in devastating losses throughout history. In 218 BC, Hannibal lost over half his army to cold-related injuries while crossing the Pyrenees Alps. The human body attempts to maintain a constant body temperature (38°C rectally and approximately 32°C at the skin). However, in many circumstances this can be difficult, especially when a person is exposed to wilderness conditions, high altitude, or substances that inhibit normal thermoregulation. Hypothermia is defined as a core body temperature of less than 35°C (95°F) and occurs in mild, moderate, and severe forms. Prevention, recognition, and treatment are essential in reducing morbidity and preventing mortality from hypothermia.

Epidemiology

Hypothermia results in approximately 700 deaths annually in the United States and is one of the leading causes of death during outdoor recreation. Hypothermia has a mortality of 50 percent for individuals with comorbid conditions. Length of exposure and ambient temperature are responsible for the greatest risk for developing hypothermia. In addition, individuals can be predisposed to developing hypothermia. Risk factors that increase the incidence of cold-related injury include extremes of age, intoxication, inadequate nutrition, certain medications, and presence of chronic disease.

Pathophysiology

The human body dissipates heat to the environment via respiration, evaporation, convection, conduction, and radiation.
- Respiration and evaporation release heat through water droplets.
- Heat is lost from the body through convection by the movement of air (wind chill) or liquids over the body surface.
- Transfer of heat from the body by direct contact with a cooler object is conduction.
- Radiation is heat loss through infrared heat emission into a cooler surrounding environment.

The hypothalamus provides thermoregulation for the body and maintains body temperature through release of neurotransmitters causing vasoconstriction and increased metabolic rate in conjunction with the endocrine system. The body also generates heat by increasing metabolic rate and shivering. This system of thermoregulation allows humans to survive temperature ranges from −50°C (−58°F) to 100°C (212°F).

Metabolic rate decreases 6 percent for every 1°C decrease in core body temperature degrading the body's ability to compensate for heat loss. This occurs between 30°C (86°F) and 32°C (90°F). In response to cold exposure, vasoconstriction occurs and the body's metabolic rate decreases, resulting in decreased end-organ perfusion, relative hypovolemia, blood sludging and, if not corrected, eventual cardiovascular collapse.

Physical findings

Clinical presentation correlates with core temperature. Hypothermia occurs in three different stages: mild, moderate, and severe.

- Mild hypothermia is a temperature of 32.2°C to 35°C (90°F to 95°F). These patients present with shivering, tachycardia, tachypnea, fatigue, decreased ability to concentrate.
- Moderate hypothermia is defined as 28°C to 32.2°C (82.4°F to 90°F). In this stage, the body begins losing the ability to compensate. Shivering stops in this stage and level of consciousness decreases. Bradycardia occurs in moderate hypothermia and J waves (Osborn waves) may be seen on the electrocardiogram (ECG).
- Severe hypothermia, core temperature decreases to 28°C (82.4°F) or lower. Patients are unresponsive and lapse into a coma. They may appear clinically "dead." In this stage, various dysrhythmias, apnea, and loss of reflexes occur.

Diagnosis

The diagnosis of hypothermia is made on a patient's core temperature and clinical findings. However, thermometers measuring peripheral temperature are inaccurate. In addition, standard thermometers used in the emergency department setting are limited to a low recorded temperature of 34.4°C (94°F). Any patient suspected of having hypothermia must have a core temperature taken. There is no specific laboratory test to confirm or exclude a diagnosis of hypothermia. However, routine labs should be drawn for all patients presenting with moderate to severe hypothermia. Electrolyte abnormalities, hemoconcentration, and coagulopathies may be seen in these patients. If specific comorbidities are suspected in hypothermic patients, laboratory testing should be directed in evaluating these conditions (i.e., thyroid functions, toxicology screening, blood cultures, etc.).

Treatment

Treatment of the hypothermic patient depends on his/her location, available assets, and his/her clinical condition. As with all serious illness, initial management of hypothermic patients begins by addressing all life-threatening conditions first (ABCs) and initiating continuous monitoring of vital signs including telemetry.

On arrival to a medical facility, hypothermic patients should be removed from the cold environment, and all wet clothing should be removed and replaced with warm blankets. Empiric administration of naloxone and thiamine should be performed and correction of any glucose abnormalities addressed in all nonresponsive patients. Responsive patients with mild to moderate hypothermia should be treated with passive external rewarming. These patients should be encouraged to drink warm liquids containing sugar and limit exertional activity until core temperature normalizes. For active external warming, a heating blanket or a system that warms the core such as the Bair Hugger™ should be utilized. Heating the peripheral areas of hypothermic patients before the core area is discouraged and may result in core temperature "afterdrop." Afterdrop occurs when the cooler peripheral blood returns to the body's core area. This may cause cardiac irritability and dysrhythmias. Direct skin contact to heated items should also be avoided.

Severe hypothermic patients with a pulse and normal cardiac activity should be treated with aggressive active internal rewarming and invasive monitoring. Active internal rewarming can be done through warmed oxygen via face mask or endotracheal tube, warmed gastric lavage, warmed bladder lavage, warmed peritoneal lavage or warmed pleural lavage with chest tube thoracostomy. Extracorporeal blood warming can be accomplished through hemodialysis, arteriovenous rewarming, venovenous rewarming or cardiopulmonary bypass.

Severe hypothermic patients with cardiac dysfunction or no pulse should be managed according to the American Heart Association Basic and Advanced Cardiac Life Support guidelines. Management of cardiac-arrest victims in this setting focuses on active core rewarming as described earlier. There are documented survival cases for both children and adults with severe hypothermia and initially no cardiac activity with extremely low temperatures (<58°C).

Resuscitation should be attempted and not be discontinued in hypothermic patients until core temperature is above 32°C (89.6°F). Handle all patients gently because many physical manipulations have been shown to precipitate cardiac dysrhythmias. If a patient has a pulse, no matter how slow, do not initiate CPR. Providers should assess breathing and pulse for 30 to 45 seconds to determine presence or absence. If breathing and pulse are absent, general advanced cardiac life support (ACLS) management should begin, including endotracheal intubation. Rescuers should then begin CPR, attempt defibrillation once, establish IV access and provide active warming techniques. IV medications and repeat defibrillation should be withheld until core temperature reaches >30°C (86°F). Management of cardiac arrhythmias, electrolyte disorders, and medication delivery should be based on current ACLS guidelines.

Hypothermia is well-recognized as an independent contributing factor for increased morbidity and mortality in trauma patients. Studies have shown hypothermia to be associated with increases in coagulopathy, multiple organ failure, length of hospital stay, and mortality. In the care of the patient with traumatic injuries, focus should be placed on prevention and correction of hypothermia, especially in the prehospital setting. Hypothermia occurs in trauma patients for a multitude of reasons. Prolonged prehospital times, cold IV fluid administration, and environmental factors all affect a patient's core temperature. In addition, trauma itself can worsen hypothermia, as a result of bleeding and resultant hypoperfusion, and impaired thermoregulation.

Key points

- The most accurate way to access a patient's temperature is by obtaining a rectal temperature.
- The body looses the ability to compensate around 30°C to 32°C.
- Humidified, warm oxygen delivery, heating blankets, Bair Hugger™ are all appropriate rewarming techniques. Warming just the extremities and not the core may lead to core-temperature afterdrop.
- Never rub cold exposed area with hands, snow, or any objects. Furthermore, do not thaw a cold injured extremity if continued need to ambulate to definitive medical care.
- Once the patient reaches definitive care, 36.7°C to 40°C (98–104°F) circulating water should be used to rewarm the cold injured areas.
- Use of alcohol, poor nutrition, inactivity, improper clothing, mental fatigue are all risk factors for developing hypothermia in patients.

Suggested readings

2005 American Heart Association Guidelines for Cardiopulmonary Resuscitation and Emergency Cardiovascular Care (2005). Hypothermia. *Circ* 112: IV–136–138.

Danzl DF, Pozos RF (1994). Accidental hypothermia. *N Engl J Med* 331: 1756–1760.

Eddy VA, Morris JA Jr, Cullinane DC (2000). Hypothermia, coagulopathy, and acidosis. *Surg Clin North Am* 80: 845–854.

Gilbert M, Busund R, Skagseth A, Nilsen PA, Solbø JP (2000). Resuscitation from accidental hypothermia of 13.7°C with circulatory arrest. *Lancet* 355: 375–376.

Otis JD, Keane TM, Kerns RD (2003). An examination of the relationship between chronic pain and post-traumatic stress disorder. *J Rehabil Res Dev* 40: 397–405.

Petrone P, Kuncir EJ, Asensio JA (2003). Surgical management and strategies in the treatment of hypothermia and cold injury. *Emerg Med Clin North Am* 21(4): 1165–1178.

Silfvast T, Pettila V (2003). Outcome from severe accidental hypothermia in Southern Finland—A 10-year review. *Resuscitation* 59: 285–290.

Stoner J, Martin G, O'Mara K, Ehlers J, Tomlanovich M (2003). Amiodarone and bretylium in the treatment of hypothermic ventricular fibrillation in a canine model. *Acad Emerg Med* 10(3): 187–191.

Ulrich A, Rathlev N (2004). Hypothermia and localized cold injuries. *Emerg Med Clin N Am* 22: 281–298.

Chapter 82

Earthquakes

Ramon W. Johnson

Why earthquakes occur

Earthquakes are sudden slippages or movements in a portion of the earth's crust accompanied by a series of vibrations. They occur in areas of the earth's surface where colliding tectonic plates cause deformations resulting in points of stress. When these points of stress or faults rupture, the release of enormous energy over a few seconds causes the propagation of shock waves. Earthquakes also can occur in association with active volcanoes and may either precede or accompany eruptions. The magnitude of an earthquake is a measure of actual physical energy release at its source as estimated from instrumental observations. The oldest and most widely used is the Richter scale, developed in 1936. The intensity of an earthquake is a measure of how severe the tremor was at a particular location and is usually strongest close to the epicenter.

Earthquake zones

A large percentage of the world's earthquakes occur in an arching band extending around the rim of the Pacific Ocean (Ring of Fire). Another band of seismic activity extends through the Middle East and southern Europe. In the United States, although Alaska has the most earthquakes, the New Madrid Fault in the central U.S. zone and the San Andreas Fault in southern California are considered the areas of greatest risk for a significant seismic event. Earthquakes can also result in a secondary disaster, catastrophic tsunami. Tsunami, a series of waves of very great length and period, are usually generated by large earthquakes under or near the oceans, close to the edges of the tectonic plates. These waves may travel long distances, increase in height abruptly when they reach shallow water, and cause great devastation far away from the source. Submarine landslides and volcanic eruptions beneath the sea or on small islands can also be responsible for tsunami, but their effects are usually limited to smaller areas. Volcanic tsunami are usually of greater magnitude than seismic ones; waves of more than 40 meters (131.2 feet) in height have been witnessed.

Factors affecting earthquake occurrence and severity

The destruction that an earthquake causes is a function of its intensity and of the resistance of structures to seismic damage. Four human activities or consequences of human activities have been known to induce earthquakes:

- The filling of large water impoundments.
- Deep well injection.
- Underground explosions of nuclear devices.
- Collapse of underground mine workings

Factors affecting earthquake mortality and morbidity

The number of casualties caused by an earthquake will depend on its magnitude, its proximity to an urban center, and the degree of earthquake disaster preparedness and mitigation measures implemented in the urban center closest to where the earthquake takes place. See Box 82.1.

> **Box 82.1 Factors affecting earthquake mortality and morbidity**
> - Natural factors
>   - Aftershocks
>   - Landslides
>   - Fires
>   - Hazardous materials
>   - Dams
>   - Weather conditions
> - Structural factors
>   - Building collapse
> - Individual risk factors
>   - Increased risk of death in the very young and very old
>   — Lack of mobility
>   — Exacerbation of underlying diseases
>   — Inability to withstand major traumatic injury
>   - Entrapment
>   - Time to rescue

Clinical consequences of earthquakes

In most earthquakes, most people are killed by mechanical energy as a direct result of being crushed by falling building materials. Deaths resulting from major earthquakes can be instantaneous, rapid, or delayed.
- Instantaneous death can be due to severe crushing injuries to the head or chest, external or internal hemorrhage, or drowning from earthquake-induced tsunamis. Rapid death occurs within minutes or hours and can be due to asphyxia from dust inhalation or chest compression, hypovolemic shock, or environmental exposure (e.g., hypothermia).
- Delayed death occurs within days and can be due to dehydration, hypothermia, hyperthermia, crush syndrome, wound infections, or postoperative sepsis.

Earthquake injury patterns

Trauma caused by the collapse of buildings produces the majority of deaths and injuries in most earthquakes.

Major injuries and illnesses requiring hospitalization:

- Skull fractures with intracranial hemorrhage (e.g., subdural hematoma).
- Cervical spine injuries with neurologic impairment.
- Intrathoracic, intra-abdominal, and intrapelvic organ injury, including pneumothorax, liver lacerations, and ruptured spleen. Most seriously injured people will sustain combination injuries, such as pneumothorax in addition to an extremity fracture.
- Crush syndrome results from prolonged pressure on limbs causing disintegration of muscle tissue (rhabdomyolysis) and release of myoglobin, potassium, and phosphate into the circulation. Systemic effects include hypovolemic shock, hyperkalemia, renal failure (occurs in up to half of all patients with crush injury), and fatal cardiac arrhythmias. Patients with crush syndrome may develop kidney failure and require dialysis.

Other possible injuries:

- Hypothermia.
- Burns.
- Secondary wound infections.
- Gangrene requiring amputation.
- Sepsis.
- Adult respiratory distress syndrome (ARDS).
- Multiple organ failure.

As with most natural disasters, the majority of people requiring medical assistance following earthquakes have minor lacerations and contusions caused by falling elements, like pieces of masonry, roof tiles, and timber beams. The next most frequent reason for seeking medical attention are simple fractures that do not require operative intervention. A large number of patients require acute care for non-surgical problems, such as acute myocardial infarction, exacerbation of chronic diseases such as diabetes or hypertension, anxiety, and other mental-health problems such as depression. Huge amounts of dust are generated when a building is damaged or collapses, and dust clogging the air passages and filling the lungs is a major cause of death for many building-collapse victims. Dust inhalation may also cause respiratory problems ranging from local irritation to fulminant pulmonary edema. Smoke inhalation from fires may also be seen.

Medical response to earthquakes

In order to save the greatest number of victims, medical care must be provided to those at risk for rapid death or delayed death as soon as possible. This should lessen the sequelae of the primary injuries. Rapid mass casualty response must be instituted and includes the four essential elements of disaster medical response.
- Rescue awareness and operations.
- Triage and initial stabilization.
- Definitive medical care.
- Evacuation.

Rescue awareness and operations

Initially, the local population near any disaster site is the immediate search-and-rescue resource that may lack the technical equipment and exper-tise to facilitate the extraction of may victims. As additional personnel or search and rescue teams are activated, they should be trained to rec-ognize hazards and understand when additional resources are needed at the scene. Because rapid rescue of trapped victims and prompt treatment of those with life-threatening injuries can improve outcome, early rapid assessment of the extent of damage and injuries is needed to help mobilize resources and direct them to where they are most needed.
- Seven phases of a rescue operation:
- Arrival and size-up.
  - Evaluate the environment and potential risks.
- Hazard control.
  - Potential hazards include poisonous or caustic substances.
  - Biological agents or germ-infected materials.
  - Swift-moving currents, floating debris or contaminated water.
  - Confined spaces such as vessels, trenches, mines, or caves.
  - Extreme heights or buildings.
  - Possible psychological instability or individual emotional trauma involving patients or the rescue crews.
- Patient access.
  - Objectively evaluate the training and skills needed to access the patient. Untrained, poorly equipped, or inexperienced rescue personnel must not put their safety and the safety of others at risk by attempting heroic rescues.
- Medical treatment.
  - Initial assessment of ABCs.
  - Management of life-threatening airway, breathing, and circulation.
  - Immobilization of the spine.
  - Splinting of major fractures.
- Disentanglement.
  - Actual release from the cause of the entrapment.
- Patient packaging.
  - Factor time based on the patient's medical condition and minimize injury to the patient.
- Removal/transport.
  - Perform ongoing assessment and treatment during transport to definitive care.

Definitive care

Unconscious patients with either upper airway obstruction or inhalation injury or any patients with correctable hypovolemia resulting from hemorrhage or burns will likely benefit from early medical intervention. Injured people usually seek emergency medical attention only during the first three to five days following an earthquake, after which hospital-case-mix patterns usually return to normal.

Medical management of crush injury

Pretreat casualties with prolonged crush (greater than four hours) as well as those who demonstrate abnormal neurologic or vascular exams with 1 to 2 liters of normal saline before releasing crush object whenever possible.

- If pretreatment with intravenous fluids is not possible before releasing the crushing object, apply a tourniquet to the crushed limb until hydration can be initiated.
- Field amputation is an operation that can be life saving, especially with entrapped earthquake victims, victims with severely crushed or mangled extremities, and in the case of prolonged limb ischemia following entrapment.

Aftershocks

Aftershocks of similar or lesser intensity can follow the main quake and results from a continued vibrational wave that is released into the surrounding ground.

Suggested readings

Briggs, SM (2006). Earthquakes. *Surg Clin N Am* 86: 537–544.

Briggs SM, ed. (2003). *Advanced Disaster Medical Response Manual for Providers.* Boston: Harvard Medical International.

Coburn A, Spence R (1992). *Earthquake Protection.* Chichester, UK: John Wiley & Sons.

Eknoyan G (1993). Acute renal failure in the Armenian earthquake. *Kidney Int* 44: 241–244.

Noji EK (1992). Acute renal failure in natural disasters. *Ren Fail* 14: 245–249.

Prager EJ (1999). *Furious Earth, the Science and Nature of Earthquakes, Volcanoes, and Tsunamis.* New York: McGraw-Hill.

Pretto E, Safar P (1993). Disaster reanimatology potentials revealed by interviews of survivors of five major earthquakes. *Prehosp Disaster Med* 8: S139.

Pretto EA, Angus DC, Abrams JI, Shen B, Bissell, Ruiz Castro VM, et al, (1994). An analysis of prehospital mortality in an earthquake. *Prehosp Disaster Med* 9: 107–124.

Stratton JW (1989). Earthquakes. In Gregg MB, ed. *The Public Health Consequences of Disasters,* pp. 13–24. Atlanta, GA: Centers for Disease Control.

Chapter 83

Flooding

John L. Hick
Jennifer Bahr

Causes of flooding

Floods are the result of water overflowing natural or artificial boundaries or barriers. Flash floods are the most dangerous due to the huge amount of water that can inundate an area with little warning to the residents of the area.

- Extreme amounts of rainfall in short period.
- Rapid snowmelt.
- Breached dam or levee, as in Estes Park, CO flood of 1976.

Flash floods are the No. 1 cause of natural-disaster-related death.

Prediction of floods is difficult in both expected timing and extent of damage or water rise. The National Weather Service issues flood watches and warnings and should be heeded for evacuation planning. These are posted at www.nws.noaa.gov.

Mechanism of injury during floods

Environmental

Environmental injuries sustained during floods include drowning, hypothermia, hyperthermia, animal bites, and insect bites.

Drowning is the most common cause of flood-related death. People who have limited mobility, limited swimming ability or underestimate current flow have higher risks of drowning. Traumatic injuries occur from being struck by debris or a victim being thrown against solid objects (trees, buildings). Immersion injury patients may aspirate contaminated water during their struggle, and this can result in serious lung damage. Surfactant is destroyed by fresh and salt water, and the resulting ventilation/perfusion (V/Q) mismatch manifests as hypoxia and dyspnea. Treatment includes oxygen and treatment of bronchospasm if needed. No benefit has been shown for prophylactic antibiotics or steroids. When pneumonia does develop, antibiotic choice should be guided by culture results after initial treatment with broad-spectrum antibiotics such as pipericillin/tazobactam to cover Gram positive, Gram negative, and anaerobic organisms.

Hypothermia is multifactorial. Water immersion is common during flood rescue, evacuation, and clean-up. Body-heat loss is drastically increased by water immersion and lack of sheltered areas. Recovering requires access to shelter, exogenous heat or insulation (depending on the degree of hypothermia), and clean food and water with which to refuel. Hypothermia from immersion should respond to usual active rewarming measures. Aggressive resuscitation of hypothermic cardiac arrest is recommended, as intact neurological outcomes have occurred despite long immersion times.

Hyperthermia can easily occur in unacclimated individuals who are doing vigorous activities such as sandbagging or debris removal. Heat-related illness was the most frequently reported injury diagnosed during the 1993 Illinois flood.

Animal bites are not infrequent as displaced domestic animals roam the street or are anxious during rescue and evacuation activities. Insect populations can also be displaced, and some species flourish in wet environments. This can lead to increased stings by *hymenoptera* producing serious allergic reactions or bites by mosquitoes carrying pathogens like malaria.

Mold growth after flooding may lead to allergic symptoms or may contribute to exacerbation of respiratory diseases.

Motor vehicle related

Only six inches of still water can stall a vehicle or cause loss of control of steering. Water moving at only 8 miles per hour exerts enough force to sweep away a vehicle and its occupants.

One-third of flood-related deaths are due to drowning inside a motor vehicle. This speaks to the difficulty of judging how deep water is and the danger of attempting to drive over flooded roadways and bridges, which may be unstable.

Motor-vehicle collisions (MVC) also occur during flood evacuation and clean-up efforts. Six percent of flood-related deaths occur due to physical trauma from MVCs.

Infectious

Food is frequently spoiled due to lack of refrigeration or contaminated by floodwaters. Normal water sources may be unavailable or contaminated by floodwaters. Gastroenteritis resulting from eating or drinking contaminated food or water spreads easily between individuals in the close quarters of an emergency shelter, so prevention is paramount.

Basic Health Safety Measures
Food safety: If in doubt, throw it out!
Water safety: Boil water for 1 minute, including water used for drinking, ice, baby formula, baby formula, dishwashing.
Hygiene: Wash hands with soap and clean water or alcohol-based sanitizer frequently.

Further Water Purification Resources
http://www.bt.cdc.gov/disasters/earthquakes/food.asp

Wounds sustained during floods can be difficult to manage. Lacerations and abrasions should be cleaned and dressed to keep out contaminants, kept dry, and treated with secondary closure or allowed to heal by secondary intention if significant contamination was present. Wounds should be closely monitored by the patient for signs of infection, and antibiotics should be dispensed if this occurs. Prophylactic antibiotics may be indicated for contaminated wounds or wounds to the hands or feet. Common bacteria responsible for cellulitis after water contact include Streptococcus, E. coli, Staphylococcus, and Aeromonas. Antibiotic choices to cover these include sulfamethoxazole/trimethoprim, fluoroquinolones, and aminoglycosides. Aeromonas is usually resistant to penicillins and cephalosporins.

Q: Do I need a tetanus shot prior to working in a flood zone?

A: No. If you get an injury that breaks the skin and your last tetanus shot was >5 years ago, you should receive a booster. All health-care workers should maintain up-to-date immunization status.

Electrical

Water and electricity are dangerous in combination as wet skin reduces resistance to current flow. Flooded home wiring can also cause an electrical short and cause fires. Power lines are frequently blown down by storm winds and are dangerous to approach. Debris may cover current sources and make them difficult to detect.

Prehospital issues

Response route planning

Floodwaters, mudslides, downed trees and power lines, damaged bridges and roadways will impact regular response routes. At the least, this will increase normal response times, at worst; it may prevent rescuers from accessing a scene at all with usual vehicles. Specialized vehicles such as high-clearance and four-wheel drive may be required. Other equipment has been used successfully for transport including front-end loaders and airboats.

Swift-water rescue

Swift water rescue teams should be trained and ready for response in flood-prone areas. This includes population areas near river deltas as well as urban areas with culvert drainage systems for storm water management. The importance of boat transport has been shown in multiple incidents. All potential rescuers need access to personal floatation devices and specialized equipment such as throw bags and ropes.

Hospital issues

Evacuation

Moving patients is required if any risk exists that the hospital may flood. Preplanning with regional health-care facilities should include contingency plans for providing care for displaced patients. Moving a significant number of patients requires a large manpower force and supplementary staff may need to be called in to help. Complete hospital evacuation is a rare event. We can learn from the Grand Forks, ND April 1997 and the Cedar Rapids, IA 2008 experiences among others. Hospital evacuation due to tropical storm and hurricane threat is more commonplace, and many of the same lessons apply. Preplanning medical-record and patient-belongings movement, interagency coordination mechanisms, and coordination of transportation assets are critical issues.

Power, oxygen, and water supply are vulnerable parts of a hospital. Telephone systems, medical records, and information technology systems may also be lost and alternate communication arrangements should be made.

Staffing

Hospitals should develop an emergency staffing plan. This may include tiered responses based on size of disaster and staffing resources required. Staff may be required to shelter and board in the hospital due to difficulty navigating the flooded community.

Hospitals also should expect that the normal prearrival notification by ambulances might be disrupted.

Wound care resources

Many patients will present for wound care, especially during the clean-up/recovery phase after the flood. Irrigation supplies, tetanus prophylaxis, and bandage supplies should be maintained at high stocking levels.

Pharmacy and food supply

Floods are long-term events lasting days to weeks and adequate supplies for hospital patients and personnel should be maintained at all times in flood prone areas.

Behavioral health

Flooding can devastate a community. Having your home and possessions destroyed is extremely stressful. The long-term nature of this stress during clean up and rebuilding can induce new psychiatric symptoms or may destabilize individuals with existing behavioral health issues. Posttraumatic stress disorders are common. Children are commonly affected psychologically, which may manifest as behavior problems. Care should be taken to address the psychological needs of victims and staff in conjunction with community and other resources.

Suggested readings

FEMA website: www.fema.gov

Jonkman S, Keltman I (2005). An analysis of the causes and circumstances of flood disaster deaths. *Disasters* 29(1): 75–97.

Nufer K, et al (2003). Different medical needs between hurricane and flood victims. *Wilderness and Environmental Medicine* 14(2): 89–93.

Sliders C, Jacobson R (1998) Flood disaster preparedness: A retrospect from Grand Forks, North Dakota. *Journal of Healthcare Risk Management* 18(2): 33–40.

Chapter 84

Heat wave

Liudvikas Jagminas

Introduction

A heat wave is a prolonged period of excessively hot weather, which may be accompanied by high humidity. There is no universal definition of a heat wave. Instead, the term is relative to the usual weather in that particular area. The World Meteorological Organization defines a heat wave as occurring when the daily maximum temperature of more than five consecutive days exceeds the average maximum temperature by 5°C (9°F), using the period from 1961–1990. An index used by some, including the American College of Sports Medicine, is the Wet-Bulb Globe Temperature (WBGT). It is an environmental heat-stress index used to evaluate the risk of heat-related illness on an individual. It is calculated using three parameters: temperature, humidity, and radiant heat. There is low risk if the WBGT is <65°F, moderate risk if it is between 65–73°F, high risk if between 73–82°F, and very high risk >82°F. Conditions that can induce heat-related illnesses include stagnant atmospheric conditions and poor air quality. Consequently, people living in urban areas may be at greater risk from the effects of a prolonged heat wave than those living in rural areas. Also, asphalt and concrete store heat longer and gradually release heat at night, which can produce higher nighttime temperatures known as the "urban heat island effect."

Terms

Heat cramps
- Muscular pains and spasms due to heavy exertion.
- Least severe form, often the first signal that the body is having trouble with heat.

Heat exhaustion
- Typically occurs with heavy exercise or work in a hot, humid place where body fluids are lost through heavy sweating.
- Blood flow to the skin increases, results in a form of mild shock.
- If not treated, the victim's condition will worsen, body temperature will keep rising and the victim may suffer heat stroke.

Heat stroke
- A life-threatening condition typically defined as hyperthermia exceeding 41°C and anhidrosis associated with an altered sensorium.
- Body temperature can rise unchecked, resulting in brain damage and death if the body is not cooled quickly.

Clinically, two forms of heatstroke are generally recognized:
- Classic Heat Stroke, which occurs during environmental heat waves:
  - Failure of the body's heat-dissipating mechanisms.
  - More common in children and in the elderly population.
  - Should be suspected in individuals who are chronically ill who present with an altered sensorium.
- Exertional Heat Stroke affects young, healthy individuals who engage in strenuous physical activity in a hot environment:
  - Characterized by hyperthermia, diaphoresis, and an altered sensorium.
  - Should be suspected in all individuals with bizarre irrational behavior or a history of syncope during strenuous exercise.

Etiology of heat-related illness

- Increased heat production
  - Increased metabolism.
  - Infections.
  - Sepsis.
  - Encephalitis.
  - Stimulant drugs.
  - Drug withdrawal.
  - Thyroid storm.
- Increased muscular activity
  - Exercise.
  - Convulsions.
  - Strychnine poisoning.
  - Sympathomimetics.
  - Drug withdrawal.
  - Tetanus.
  - Thyroid storm.
- Decreased heat loss
  - Reduced sweating.
  - Dermatologic diseases.
  - Drugs.
  - Burns.
- Reduced central nervous system (CNS) responses
  - Advanced age.
  - Toddlers and infants.
  - Alcohol.
  - Barbiturates.
  - Other sedatives.
- Reduced cardiovascular reserve
  - Elderly persons.
  - Beta-blockers.
  - Calcium channel blockers.
  - Diuretics.
- Drugs
  - Anticholinergics.
  - Neuroleptics.
  - Antihistamines.
- Exogenous factors
  - High ambient temperatures.
  - High ambient humidity.
- Reduced ability to acclimatize
  - Children and toddlers.
  - Elderly persons.
  - Diuretic use.
  - Hypokalemia.

Evaluation

- Blood studies:
  - Hypoglycemia found in patients with fulminant hepatic failure.
  - Hypernatremia: observed early in dehydration.
  - Hyponatremia: found with excessive free water intake.
- Calcium: hypocalcemia secondary to increased binding with damaged muscle.
- Magnesium: commonly observed and must be repleted.
- Phosphorus:
  - Hypophosphatemia secondary to phosphaturia.
  - Hyperphosphatemia due to rhabdomyolysis.
- Lactic acid: elevated levels are associated with poor prognostic outcome.
- Liver function tests:
  - Aspartate transaminase (AST) & Alanine transaminase (ALT) commonly rise during early phases of heat stroke and peak at 48 hours.
  - Jaundice may be noted 36–72 hours after the onset of liver failure.
- Creatinine kinase, lactic dehydrogenase (LDH) and myogloblin are commonly released when muscle necrosis occurs and can be found in patients with exertional heat stroke.

Imaging studies

- Computerized tomography scans may be helpful in ruling out CNS injury in patients with altered mental status.
- Chest radiographs may show atelectasis, pneumonia, pulmonary infarction, or pulmonary edema.

Treatment

Rapid reduction of the core body temperature is the cornerstone of treatment because the duration of hyperthermia is the primary determinant of outcome. Once heatstroke is suspected, cooling must begin immediately and must be continued during the patient's resuscitation. The basic premise of rapidly lowering the core temperature to about 39°C (avoid overshooting and rebound hyperthermia) remains the primary goal.

- Remove restrictive clothing.
- Spray water on the body.
- Cover the patient with ice-water--soaked sheets, or place ice packs in the axillae and groin.
- Reduce the temperature by at least 0.2°C/min to approximately 39°C. Stop cooling at 39°C to prevent overshooting, which can result in iatrogenic hypothermia.
- Patients who are unable to protect their airway should be intubated.
- Intravenous lines may be placed in anticipation of fluid resuscitation and for the infusion of dextrose and thiamine if indicated.
- Hypoglycemia is a common occurrence in patients with EHS and may be a manifestation of liver failure.
- Insert a thermistor probe to monitor temperature continuously.
- Insert a nasogastric tube to monitor for gastrointestinal bleeding and fluid losses.
- Place a Foley catheter to monitor urine output.
- Agitation and shivering should be treated immediately with benzodiazepines.
- Convulsions must be controlled; benzodiazepines and, if necessary, barbiturates are the recommended agents.
- Phenytoin is not effective in controlling convulsions in heat stroke.
- Convulsions refractory to benzodiazepines and barbiturates should be paralyzed and provided mechanical ventilation. Electroencephalographic monitoring is recommended in all such patients, and anticonvulsant medications should be adjusted accordingly.

Consultation

- Consider consultation with a nephrologist as soon as renal failure occurs.
- Consultation with a surgeon is indicated when compartment syndrome is suspected.
- Consider consultation with a liver transplant service for patients with fulminant liver failure.

Prognosis

Indicators of poor prognosis during acute episodes include the following:

- Initial temperature measurement higher than 41°C, any temperature higher than 108°F or a temperature persisting above 102°F despite aggressive cooling measures.
- Coma duration longer than two hours.
- Severe pulmonary edema.

- Delayed or prolonged hypotension.
- Lactic acidosis in patients with classic heatstroke.
- ARF and hyperkalemia.
- Aminotransferase levels greater than 1000 IU/L during the first 24 hours.

Prevention

Heatstroke is a preventable illness, and education is the single most important tool for its prevention.

Recognition of host risk factors and modification of behavior (e.g., limiting alcohol and drug intake, avoiding use of medications and drugs that interfere with heat dissipation) and physical activity also can prevent heatstroke.

The media, public education, public-health programs, and athlete- safety programs can play a pivotal role in increasing the public's awareness of the dangers of heat during heat waves and advising the public on methods of remaining cool.

Drinking fluids on schedule (and not based only on thirst), frequent cooling breaks, and frequent visits to air-conditioned places are very important because even short stays in an air-conditioned environment may drastically reduce the incidence of heatstroke.

Suggested readings

Bouchama A, Dehbi M, Chaves-Carballo E (2007). Cooling and hemodynamic management in heatstroke: Practical recommendations. *Critical Care 11* (3): 1–17.

Bouchama A, Knochel JP (2002). Heat stroke. *N Engl J Med 346*(25): 1978–1988.

Centers for Disease Control and Prevention. Heat waves. Available at http://www.cdc.gov/climate-change/effects/heat.htm

Centers for Disease Control and Prevention. Extreme heat: A prevention guide to promote your personal health and safety. Updated July 31, 2009. Available at http://emergency.cdc.gov/disasters/extremeheat/heat_guide.asp

Heled Y, Rav-Acha M, Shani Y, Epstein Y, Moran DS (2004, March). The "golden hour" for heatstroke treatment. *Mil Med 169*(3): 184–186.

Moran DS, Squire DL (2007). Heat-related illnesses. In Auerbach P, ed. *Wilderness Medicine: Management of Wilderness and Environmental Emergencies*, 5th ed. St. Louis, Mo: Mosby.

Vassalo SU, Delaney KA (2006). Thermoregulatory principles. In Goldfrank, ed., *Toxicologic Emergencies*, 8th ed., pp. 285–307. Stamford, CT: Appleton & Lange.

Hurricane disasters

Michelle A. Fischer

Introduction

- Definition: A tropical storm system with low-pressure center and surrounding spiral heavy rain with winds greater than 120 km/hr (74 mph).
- Destruction caused by: massive rain, flooding, high winds, tornadoes, and storm surge.
- Wind direction is counterclockwise in the Northern Hemisphere and clockwise in the Southern Hemisphere.
- Alias: typhoon (western Pacific), cyclone (Indian Ocean).
- Duration of several hours to days depending on location and speed.
- Season lasts June to November with peak in August and September.
- Five categories based on wind speed, central pressure and damage potential (see Table 85.1, the Saffir-Simpson Hurricane Scale).
- Categories 3, 4, and 5 are considered major storms.
- Costliest mainland U.S. hurricane was Katrina in 2005 (category 3 with over $81 billion in damage. Third deadliest with 1,500 deaths).

Formation of a hurricane

A self-propagating, spiral-wind cycle is created when warm moist air from the ocean surface rises and contacts the cooler air above forming condensation. This condensation process releases heat into cooler air above, allowing even more moisture to accumulate.

Table 85.1 Saffir Simpson Hurricane Scale

Category	Sustained Wind (mph)	Damage	Surge (ft) above normal
1	74–95	Minimal—unanchored mobile homes, vegetation, signs	4–5
2	96–110	Moderate—all mobile homes, roofs, small crafts, flooding	6–8
3	111–130	Extensive—small buildings, low-lying roads cut off	9–12
4	131–155	Extreme—roofs destroyed, trees down, roads cut off, beach homes flooded	13–18
5	>155	Catastrophic—most buildings and vegetation destroyed, major roads cut off, homes flooded	>18

Preparation for a hurricane

In the United States, the National Hurricane Center in Miami, Florida tracks all storm systems from their inception. The purpose is to accurately predict the power and the anticipated landfall location of active storms. This advanced warning allows potentially affected communities to prepare for the storm. This may include the accumulation of essential supplies such as batteries, flashlights, fuel, water, food, prescription medication, and the preparation of their homes by securing items such as mobile homes, lawn furniture, and vehicles.

For predicted major storms (category 3 and higher), evacuation and disaster plans should be executed and must take into account those who are unable to evacuate themselves such as: hospitalized, nursing home, hospice patients, and those healthy individuals without transportation. Dialysis patients should receive dialysis immediately prior to the storm, allowing them three days after the storm to receive their subsequent dialysis. Keep in mind that as the storm approaches, emergency medical services disappear. Operation of high-profile ambulances becomes risky at wind speeds over 45 mph, and fire units cannot be dispatched at winds over 55 mph. Therefore, once the weather becomes this severe, individual with serious injuries or illnesses cannot be transported. Medical stations should plan and prepare to be self-sustaining and functional for at least a 72-hour period. A plentiful supply of tetanus, antibiotics, insulin, and chronic maintenance medications such as antihypertensive and pain medications should be kept on hand. See Table 85.2 for a list of suggested supplies.

Only a few injuries are a direct result of the hurricane, most occur during the clean up or recovery phase. Most acute medical conditions will fall into one of the following four groups: orthopedic or soft- tissue injury, gastrointestinal illness, respiratory illness or cardiovascular disease. Carbon monoxide poisonings and gasoline burns are likely secondary to the use of generators. Supplies will be necessary to care for patients with chronic medical conditions like diabetes or hypertension, who are without medications and supplies. See Table 85.3 for the most frequent conditions treated posthurricane at evacuation centers. Accountability is a medical necessity, and the performance of essential functions such as record keeping, supply replenishment, and communication must be continued as best as possible, despite austere circumstances.

Table 85.2 Suggested supplies for medical stations

Sheets, gowns, exam tables, crutches, wheelchairs, walkers	BP cuffs, otoscope, penlight, angiocaths, IV tubing, needles, syringes, thermometers, glucometer
Local anesthesia, soap, antiseptics	Gloves, alcohol pads, hand sanitizer, wipes, tongue blades
Nebulizer, tubing, oxygen	Suture kits, sharps container

Table 85.3 Top 10 conditions: From limited needs assessments among persons staying in Hurricane Katrina evacuation centers, Sept. 10–12, 2005

Condition	Incidence per 1,000 residents
Hypertension/Cardiovascular	108.2
Diabetes	65.3
New Psychiatric Condition	59.0
Preexisting Psychiatric Condition	50.0
Rash	27.9
Asthma/COPD	27.5
Flu-like Illness of Pneumonia	26.3
Toxic Exposure	16.0
Other Infections (pertussis, varicella, hepatitis, TB, rubella)	15.6
Diarrhea	12.8

Hazards of a hurricane

The damage created by the hurricane is directly related to the terrain it strikes, population density, structural integrity of the buildings, tide at the time the hurricane comes ashore and the amount of flooding. A major portion of hurricane-related death and damage is associated with large storm surge and flooding. Disaster consequences include population displacement (common), injury, death, communicable disease outbreaks, and food/supply scarcity. Expect outages for power, telephone, and cell-phone towers. Generators can lessen the impact with temporary power, but communication will be affected and cause additional anxiety and chaos.

Response to a hurricane

The initial post-storm response is typically performed by local authorities. This entails:

- Rapid damage assessment.
- Restoration of power outages.
- Road clearing for traffic and medical personnel and law enforcement presence.
- Victims removed from danger and placed in predetermined safe areas or collection points. These areas should plan for basic-needs medical care and be adequately staffed and equipped.

Mass casualty triage must be used effectively with the goal to treat the greatest number of patients as rapidly as possible with limited resources based upon injury severity.

Hospital disaster plans should include a process to discharge or transfer nonacute patients to other facilities. Critically ill patients are usually left in place secondary to their acuity. Transportation is a difficult issue poststorm, secondary to road debris, flooding, and communication. When generators are utilized, hospitals typically carry enough fuel for a minimum of 24 hours of continuous operation. Gasoline availability and shortages will occur, and it may be necessary to secure a source from another region.

The state becomes involved when the local resources are exhausted or overwhelmed. During this time, the governor, as the state's chief executive officer, is responsible for allocating the state's resources. When it is felt that the state's resources are exhausted or exceeded, the governor may request federal assistance. Direct assistance to individuals and families may come from a number of organizations such as the American Red Cross, Salvation Army, and other volunteer organizations that offer food, shelter, supplies, and clean-up assistance.

Recovery from a hurricane

Lack of power causes problems such as no refrigeration for medication; power for medical equipment, lighting, and air conditioning. Many victims displaced from their homes are without their daily medications, forcing them to seek urgent medical attention for their chronic medical conditions. Medical needs poststorm are coordinated through local and state Emergency Operation Centers. Federal assistance is implemented via the National Response Plan (NRP) based on the National Incident Management System. This includes Disaster Medical Assistance Teams (DMAT) that can serve as functional field hospitals if necessary. Military assets can also be utilized for medical care, transport, supplies, manpower, and law enforcement.

Pitfalls

- Preparation is critical and can minimize death and disability—perform drills, scenarios, execute evacuation-response plans, and keep emergency supplies up to date.
- Be prepared to treat chronic medical conditions such as hypertension, diabetes, pulmonary disease, and psychiatric illnesses.
- Expect communication and transportation issues.

Suggested readings

Currier M, King DS, Wofford MR, et al. (2006). A Katrina experience: Lessons learned. *Am J Med 119*: 986–982.

Federal Emergency Management Agency. Available at http://www.nhc.noaa.gov/pdf/NWS-TPC-5. pdf Accessed October 21, 2008.

Greenough PG, Lappi MD, Hsu EB, et al. (2008). Burden of disease and health status among Hurricane Katrina—Displaced persons in shelters: A population-based cluster sample. *Ann Emerg Med 51*: 426–432.

Llewellyn, M (2006). Floods and tsunamis. *Surg Clin N Am 86*: 557–578.

National Weather Service National Hurricane Center. Available at http://www.nhc.noaa.gov/ Accessed September 5, 2008.

Shatz VF, Wolcott K, Fairburn JB (2006). Response to hurricane disasters. *Surg Clin N Am 86*: 545–555.

Landslides and mudslides

Melissa White

Introduction

Landslides and mudslides are geologic disturbances that occur throughout the world and cause up to $2 billion in property losses and 25 deaths per year. Landslides occur when earth, debris, or rock move down a slope. Mudslides are usually fast-moving landslides that may flow in channels and are typically due to heavy rainfall or a rapid snow melt.

Causes
- Earthquakes.
- Storms.
- Volcanic activity.
- Fires.
- Extreme fluctuations in climate temperatures, http://fema.gov/hazard/landslide/index.shtm.09/08

Areas at risk

- Steep hillsides.
- Bases of slopes.
- Existing old landslide sites.
- Drainage channels from streams or rivers.
- Areas containing leach field septic systems.
- Areas of land devoid of vegetation due to natural or man-made disasters.
- Areas where surface runoff is directed.
- Embankments along roadsides with fallen rock or debris. http://www.bt.cdc.gov/disasters/landslides.asp

Warning signs

- New cracks in pavement/foundation.
- Broken water lines.
- Unequal fence lines.
- Leaning trees, walls, and/or utility posts.
- Soil receding from foundations.
- Rumbling sounds present to suggest the movement of debris flow.
- Sudden decrease or increase in the water level of a lake, stream, or channel.
- Water flow from a stream or channel changing from clear to muddy. http://landslides.usgs.gov/learning/prepare

Prevention and planning

- Investigate landslide risk in your area via geologic surveys.
- Utilize information from the National Landslide Hazards Program (LHP).
- Identify hazard locations:
  - Obtain site analysis of your property if high risk.
  - Correct recommended measures.
  - Consult with an insurance agent to determine if landslides/ mudslides are included in a flood policy.
  - Develop an evacuation plan. http://www.redcross.org/services/ disaster/landslide.09/08

Actions during a landslide or mudslide

- Evacuate from the oncoming path.
- Inform local emergency services: fire, police, emergency medical services, hospitals, and public works.

Suggested readings

http://fema.gov/areyouready/landslide.shtm.09/08
http://www.ready.gov/america/beinformed/landslides.html.09/08

Chapter 87

Lightning strikes

Deborah L. Korik

Richard D. Zane

Incidence and epidemiology

On average, 62 people are killed by lightning every year in the United States. Of those struck by lightning, the mortality is as high as 30 percent although some recent literature suggests mortality may be lower (5–10%). The morbidity among survivors though is 70 percent and includes a large number of persistent neurologic deficits as well as vision and hearing problems.

Mechanisms of injury

- Direct:
  - Direct strike.
  - Splash injury (current jumps from object initially struck—mechanism by which injury occurs when using a connected appliance while indoors).
  - Contact injury (person is touching an object that is struck by lightning).
- Blunt injury:
  - Concussive.
  - Being thrown.
- Indirect:
  - House fires.
  - Forest fires.

Making the diagnosis

- Diagnosis can be challenging if lightning strike was unwitnessed.
- Lightning strikes cannot occur without storm activity (sunny day).
- For unwitnessed strikes, elicit as much history as possible.
- Careful physical exam may reveal typical injury pattern although rare.

Examination findings

Cardiopulmonary

- Cardiac arrest:
  - Primary cause of death from lightning strikes.
  - Asystole is the most common cardiac dysrhythmia.
- Respiratory arrest:
  - Caused by paralysis of respiratory center.
  - May persist after return of spontaneous circulation.
- Hypertension (often transient); tachycardia.
- Nonspecific EKG changes (prolonged QT possible).
- Acute arrhythmias uncommon.
- May have nonpalpable peripheral pulses due to arterial spasm (check femoral, carotid, or brachial pulses).
- Important to differentiate true hypotension versus arterial spasm and sympathetic instability.

Neurologic

- Altered level of consciousness including confusion, loss of consciousness, and amnesia (common).
- Paresthesias.

Integumentary

- Burns (usually superficial and may take a few hours to develop):
  - Can be linear or punctate.
  - Feathering burns (ferning pattern) are pathognomonic but not commonly seen (Figure 87.1).

Figure 87.1 Lightning strike with characteristic feathering burns

Musculoskeletal
- Keraunoparalysis (paralyzed and pulseless extremities).
- Spinal cord injury.
- Fractures uncommon.
- Blunt trauma from being thrown.

Ears
- Tympanic-membrane rupture.
- Temporary deafness.
- Hemotympanum indicative of basilar skull fracture.

Eyes
- Cataracts can be present on initial presentation.
- Pupils can be dilated or nonreactive (even in absence of brain death).
- Transient blindness.

Gastrointestinal
- Absent bowel sounds possible secondary to ileus or acute traumatic injury.

Renal
- Myoglobinuria rare.
- Renal failure exceedingly rare.

Differential Diagnosis

Victims of lightning strikes may be difficult to diagnose if the strike was unwitnessed.

Possible alternative diagnoses include:
- CVA.
- Seizure disorder.
- Spinal cord injury.
- Closed head injury.
- Hypertensive encephalopathy.
- Cardiac arrhythmia.
- Myocardial infarction.
- Toxic ingestion.
- Malingering.
- Conversion reaction.

Investigations

- EKG.
- Urinalysis (evaluate for myoglobin).
- Cardiac biomarkers.
- CBC, Electrolytes, BUN, Creatinine (in severely injured patients).
- CT scan as dictated by associated trauma.
- Other imaging depends on history and physical examination findings.

Management/treatment

Victims of lightning strikes are not "charged" and are safe to treat.

Triage

- Ensure scene safety.
- Triage those in cardiac arrest as most emergent because patients who survive initial strike or who are resuscitated immediately have excellent chance of survival.

Immediate management at scene

- Immediate CPR and initiation of Advanced Cardiac Life Support measures (ACLS) if in cardiac arrest.
- Endotracheal intubation for respiratory arrest.
- Respiratory arrest may persist after return of spontaneous circulation due to paralysis of respiratory center. It is important to continue to support respirations to avoid secondary cardiac arrest.

Continuing management

- Remove wet clothing; keep patient warm.
- Fluid therapy for hypotension (normal saline or Ringer's lactate).
  - Avoid overhydration, which can result in cerebral edema.
  - Restrict fluid therapy in those who are normotensive or hypertensive.
- Compartment syndrome unlikely.
  - Avoid fasciotomies unless no sign of improvement over several hours and documented elevated intracompartmental pressures.
- Tetanus prophylaxis (if burns or lacerations are present).
- Antibiotics not generally indicated (exceptions include open dural wounds and open extremity fractures).
- Local wound care for deep burns (rare).
- Rhabdomyolysis and renal failure (rare); if present, should be treated with IV hydration, forced diuresis, and alkalinization of urine.
- Persistent hypotension—consider other organ damage (possibly due to blunt injury sustained after strike).
- Fetal monitoring in pregnant victim; survival of fetus is unpredictable.

Disposition

Admit for:

- Confusion.
- Loss of consciousness.
- Post-cardiac or respiratory arrest.
- Chest pain.
- Focal neurologic deficit.

Determining death

- Fixed and dilated pupils not necessarily indicative of brain death.
- No indication for prolonged resuscitation. If no return of spontaneous circulation after 20–30 minutes of treatment, it is acceptable to stop resuscitation efforts.
- Cannot declare patients dead if they are hypothermic.

Differences from other high-voltage injuries

Injuries due to lightning strikes are often markedly different from those caused by other high-voltage sources and require different evaluation and management.

Lightning strikes
- Instantaneous (flashover).
- Higher energy level.
- Compartment syndrome unlikely.
- Renal failure unlikely.
- Myoglobinuria unlikely.
- Usually superficial burns.

High voltage
- Prolonged exposure to voltage.
- Renal failure more common.
- Compartment syndrome more likely.
- Deep burns more likely.

Complications

Acute
- Adult Respiratory Distress Syndrome (ARDS).
- Multi-organ system failure.

Chronic
- Headaches (can be severe).
- Cataracts.
- Hearing loss (due to tympanic-membrane or ossicle damage).
- Neurologic complications include long-term cognitive deficits (particularly memory deficits, difficulty with concentration and complex calculations), peripheral neuropathy, chronic-pain syndromes, and autonomic dystrophies.
- Emotional lability.
- Fatigue, energy loss.
- Psychological dysfunction (depression, suicidality, behavioral issues).
- Impotence, ↓libido.
- Victims of lightning strikes should seek early attention for psychosocial complications.
- Victims may require treatment with antidepressants.

Box 87.1 Consider referring survivors of lightning strikes to Lightning Strike and Electric Shock Survivors, International (LSESSI) organization
- www.lightning-strike.org
- 910-346-4708

Prevention

- Wearing or carrying metal or metal objects does not increase the risk of being struck by lightning.
- Avoid water activities during thunderstorms.
- Avoid isolated trees during thunderstorms.
- Avoid corded phones, computers, and open windows when indoors.
- Take shelter in a substantial building or in a car with a metal top.
- If caught outside without shelter during a storm, assume a crouched position with hands over ears.
- 30-30 rule: Seek shelter when time between hearing thunder and seeing lightning is less than 30 seconds. Stay indoors until 30 minutes after cessation of lightning and thunder.

Suggested readings

Circulation (2005). 112-IV-154-IV-155. Available at http://circ.ahajournals.org/cgi/content/full/112/24_suppl/IV-154

Cooper M, Andrews C, Holle R (2007). Lightning injuries. In P. Auerbach, ed. *Wilderness Medicine*, 5th ed., pp. 67–108. Philadelphia, PA: Mosby Elsevier.

National Weather Service website. Available at www.nws.noaa.gov

O'Keefe Gatewood M, Zane R (2004). Lightning injuries. *Emerg Med Clin N Am* 22: 369–403.

Influenza pandemic

Alexander P. Isakov

Overview

A pandemic is a global disease outbreak. An influenza or flu pandemic is the outbreak of an influenza strain that is sufficiently novel in its genetic make-up that there is virtually no immunity in the human population. If the virus is capable of causing serious disease in humans and is also easily transmissible, influenza pandemic ensues.

Seasonal influenza, the winter flu, is a highly contagious respiratory illness which affects 5–20 percent of the U.S. population annually. It results in over 200,000 hospitalizations and 36,000 deaths in the United States every year. A seasonal flu epidemic is caused by influenza viruses that were circulating the previous season or ones with slight antigenic changes (antigenic drift). A pandemic viral strain contains a surface protein for which no previous human immunity exists, often occurring as a result of a gene mutation or gene reassortment (antigenic shift). Differences between the familiar winter flu and a pandemic flu include:

- Winter flu occurs every year; pandemic flu occurs 3–4 times per century and is not restricted to the winter months.
- Winter flu affects 5–20 percent of the population; pandemic flu is projected to make approximately 15–40 percent of the world's population ill.
- Winter flu kills approximately 36,000 annually in the United States and 500,000 to 1 million worldwide; the 1918 pandemic killed 500,000 in the United States and over 50 million worldwide.
- Most people recover from winter flu in a week to ten days; pandemic flu may be more severe, resulting in longer recovery periods and higher death rates.
- Winter flu deaths are usually confined to individuals with preexisting illness or those at the extremes of age; a pandemic strain has a much greater likelihood of affecting young, healthy individuals who make up a large portion of the workforce.
- Effective vaccines exist for seasonal flu; there would be no vaccine at the onset of a pandemic and it is estimated it would take several months for the first vaccines to become available.

History

The world has been witness to three pandemics in the last century and one in this century. The pandemics of the twentieth century include the following Influenza A subtypes, 1918 (H1N1), 1957 (H2N2), and 1968 (H3N2). The 1918 pandemic is regarded as the deadliest disease on record. It affected approximately 25–30 percent of the world's population, striking every continent and is estimated to have killed 500,000 in the United States and 50–100 million people worldwide. A disproportionate number of them were young, healthy adults with most of the deaths occurring in the period of six months. The population in 1918 was 1.8 billion, roughly 28 percent of the over 6 billion inhabitants today. If 1918 mortality data were extrapolated to today's population, 1.7 million Americans could die, with global estimates reaching 180–300 million deaths.

The 1957 pandemic caused approximately 70,000 U.S. deaths and 1–2 million worldwide. The 1968 pandemic caused about 34,000 U.S. deaths and 700,000 worldwide. By comparison, these pandemics were mild. However, given the growth in the world's population, the World Health Organization estimates that a mild pandemic similar to the one in 1968 would kill an estimated 2–7.4 million individuals worldwide. The CDC predicts a mild pandemic could kill between 89,000 and 207,000 Americans.

Clinical considerations during a pandemic

Clinical presentation

The particular clinical characteristics of a novel circulating influenza virus responsible for a human pandemic will only be revealed during the course of the disease outbreak. Influenza viruses cause respiratory illness with typical symptoms including fever, cough, sore throat, myalgias, fatigue, sinus congestion, and headache. Some will also experience nausea, vomiting, and diarrhea, though this is more common in children than adults.

In the case of pandemic, patients are likely to be evaluated and treated based on a clinical presentation of "influenza-like illness" (ILI) because confirmatory testing will not likely be available at the point of care.

- Influenza-like Illness (ILI)
  - Nonspecific respiratory syndrome:
    — Defined by the CDC as fever (>/= 100°F) AND (cough or sore throat) in the absence of a known cause other than influenza.
  - ILI symptoms may be caused by a host of viruses including rhinovirus, respiratory syncytial virus (RSV), coronavirus, parainfluenza virus, influenza virus, and others.
  - In the context of an influenza pandemic, patients presenting with ILI will be considered at risk for having the novel virus.
- The natural course of the novel virus will only be revealed after onset of the pandemic but typical characteristics of influenza viruses include:
  - Acquired when mucous membranes (eyes, nose, mouth) of a susceptible host are exposed to large-particle respiratory droplets carrying the virus. Transmission could be by coughing, sneezing, and direct contact.
  - The incubation period is typically 1–4 days (average 2).
  - The duration of uncomplicated illness is typically 3–7 days with some symptoms lasting as long as 2 weeks.
  - Individuals are typically contagious 1–2 days before symptoms develop and 5–7 days after onset of illness.
  - May cause primary viral pneumonia, predispose to secondary bacterial pneumonia, and other co-infections; may exacerbate underlying medical conditions.
- Certain underlying medical conditions will be recognized to increase the likelihood of complications and more severe illness. These conditions will not be revealed until after onset of the pandemic, but for influenza viruses typically include those shown in Box 88.1.

Influenza virus testing

- The reference standard for laboratory confirmation is reverse transcription-polymerase chain reaction (RT-PCR) testing or viral culture.
  - Provides information on specific influenza subtypes and antiviral susceptibility.
  - Only available in special laboratory settings.
  - Not available as a point of care test.

Box 88.1 Factors increasing risk of flu-related complications
- Age
- Pregnancy
- Respiratory illness (asthma, COPD, cystic fibrosis)
- Cardiac illness (CHF, coronary artery disease, congenital heart disease
- Diabetes Mellitus
- Immunocompromised (HIV, AIDS, cancer, transplant patients, long-term steroid use)
- Neurological disorders
- Morbid obesity

- Rapid Influenza Diagnostic Tests (RIDTs) are immunoassays, which can detect influenza A and B in respiratory specimens.
  - Advantages:
    — Are available as point-of-care tests that yield information in a clinically relevant timeframe.
    — Highly specific, will not often produce false positive results.
  - Disadvantages:
    — Poor sensitivity (false negatives are common) – a negative RIDT does not rule out influenza infection.
    — Could be used to identify presence or absence of Influenza A or B – but not to identify the novel subtype.
- Testing is not needed for making treatment decisions for patients presenting with ILI symptoms, especially in the context of documented influenza activity in the community.
  - Testing guidance, including recommendations for who should be tested, will be available from the public-health authority (local, state, and federal public-health agencies) and/or your institution's laboratory.

Prevention
- Vaccination:
  - The most effective way to prevent influenza virus infection.
  - Reduces the likelihood of becoming ill from influenza virus and reduces likelihood of transmission to others.
  - Vaccine for seasonal influenza is broadly available in two forms:
    — Trivalent inactivated influenza vaccine (intramuscular injection).
      - Appropriate for age > 6 months, chronic medical conditions and pregnancy.
    — Live, Intranasal influenza vaccine.
      - Appropriate for healthy, nonpregnant individuals age 2–49 years old.
  - CDC recommends vaccination for all above 6 months of age who do not have contraindications.
  - Seasonal flu vaccination provides protection against three main flu viruses that are predicted to cause the most illness in a season.

- After onset of a pandemic, manufacturers will race to develop vaccine effective against the novel virus, but it may not be available until several months after recognition of the outbreak.
- Antibody development in adults takes about two weeks after vaccination and may take longer for children.
- Infection-Control Measures
  - Minimize exposure:
    — Screen patients to identify influenza-like illness.
    — Implement respiratory hygiene and cough etiquette.
    — Implement hand hygiene.
    — Apply a surgical mask to individuals who are coughing to contain their respiratory secretions.
    — Encourage coughing individuals to sit at least three feet from one another in common areas.
  - Adhere to recommended infection-control posture.
    — Standard Precautions:
      - Hand hygiene—before and after every patient contact, before and after handling personal protective equipment, after handling potentially infectious material.
      - Gloves.
      - Gown—when anticipating contact with secretions.
    — Droplet precautions:
      - Surgical masks will prevent transmission of illness via large respiratory droplet.
      - Droplet precautions are recommended for contact with seasonal influenza patients in the health-care setting.
    — Aerosol precautions:
      - NIOSH approved, fitted N-95 respirators (TB masks) will prevent transmission of illness via infectious respiratory aerosol.
      - Certain procedures increase the likelihood of generating higher concentration of aerosol, and fitted N-95 respirators are recommended to decrease the likelihood of exposure to infectious aerosols. See Box 88.2.

Specific infection-control guidance for a novel influenza virus will be recommended by the Centers for Disease Control, state and local public-health authorities, and your institution's infection-control authority. Recommendations will be based on the best evidence available about transmission of the novel virus. In the absence of data regarding virulence

---

Box 88.2 Examples of aerosol generating procedures
- Bronchoscopy
- Sputum induction
- Intubation
- Open suctioning
- CPR
- Positive pressure ventilation (BiPAP, CPAP)
- Nebulized medication delivery
- High-frequency oscillatory ventilation

and transmission of the novel virus early in the course of the pandemic, it should be expected that infection-control recommendations would be more conservative.

- Chemoprophylaxis:
  - Although vaccination is the most effective way to prevent illness from influenza virus, until vaccine effective against the novel virus is available, chemoprophylaxis with antiviral medications may be effective in preventing infection. Antiviral medications are 70–90 percent effective in preventing seasonal influenza.
  - Advantages:
    — May assist in prevention of the flu until vaccine becomes available.
    — May assist in control of outbreaks among persons at high risk for complications secondary to flu.
  - Disadvantages:
    — Antiviral medications must be taken each day for the duration of possible exposure to influenza virus.
    — Antiviral medications may not be available in sufficient quantity in the community.
    — The novel virus may be resistant to available antiviral medications.
    — Widespread or routine use of antiviral medications may contribute to emergence of resistant viruses.

Treatment

Treatment for influenza infection is primarily supportive. All persons should be vigilant for complications of influenza illness, especially for those with underlying medical conditions that put them at greater risk. Therapy will be dependent on the clinical manifestations of the disease that may come from direct effects of the influenza virus, complications associated with pregnancy, or complications associated with underlying respiratory, cardiac, or other chronic medical conditions. For example, influenza can be complicated by bacterial pneumonia, necessitating treatment with antibiotics.

- Supportive therapy:
  - Adequate hydration.
  - Antipyretics.
  - Antitussives.
  - Analgesics.

Antiviral medications may also be used to treat influenza infection. Use of these medications may reduce illness severity and shorten duration of symptoms. They may also reduce the risk of serious complications associated with influenza-like respiratory failure and death. When indicated, antiviral treatment should be started as soon as possible after onset of symptoms. They have been shown to be most effective if treatment is started within two days of onset of illness, but they may still be beneficial for patients with risk factors for complications or severe illness if given later. The public-health authority (CDC, state, local) will make recommendations for use of antiviral medications for treatment of influenza in the context of pandemic. Recommendations for use of antiviral medications for treatment of seasonal influenza are routinely available.

Health-system considerations

Pandemic influenza has potential to cause significant illness and death and cause significant social and economic impact. Health-care resources and operations are at particular risk for being impacted. The following are a number of considerations for health systems in response to a pandemic.

Surveillance—monitor influenza activity

Pandemic influenza activity is global, but not uniform. Communities will be impacted at different times as the influenza spreads across the globe. Mechanisms should be in place to recognize increase in influenza activity in the community as well as in the health system. This situational awareness will guide system communications, testing and treatment guidance, and implementation of mitigation strategies for patient surge. The surveillance can be both syndromic (number of ILI patients presenting for evaluation to the clinic or emergency department) or laboratory based (number of samples positive for influenza).

Communications

Mechanisms should be in place to communicate with health-system administrators, staff, patients, and visitors regarding the impact of the pandemic on the health-care facility. Communications will include guidance and education on prevention and control of influenza transmission, role of vaccine and antivirals in preventing and reducing the impact of disease, work and sick leave policies, and other pertinent information.

Visitor access

Visitation rights for patients' families are important for their well-being and recovery. To decrease likelihood of influenza transmission, visitor-restriction policies may be instituted. Visitors may be screened for presence of ILI, may be limited in number, and may receive flu-prevention guidance such as hand hygiene, cough etiquette, and use of PPE.

Monitor workforce illness

Health-care providers will be discouraged from coming to work if they develop signs and symptoms of ILI during pandemic. Guidance for when a health-care worker is suitable to return to work will be provided based on consideration of infectivity and patient contact. Persons may be excluded from work for some period after which they are no longer febrile. Further restrictions may be recommended for health-care workers with exposure to immunocompromised patients. Sick-leave policies should facilitate adherence to the recommended guidelines. Guidance will be available from public-health authorities and adopted by health-care administration and occupational health.

Absenteeism

Health systems should anticipate workforce shortages secondary to illness and time needed for recovery. Absenteeism may also result from child-care responsibilities aggravated by school and daycare closures as well as sick family members. Monitoring of absences will assist in determining the impact on operations. Mitigation strategies may include cross-training of individuals in advance to perform critical functions.

Environmental and engineering controls

Special provisions may be made to prevent transmission of influenza virus in the health-care setting. This will include special attention to cleaning and disinfection procedures, physical barriers between patients in common areas, special care in areas where aerosol-producing procedures are performed and possibly also areas with special-air-handling capacity.

Stockpiling

Pandemic influenza may impact supply-chain logistics resulting in shortages of essential consumable medical supplies and pharmaceuticals. Health systems may choose to increase their on-hand inventory. Items may include respirators (face masks) and other PPEs, antiviral medications, ventilators, and so forth. Resources may be released from state and federal inventories, such as the Strategic National Stockpile.

Surge capacity planning

Depending on the severity of the pandemic, health systems may become overwhelmed with patients seeking evaluation and those requiring treatment or hospitalization. In addition to making provisions to care for more patients in the clinical setting, mitigation strategies may also include public-service messaging about need to seek medical evaluation, web-based self assessment, nurse-advice call lines, and point-of-entry triage strategies that direct patients to the appropriate level of care, hospital, clinic, or self-care at home.

Summary

Influenza pandemics impact large portions of the global population and can cause significant illness and death. Mitigation of an influenza pandemic will be dependent on good public health response measures, adherence to sound infection control practices, availability of vaccine, and antiviral medications, and capacity to manage the health-care consequences.

Updated information about pandemic influenza can be found at:
- http://www.cdc.gov/flu/pandemic/
- http://www.pandemicflu.gov/
- http://www.who.int/csr/disease/influenza/pandemic/en/
- http://www.cidrap.umn.edu/cidrap/content/influenza/panflu/index.html

Suggested readings

Centers for Disease Control and Prevention. Clinical signs and symptoms of influenza. Available at http://www.cdc.gov/flu/professionals/acip/clinical.htm Accessed November 5, 2010.

Centers for Disease Control and Prevention. Guidance for clinicians on the use of rapid influenza diagnostic tests for the 2010–2011 influenza season. Available at http://www.cdc.gov/flu/pdf/professionals/diagnosis/clinician_guidance_ridt.pdf Accessed November 5, 2010.

Centers for Disease Control and Prevention. People at high risk of developing flu-related complications. Available at http://www.cdc.gov/flu/about/disease/high_risk.htm Accessed November 5, 2010.

Centers for Disease Control and Prevention. 2010–2011 Influenza antiviral medications: Summary for clinicians. Available at http://www.cdc.gov/flu/professionals/antivirals/summary-clinicians.htm Accessed December 5, 2010.

Osterholm M (2005, July/Aug). Preparing for the next pandemic. *Foreign Affairs.*

Tornadoes

Bryan F. McNally

Background

A tornado is one of the most dramatic manifestations of severe weather. Physically, it is a rotating column of air that travels in contact with a cloud and the earth's surface. They are capable of causing significant morbidity and mortality, in addition to causing property damage and imposing an economic burden on affected communities.

- Tornadoes typically form in the context of a thunderstorm class known as supercells, where cold and warm air currents meet.
- They often appear as a funnel of condensation, surrounded by debris and dirt.
- At their extremes, they can be 2–3 kilometers wide, achieve ground speeds in excess of 450 km/h, and travel for hundreds of kilometers.

Incidence

Accurate measurements of incidence are limited by underreporting and lack of monitoring ability in unpopulated or resource-constrained settings.

- Tornadoes are reported worldwide, but are most common in the United States, where approximately 1,200 are confirmed annually.
- Recent data from Europe suggests an average annual incidence of 170.
- The increased frequency in the United States stems from particular geographic conditions, as dry air descending from the Rocky Mountains meets warm moist air from the Gulf of Mexico, creating fertile conditions for tornado formation.
- The central plains of North America have been dubbed "Tornado Alley" due to the frequency of tornadoes in the region.
- Although tornadoes can occur at any time of year and at any time of day, peak incidence in North America is in spring and fall, and tornadoes are most common in the late afternoon and early evening.

Intensity

Several indices have been developed to describe tornado strength, including the Fujita, Enhanced Fujita (EF), and TORRO scales. The EF scale is the most recently developed and perhaps in widest use.

- The EF scale classifies tornadoes using a six-point scale, on the basis of their ability to cause structural damage.
- The potential for damage and serious injury increases with class, although tornadoes from each EF level have caused deaths.
- An EF0 tornado causes damage to trees and superficial structures; an EF5 tornado can destroy well-engineered buildings and subterranean storm shelters.
- Approximately 80 percent of tornadoes are lower intensity (EF0 and EF1); less than 0.1 percent of tornadoes are classified as EF5.
- EF4 and EF5 tornadoes cause a disproportionate fraction of all tornado-related injury and property damage.

Patterns of injury

Most tornado-related injuries result from victims becoming airborne, solid objects becoming airborne, or structural collapse. Both blunt and penetrating mechanisms of injury are described.

- Soft tissue wounds are the most commonly reported injury, including contusions, lacerations, puncture wounds, and abrasions.
- Wounds are often deep and contaminated; many will require surgical debridement. Contamination and any subsequent infection is polymicrobial. Foreign bodies such as glass and organic debris will be present in many wounds.
- Fractures are the second most common type of injury encountered. In some reports, up to 30 percent of victims presenting for care had fractures, with over 20 percent open fractures.
- Closed head injuries are one of the most common mechanisms of severe injury, and they contribute to mortality after a tornado. In addition to intracranial injuries, scalp lacerations and skull fractures are frequently encountered.
- Death from tornadoes typically occurs on scene, and is associated with severe head injuries, cervical spine injury, or crush injury to the chest.
- Tornadoes can damage the power supply, leading to the possibility of electrical injury. Occasionally, posttornado fires and burns have been reported.
- Prehospital providers should recognize the risk of injury in search and rescue operations, particularly if structures have collapsed or if there are fires or downed wires.

Risk factors for injury

Risk factors for injuries after a tornado have been established by retrospective analysis of victims.

- Individuals who seek shelter from a tornado are consistently found to have lower rates of injury than those who do not.
- The most effective shelters are in cellars of houses or buildings with foundations, away from windows or other glass.
- Residents of mobile homes are at particularly high risk for increased rates of both injury and severe injury, as are individuals in motor vehicles.
- Both the absence of a tornado warning, and a shorter duration of warning are associated with more significant injuries.
- Older adults are at increased risk of injury, likely, in part, due to comorbidities and decreased mobility.

Prehospital and emergency department response

Tornadoes present several challenges to prehospital providers and the staff of emergency departments (EDs) that will treat victims.

- The search for and transportation of victims may be obstructed by debris and blocked roads. Patients may be taken to the most accessible hospital, rather than closer but inaccessible facilities. EDs should prepare accordingly.
- Victims may be scattered over a wide area of the tornado's path.
- Because of typical injury patterns, prehospital interventions may have little impact on long-term patient outcomes. Rapid transportation to definitive care is preferred, in accordance with regional trauma and disaster protocols.
- Scene response by physicians or nurses has little impact on morbidity or mortality. Health-care personnel with field-medicine experience may be of assistance in triage of victims to specialized receiving facilities.
- Communication between scene responders and EDs may be limited by damage to infrastructure assets.
- All hospitals should have a disaster plan that includes a response to natural disasters. Plans should have provisions to both minimize damage to the facility and personnel and accommodate the arrival of casualties.
- EDs should anticipate a surge of patients following a tornado and must consider activating their disaster plan.
- Many patients, including the initial wave of patients, may present by private vehicle, rather than ambulance. Patients with more severe injuries may arrive in a second wave, 1–4 hours after the tornado.
- Supplies for wound management, including dressings, equipment for irrigation and closure, and tetanus toxoid will be among the principal needs.
- Tornado-related wounds have a high rate of infection when closed primarily in the ED. Providers should strongly consider delayed primary closure. Limited, retrospective data does not support the use of empiric broad-spectrum antibiotics for prevention of infections.

Injury prevention

Relatively simple interventions can minimize tornado-related injuries. Government and public health agencies can contribute to injury prevention through education, meteorological monitoring, and dissemination of tornado warnings.

- Efforts to minimize morbidity and mortality from tornadoes should focus on encouraging individuals to seek adequate shelter in basements or cellars.
- Occupants of mobile homes and other motor vehicles should be counseled to seek more substantive shelter. Mobile home parks, particularly in tornado-prone regions, should provide a communal shelter for residents.
- Individuals in a motor vehicle who cannot access other shelters should exit their vehicles and lie low in a ditch or other low ground with their heads covered.
- Tornado warnings should be issued through any available media outlets, including radio, television, and the Internet. Earlier warnings are more likely to be effective.
- Community members should consider contacting older adults, who may be less likely to receive warnings.

Resource-limited settings

Although the majority of tornadoes occur in nations with advanced weather tracking, communication systems, and health-care facilities, tornadoes occur worldwide. Some of the recorded tornadoes with the greatest impact on humans and human settlements have occurred in underresourced settings. Retrospective analysis of tornadoes has yielded several insights:

• Patterns of injury after a tornado appear similar, regardless of location.
• Obtaining shelter is protective against injury and death.
• Structural collapse of a shelter, and some elements of construction materials, such as tin roofs, may be risk factors for injury. Older age is another risk factor for injury.
• Seeking and accessing medical care after injury helps prevent disability and mortality by ensuring wound care and fracture management.
• Efforts to identify and transport victims may be complicated by infrastructure limitations.
• Identifying conditions for tornadoes and distributing warnings to affected populations is an area of opportunity for public health research and practice.

Suggested readings

Bohonos JJ, Hogan DE (1999). The medical impact of tornadoes in North America. *J Emerg Med* 17(1): 67–73.

Comstock RD, Mallonee S (2005). Comparing reactions to two severe tornadoes in one Oklahoma community. *Disasters* 29(3): 277–287.

Comstock RD, Mallonee S (2005). Get off the bus: Sound strategy for injury prevention during a tornado. *Prehosp Disaster Med* 20(3): 189–192.

Daley WR, Brown S, Archer P, Kruger E, Jordan F, Batts D, Mallonee S (2005). Risk of tornado related death and injury in Oklahoma, May 3, 1999. *Am J Epidemiol* 161(12): 1144–1150.

Hogan DE, Askins DC, Osborn AE (1999). The May 3, 1999 tornado in Oklahoma City. *Ann Emerg Med* 34(2): 225–226.

Kunii O, Kunori T, Takahashi K, Kaneda M, Fuke N (1996). Health impact of 1996 tornado in Bangladesh. *Lancet* 348 (029): 757.

May AK, McGwin G, Lancaster LJ, Hardin W, Taylor AJ, Holden S, Davis GG, Rue LW (2000). The April 8 1998 tornado: Assessment of the trauma system response and the resulting injuries. *J Trauma* 48(4):666–672.

Noji EK (2000). The public health consequences of disasters. *Prehosp Disaster Med* 15(4): 147–157.

Sookram S, Borkent H, Powell G, Horgarth WD, Shepherd L (2001). Tornado at Pine Lake, Alberta—Assessment of the emergency medicine response to a disaster. *CJEM* 3(1): 34–37.

Sugimoto JD, Labrique AB, Ahmad S, Rashid M, Shamim AA, Ullah B, Klemm RD, Christian P, West KP (2010, Nov). Epidemiology of tornado destruction in northern Bangladesh: Risk factors for death and injury. *Disasters* Epub ahead of print.

Weir E (2000). Tornadoes and disaster management. *CMAJ* 163(6): 756.

Tsunami

Lori L. Harrington

Introduction

A tsunami is defined as a series of waves, generated by an offshore disturbance. A tsunami reaches land with enormous destructive force. The energy created and then dispersed by the wave leads to extensive destruction of infrastructure and risk to human life. The word *tsunami* comes from the Japanese language, meaning harbor wave, not the often misnamed "tidal wave."

Physics
- Most commonly caused by offshore/underwater earthquake.
- Uncommonly caused by underwater sediment slide, landslide, volcanic collapse, asteroid impact.
- Generated by vertical displacement of a large volume of water from an underground disturbance.
- Very large volume of water from the floor of ocean to the surface, not just surface waves.
- Often not felt in the open ocean by ships.
- Travels extremely fast in deep water (450–600 mph) and slows as it reaches land.
- Waves travel across the ocean without diminution of power.
- Propagation from low-amplitude, high-wavelength waves in deep water to high-amplitude, lower-wavelength, high-energy waves in shallow water.
- Destruction can occur distant from the waves' origin.
- Wave landfall leads to massive destruction of infrastructure, extensive debris, utility interruption, loss of life, and injury.

Recent history
Tsunamis most commonly occur in the "Ring of fire" in the Pacific Ocean due to frequency of earthquakes and volcanic activity. Damaging tsunamis occur 1–2 times yearly. Recent history has shaped the understanding of tsunami including:
- 1946 Aleutian Islands tsunami struck Hawaii killing 150 people, prompting the development of tsunami warning systems.
- 1949 Pacific Tsunami Warning Center established.
- 1960 Chilean tsunami, resulted from the largest earthquake recorded (9.5 on the Richter scale) off coast of Chile. 2,000 deaths in Chile, 61 deaths in Hawaii, 122 deaths in Japan.
- 1964 great Alaskan earthquake, 122 deaths attributed to tsunami.
- 1967 West Coast/Alaskan Tsunami Warning Center established.
- 1998 Papua, New Guinea 2,200 deaths, 700 injuries.

Current experience
- 2004 Indian Ocean Southeast Asian tsunami
  - Caused by 9.2 magnitude earthquake off coast of Sumatra, Indonesia.
  - Directly affected 14 countries including India, Indonesia, Malaysia, the Maldives, Somalia, Sri Lanka, and Thailand.
  - Catastrophic destruction and loss of life.
  - Largest tsunami in written human history.

- Largest number of recorded deaths from a tsunami, estimated at 230,000 deaths.
- Estimated 1.7 million people displaced.
- Estimated economic loss to the region $9.9 billion.
- Increased risk of destruction and human loss due to increased population density along coasts and beach tourism.
- 2011 Japanese tsunami
  - Caused by 9.0 magnitude earthquake off east coast of Japan.
  - 20,000 dead or missing, hundreds of thousands displaced.
  - Massive 40 meter waves traveled up to 10km inland.
  - 125,000 buildings destroyed
  - Caused a 2nd catastrophic disaster from damage to Fukushima Nuclear Power Plant complex and resulting level 7 meltdown at 3 nuclear reactors.

Medical care after tsunami

Disease patterns and injuries noted after tsunamis are comparable to those occurring as a result of floods and earthquakes. Much of the current data regarding clinically important diseases and injuries resulting from tsunami disasters was acquired after the tsunami that struck Southeast Asia on December 26, 2004.

- Majority of morbidity and mortality:
  - Traumatic injuries with associated wound infections.
  - Drowning or near drowning complicated by aspiration pneumonia.
- Exacerbation of chronic illness proved a significant complaint among patients.
- Communicable diseases not a significant cause of morbidity and mortality with this disaster, but should be considered.

Traumatic injury

The most common traumatic injuries as a result of the 2004 tsunami were minor injuries; major wounds with wound infections were the second most common health problem among tsunami survivors. There were a significant number of fractures as well. Injuries were described in multiple areas of the body, with the lower extremities being the most common. Wounds were often grossly contaminated with sand, mud, and debris. Surgical debridement was required in 90 percent of cases in one study.

- Most common mechanism of injury was blunt trauma from floating debris or crush injury from compression into large stationary or mobile masses.
- Approximately one-third of fractures sustained were open.
- Delayed surgical debridement led to infection.
- Gram-negative bacilli were most commonly isolated when wound cultures were performed. See Box 90.1.
- Some pathogens were highly resistant.

Management

Extremity fractures should be splinted as with basic orthopedic care. These patients should be transported to a facility for definitive care as soon as possible. All wounds should be considered highly contaminated. They should be aggressively irrigated and debrided as indicated as soon as possible.

- Wounds should be left open.
- Broad-spectrum antibiotics to cover treatment of Gram negatives and polymicrobial infections.

Box 90.1 Commonly isolated organisms

- Aeromonas species
- Escherichia coli
- Klebsiella pneumoniae
- Pseudomonas aeruginosa
- Acinetobacter baumanii

- Consider the possibility of mixed infection and include coverage for anaerobic bacteria for wounds that are deep, heavily contaminated and/or have a foul-smelling discharge.
- Wounds should be re-assessed at 48 hours for exploration and debridement as needed.

Drowning and near drowning

"Near drowning" is defined as a submersion episode of sufficient severity to warrant medical attention. Drowning is death from asphyxia within 24 hours of submersion. The majority of patients experiencing near-drowning events are young and otherwise healthy. The case fatality rate associated with pneumonias caused by near drowning is 60 percent. See Table 90.1.

Aspiration is an important determining factor about whether pneumonia develops. Seventy percent of drowning victims aspirate mud, sand, and fragments of aquatic vegetation.

- Involuntary breathing causes aspiration of water.
- Victims of near-drowning, while in a panic state, often swallow large amounts of water, placing them at significant risk for vomiting, particularly during resuscitation, increasing aspiration risk.
- Submersion in contaminated water increases the risk of developing pneumonia due to inflammatory changes and damage to lung parenchyma.
- Bacteria are endemic to particular areas and bodies of water, a fact that should be kept in mind in determining antibiotic therapy.
- "Tsunami lung" is a term coined to describe a necrotizing pneumonia found in survivors of the Asian tsunami.
  - Subacute presentation (approx 4 weeks after event) with fluctuating fever, chronic, nonproductive cough, and radiologic evidence of bilateral asymmetric, necrotizing pneumonia with cavitation.
  - Not responsive to first-line therapy.

Table 90.1 Common pathogens causing near drowning infections.

	Description	Disease	Located	Special Considerations
Aeromonas species	Gram negative	Commonly causes pneumonia	Freshwater and saltwater	
Burkholderia pseudomallei	Gram negative	Meliodosis, post immersion pneumonia	Soil and water, endemic in Southeast Asia	Short incubation period and severe disease, healthy host
Pseudallescheria boydii and Aspergillus	Fungi	Pneumonia, disseminated disease, CNS manifestation		Severe disease in immuno-competent host

Management
- Low threshold for starting empiric antibiotics.
- Initial regimen should include an extended spectrum penicillin/beta-lactamase inhibitor.
- Add an aminoglycoside for ill patients.
- Empiric antifungal therapy should generally be avoided except in patients slow to respond to antibiotic therapy. In patients developing pneumonia several weeks after the near-drowning event, or developing CNS infection, antifungal therapy should be considered.

Skin infection

Natural disasters can have an effect on human skin. One study found the most prevalent skin problems after the tsunami were infectious infestations, with superficial fungal infections, such as tinea corporis and tinea pedis, being the most common. Eczemas were the second most common, which were mostly comprised of irritant contact dermatitis. Traumatic skin disorders were the third most common in this study, however, the findings may be biased because data collection did not begin until 10 days after the event.

Vector-borne disease

Malaria and other vector-borne disease outbreaks, such as dengue, were a public-health concern following the tsunami. This was of particular concern in Sri Lanka, because there had been an outbreak of dengue hemorrhagic fever with the loss of 300 lives earlier in 2004. However, one study examining the conditions in Sri Lanka, an area hit hard by the tsunami, concluded that the actual risk of malaria outbreak was relatively low. This risk assessment was supported a year later when the same study group returned to the region to assess the incidence of malaria. They found that the incidence of malaria had decreased in 2005 as compared to 2004 in most districts in Sri Lanka, including the ones hardest hit by the tsunami. They concluded that there was no evidence that the tsunami affected the incidence of malaria. However, monitoring for outbreaks of vector-borne disease should be conducted with continual surveillance in endemic areas.

Management
- Prevention is paramount in reducing the transmission of malaria and other vector-borne illness.
- Remove standing pools of water and other known breeding grounds for the insect vector.
- Provide external protection, such as chemically treated mosquito netting or chemically impregnated coverings for temporary shelters to prevent bites.
- Use barrier protection such as DEET on exposed skin.
- Distribute appropriate chemoprophylaxis to those living and working in temporary camps in conjunction with the host nation's local ministry of health.

Communicable disease

Crowded, unsanitary conditions that are typical in the immediate post-disaster period increase the risk of infectious -disease outbreaks. This risk is not particular to tsunami, but can occur wherever disaster strikes. The primary goal of emergency health intervention is to prevent epidemics of disease and improve deteriorating health conditions in the affected population. Diseases such as cholera, measles, and meningitis are highly communicable and can cause significant morbidity and mortality in vulnerable populations. Children are at particular risk. As such, diarrheal illness, respiratory illness, and febrile illnesses are closely monitored.

Diarrheal disease

In some reports, diarrheal diseases have accounted for up to 40 percent of deaths in the acute phase of an emergency, with over 80 percent of those deaths occurring in children.

- Common sources of infection include polluted water sources, contamination of clean water thorough soiled hands, scarcity of soap, and contaminated foods.
- Treatment involves providing clean water resources and education regarding good sanitation practices.

Measles

Measles epidemics have been a major cause of mortality in camp settings, especially in children. In complex emergency settings, the case fatality rate has been reported as high as 33 percent, whereas it is only 1 percent in stable populations. This is likely due to transmission of a higher infectious dose in the setting of overcrowded conditions.

- Rapid immunization of children 6 months to 14 years is now routinely implemented in emergency camp settings.
- Repeat vaccination is encouraged in populations having a high rate of one-dose measles coverage.
- Supplementation with vitamin A during measles vaccination campaigns acts as a protective factor for acute respiratory infections independently of measles.
- Maintain standard respiratory precautions (i.e., covering your mouth when coughing, good hand washing, etc.).

Respiratory illness

Acute respiratory infections can be a major cause of morbidity and mortality in emergency settings and account for up to 20 percent of all deaths in children younger than 5 in emergency camps.

- Acute respiratory infections amplify the transmission risk for meningococcal disease through droplet transmission.
- Early recognition and management of pneumonia are keys to preventing an outbreak.

Public-health response

After all natural disasters including tsunamis, public-health needs of the population must be quickly evaluated by a rapid needs assessment to provide an understanding of the disaster's impact on the affected population. The needs assessment is a continuous and ongoing process during all stages of disaster management. Public-health needs assessment should occur concurrently with medical needs assessment and provision of medical care. See Box 90.2.

The peak need for assistance comes in the first few hours to days before outside agencies are available. Therefore, local resources are often the first and only available.

Public-health agencies including private outside aid organizations, non-governmental organizations (NGOs), and foreign governments must work with the local people and agencies to develop and coordinate strategies for continued response and recovery. Coordination of outside aid agencies is essential in avoiding inappropriate and ovelapping aid. Outside aid must involve local peoples in order to overcome cultural and linguistic barriers.

- In addition to addressing immediate basic human needs, public- health agencies, both local and outside, must also address:
- Ongoing disease surveillance.
- Record keeping including relocation records, IDP camp census.
- Infrastructure redevelopment.
- Reinstitution of social norms (e.g., children returning to school, adults returning to work).
- Environmental implications of disaster, including:
  - Disposal of solid waste, debris, and hazardous materials.
  - Contamination of soil and water supply, including salination of fresh water supply.
  - Contamination of fishing grounds.
  - Loss of natural barriers of coastal land.

Box 90.2 Public-health needs assessment
- Water
- Food
- Shelter
- Sanitation
- Security
- Transportation
- Communication
- Patient and family tracking
- Morgue facility needs
- Disease and vector control

Mental-health considerations

Mental health is often considered secondary to immediate medical needs of a population and is often not evaluated as part of a needs assessment. However, after experiencing such an incomprehensible tragedy as occurred in the Southeast Asian tsunami, mental-health workers determined there was a very large burden of psychological distress among vulnerable individuals. In general, mental-health problems improve over time through a natural period of recovery. Returning to normal social structures is essential in early recovery to relieve psychosocial stressors.

- Both displaced and nondisplaced survivors of the tsunami experienced psychology symptoms.
- Symptoms of depression, anxiety, and posttraumatic stress disorder (PTSD) were experienced.
- Younger persons were more likely to experience higher levels of psychological distress. Persons who were closer to the coast and those in more highly damaged zones were also more likely to have symptoms.
- High levels of psychosocial distress are clearly evident after large disasters. Therefore, mental-health response should be part of the health care offered through aid agencies, both for immediate care and long-term recovery. Incorporating local resources is especially important in providing mental-health care to ensure culturally competent and appropriate care.

Box 90.3 Stressors experienced by survivors of the 2004 tsunami
- Fear of dying
- Fear of losing a loved one
- Exposure to dead bodies
- Loss of loved ones
- Community disruption
- Economic hardship
- Physical hardship

Mortality

Deaths frequently exceed the number of injuries in tsunami, unlike most disasters where there are more injured than dead. Death disproportionately affects more vulnerable populations including elderly, children, physically disabled, and even women secondary to decreased physical strength and stamina.

Causes of death
- Trimodal model: pattern of death in mass-casualty incidents.
  - First and largest mortality peak occurs at the time of injury (death from severe trauma, drowning).
  - Second mortality peak occurs minutes to hours after initial insult (death from blunt or penetrating chest or abdominal injury, intracranial injury, blood loss, hypoxia from aspiration).
  - Final mortality peak occurs in weeks (sepsis, respiratory failure, multi-organ system failure).
- Most common cause of death is drowning, second most common cause is trauma.

Morgue facilities
- Hospital morgues are not of sufficient size to handle the number of dead bodies in a large tsunami.
- Due to limited availability of morgue facilities, during the 2004 Asian tsunami, bodies were left on the grounds of hospitals, in hallways, and in wards, disrupting normal hospital operations.
- Alternative temporary morgue facilities must be established, including refrigeration units as available and infection-control protocols, to allow time for victim identification.

Disaster victim identification
All bodies should be tracked using a unique identifier or tracking number, linked to potentially identifiable information: photographs, fingerprints, dental records, DNA, belongings, basic descriptions, and specific identifiers (tattoos, scars). Computer-based patient-tracking systems exist for mass casualty patient tracking and can be used for tracking bodies as well. Alternatively, paper logs can be used to track all victims. An analogous log should be kept from family members seeking potential victims, which can then be correlated to the identified victims.
- Disaster victim identification of bodies is difficult in tsunami owing to the rapid decomposition from water immersion.
- Traditional identifiers can be used such as fingerprints, dental records, and photographs, and if possible DNA samples.
- Identification of all bodies should be attempted prior to burial if possible.
- Limited morgue facilities may necessitate earlier burial without traditional rituals.
- The dead still must be treated with dignity and respect.

Future warnings

Tsunami warning systems
- In place since 1940s in Pacific Ocean.
- Monitors earthquake activity and potential tsunami waves at tide gauges.
- Allows for potential monitoring of tsunami generation, but cannot predict information about size, extent, or location of potential tsunami landfall.
- Newer real-time deep-ocean tsunami detectors, known as tsunameters, have been more successful at using measured data and model estimates to predict tsunami impact.
- Predicting tsunami occurrence is nearly impossible because earthquakes are not predictable.
- Once generated, the tsunami's arrival and impact can be followed.

Preparedness
- Risk reduction and preparedness is the key to reducing future tsunami disasters.
- Recognition of tsunami as a potential hazard.
- Tsunami-safe construction.
- Education programs for locals and tourists.

Recovery

The goal of postdisaster recovery is to return a population to its predisaster state. Long-term recovery from a tsunami takes many years. Stakeholders must recognize the difference between meaningful short-term recovery and the ultimate long-term goal. Long-term recovery plans must consider the constraints of the predisaster social situation including baseline economic characteristics and political conflicts and requires the involvement of local people and political structure as the key central stakeholders.

- Building schools, homes, hospitals, roads.
- Sanitation infrastructure.
- Environmental recovery.
- Long-term health care needs, preventative care, immunization programs.
- Return to local economic strengths for the Asian tsunami included fishing, agriculture, and return of tourism.
- May be an opportunity for growth of policies addressing predisaster conflict and inequality.

Suggested readings

Allworth A (2005).Tsunami lung: A necrotizing pneumonia in survivors of the Asian tsunami. *MJA* 7: 364.

Briet O, Galappaththy G, Amerasinghe P, Konradsen F (2006). Malaria in Sri Lanka: One year post tsunami. *Malaria Journal* 5: 42.

Ender P, Dolan M (1997). Pneumonia associated with near-drowning. *Clin Infect Dis* 25: 896–907.

Frankenberg E, Friedman J, et al. (2008). Mental health in Sumatra after the tsunami. *Am J Pub Health* 98: 1671–1677.

Hiransuthikul N, Tantisiriwat W, Lertutsahakul K (2005). Skin and soft-tissue infections among tsunami survivors in southern Thailand. *Clin Infect Dis* 41: e93–96.

Johnson LJ, Travis AR (2006). Trimodal death and the injuries of survivors in Krabi Province Thailand, post-tsunami. *ANZ J Surg* 76: 288–289.

Kaewlai R, Srisuwan T, Prasitvoranant W, et al. (2007). Radiologic findings in tsunami trauma: Experience with 225 patients injured in the 2004 tsunami. *Emerg Radiol* 14: 395–402.

Lee S, Choi C, Eun H, Kwon O (2006). Skin problems after a tsunami. *European Academy of Dermatology and Venereology* 20: 860–863.

Maegele M, Gregor S, Yuecei N, et al. (2006). One year ago not business as usual: Wound management, infection and psychoemeotional control during tertiary medical care following the 2004 tsunami disaster in southeast Asia. *Crit Care* 10: 1–9.

Prasartritha T, Tungsiripat R, Warachit P (2008). The revisit of 2004 tsunami in Thailand: Characteristics of wounds. *International Wound Journal* 5: 8–19.

Sechriest V, Lhowe D (2008). Orthopaedic care abord the USNS Mercy during operation unified assistance after the 2004 Asian tsunami. *J Bone Joint Surg Am* 90: 849–861.

Souza R, Bernatsky S, Reyes R, de Jong K (2007). Mental health status of vulnerable tsunami-affected communities: A survey in Aceh Province, Indonesia. *J Trauma Stress* 20: 263–269.

Telford J, Cosgrave J (2006). *Joint evaluation of the international response to the Indian Ocean tsunami: Synthesis report*. London: Tsunami Evaluation Coalition.

Wilder-Smith A. (2005) Tsunami in South Asia: What is the risk of post-disaster infectious disease outbreaks? *Annals Academy of Medicine* 34:625–631.

Warling S, Brown B (2005). The threat of communicable disease following natural disasters: A public health response. *Disaster Manag Response* 3: 41–47.

Yamada S, Gunatilake R, Roytman T, et al. (2006). The Sri Lanka tsunami experience. *Disaster Manag Response* 4: 38–47.

Volcanic eruption

Siri Daulaire

Background

Historical relevance

Volcanoes are openings in the planet's crust that allow hot magma, ash, and gases to reach the surface. More than three-quarters of the earth's surface is volcanic in origin. Volcanic eruptions and the resulting damage are estimated to have caused approximately 1 million deaths in the last 2000 years. More than six hundred volcanoes have erupted in human history and are considered active, with additional thousands still lying dormant. Globally, there are approximately 50 eruptions annually. The highest risk areas for volcanic disaster include: Southeast Asia, the Pacific Rim, western South America, the Middle East, western Africa, the western United States, the Hawaiian Islands, and Iceland. See Table 91.1.

Table 91.1 Historical volcanic disasters

Year	Volcano	Country	Mortality	Other Effects
79 AD	Mt Vesuvius	Italy	Unknown death toll, ~1500 remains found	Still an active volcano, in the most densely populated volcanic region in the world
1883	Krakatau	Indonesia	36,000 deaths	
1815	Tambora	Indonesia	92,000 deaths	Lowered global temperatures by 3°C
1908	Mt Pele	Martinique	28,000 deaths	200 square miles of deforestation, within minutes
1985	Mt Nevado Del Ruiz	Columbia	22,000 deaths	
1986	Lake Nyos	Cameroon	1700 deaths, 1000s displaced	CO_2 gas release caused most deaths
1991	Pinatubo	Philippines	300–800 deaths	15 to 30 million tons of sulfur dioxide, blocking sunlight and leading to global cooling by 0.5°C
2010	Eyjafjallajokull	Iceland	500 people evacuated, no deaths	Ash cloud caused the greatest disruption of air travel in Europe since WWII

Definitions

Types of eruption

- Effusive eruption: outpouring of lava without significant explosion.
- Explosive eruption: gas driven explosions that propels magma and tephra.

Types of volcano

- Shield volcano: broad based volcano built of layered viscous lava flows.
- Composite volcano (stratovolcano): tall conical volcano built of periodic explosive eruptions.
- Cinder cone volcano: steep conical hill of volcanic rocks accumulating downwind from a volcanic vent. See Table 91.2.

Table 91.2 Subtypes of volcanic eruptions

Hawaiian	Effusive	lava fountains and fluid lava flows with a very low volume of ejected material
Strombolian	Explosive	Bursting of gas bubbles within magma throwing magma high into the air, generally short lived
Vulcanian	Explosive	Built up gas pressure in viscous magma breaking through a solid "cap" with intermittent explosive events
Pelean	Explosive	Large amount of gas, dust, ash, and lava blown out of the central crater; generally the most dangerous type
Plinian (aka Vesuvian)	Explosive	Dissolved volatile gases in magma expand as they rise then explode, forcing magma up an eruption column at high speeds for sustained time period
Surtseyan	Explosive	Rising magma contacts shallow water which flashes to steam and expands, fragmenting lava

Mechanisms of injury

Volcanic eruptions cause significant damage to their surrounding environment, and they have myriad health impacts on the population in the vicinity. The direct effects of volcanic eruption cause much less morbidity than the indirect effects of starvation, water contamination, exposure, and the broader concerns of a displaced populace. Mechanical trauma is the most significant direct cause of injuries, with chemical exposure and inhalation injuries making the bulk of the rest. Volcanic eruptions are also a major cause of tsunamis and can trigger earthquakes leading to greater damage.

Pyroclastic flows

A hot mix of gas, ash, pumice, and rock, which burst at high speeds.
- The most common cause of death associated with volcanoes.
- Move at high speeds (may be >100 kph).
- Cause injury by blunt or penetrating trauma in the blast effect, thermal injury, and asphyxia.

Lava flows

Streams of molten rock erupting or oozing from a volcanic vent.
- Magma flow will destroy everything in its path.
- Speed of flow is defined by the type of lava, the steepness of the ground, and whether it is confined or spreading to the sides.
- Generally slow-moving but may become pyroclastic.
- Cause injury by blunt trauma and thermal injury when escape routes are blocked by other flows.

Lahars (volcanic mud flows)

Hot or cold mix of rock, ash, and water moving down a slope or river valley.
- Appearance is that of fluid concrete.
- Varies in size and speed.
- Major damage to property, bridges, and roads.
- Cause injury by blunt trauma and thermal injury.
- Be aware of crush syndromes in patients requiring long extrications.

Volcanic ash

Shattered solid rock that is hard, abrasive, corrosive, not dissolvable in water, and conducts electricity when wet. When fragments are greater than 2 mm they are called tephra.
- Composed of shattered rock in the explosion (not a product of combustion).
- Limits visibility over significant distances.
- Clogs engines, electric generators and building-wide air filters.
- Shorts out exposed electrical insulation causing power failure.
- Negatively charged ash causes electrical storms when interacting with positively charged gases also released by the volcanic eruption.

- Settles on buildings with weights up to 5 tons/m², causing potential collapse.
- Causes injury by:
  - Irritation to the respiratory tract, causing bronchitis and asthma exacerbations.
  - irritation to eyes, causing corneal abrasions and conjunctivitis.

Silicosis

Free silica is found in volcanic ash in varying amounts. Exposure to significant amounts of free silica may cause a pulmonary disease characterized by lung inflammation and eventual pulmonary fibrosis.

Toxic gases

Many products of combustion may be released into the air in a volcanic eruption, the most dangerous of which are carbon dioxide, sulfur dioxide, and hydrogen fluoride. See Table 91.3.

Table 91.3 Toxic gases in volcanic eruption

Gas	Physical characteristics	Signs and Symptoms	Environmental impact
CO_2	Colorless and odorless gas that rapidly disperses	Tachypnea, dyspnea, headache, dizziness, impaired coordination, muscle contractions, coma, seizures, death	Settles in low lying areas because it is heavier than air
SO_2	Colorless pungent gas	Skin and mucus membrane irritation, upper-respiratory inflammation, bronchitis	Causes acid rain and smog that may trigger worldwide climate changes, depletes the ozone layer
HCl	Caustic colorless gas, forming white fumes of hydrochloric acid when in contact with humid air	Mucus membrane irritation, pulmonary edema, laryngeal spasm	Causes acid rain and long term crop failure
H_2S	Colorless, flammable gas with "sewer gas" odor	Headache, dizziness, upper airway irritation, bronchitis, altered mental status, pulmonary edema	May cause asphyxiation
HF	Pale yellow gas	Mucus membrane irritation, conjunctivitis, bone and tooth degeneration	Attaches to fine ash particles and grass, causes death and injury to livestock who eat grass

Public health and preventive measures

A volcanic eruption may range from gradual and minor activity, as in the slow-moving magma flows of Hawaii, to the grand scale of devastation evident in the eruption of Mt Vesuvius. The intensity of the eruption and site-specific factors (e.g., population density and vulnerability, local infrastructure, availability of early warning systems) defines the extent of damage after a volcanic eruption. Coordinated local disaster and evacuation plans are necessary to mitigate the potential damage. Prediction of volcanoes is challenging, because many erupt with no warning. Even in those that are predicted, the type and timing of eruption is rarely accurately determined.

General concerns
Considerations in preparation for volcanic emergencies should include:
- Ash removal protocol for hospitals, EMS, and other critical structures.
- Ash removal and maintenance of access and egress routes.
- Hazardous driving protocols for search and rescue and EMS.
- Respiratory and eye protection for first responders, local inhabitants and others.
- Search and rescue team availability with appropriate personal protective equipment.
- Evacuee welfare and shelter.
- Local hospital emergency plans with mass-casualty capabilities.
- Specialized equipment for ash collection and analysis.
- Respiratory protection with masks capable of filtering particles to submicrometer size.
- Air monitoring for toxins.
- Local population should be instructed to:
  - Stay indoors with sealed windows and doors.
  - Wear a damp cloth or mask over nose and mouth.

Transportation
Both air and ground transport may be damaged by volcanic eruption. Air transport is limited by visibility and ash, which may clog engines. Ground transport relies on roads that may be damaged or destroyed by an eruption. Accumulations of ash and other debris lead to hazardous road conditions and motor vehicle accidents. Planning for emergency evacuation and safe ground transport for rescue personnel is one of the highest priorities in mitigating a volcanic disaster.

Water
Potable water may be lost, either secondary to mechanical damage to reservoirs or by contamination of ash and other toxic substances released in a volcanic explosion. Adequate chlorination and decontamination of drinking water is critical.

Sewage
Sewage treatment facilities and sewer lines may be damaged in the setting of an eruption, contaminating drinking water and leading to an increase in

infectious diseases. Clean up activities must take place prior to allowing citizenry to return to a site after an eruption.

Infectious diseases

Rates of infection of both fecal-oral contaminants and environmental contaminants increase after a volcanic eruption. Disaster response will require adequate control of drinking water, sewage cleanup, and awareness of local concerns such as malaria.

Shelter and food

Many deaths after volcanoes occur as a result of environmental exposure and starvation. The availability of shelter at an appropriate distance from the volcano site after an explosion must be considered early in the planning of disaster relief. Food must be managed and stored properly to mitigate the risks of exposure to possible environmental toxins as well as spoilage.

Hospital treatment

Prevention of injury and adequate preparation for volcanic eruptions are the greatest resource for helping the population in the area of a volcanic disaster. In a massive explosion the number of victims immediately killed is much greater than those requiring immediate medical care. However, local hospitals should be prepared for the myriad injuries and complaints brought about by a volcanic eruption.

Trauma

Major blunt and penetrating trauma of any type may be seen after an eruption, from the damage to surrounding structures, injury in the explosion itself, or car accidents in the evacuation attempt. Care should be managed by following the current Advanced Trauma Life Support guidelines, starting with monitoring of the airway, breathing, and circulation (ABC). Major burn care is also a likely component of trauma following a volcanic eruption and adequate burn facilities should be available. Hospitals should be well-stocked with wound care supplies, pain medication, antibiotics, and tetanus immunizations and boosters.

Respiratory tract injury

Volcanic eruptions cause respiratory injury through trauma, thermal injury, and in the expulsion of ash and toxic gases. Treatment of airway injury should include prompt use of oxygen and early intubation in patients with thermal injury. Those patients with underlying lung disease such as asthma and COPD are at higher risk for significant injury and bronchodilators may be necessary. In the longer term, presentations of bronchitis and asthma exacerbations are much higher after a volcanic eruption, and local physicians should be aware of their patients with underlying disease.

Toxic exposure

Many toxic gases may be present following a volcanic eruption. Prompt decontamination, prior to entry into the Emergency Department, is necessary in any patient suspected to be exposed to a toxin. Oxygen should be administered for respiratory complaints. The possibility of multiple presentations over a period of time following the eruption should be expected, as these gases can travel over large distances and may not dissipate for a long period of time.

Suggested readings

Baxter P, et al. (1986). Preventive health measures in volcanic eruptions. *Am J Public Health* 76: 84–90.

EPA. Available at http://www.epa.gove/naturalevents/volcanoes.html

Smithsonian Institute. Available at http://www.volcano.si.edu

U.S. Geological Survey. Available at http://volcanoes.usgs.gov/hazards

Part 7

Post-disaster
Considerations

Survivor mental health

Christian Arbelaez

Helen Ouyang

Essential concepts

The mental health of disaster survivors is a crucial, yet often neglected, aspect of humanitarian assistance and reconstruction, as the physical well-being in the acute postdisaster setting often takes precedence. The lasting effects of disasters can often perpetuate for years, even a lifetime. Some research has been done on the mental health of survivors after disasters, wars, acts of terrorism, and domestic violence that has shed light on the needs and interventions needed for relief response teams. However, outcomes-based research is lacking and most likely the prevalence of mental health disease is underreported. There is some agreement around the basic concept that any exposure to an extreme stressor after a disaster is a risk factor for social and mental-health problems by disrupting social structures and impeding access to care for those who need it.

For these reasons, disaster relief workers must:
• Maintain a high index of suspicion for mental health issues.
• Be sensitive to the mental-health issues of disaster survivors, regardless of whether the relief worker is directly involved in developing psychosocial programming.
• Ensure highly trained and experienced mental-health experts are involved in every aspect of such efforts.
• Consider the societal norms and cultural practices of the community along with the available mental-health infrastructure and capacity.
• Be aware of deep-seated stigma and discrimination against individuals with mental-health conditions that may be a barrier to receiving appropriate services and health care.

Because of the expected high prevalence of mental health, the lack of outcomes-based research, the shortage of trained mental-health providers, and the challenges associated with disasters, the mental health of survivors is a critical component of any relief efforts. This chapter is intended to serve as a resource to help address the acute and persistent psychosocial effects of a disaster on survivors.

Clinical implications

Acute medical conditions

It is important to note that a disaster may directly or indirectly lead to an acute medical condition that may also co-exist with an acute stress disorder. On the other hand, practitioners also need to be aware that some acute medical conditions may manifest, and often are confused with, an acute mental illness. Providers need to make sure that acute active medical problems have been excluded. In cases where there may be an active acute medical problem, providers need to have a high index of suspicion for an acute stress disorder.

Some examples include:
- Acute traumatic injury caused from the disaster.
- Acute exacerbation of a chronic medical problem.
  - May result from lack of access to care and medications.
- Acute infection from endemic or epidemic outbreaks.
- Acute delirium.
- Acute toxin overdose or withdrawal.

Psycho-social stressors

Disasters are often associated directly or indirectly with psychosocial stressors that may result in ongoing insults on survivors that may ultimately lead to mental-health consequences. Some of these factors, such as loss of family members, may be quite devastating. Another important fact is that, although there is an increase in the prevalence of mental illness, there may be a parallel increase in the rates of domestic violence and substance abuse.

Sources of psychosocial suffering include:
- Loss of loved ones.
- Family separation.
- Displacement.
- Lack of protection.
- Loss of possessions.
- Personal attacks.
- Gender-based violence.

Predictive and protective factors

Along with these sources of psycho-social stressors are factors that put the survivor at risk for developing mental-health illness after being confronted with a new stressor:
  - Exposure and severity of exposure to prior trauma or disasters.
- History of mental disorder (i.e., prior posttraumatic stress disorders [PTSD]).
- Disruption of community.

- Lack of or poor social support.
- Vulnerable populations: children, minority groups, displaced individuals.
- Substance abuse.

In contrast, there may be protective factors that help minimize or prevent a disaster survivor from developing an acute mental disorder:
- Individual and community resilience.
- Community social support networks.
- Early recognition by relief workers.

Clinical manifestations: acute and posttraumatic stress disorders

After a disaster, survivors may suffer from the clinical manifestations of acute stress disorder (ASD) and posttraumatic stress disorder (PTSD). Studies have estimated that nearly half of all disaster survivors develop psychological sequelae, and this number is higher in children. Thus, it is critical that relief workers coming in contact with these individuals be able to recognize some of the key characteristics.

Psychological distress or acute mental distress
- This term is used to describe symptoms of mental distress that are experienced by the general population and not just individuals.
- Common symptoms are anxiety, anger, and insomnia.
- Expected during and postdisasters.
- Nonpathological.

Acute stress disorder (DSM-IV)
Definition: The person has been exposed to a traumatic event in which both of the following were present:
- The person experienced, witnessed, or was confronted with an event or events that involved actual or threatened death or serious injury, or a threat to the physical integrity of self or others.
- The person's response involved intense fear, helplessness, or horror.
  - Either while experiencing or after experiencing the distressing event, the individual has three (or more) of the following dissociative symptoms:
  - Subjective sense of numbing, detachment, or absence of emotional responsiveness.
  - Reduction in awareness of his or her surroundings (e.g., "being in a daze").
  - Derealization.
  - Depersonalization.
  - Dissociative amnesia (i.e., inability to recall an important aspect of the trauma).
- The traumatic event is persistently re-experienced in at least one of the following ways: recurrent images, thoughts, dreams, illusions, flashback episodes, or a sense of reliving the experience; or distress on exposure to reminders of the traumatic event.
- Marked avoidance of stimuli that arouse recollections of the trauma (e.g., thoughts, feelings, conversations, activities, places, people).
- Marked symptoms of anxiety or increased arousal (e.g., difficulty sleeping, irritability, poor concentration, hypervigilance, exaggerated startle response, motor restlessness).
- The disturbance causes clinically significant distress or impairment in social, occupational, or other important areas of functioning or impairs the individual's ability to pursue some necessary task, such as obtaining necessary assistance or mobilizing personal resources by telling family members about the traumatic experience.

- The disturbance lasts for a minimum of two days and a maximum of four weeks and occurs within weeks of the traumatic event.
- The disturbance is not due to the direct physiological effects of a substance (e.g., a drug of abuse, a medication) or a general medical condition, is not better accounted for by Brief Psychotic Disorder, and is not merely an exacerbation of a preexisting mental (Axis I or Axis II) disorder.

Posttraumatic stress disorder (DSM-IV)

Definition: The person has been exposed to a traumatic event in which both of the following have been present:

- The person experienced, witnessed, or was confronted with an event or events that involved actual or threatened death or serious injury, or a threat to the physical integrity of self or others.
- The person's response involved intense fear, helplessness, or horror.

The traumatic event is persistently re-experienced in one (or more) of the following ways:

- Recurrent and intrusive distressing recollections of the event, including images, thoughts, or perceptions.
- Recurrent distressing dreams of the event.
- Acting or feeling as if the traumatic event were recurring (includes a sense of reliving the experience, illusions, hallucinations, and dissociative flashback episodes, including those that occur upon awakening or when intoxicated).
- Intense psychological distress at exposure to internal or external cues that symbolize or resemble an aspect of the traumatic event.
- Physiological reactivity on exposure to internal or external cues that symbolize or resemble an aspect of the traumatic event.

Persistent avoidance of stimuli associated with the trauma and numbing of general responsiveness (not present before the trauma), as indicated by three (or more) of the following:

- Efforts to avoid thoughts, feelings, or conversations associated with the trauma.
- Efforts to avoid activities, places, or people that arouse recollections of the trauma.
- Inability to recall an important aspect of the trauma.
- Markedly diminished interest or participation in significant activities.
- Feeling of detachment or estrangement from others.
- Restricted range of affect (e.g., unable to have loving feelings).
- Sense of a foreshortened future (e.g., does not expect to have a career, marriage, children, or a normal life span).

Persistent symptoms of increased arousal (not present before the trauma), as indicated by two (or more) of the following:

- Difficulty falling or staying asleep.
- Irritability or outbursts of anger.
- Difficulty concentrating.
- Hypervigilance.
- Exaggerated startle response.
- Duration of the disturbance is more than one month.

The disturbance causes clinically significant distress or impairment in social, occupational, or other important areas of functioning.
- Time specificity:
  - Acute: if duration of symptoms is less than three months.
  - Chronic: if duration of symptoms is three months or more.
  - Delayed Onset: If onset of symptoms is at least 6 months after the stressor.
- Epidemiology
  - Over 80 percent of people with ASD have PTSD six months later.
  - Those who do not get ASD can still develop PTSD later on.
  - Small number (4–13%) of survivors who do not get ASD in the first month after a trauma will get PTSD in later months or years.
- ASD and PTSD differ in two fundamental ways:
  - Diagnosis of ASD can be given only within the first month following a traumatic event. If posttraumatic symptoms were to persist beyond a month, the clinician would assess for the presence of PTSD. The ASD diagnosis would no longer apply.
  - ASD has a greater emphasis on dissociative symptoms. An ASD diagnosis requires that a person experience three symptoms of dissociation (e.g., numbing, reduced awareness, depersonalization, de-realization, or amnesia), whereas the PTSD diagnosis does not.

Interventions: A comprehensive mental health approach

The overall goals of providing survivor mental health services are to:
- Promote a sense of safety.
- Promote calming.
- Promote connectedness.
- Promote hope.
- Promote sense of self- and collective efficacy.
- Promote returning to social norms and routine.
- Promote social interventions.
- Promote multisector approaches.

Current guidelines

There are several leading mental-health field manuals that provide guidance:
- *The Sphere Handbook,* revised 2004
- The WHO *Mental Health in Emergencies Handbook,* 2003.
- *IASC Guidelines on Mental Health and Psychosocial Support in Emergency Settings.* IASC, 2003.
- *Field Manual for Mental Health and Human Service Workers in Major Disasters.* SAMHSA, 2001.
- *Mental Health of Refugees.* WHO/UNHCR, 1996.

Key principles for interventions

Table 92.1 provides an overview of the principles of mental health and psychosocial support in disasters.

Table 92.1 Disaster mental health: basic principles

Principle	Explanation
1 Contingency planning	Before the emergency, national-level contingency planning should include (a) developing interagency coordination systems, (b) designing detailed plans for a mental health response, and (c) training general health care personnel in basic, general mental health care and psychological first aid.
2 Assessment	Assessment should cover the sociocultural context (setting, culture, history and nature of problems, local perceptions of illness, and ways of coping), available services, resources and needs. In assessment of individuals, a focus on disability or daily functioning is recommended.
3 Long-term perspective	Even though impetus for mental health programmes is highest during or immediately after acute emergencies, the population is best helped by a focus on the medium- and long-term development of services.
4 Collaboration	Strong collaboration with other agencies will avoid wastage of resources. Continuous involvement of the government, local universities or established local organizations is essential for sustainability.
5 Integration into primary health care	Led by the health sector, mental health treatment should be made available within primary health care to ensure (low-stigma) access to services for the largest number of people.
6 Access to service for all	Setting up separate, vertical mental health services for special populations is discouraged. Nevertheless, outreach and awareness programmes are important to ensure the treatment of vulnerable groups within general health sevices and other community services.
7 Thorough training and supervision	Training and supervision should be carried out by mental health specialists (or under their guidance) for a substantial amount of time, in order to ensure lasting effects of training and responsible care.
8 Monitoring indicators	Activities should be monitored and evaluated through key indicators that need to be determined, if possible, before starting the activity. Indicators should focus on inputs (available resources, including pre-existing services), processes (aspects of programme implementation), and outcomes (e.g., daily functioning of beneficiaries).

Reprinted with permission from Van Ommeren et al. Mental and Social Health during and after Acute Emergencies: Emerging Consensus? *Bull World Health Organ.* 83 (1): (2005) 71–75.

Postdisaster programming strategies

Contingency planning
If a contingency plan is available, make sure it is context-appropriate for the specific situation and that it is fully implemented.

Needs assessment
- Early identification of individuals with preexisting mental health by first responders and shelter personnel will allow initiation of referrals to mental-health clinicians who can assess for high-risk behaviors, such as suicidal or homicidal ideation.
- Based on the different time points, there may be associated needs.
- Pre-emergency mental and psychosocial issues.
- Emergency-induced mental and psychosocial issues.
- Aid-induced mental and psychosocial issues.
- For the general population, the use of brief screening tools for diagnostic evaluations.
- Development of an ongoing surveillance system.
- Tailor validated tools to local context:
  - Patient Health Questionnaire-2 (PHQ-2) for depression.
  - CAGE questions for alcohol abuse.
  - OK Integrated Mental Health and Substance Abuse Screen for Adults.
  - Generalized Anxiety Disorder-7 Item (GAD-7) for anxiety.
  - Pediatric Symptom Checklist-17 (PSC-17) for youths ages 11–17.
  - Massachusetts Youth Screening Instrument (MAYSI-2) for alcohol and drug abuse, depression, and traumatic experiences in youths.
  - Be cognizant of gender differences.

Capacity assessment
- Evaluate the current access to primary care and specialized mental-health care.
  - Understand the capacity for inpatient and outpatient management.
- Evaluate the ability for patients to have access to medications needed.
  - Understand the types of medications used by the country.

Collaboration and integration
- A team-based approach to the diagnosis and management of acute medical and psychiatric conditions.
- In synergy with current health-care system.
  - Aim for programs that are community based and managed.
- Operational considerations and challenges:
  - Use of interpreters from the community.
  - Resource utilization.
  - Establish modes of communication with the community and providers.
- Often, because of limited resources and available trained personnel, it is necessary to triage services according to need and available resources and trained personnel.

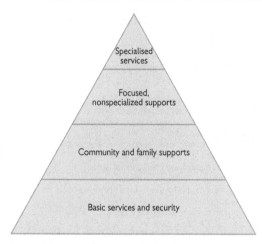

Figure 92.1 Intervention pyramid for mental-health and psychosocial support in emergencies. Source: Inter-Agency Standing Committee (IASC). Mental Health and Psychosocial Support: Checklist for Field Use 2008.

- Integration of mental-health assessments into the primary points of medical access to increase screening and decrease stigma.
  - Ideally professionals trained in both mental-health and disaster response.
  - Health-care providers who receive ad-hoc training in mental health.
  - Nonmedical aid workers.
- Education and training of community through empowerment.
  - If hiring local personnel, try to check references.
  - Community leaders.
  - Existent family and social networks.
- Shelter workers.
- Referral of more complex cases to specialized mental health services.
  - Local mental health workers.

Types of mental-health services
Ensure that there is close supervision and monitoring after each intervention.
- Psychotherapeutic interventions.
  - Teaching of coping skills and anxiety reducing techniques.
  - Critical Incident Stress Debriefing (CISD).
  - Disaster Focused Interventions.
- Outreach programs for the survivor and community.
  - Family locator system and family assistance centers.
  - Substance abuse programs.

- Pharmacological interventions.
  - Based on available medications.
  - In consultation with psychiatrist if possible.
  - Anxiolytic therapy.
- Consider linking services to outcomes measures that help track success.

Recommended locations and sites for providing services

- Depends on the type of disaster, resources available, and pre-existing facilities.
- Areas that are sensitive to privacy and confidentiality.
- Minimize the stigma associated with seeking services.
- Triage area at the site of disaster.
- Camps for internally displaced persons and refugees.
  - Formal and informal resettlement areas.
- Hospital, clinic, community health center, and medical tent areas.
- Areas where the community gathers.
  - Religious sites, if culturally appropriate.
  - Schools.

Time line for delivery of services

Acute-Term Phase: The WHO manual recommends providers:

- Conduct mostly social interventions that do not interfere with acute basic needs.
- Disseminate reliable information on the emergency, relief efforts, and location of relatives at the level of local 12-year olds.
- Brief field officers on the issues of grief and disorientation.
- Provide religious, recreation, and cultural space in camps.
- Discourage unceremonious disposal of corpses; contrary to myth, dead bodies carry very limited risk of communicable disease.
- Facilitate with grieving rituals.
- Encourage activities that include orphans and widows into social networks.
- Organize recreational and educational activities for children.
- Establish contact with healthcare providers to and ensure availability of psychotropic medications.

Midterm phase and long-term phase: The WHO manual recommends providers:

- Continue with all the previous social interventions.
- Organize outreach and psycho-education and educate the community on availability of mental health care.
- Four weeks after the acute phase, educate on the difference between psychopathology and normal psychological distress.
- Encourage economic development initiatives such as income-generating activities.
- Facilitate creation of community-based self-health groups that are self-sustainable.
- Continue ensuring provision of psychotropic medications as needed.
- Continue to educate other aid workers and community leaders in core psychological care skills.

Special populations

Children
- In a study done on children affected by Hurricane Katrina, researchers found that 60 percent of children screened positive for PTSD symptoms.
- Most have atypical presentations and it may be difficult to obtain a history.
- Input from parents/guardians helpful.
  - Understand familial context and ongoing distress.
  - Understand parental coping capabilities.
  - Recognize that children may be emulating parents behaviors.
- Orphans need to be included into social networks as soon as possible.
- Encourage children to return to normal activities such as school and recreational activities as soon as possible.

Gender-based violence survivors
- May be difficult to screen for these patients because they may not disclose.
- Health-care workers may need training.
- Collaborate with sexual assault workers who are addressing the physical effects.
- Documentation especially important as survivors may pursue legal redress.

Health-care worker survivors and disaster-relief providers
- Will typically work long hours providing health care.
- Are at risk of ongoing trauma from their patients stories and services provided.
- Family of providers also at risk for acute mental-health conditions.
- Disaster relief workers will have needs based on time period.
  - Predeployment, deployment, and postdeployment considerations.

Other vulnerable populations may include women, disabled, and the elderly.

Common pitfalls to avoid

The longer one's engagement in humanitarian work, the greater one's appreciation of its complexity, the potential for harm, and the need to address a number of important issues, including:

- Contextual insensitivity to the cultural, structural, and political aspects of emergency situations.
- Excessive focus on deficits such as mental-health problems without sufficient attention to resilience and coping.
- Over-reliance on individualistic approaches.
- Power abuses such as the imposition of outsider approaches.
- Provision of inadequate training and supervision for staff.

Common mistakes

- Don't assume that everyone needs help.
- Don't assess without making sure you can provide services and follow-up.
- Don't organize programs that undermine local efforts.
- Don't create parallel services for segments of the population.
- Don't institutionalize anyone unless it is a last resort.
- Don't leave use of psychotropic medications unmonitored.
- Don't create dependency through programs that use a charity model.
- Don't forget to coordinate your efforts.
- Don't forget about sustainability and an exit strategy.
- Don't neglect the mental health of providers and aid workers.
- Don't violate the sociocultural norms.
- Don't forget the importance of security for survivors and aid workers.

Public-health implications

The importance of mental-health assessment, practical interventions, and policy development after a disaster cannot be emphasized enough as a public-health priority. Although there is consensus on the need for these interventions, there is controversy around which strategies are most effective and how best to deploy them. Furthermore, best practices for surveillance for mental-health problems and substance abuse during disasters remain largely undeveloped. Meeting these challenges will require making the capacity to address mental-health issues a central component of disaster preparedness and response.

Summary

The mental health of postdisaster survivors and communities is a critical component of any comprehensive humanitarian assistance effort. Despite the lack of well-designed outcomes-based research on postdisaster mental health, there are expert-based consensus guidelines that serve as manuals for relief response teams. We hope that this chapter serves as a quick reference for relief workers who might help address the acute and persistent psychosocial effects of a disaster on survivors.

Suggested readings

Hobfoll SE, et al (2007). Five essential elements of immediate and mid-term mass trauma interventions: Empirical evidence. *Psychiatry 70*(4): 283–315.

Hoven CW, et al (2009). Parental exposure to mass violence and child mental health: The first responder and WTC evacuee study. *Clin Child Fam Psychol Rev 12*(2): 95–112.

The International Society for Traumatic Stress Studies (2001). 50,000 Disaster Victims Speak. Washington, D.C.: The National Center for PTSD and the Center for Mental Health Services.

IASC (2007). IASC Guidelines on Mental Health and Psychosocial Support in Emergency Settings.

Jaycox LH, et al (2010, April). Children's mental health care following Hurricane Katrina: A field trial of trauma-focused psychotherapies. *J Trauma Stress 23*(2): 223–231.

Milligan, McGuinness (2009). Mental health needs in a post-disaster environment. *J Psychosoc Nurs Ment Health Serv 47* (9): 23–30.

Morris, et al (2007). Children and the sphere standard on mental and social aspects of health. *Disasters 31* (1): 71–90.

Pender DA, Prichard KK (2008). Group process research and emergence of therapeutic factors in critical incident stress debriefing. *Int J Emerg Ment Health 10*(1): 39–48.

The Sphere Project (2004). *Humanitarian Charter and Minimum Standards in Disaster Response* Geneva Switzerland

Van Ommeren M, et al (2005a). Aid after disasters. *BMJ 330* (7501): 1160–1161.

Van Ommeren M, et al (2005b). Mental and social health during and after acute emergencies: Emerging consensus? *Bull World Health Organ 83* (1): 71–76.

Wessells M (2009). Do no harm: Toward contextually appropriate psychosocial support in international emergencies. *Am Psychol 64* (8): 842–854.

WHO (2003). *Mental Health in Emergencies Handbook.* Geneva, Switzerland.

WHO/UNHCR (1996). *Mental Health of Refugees.* Geneva, Switzerland.

Yun, N, et al (2010). Moving mental health into the disaster-preparedness spotlight. *NEJM 363*: 1193–1195.

http://www.ptsd.va.gov/public/pages/acute-stress-disorder.asp

http://sbirt.samhsa.gov

Displaced populations

Deepti Thomas-Paulose
John D. Cahill

Introduction

The displacement of people from their homes, neighborhoods, livelihoods, and families as a result of a disaster makes them particularly vulnerable to physical and psychological stress. Families are often separated; without a way to make a living and provide for their loved ones people loose their sense of identity and purpose and the more vulnerable segments of the population (women, children, the elderly and disabled) are further marginalized. In some settings they are subjected to human-rights abuses and gender-based violence. Displaced populations come from diverse backgrounds and have many different needs but, in general, fall under two broad categories: refugees or internally displaced populations.

Definitions

Refugees

A refugee is defined as a person residing outside his or her country of nationality, who is unable or unwilling to return because of a "well-founded fear of persecution on account of race, religion, nationality, membership in a political social group, or political opinion." Those recognized as refugees have a clear international legal status and are afforded the protection of the United Nations High Commissioner for Refugees (UNHCR). The vast majority of refugees are in the world's poorest countries particularly in Asia and Africa. Current figures estimate a worldwide refugee population of 15.2 million at the end of 2009.

Internally displaced persons (IDPs)

Internally displaced persons (IDPs) are persons or groups of persons who have been forced or obliged to flee or to leave their homes or places of habitual residence, in particular as a result of or in order to avoid the effects of armed conflict, situations of generalized violence, violations of human rights or natural or human-made disasters, and who have not crossed an internationally recognized state border.

There is no specifically mandated body to provide assistance to IDPs, as there is with refugees. However, UNHCR has increasingly provided more protection to IDPs in recent years under the United Nations (UN) "cluster" approach. Often persecuted or under attack from their own governments, they are sometimes in a more dire situation than refugees and outnumber them two to one.

At the end of 2009, there were estimated to be 27.1 million IDPs worldwide.

Standards in humanitarian response

The Sphere Project's *Humanitarian Charter and Minimum Standards in Disaster Response* established, for the first time, the humanitarian assistance people affected by disasters have a right to expect. The *Charter* is concerned with the most basic requirements for sustaining the lives and dignity of those affected by calamity or conflict, as reflected in the body of international human rights, humanitarian, and refugee law. It is on this basis that agencies offer their services. The *Charter* reaffirms the fundamental importance of three key principles:

- The right to life with dignity.
- The distinction between combatants and noncombatants.
- The principle of nonrefoulement (to not forcibly return refugees to the place from which they were fleeing).

The three phases of an emergency

- The emergency phase: often defined as the period when crude mortality rates (number of deaths/10,000 population/per day) are at least two times higher than baseline.
- The postemergency phase begins when the basic needs of the population (food, water, shelter, health care, etc.) have been met and the crude mortality rates are comparable to those of the surrounding population. In the postemergency phase, humanitarian efforts seek to maintain the health and well-being of the population through the following:
  - Enhancement / extension (improved coverage, greater depth of services) of the interventions described for the emergency response.
  - Family tracing and reunification.
  - Social services: schools, community/youth centers.
  - Community-health programs.
  - Continuation of preventative health services for incoming displaced populations.
- The durable solution phase happens when a permanent solution has been found for the refugee population. Often, individuals consider refugee status to be a temporary matter, when, in reality, it can go on for years to decades. Whole new generations have been born in refugee camps, with no identity of their original country. There are generally three options:
  - Repatriation: returning refugees to their communities in their country of origin.
  - Reintegration: integrating refugees permanently into new communities in host countries or their country of origin.
  - Resettlement: integrating refugees permanently into new communities in a third country.

Priorities for a displaced population

Many different actors may be involved in managing a displaced population:
- Governments (including multiple countries, states, or local).
- Military.
- NGOs.

Members of the local community should be involved in the process.

Initial assessment

Understanding the context of the displacement will allow for (1) the appropriate allocation and management of resources and (2) to put in place a system of monitoring and evaluation to determine the effectiveness of the humanitarian response. Displacement due to conflict will demand a different set of resources than that due to a flash flood. The context also includes understanding the location in which displaced individuals will settle; its accessibility through roads, bridges, landing strips, railways, and ports; as well as availability of food, water, building materials, and other equipment.

Rapid assessment surveys, initial registration data, health records, census records or speaking with local authorities can be undertaken in the first few days to understand the demographics and health needs of a population.

Basic essential data include:
- Size of the population.
- Sex.
- Age distribution.
- Family members.
- Cultural make up (religion, ethnicity, etc.).
- Medical health/disease prevalence/vaccine status.
- Identification of potential vulnerable groups.

Table 93.1 Top 10 priorities for displaced populations

Initial assessment
Measles immunization
Water and sanitation
Food and nutrition
Shelter and site planning
Health care in the emergency phase
Control of communicable diseases and epidemics
Public-health surveillance
Human resources and training
Coordination

Source: Refugee Health: An approach to emergency situations, MSF, 2008.

The security of both the population and those responding to the crisis is also an important concept and one that deserves full attention so that the efforts of the humanitarian response are not undermined.

Measles

Measles continues to be a major cause of morbidity and mortality throughout the world. The pediatric population is at highest risk, and mass vaccination should be highest priority in children from 6 months to 15 years of age. Measles is an RNA paramyxovirus that is highly contagious and spread through secretions in the respiratory tract. Approximately 90 percent of susceptible individuals will contract the disease after exposure to an infected individual. Vitamin A deficiency can cause more severe and complicated cases of measles.

Water and sanitation

Water should be a top priority in any disaster situation. It is the cornerstone in the foundation of emergency response. The absolute minimum requirement of water is 5 liters/person/day; this should be increased as soon as possible to reach a level of 15–20 liters/person/day. Other aspects to consider about water include: accessibility, location, availability of carrying containers, and protection of water points. Different sources of water include: surface water, well, bore hole, and springs. Water for consumption should contain less than 10 fecal forms per 100 ml. As seen in Table 93.2, a number of waterborne diseases arise from drinking contaminated water. The treatment of water to make it suitable for drinking will likely require additional expertise.

Besides water, sanitation and hygiene are top priorities in the emergency response. These measures are the first barrier to preventing the spread of diseases by the fecal/oral route. When considering a sanitation system, one needs to be culturally sensitive to the population that is being served. The distribution of soap can be a key intervention to reduce the incidence of diarrheal illness.

Food and nutrition

The daily minimum nutritional requirement is 2,100 kilocalories/person/day. At least 10 percent of the calories in the general ration should be in the form of fats and at least 12 percent should be derived from

Table 93.2 Waterborne diseases from contaminated water ingestion

Disease	Morbidity per annum	Mortality per annum
Diarrhea	1000 million	3.3 million
Typhoid	12.5 million	>125,000
Cholera	>300,000	>3,000
Ascaris infection	1 billion	Negligible

This table was published in Cahill J, Displaced populations. Ciottone G [ed.]. *Textbook on Disaster Medicine*, pp.313–317. Copyright Elsevier 2006.

proteins. For children, the caloric requirements range from 1,290 kcal for 0–4 years of age to 2,420 kcal for 15–19 year olds. Children up to 2 years of age should derive 30–40 percent of their calories from fats. The caloric demand may be higher based upon: underlying nutritional status of the population, shelter, environment, and burden of disease. An important aspect of feeding large populations is food distribution. Ideally, this should be done in a community-based setting in an organized and secure manner. Feeding centers may be established for the severely malnourished.

A food basket for distribution may include: wheat flour, rice, sugar, vegetable oil, salt, and possibly local fish or meat. It is preferable to use local food when available. Cultural practices and diet also need to be considered. Utensils and fuel for cooking need to be supplied. Breastfeeding should be encouraged and bottle feeding avoided. Nutritional screening of the population should be performed to assess particular needs. In general, the incidence of malnutrition in children less than 5 years of age is used as the general indicator of malnutrition for the population. The weight-to-height index, evidence of edema, and the mid-upper-arm circumference are means to do a nutritional survey.

Shelter

With small populations, it might be possible to house individuals with the local population in their homes. Another option is to use existing structures such as factories, schools, warehouses, and other public buildings (shelter in place). When a camp is being built, considerations on shelter and the site will be based on a number of factors: type of disaster, size and demographics of the population, anticipated time of displacement, environmental health risks, terrain, accessibility, available existent structures and infrastructure, climate, security (ideally away from borders), local building materials, and cultural considerations.

Health care

The immediate medical needs in a displaced population will center around the most common communicable diseases, which include diarrhea, respiratory-tract infections, measles, and malaria. Chronic disease, malnutrition, conflict-related traumatic injuries, and maternal health are also issues that need to be addressed shortly thereafter. Local health authorities must be contacted when planning health programs. Ideally, the existing facilities of the host country should be utilized. The four-tier health-care model has been used repeatedly with success in reducing excess mortality. The levels include:

- A referral hospital.
- A central health facility (one for every 10,000 to 30,000 persons in a camp).
- A peripheral health facility (one for every 3,000 to 5,000 persons).
- Home visits/assessments.

"Essential" medical kits have been developed and are available from a number of organizations. Treatment protocols for common illnesses are also effective in the emergency setting. At all levels of care, a system of surveillance should be established to collect data to anticipate resources for ongoing health activities and to monitor for outbreaks of disease.

Malnutrition

In the context of emergencies, malnutrition also refers to protein-energy malnutrition (PEM), which signifies an imbalance in the supply of protein and energy and the body's demand for them to ensure optimal growth and function. Inadequate energy intake of this kind can lead to wasting and stunting. Malnutrition is a significant cause of morbidity in mortality in many disasters. It is important to not only remember the direct complications of malnutrition and disease states, but to understand that many diseases increase in severity secondary to malnutrition. In the pediatric population, some of the main causes of death (diarrhea, pneumonia, HIV, tuberculosis, malaria, measles, hypoglycemia, and hypothermia) run parallel with malnutrition. In displaced settings, where food is scarce and where people are dependent on food rations, micronutrient deficiency diseases can emerge. See Table 93.3.

Famine

Famine is a complex emergency that can result from natural and human-caused disasters. It is the most severe form of lack of access to food and nutrition, and it results in significant morbidity and mortality. Drought, flooding, crop failure, domestic animal disease, human conflict and economic disaster have all been associated with famine. Famine is more likely to occur under these conditions of a population is already stressed by poverty and preexisting malnutrition.

Table 93.3 Malnutrition/micronutrient deficiencies

Disease	Deficiency
Anemia	Iron/B12
Goiter/Cretinism	Iodine
Scurvy	Vitamin C
Rickets/Osteomalacia	Vitamin D
Beriberi	Vitamin B1 (Thiamin)
Pellagra	Niacin
Ariboflavinosis	Vitamin B2 (Riboflavin)
Nightblindness/Xeropthalmia	Vitamin A
Kwashikor	Protein

This table was published in Cahill J, Displaced populations. Ciottone G [ed.]. *Textbook on Disaster Medicine*, p.313–317. Copyright Elsevier 2006.

Malaria

Malaria is a parasitic disease caused by the protozoa species Plasmodium and transmitted by the bite of the female Anopheles mosquito. Malaria continues to contribute to high morbidity and mortality rates in endemic regions of the world, particularly in young children and pregnant women. The severity of these outbreaks has been exacerbated by the rapid drug-resistance developed by this parasite. Measures to decrease exposure should be implemented whenever possible including the use of permethrin-impregnated mosquito nets or housing structures. Rapid diagnosis dipsticks are easy to use with a simple fingerstick; results are available within 20 minutes. Treatment of malaria should never be withheld if the diagnosis is suspected, because it can be rapidly fatal.

War-related injury/trauma

In recent wars, civilians have become major targets of war-related violence. In settings where infectious disease is not endemic and where health care and population health status prior to conflict is relatively good, the leading cause of mortality among affected populations have been the injuries/traumas that have resulted from war-related violence.

Complications of chronic disease

There is evidence to suggest that there is an increased incidence of acute complications from chronic diseases associated with disasters. These complications are generally due to disruptions of ongoing treatment regimens. However, a variety of other stressors associated with disasters may also precipitate an acute deterioration of chronic medical conditions.

Reproductive/maternal health

In times of upheaval the incidence of sexual violence increases. Gender-specific provisions of humanitarian law were strengthened by recent affirmations of rape as a specific war crime and as an element of other international crimes.

Reproductive-health services, including prenatal care, assisted delivery, and emergency obstetric care, are often unavailable. Young people become more vulnerable to sexual exploitation, and many women lose access to family-planning services, exposing them to unwanted pregnancy in perilous conditions. Approximately 25 percent of all refugees worldwide are women of reproductive age (15–49 years) and one in five is likely to be pregnant. In refugee settings where emergency obstetric services are not available, complications of pregnancy and childbirth can be a major cause of mortality. United Nations High Commission for Refugees (UNHCR), together with other organizations, has defined a Minimal Initial Services Package (MISP) to be implemented as soon as possible to address some aspects of reproductive health in the emergency phase, including making condoms available and handing out clean delivery kits to all visibly pregnant women.

Special issues

Military forces have taken a stronger role in the humanitarian effort in recent years. Although they are very organized units that can help aid a population in a timely and efficient manner, there are also a number of security concerns with their presence that threaten the perception of impartiality and neutrality.

Suggested readings

The Sphere Project (2004). *Humanitarian Charter and Minimum Standards in Disaster Response*. Geneva, Switzerland.

UNFPA (2001). *Reproductive Health for Communities in Crisis: Emergency Response*. Geneva, Switzerland.

UNHCR (2010). 2009 Global Trends: Refugees, Asylum-Seekers, Returnees, Internally Displaced and Stateless Persons. Geneva, Switzerland.

WHO (2000). *The Management of Nutrition in Major Emergencies*. Geneva, Switzerland.

Lessons learned

Adam C. Levine

General lessons

Given the great diversity of disaster types and settings, it may be impossible to develop a comprehensive list of lessons that can be applied to all future disasters. However, there are several common recurrent themes that have been identified from interviews with responders and victims after a wide variety of different disasters. This chapter focuses on the lessons gleaned from several major natural and human-generated disasters occurring over the past two decades. Although not all these lessons will be applicable in all settings, they can provide some guidance to future disaster planners in order to avoid repeating the mistakes made in the past. A summary of the most important lessons is listed in the following section.

Major lessons learned

Coordination
- Prioritize both intra-agency and interagency coordination, because lack of it consistently ranks as the greatest obstacle to an effective disaster response.
- Create an Incident Command System (ICS) and ensure all staff are well trained in it. Create protocols in advance of a disaster for resource and data sharing between different organizations and government agencies.

Communication
Don't rely on one or even two major systems of communication, because all systems are fallible in a major disaster.
- Hold town-hall-style meetings on a daily basis to keep staff up to date.
- Establish clear and consistent messaging for both disaster victims and the media that is released at set times and in set ways.

Logistics
- Have several back-up systems in place for providing fuel and electricity.
- Prepare necessary food and supplies in advance that can be rapidly deployed or used in a disaster.
- Maintain lists of "on call" disaster responders who receive regular training during the year in disaster response.

Health
- Prepare systems for hand hygiene and sanitation that don't rely on public water or sewer supply.
- Ensure adequate protective equipment and training for disaster responders.
- In general, expect the diseases prevalent in an area prior to the disaster to be the ones most in need of addressing after a disaster.

Perform a rapid-needs assessment at the start of a disaster and conduct ongoing surveillance to detect disease outbreaks.

Prepare for the mental-health needs of both disaster victims and responders through psychological counseling and a rapid return to normal activities.

Coordination

By their very nature, disasters tend to be chaotic situations, with a mix of local government agencies, local NGOs, foreign governments, international NGOs, UN agencies, and individual citizens rushing in to help. The need to ensure adequate coordination, both within organizations and between different organizations, is repeatedly cited as one of the most important lessons learned from a variety of disaster situations, ranging from the recent earthquakes in Pakistan and Haiti to domestic disasters like Hurricane Katrina and the California wildfires. Poor coordination can lead to the duplication of efforts in some areas, underutilization of resources in other areas. It can also result in groups and individuals working at cross-purposes. Overall, lack of coordination can undermine the humanitarian response and lead to many more lost lives.

Intra-agency coordination

Most organizations are designed with multiple channels of authority and a variety of departments and committees that work in parallel to accomplish their day-to-day tasks and overall mission. Although these usual mechanisms clearly serve the organization well during normal operations, they are typically too slow, unwieldy, and unfocused to respond adequately to the increased needs and rapid situational changes occurring after a large disaster.

One of the most important take-home points from prior disasters is that each organization should have an Incident Command System (ICS) in place prior to the onset of a disaster that establishes clear lines of authority for use during a disaster situation. The ICS should list an incident commander who will have final decision-making authority for the organization during the course of a disaster and a series of people working directly under him or her in charge of various operations, such as clinical care, logistics, sanitation, and so forth. The ICS should also clearly describe the duties of individual staff members working in different areas, the expected lines of communication among staff members, and the means for rapidly resolving the conflicts that inevitably arise.

Equally important to the creation of an ICS is ensuring that all staff members in the organization understand how it functions. An ICS is completely useless if the majority of staff members within the organization is unaware of its existence, and it can begin to break down if even a handful of staff members are not well trained in its basic structure. In order to ensure the smooth operation of an ICS, regular disaster simulations may be helpful for organizations that experience disasters infrequently. International NGOs deploying humanitarian- aid workers to a disaster situation should, at a minimum, hold a pre-departure briefing detailing the organization's ICS and each individual's expected role within it.

Interagency coordination

A significant disaster may overwhelm even the largest and richest nation's capacity to respond effectively. Local NGOs, international NGOs, foreign governments, and UN agencies can, and often do, fill in the gaps in emergency response by providing for a rapid influx of "surge capacity." However, without adequate coordination between these different organizations and local government agencies, there can be a great deal of redundancy and inefficiency. A great deal has been learned about the various barriers to coordination between disaster response organizations; more recently, improved methods for interagency coordination have been developed and piloted, which could lead to a more efficient disaster-response system.

Logistical barriers

In the rush to provide services in the aftermath of a disaster, efforts at coordination are often little more than an afterthought for many organizations. In addition, poor communication and transportation infrastructure on the ground may stymie the efforts of organizations to coordinate effectively with each other. However, over the past two decades, humanitarian organizations and governments alike have begun to learn the importance of creating standing systems for coordination with established protocols that can easily be implemented in the setting of a disaster. The UN cluster system is an example of one such system for interagency coordination at the global level (see Box 94.1).

Box 94.1 UN cluster system

The UN cluster system is perhaps the largest and most well established system for interagency coordination during a disaster. The cluster system was first developed in 2005 by the UN Office for Coordination of Humanitarian Affairs (OCHA) in a response to a UN review finding major deficiencies in the global humanitarian- response system. Essentially, the cluster approach brings together UN agencies and international NGOs by grouping them into 11 different clusters, including agriculture; camp management; early recovery; education; shelter; telecommunications; health; logistics; nutrition; protection; and water, sanitation, and hygiene. Each cluster has a specific lead agency at the global level to aid in disaster preparedness and build response capacity across the humanitarian system. In addition, within 24 hours of a major disaster, the UN Emergency Relief Coordinator (the Director of UN OCHA) designates a specific lead organization for each cluster, which takes on the role of coordinating all organizations working within that cluster in the aftermath of the disaster.

The cluster system was first used in October 2005 during the Pakistan earthquake. Since its inception, there have been a variety of critiques of the cluster system, including a lack of involvement of local NGOs in the process, failure to provide translators during cluster meetings, "meeting fatigue," lack of communication between NGO representatives taking part in the cluster meetings and their operatives in the field, a poor understanding of the role of donors in the cluster process, and lack of media awareness of the cluster system and the way it operates. In addition, the cluster system does not address many of the underlying structural issues that lead to poor coordination, such as competition among NGOs for media attention and donor funding. Clearly, much work needs to be done to continue to improve coordination among global agencies during future humanitarian disasters.

In addition, many governments have also worked to establish protocols through which their various agencies work together more smoothly during a disaster, such as the Standard Emergency Management System established in the aftermath of California wildfires during the 1970s, which eventually led to the creation of the National Incident Management System (NIMS) by the U.S. government in 2003. NIMS requires all local, state, and federal agencies to comply with common protocols, which allow for interagency coordination during a disaster as a condition for receiving federal funding.

Financial barriers

In addition to logistical barriers, competition among NGOs for donor funding can create perverse incentives for NGOs not to coordinate with each other. Instead, each NGO's attempts to "plant its flag" in a particular area and work to maximize media attention toward its own individual efforts, thereby maximizing its ability to garner donations from both public and private entities. One way of addressing this problem at the global level has been the UN consolidated-appeals process, by which a single, large appeal for funding is made by the UN to donor governments at the start of a disaster, which is then apportioned to organizations working on the ground. Efforts to strengthen this process and apply it to private donations in addition to government funding may be helpful in reducing the financial barriers to coordination during disasters.

Data barriers

Data sharing between organizations during a disaster may be as important, if not more so, than sharing resources. However, many barriers exist to sharing data in the field, including the use of different data-collection forms, storing data in formats that are not easily transferable, and fear that data will be used inappropriately by another organization. Lack of data sharing can result in misdistribution of resources, as well as direct harm to victims. During the cholera outbreak in Goma in 1994, for instance, the UNHCR coordinating team had been provided with the antibiotic sensitivity patterns of the major cholera strains, whereas many NGOs continued to provide doxycycline and tetracycline to victims, unaware that those cholera strains were largely resistant.

The development of the Sphere Project's Humanitarian Charter and Minimum Standards for Disaster Response have helped to address the issue of data sharing by creating a common set of indicators and targets which agencies can use in monitoring outcomes during a disaster situation.

Communication

Methods of communication

In interviews with disaster responders, communication is consistently rated as one of the most important problems encountered during a disaster situation. Normal communication systems are often disrupted by the disaster itself, and many back-up communication systems may also not function when needed. See Box 94.2.

Types of communication

- *Among disaster responders*
  - Vital to ensure staff safety and prevent duplication of efforts or even working at cross-purposes.
  - All staff should receive as much information and training as possible prior to the disaster in the form of regular trainings for hospital staff or predeployment briefings for disaster responders.
  - Once or twice daily town-hall-style meetings are an effective means to communicate important information to responders on a regular basis.
- *Among responders and victims*
  - Important to both to ensure an orderly response and also to reduce anxiety and psychological stress among disaster victims.
  - Consistency of messaging to victims is important.
  - Radio announcements may be effective.
  - Station staff at entrance to hospital or at displaced-persons camp to provide necessary information verbally or through written flyers.
  - Public message board in hospitals or at displaced-persons camps can provide updated information and does not require electricity.
- *Communication with outside media*
  - Media can aid with communication to victims and the outside world, but they can also overutilize resources needed for the disaster response.
  - Regular press briefings involving a limited number of disaster responders and victims can be one method to manage these trade-offs.
  - Early coordination with media to ensure that disaster responders have first access to transportation, and that satellites are left open for specified periods of the day to allow responders to use the bandwidth may prevent tensions from arising later.

Box 94.2 Improvised communication methods

In some cases, especially when power is unavailable for long periods, all technological methods of communication might fail, and it will be necessary to resort to human-based methods. During Hurricane Katrina, when all phone lines were down, staff at Charity Hospital communicated with staff at nearby Tulane University Hospital by posting someone with a bullhorn on the roof of each hospital to relay messages back and forth. On September 11, 2001, staff at St. Vincent's Hospital relied on the hospital tube system, hard wired intercoms, and volunteer runners to transmit messages when all phone lines were jammed.

Logistics

The logistical challenges faced in responding to disasters include a diverse array of challenges, which, in turn, will vary greatly depending on the remoteness of the disaster area and the severity of the disaster itself. Several important areas have been identified as key logistical constraints in the context of a wide variety of different disasters over the past two decades.

Energy

One of the most important lessons is to ensure the availability of fuel and energy supplies. Nearly all operations in a disaster will require power, including transportation, communication, health, and sanitation. Loss of power can be a major limitation in providing services after a disaster. In the aftermath of Hurricane Katrina, not only was power lost for the city of New Orleans as a whole, but the back-up generator for Charity Hospital, located on the first floor, was destroyed by the flooding. Loss of power had a profound impact on hospital operations, both in anticipated ways, such as the loss of power for ventilators and other equipment, and also in unanticipated ways, such as the failure of most hospital telephones, which were controlled by a hospital-based switchboard, as well as the inability to recharge cellular phones. Fortunately, the hospital had just purchased a series of portable generators, which could be brought up to each floor to provide power. In addition to back-up generators, battery-powered flashlights and other equipment can be used in settings where power is lost, although it is important to ensure an adequate supply of replacement batteries if this strategy is utilized. Fire departments may also be able to provide temporary power in a disaster. Finally, when possible, back-up equipment that does not require electricity, such as wind up radios, should also be available.

Transportation

Transportation is important for the delivery of supplies, food, fuel, and human resources into a disaster context, and also for the evacuation of patients and victims out of a disaster area. In the aftermath of a large disaster, not only will most public transportation systems be shut down, but even private cars and trucks may face difficulties reaching disaster-affected areas. Both after Hurricane Katrina and the tsunami in Sri Lanka, roads became largely impassable due to flooding. As a result, helicopters were essentially the only means of long-distance transportation.

At Charity Hospital in New Orleans, a special system had to be created to manage helicopters landing on the single functioning helipad on the roof of the nearby parking garage in order to efficiently load patients being evacuated to other hospitals outside New Orleans. Even transporting patients within the hospital became a logistical challenge when power was lost and the elevators ceased functioning. Special protocols had to be developed to hand-carry bed-bound patients using the stairwells. This was especially difficult for patients attached to heavy equipment such as ventilators.

Food and supplies

Each new disaster brings with it a flood of donated supplies from well-meaning families and religious groups in the developed world, from culturally inappropriate clothing to expired medications to crates of canned food that could easily be purchased fresh in local markets. Private citizens are encouraged to donate money rather than food and supplies in the setting of a major disaster. It is important for organizations responding to disasters to ensure that they have arranged for purchase and transportation of critical supplies to the disaster area. An example of failure of such preparation was in the aftermath of the Haiti earthquake, when several surgical teams arrived to help, without an operating theatre to work in or the proper surgical tools to complete their operations or methods of disinfecting those tools in between operations.

In general, the most well-prepared organizations will have large, pre-assembled kits containing everything necessary to perform a certain function in the aftermath of a disaster. Such kits have diverse functions, including sterilization of drinking water, delivery kits for newborn children, and measles-immunization kits. These kits should be kept fully assembled and ready to transport rapidly in the event of a disaster, and disaster responders should be pretrained in their assembly and functioning. The Israeli Field Hospital, recently deployed to assist after the earthquake in Haiti, is an example of an entire "hospital in a box" that has been used effectively in a variety of disaster settings (see Box 94.3).

Security

In desperate situations, human beings tend to resort to desperate measures. Looting, especially of food and other essential supplies, has been a recurring problem in the aftermath of many large disasters. It is important that organizations arrange for secure storage facilities for food, supplies, equipment, and adequate security personnel to protect their staff. In addition, organizations should create specific plans for volunteer safety, such as curfews and other restrictions on responder movement.

Human resources

Perhaps no single resource is more important to an effective disaster response than human resources. Unfortunately, recruitment of personnel in the aftermath of a disaster can often be haphazard and inefficient. Disasters that are well publicized and easily accessible, such as the recent earthquake in Haiti, can generate a flood of volunteers, some of whom self-deploy and most of whom will lack adequate training and resources to do their job effectively.

However, the experience in Haiti also showed that professionals, including doctors, nurses, physical therapists, technicians, and others, can be effective in a disaster situation when provided with adequate training and support. The Chicago Medical Response is an example of a collaboration among six academic medical centers in Chicago and several NGOs on the ground in Haiti, which together coordinated the deployment of several hundred medical volunteers to assist with care during the earthquake.

Box 94.3 IDFMC field hospital

Within 89 hours of the earthquake that stuck Haiti in January 2010, the Israeli Defense Force Medical Corps (IDFMC) Field Hospital was deployed, transported nearly 6,000 miles, assembled, and began admitting its first patients in a soccer field near the main airport in Port-au-Prince. 121 medical personnel and 109 support personnel staffed the 72-bed hospital, which included several operating theatres; an intensive care unit; adult, pediatric, orthopedic, and obstetric wards; an ambulatory care tent; a laboratory; an imaging department; and kitchen and sanitation facilities. The hospital treated over 1,100 patients in the first two weeks after the earthquake, two-thirds of whom had suffered earthquake-related trauma and many of whom were seriously ill patients referred by other clinics and NGOs operating in the area.

The IDFMC is composed of a cadre of professionals in various medical disciplines, most of whom have regular jobs in the government or private medical sector. The "on call" nature of the IDFMC, along with its high level of preparedness and regular training in disaster response, ensure that it can respond effectively and rapidly to any disaster situation. The entire field hospital is contained in crates at Ben Gurion International Airport in Tel Aviv in order to be rapidly deployed by cargo plane anywhere in the world. The IDFMC has previously been deployed to a variety of disaster situations over the past two decades, including Turkey, India, Rwanda, and the Balkans.

Within two days of its arrival, the IDFMC field hospital was operating at full capacity, with every bed filled and 3–4 operating rooms running around the clock. In order to maximize its efficiency, the field hospital instituted a number of special protocols, including limiting care to those with the greatest chance of survival or benefit and requiring that any facility transporting patients to them for a higher level of care had to accept a stable postop patient in return.

In order to increase the capacity of medical volunteers to respond to future disasters, government agencies, NGOs, academic medical centers, and even private sector entities, such as hospital systems, can collaborate to maintain lists of personnel with needed skills. In addition to keeping the professional qualifications, certifications, language capacity, and other particulars of these personnel on file, the collaborations should provide for the regular training of volunteers in skills pertinent to disaster response, similar to the DMAT system in the United States.

Health

Hygiene

Perhaps the first major lesson in disaster hygiene and sanitation is to be prepared for the loss of the public water system. In rural areas in the developing world, there may not be a public water system to begin with, but even in urban areas in the developed world, public water and sewage systems may be easily be disrupted by a large- scale disaster.

Alcohol-based hand sanitizers, already becoming more prevalent in hospitals throughout the United States, can be an excellent way to maintain hand hygiene without running water.

Sanitation

Latrines are the mainstay for dealing with sanitation in a postdisaster setting, though they have to be carefully adapted to the situation at hand. For instance, latrines (port-a-potties) functioned poorly in the indoor environment of Charity Hospital in the aftermath of Hurricane Katrina. Hospital staff found that utilizing red waste bags over bedside commodes or bedpans were an effective means of waste disposal for both patients and staff.

One of the largest cholera epidemics in history occurred in Goma, Zaire in 1994 due to the lack of adequate sanitation. The hard volcanic rock in the region made it difficult to dig holes in the ground for latrines, and people used the nearby lake (also the only supply of fresh water) for waste disposal. Nearly 30,000 people died of cholera as a result. In situations such as this, above-ground latrines may work better.

Health care

One of the most important lessons learned with regards to the provision of health care in disaster settings is to expect that the diseases common in that setting prior to the disaster will be the diseases seen most frequently in the aftermath of the disaster. Despite media warnings about the outbreak of cholera after the Hurricane Katrina, a cholera epidemic in New Orleans was unlikely, and, indeed, never materialized. Instead, health facilities were overwhelmed largely by patients presenting with exacerbations of their chronic conditions, such as diabetes or hypertension, in a setting in which they were unable to get access to their usual medications.

Equally important is a comprehensive needs assessment, which can determine the major health-care needs of a population early in a disaster situation. In addition, ongoing surveillance data should be collected from hospitals, shelters, and camps in the weeks and months following a disaster in order to rapidly detect outbreaks of disease.

Contrary to common misperceptions, corpses do not generally lead to the spread of disease in the aftermath of a disaster. In Sri Lanka, large numbers of tsunami victims were unnecessarily buried hastily in mass graves, depriving families of the opportunity to identify loved ones and give them a traditional funeral ceremony. However, arrangements do need to be made for the storage of dead bodies after a major disaster, which can rapidly overwhelm the capacity of local morgues.

Mental health

Across a wide variety of different disasters occurring in both developed and developing countries, issues regarding the provision, or lack of provision, of mental-health care arise frequently. Disaster responders should expect a significant amount of mental trauma following a large disaster, and they should have systems in place for addressing the mental-health needs of both victims and responders.

At an even more basic level, disaster responders can reduce psychological trauma after a disaster through the provision of up-to-date information to disaster victims. Often, the confusion and uncertainty after a disaster can be more psychologically damaging than the experience of the disaster itself. In addition, in shelters or displaced persons camps, it is important to rapidly restore normal activities. This means giving children the opportunity for play (such as through the creation of a soccer pitch, for instance) and for schooling, while giving adults the opportunity to contribute through meaningful work.

Occupational health

Another important lesson that has been learned over the past several decades is the importance of providing for the physical and mental- health needs of disaster responders. In the rush to help, disaster responders will often put their own health at risk.

After the September 11, 2001 attacks, lack of communication among multiple agencies conducting hazard assessments, mistrust created by inconsistencies among different federal and state agencies in the reporting of safe thresholds for various pollutants, and lack of training in the use of personal protective equipment among some responders all contributed to a greater-than-necessary exposure by workers to health-hazards after the clean-up.

In addition to the need to prepare disaster responders for the physical health hazards they are likely to encounter in a particular situation, efforts should also be made to address the mental-health needs of responders. This can include psychological counseling, either before, during, or after responding to disaster situation. However, far more basic methods can be used to maintain well-being among responders, such as assuring adequate time for rest between shifts, ensuring mandatory days off each week, and providing regular updates (such as through the daily town-hall meetings described earlier).

Good disaster planning should also include predeployment medical reviews for disaster responders. These reviews should address chronic health conditions, disabilities, need for refrigerated medications, physical fitness, psychological flexibility, stress tolerance, and coping mechanisms, particular hazards associated with assigned work-load, and possession of requisite training and skills.

Suggested readings

Kreiss Yitshak, Merin Ofer, Peleg Kobi, Levy Gad, Vinker Shlomo, Sagi Ram, Abargel Avi, Bartal Carmi, Lin Guy, Bar Ariel, Bar-On Elhanan, Schwaber Mitchell J, Ash Nachman (2010). Early disaster response in Haiti: The Israeli field hospital experience. *Ann Intern Med* 153: 45–48.

McSwain Norman E (2010). Disaster response. Natural disaster: Katrina. *Surg Today* 40: 587–591.

Rebmann Terri, Carrico Ruth, English Judith F (2008). Lessons public health professionals learned from past disasters. *Public Health Nursing* 25(4): 344–352.

International disaster response Organizations

Lawrence Proano

Robert Partridge

Introduction

International disaster medical response is a complex and evolving field. In the global setting, disaster medicine encompasses natural disasters, warfare, and more recently medical response after terrorism and pandemic illness. Worldwide in 2004, more than 1.6 million deaths (2.8% of all deaths) were attributed to disasters. Experience with successive disasters has highlighted the need for a structured, organized approach to meet the needs of a major crisis. Appropriate resources must be deployed in a planned and coordinated manner with careful attention to previous lessons learned if success is to be achieved in any disaster scenario.

Worldwide experience with frequent disasters causing significant impact on the health, economy, and environment of the affected population has improved the ability of multinational, national, and nongovernmental organizations to provide a rapid, effective, and coordinated response. The number of responding organizations, degree of response, coordination, and length of response will be dependent on the nature of the disaster, numbers of casualties, geographic location, financial support, and other variables including political constraints in the involved region or country.

It is important for clinicians and other disaster responders to understand who the major participants are, the type and extent of support they provide, the timing of their response, and how they coordinate with other major and minor disaster-relief organizations.

United States organizations

The United States is a major provider of international disaster relief. Direct relief efforts are coordinated through U.S. government agencies, listed below. Significant disaster relief is also provided through funding, supply, and support of private and nongovernmental organizations.

- Department of State (DoS) The U.S. DoS is the lead agency for leading responses to disasters that affect U.S. interests.
- Department of Defense (DoD). The DoD assists in humanitarian responses both by military transport of relief supplies, and occasionally by peacekeeping efforts when deployed under UN mandate.
- International Medical Surgical Response Team (IMSuRT). IMSuRT is a civilian medical and surgical unit staffed by professionals that can be rapidly mobilized to a mass casualty site domestically or overseas. IMSuRT works in cooperation with local authorities to provide rapid assessment and medical stabilization of injured persons.
- Disaster Assistance Resource Team (DART) A disaster assistance response team provides specialists, trained in a variety of disaster relief skills, to assist U.S. embassies and USAID missions with the management of U.S. government response to disasters. The United States and Canada have specialized teams trained in search and rescue, logistics, and delivery of medical assessment and care, deployable on short notice.
- U.S. Agency for International Development (USAID). The USAID provides technical and financial assistance to countries and regions after a disaster, after a request for such assistance by the affected entity. This support is not only provided in the immediate response phase, but also in the recovery phase of a disaster.
- Bureau for Democracy, Conflict, and Humanitarian Assistance (DCHA).
- Office of Foreign Disaster Assistance (OFDA). OFDA is under the direction of the DCHA, and both are agencies within USAID. In a disaster, OFDA typically will deploy advisors or a DART team to provide a needs assessment.

The organizational structure of the agencies within USAID is represented in Figure 95.1.

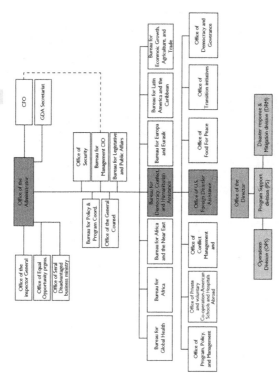

Figure 95.1 U.S. Agency for international development. This figure was published in Coppola D., *Introduction to International Disaster Management.* Copyright Elsevier 2006.

Multinational organizations

Multinational organizations have developed mechanisms of disaster response over many decades to offer rapid, coordinated, and effective assistance to disaster events. These organizations can be regional in scope, such as the North Atlantic Treaty Organization (NATO), or global, such as the World Bank and the United Nations (UN).

United Nations

The UN is the largest multinational umbrella organization that coordinates disaster-response efforts (Figure 95.2).
- United Nations Development Program (UNDP):
  - This agency assists countries in their development, offering technical and some financial support. Its role in disasters is mainly in the recovery phase.
- United Nations High Commissioner for Refugees (UNHCR):
  - The UNHCR is an agency that focuses on relief and support of refugees involved in a humanitarian crisis.
- Office for the Coordination of Humanitarian Affairs (OCHA):
  - OCHA is a result of a 1998 reorganization of the Department of Humanitarian Affairs (DHA). It coordinates major disasters and humanitarian crises. OCHA is an interagency body, and works with UN agencies as well as NGOs in humanitarian efforts. Its "Consolidated Appeals Process" is a tool to deliver humanitarian assistance in a disaster setting.
- U.N. Disaster Assessment and Coordination Team (UNDAC):
  - A UNDAC team is the UN's version of a DART team, deployed within hours, to provide a needs assessment of a disaster situation.

Other multinational organizations
- International Search and Rescue Advisory Group (INSARAG).
- World Health Organization (WHO).
- International Committee of the Red Cross (ICRC).
- International Federation of Red Cross and Red Crescent Societies (IFRC).
- World Food Program (WFP).

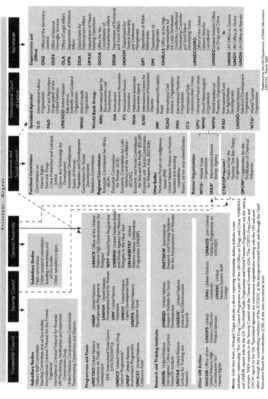

Figure 95.2 The United Nations system. From UN Department of Public Information DPI/2342, © 2004 United Nations. Reprinted with the permission of the United Nations.

Nongovernment organizations (NGOs) and private voluntary organizations (PVOs)

Some of the larger and well known NGOs include:
- International Rescue Committee (IRC).
- Medecins sans Frontieres (MSF).
- International Medical Committee (IMC).

There are numerous other NGOs that can be resourced for disasters. A resource list of such organizations and their web sites and contact information is listed in Box 95.1.

Historically there has been a lack of cooperation between NGOs, for fear of loss of independence and usurpation of power. However, in recent times, there have been more efforts at collaboration, as these organizations recognize the synergy such cooperative efforts bring.

Many humanitarian agencies utilize the military for delivery of materials and for safe transport to areas in need. However, to secure the trust of military and government forces in countries where there is ongoing conflict, they must retain neutrality on a consistent basis to maintain their security. This symbiotic interaction with sometimes hostile forces requires relationship and trust building. Agencies such as the ICRC have become adept at achieving such working relationships.

It is only through developed coordination and collaboration among agencies and groups in the United States, multinational organizations, funding bodies, NGOs, and PVOs, that response to disaster assistance has evolved to the level of sophistication that has been currently achieved. Disaster-response efforts will continue to evolve. Awareness of these constructs, and the roles and working relationships of all these bodies is important for those involved in disaster response.

Box 95.1

InterAction:
www.interaction.org/members/

Relief Web:
http://www.reliefweb.int/rw/dbc.nsf/doc100?OpenForm

NGO Voice:
www.ngovoice.org/members/index.html

AlertNet:
www.alertnet.org/member_directory.htm

One World:
www.oneworld.net/section/partners

International Council for Voluntary Organizations:
http://www.icva.ch/membership.html

Suggested readings

Blair I (2010). Defending against disasters: Global public health emergencies and opportunities for collaboration and action. *Asia Pacific Journal of Public Health* 22(3): 222S–228S.

Coppola, D (2007). *Introduction to International Disaster Management.* Amsterdam: Elseviere.

Dara SI, Ashton RW, Farmer JC, Carlton PK (2005). Worldwide disaster medical response: An historical perspective. *Crit Care Med 33*(1): S2–S6.

Hanling D, Llwewellyn C, Burkle, F (2006). International disaster response. In Ciottone G ed. *Disaster Medicine.* Amsterdam: Elsevier.

Future humanitarian crises

Frederick M. Burkle, Jr.

Future humanitarian crises

The discipline of disaster medicine and public-health preparedness differ from others in that it is multidisciplinary. Tremendous advances have been made over the last three decades, especially in research methodologies, education, training, response, and management schemes, but much remains lacking in prevention and preparedness. Increasing population numbers living in disaster-prone areas, unmanageable population densities, destructive climate changes, unconventional warfare, and major scarcities of water, energy, and food are but a few challenges impacting disaster medicine and preparedness for the coming decades. In fact, many of these humanitarian crises are currently active and beyond the tipping point of recovery.

Common characteristics of future crises:
• Share the common thread of being public-health emergencies.
• Preponderance of excess or indirect mortalities and morbidities dominate the health and public-health consequences (see Chapter 16, Complex Humanitarian Emergencies).
• Advances to date are often ad hoc, unmonitored, and arise from the work of individual nations or regions.
• Solutions require unprecedented global cooperation and collaboration in research, practice, policy, strategic planning, international surveillance, and human security.

Unconventional hostilities

The incidence of conventional warfare is the lowest in three decades, but the number of people living in some level of postconflict intensity, including easy availability of weapons and economic and social and public health stagnation, is unprecedented (see Fig. 96.1). The transition phase, before sustainable development, is the most dangerous, especially for vulnerable of populations such as women, children, and those with psychosocial and behavioral risk. The transition phase may last for years or never be resolved.

Violent events continue, but they no longer gain the attention of the international community. Many flee their surroundings to refugee camps of neighboring countries (camps surrounding Nairobi, Kenya are from eight different African countries) or are internally displaced to the false security of rapidly growing urban conclaves.

Seventeen African countries have defied expectations putting behind them the conflict, stagnation, and dictatorships of the past and replacing them with steady economic growth, deepening democracy, improved governance, and decreased poverty. Whereas Millennium Development Goals (MDG) made great progress in countries that qualify, little progress has been made in human security in the least developed and most fragile countries. In the latter, there is no reason to expect that internal unconventional conflicts and warring will decline.

Disaster medicine traditionally participates in organized emergency response initiatives through national and international nongovernmental organizations, but has limited presence during the transition phase or in long-term planning and programs of post-conflict environments.

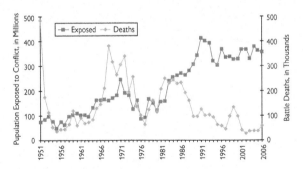

Figure 96.1 Populations living in areas of conflict and battle deaths, 1951–2006. Reproduced from Garfield RM, Polansky J, Burkle FM Jr. Changes in size of populations and level of conflict since WWII: implications for health and health services. Unpublished research.

Biodiversity crises

Biodiversity systems are areas throughout the world where major life forms (large majority of crucial vascular plants and original vertebrates) sustain our global biology. Biodiversity hotspots are 34 regions of the world with uniquely rich levels of endemic species that are most threatened.

- Dense human habitation tends to occur near biodiversity hotspots, most of which are large forests or located in the tropics.
- 80 percent of the major wars and conflicts of the last three decades occurred in 23 of the 34 biodiversity hotspots.
- Sudan's ecological collapse directly contributes to the ongoing political and social disarray.
- In Iraq, the combined ongoing war, drought, increasing sand storms, loss of marsh wetlands, and diverting of the Tigris and Euphrates Rivers by Syria and Turkey have resulted in a 70 percent volume loss of water and agricultural collapse and an unmatched environmental disaster.
- Biodiversity areas are increasingly the focus of "land grabbing" from individual countries that must import food (Asia, Middle East, and Russia).
- War money comes from timber harvesting (Cambodia, Congo), overharvesting and excess soil degradation from growing illicit drugs in Afghanistan, South East Asia, Latin America, and wide proliferation of small arms in the overhunting of vital vertebrate populations (small animals and bush meat).

These unique biodiversity areas must be recognized as global resources, not a commodity that can be owned by any one nation.

If the past is any guide to the future, areas of exceptional biodiversity loss and losses in ecosystem services are likely to be those with humanitarian crises. In coming years, there will be more resource-based conflicts, many brought about by climate change and resultant population migrations, and eminent domain debates as countries sell or lease off land and other resources to the highest bidder.

Climate change

Evidence shows that both natural climate trends, which have shown increasing influence over many decades, exist along with man's hand in accumulation of carbon emissions that will not be absorbed or disappear from the environment. Crossing one environmental boundary affects stability of the others and the entire Earth system. These factors directly impact boundary thresholds that exist for seven environmental indicators:

1. Climate change.
2. Biodiversity.
3. Global cycles of nitrogen and phosphorus.
4. Fresh-water availability and use.
5. Ocean acidification.
6. Stratospheric ozone depletion.
7. Change of land use.

A highly respected eight-year-long Oregon Ocean Study published in 2010 confirmed more acidic warmer ocean temperatures resulting in lethally low oxygen levels and increasing levels of dissolved carbon dioxide. This has already killed many bottom dwellers (e.g., crabs) and forced many fish to swim at the surface where there is more oxygen.

By 2050, 75 million islanders will be forced to relocate. Pacific island nations (e.g., Kiribati, Maldives) are currently migrating populations because of rising ocean levels and loss of food-sustaining coconut palms, taro plants, disappearing reef systems, and freshwater sources. Countries are called upon to identify vulnerabilities and to "adapt." If these measures do not work, strong migration policies must be in place. Migration patterns arising from scarcity to date have remained regional (e.g., Africans moving to the Mediterranean countries; Pacific island nations migrate primarily to Australia and New Zealand, which offer phased-in education and training programs).

Rapid urbanization

Urbanization per se is necessary for the wealth and economy of a nation when adequately sustained by production of food, resources, and services from *somewhere else*. However, the resource base that is sustaining urban populations is in steady decline.

In contrast, **rapid urbanization** is unsustainable and occurs when:

- Population increases beyond capacity of public-health infrastructures and system protections (e.g., food, water, sanitation, shelter, fuel, security).
- Increasingly, internally displaced and regional refugees flee to urban conclaves because of lack of security, economic stagnation, and lack of public-health protections.
- Extreme poverty of those migrating to cities remains or worsens.

Characteristics of rapidly urbanized settings:

- Highly dense populations: Up to 1 million people/SqKm.
- Population numbers and demographics relatively unknown.
- Limited access and availability of health facilities and public-health infrastructures and systems.
- Sanitation ignored; infectious diseases more prevalent.
- Alarmingly high under-age-5 mortality rates (U5MR) and infant mortality rates (IMR).
- Most vulnerable populations move to disaster-prone areas (cyclones, flooding, earthquakes).
- Major security issues prevail; rape epidemics.
- Increasing gap between the have and have-not populations.
- Poor or no representation by international humanitarian community.

Rapidly sprawling urban settings may:

- Determine their own climates when there is large asphalt and concrete conversions and urban topography is devoid of forests/parks.
- Each percentage point in urban growth correlates with decrease of 2.44 mm of rainfall.
- Lead to major air and water pollution and acute and chronic respiratory disease (e.g., mainland China).

Emergencies of scarcity

These emergencies differ in that they are driven by an increasing world-wide demand of:
- Energy (rise of 45% by 2030).
- Food (50% by 2030).
- Water (25% by 2025).

Inextricably linked to biodiversity hotspots, climate threats, scarcity of remaining forests and arable lands, most of which lie in developing countries. Resource competition hostilities, referred to as "distributional conflicts" are already emerging. Demands for food, energy, and water risk are becoming the major "weapons" of future wars. There is enough food to feed the existing population, yet >1 billion lack sufficient food for health. In the past, disasters defined the public health of a country and exposed their vulnerabilities. In the future, global scarcity of energy, water, and food will define the public- health status of nations.

Health-care worker scarcities:
- 57 countries face major health-care worker crises.
- Direct correlation between lack of health-care workers and worsening health indices (e.g., crude mortality rate, U5MR, IMR).
- Current solutions tied to increasing "task shifting" and use of WHO initiatives to train nonphysicians to relieve the burden of surgical disease.

Pandemics and epidemics

Contributing factors to increasing transmission of the 70 or more new and re-emerging diseases arise from:

- Easy access to worldwide travel.
- Increasing density of populations leading to rapid transmission of viral or bacterial agents.
- Poor surveillance and management capacities among nations most at risk for viral emergence and transmission.
- Uneven vaccine coverage.

The implementation of the International Health Regulations during the 2002–3 SARS pandemic that became a Treaty in 2007 provides WHO with unprecedented powers to improve national, regional, and global surveillance, investigation, and control of emerging diseases. Provisions provided under the IHR, such as deployment of WHO Emergency Response Teams have improved control and investigation of outbreaks of avian influenza and H1N1.

Concerns impacting future outbreaks:

- Decisive action and interventions taken by public-health authorities in early stages helped contain H1N1.
- H1N1 revealed improved preparedness but overall public education remains poor.
- Cannot predict a pandemic nor how severe it may be.
- Current technologies for making a vaccine take too long (6+months).
- Legal issues slow implementation of seroprevalence studies and delay in obtaining ethical clearance.
- Immunization of children confers significant protection (61%) against the unvaccinated community members.
- When vaccination shortages occur, vaccination of children should be high priority

Conclusions

- Humanitarian community is not prepared to protect the urban public-health infrastructure or systems. It is not prepared to handle emergencies of scarcity.
- Public-health solutions must include reduction in population growth rates, which are not possible without empowering women and ensuring social protections worldwide.
- Present global health research is too narrow in its content; must include other disciplines from medicine, engineering, law, social sciences, and economics.
- Public health must be seen as a strategic and security issue that deserves an international monitoring system.
- Can the global community make what works for the IHR Treaty and infectious-disease control applicable for water, food, energy, and climate threats.
- These crises transcend any one nation's capacity. As was done with WHO for pandemics, an UN-OCHA-like body must be the designated lead agency, and provided with authority, funding, and resources to manage these events.
- Disaster medicine, as a discipline, must begin to address these new challenges in health, public health, prevention, and preparedness.

Suggested readings

Burkle FM Jr (2009). Pandemics: State fragility's most telling gap. In Cronin P (ed.), *Global Strategic Assessment 2009: America's Security Role in a Changing World*, pp 105–108. Washington, DC: Institute for National Strategic Studies, National Defense University, US Government Printing Office.

Burkle FM Jr (2010, May/June). Future humanitarian crises: Challenges for practice, policy, and public health. *Prehosp Disaster Med* 25(3): 191–197.

Chivian ES, Bernstein AS (2008). How is biodiversity threatened by human activity? In *Sustaining Life: How human health depends on Biodiversity*. New York: Oxford University Press.

McQueen KA, Parmar P, Kene M, et al. (2009, July/August). Burden of surgical disease: Strategies to manage an existing public health emergency. *Prehosp Disaster Med* 24(2): s228–231.

Index